Developmental and Behavioral Pediatrics

A Handbook for Primary Care

Developmental and Behavioral Pediatrics

A Handbook
for Primary Care
Second Edition

Edited by

Steven Parker, M.D.

Associate Professor of Pediatrics, Boston
University School of Medicine; Director,
Division of Developmental and Behavioral
Pediatrics, Boston Medical Center, Boston

Barry Zuckerman, M.D.

Joel and Barbara Alpert Professor of
Pediatrics, Boston University School of
Medicine; Chief, Department of Pediatrics,
Boston Medical Center, Boston

Marilyn Augustyn, M.D.

Associate Professor of Pediatrics, Boston
University School of Medicine; Director of
Training, Division of Developmental and
Behavioral Pediatrics, Boston Medical
Center, Boston

 LIPPINCOTT WILLIAMS & WILKINS
A **Wolters Kluwer** Company
Philadelphia · Baltimore · New York · London
Buenos Aires · Hong Kong · Sydney · Tokyo

Acquisitions Editor: Anne M. Sydor
Developmental Editor: Lisa R. Kairis
Marketing Manager: Kathy Neely
Production Editor: David Murphy
Compositor: Maryland Composition, Inc.
Printer: Edwards Brothers

© 2005 by LIPPINCOTT WILLIAMS & WILKINS

530 Walnut Street
Philadelphia, PA 19106 USA
LWW.com

First Edition 1995 Copyright © 1995 by Steven Parker and Barry Zuckerman

Printed in the USA

Library of Congress Cataloging-in-Publication Data
Developmental and behavioral pediatrics: a handbook for primary care / [edited by] Steven Parker, Barry Zuckerman, and Marilyn Augustyn.—2nd ed.
     p. ; cm.
Rev. ed. of Behavioral and developmental pediatrics. 1st ed. c1995.
Includes bibliographical references and index.
ISBN 0-7817-1683-7
1. Behavior disorders in children—Handbooks, manuals, etc.
2. Child development deviations—Handbooks, manuals, etc.
3. Pediatrics—Psychological aspects—Handbooks, manuals, etc.
4. Primary care (Medicine)—Handbooks, manuals, etc.   I. Parker, Steven. II. Zuckerman, Barry S. III. Augustyn, Marilyn. IV. Behavioral and developmental pediatrics.
     [DNLM: 1. Developmental Disabilities—diagnosis—Handbooks.
2. Developmental Disabilities—therapy—Handbooks. 3. Child Behavior Disorders—disorders—Handbooks. 4. Child Behavior Disorders—therapy—Handbooks.
WS 39 D489 2004]
RJ47.5.B37 2004
618.92'89—dc22
                                                        2004015203

10 9 8 7 6 5 4 3 2 1

Dedication

To Ann, Hyman, Philip and Karen Parker and to Anne, Leo, Elliot, Diana, Pamela, Jake and Katherine Zuckerman and to George, Henry and Clare Westerman and Audrey, Henry, Joan, Ann, Kate and George Augustyn. Our enduring interest in the well-being of children and families, and our commitment to helping them through teaching and clinical care, has been fueled by the example, nurturance and support we have received from our families. It is to them, with great love and thanks, that we dedicate this book.

Contents

III
Family Issues 373

Contributing Authors

J. Stuart Ablon, PhD

Assistant Professor of Psychiatry, Harvard Medical School, Boston Massachusetts; Director, CPS Institute, Massachusetts General Hospital, Boston, Massachusetts
21. The Aggressive, Explosive Child

Travis Robert Adams, PhD

Clinical Fellow in Psychology (Psychiatry Service), Harvard Medical School, Boston, Massachusetts; Massachusetts General Hospital, Boston, Massachusetts
23. Anxiety Disorders

Marie E. Anzalone, ScD, OTR, FAOTA

Assistant Professor of Clinical Occupational Therapy, College of Physicians and Surgeons, Columbia University, New York, New York
67. Sensory Integration Disorder

Marilyn Augustyn, MD

Associate Professor of Developmental and Behavioral Pediatrics, Department of Pediatrics, Boston University School of Medicine; Director of Training, Boston Medical Center, Boston, Massachusetts
27. Bad News in the Media
41. Fears

Christine E. Barron, MD

Assistant Professor of Pediatrics, Brown University School of Medicine, Providence, Rhode Island; Clinical Director, Child Protection Program, Hasbro Children's Hospital, Providence, Rhode Island
58. Physical Abuse
69. Sexual Abuse

Joseph Biederman, MD

Professor of Psychiatry, Harvard Medical School, Boston Massachusetts; Chief of Pediatric Psychopharmacology, Department of Child and Adolescent Psychiatry, Massachusetts General Hospital, Boston, Massachusetts
28. Bipolar Disorder in Children

James A. Blackman, MD, MPH

Professor of Pediatrics, University of Virginia School of Medicine, Charlottesville, Virginia
61. Prematurity: Primary Care Follow-up

Peter A. Blasco, MD

Associate Professor of Pediatrics, Oregon Health and Science University, Portland, Oregon; Director of Neurodevelopment Program, Child Development and Rehabilitation Center, Portland, Oregon
54. Motor Delays

Stephanie Blenner, MD

Instructor in Pediatrics, Department of Pediatrics, Boston Medical Center, Boston, Massachusetts; Fellow in Developmental and Behavioral Pediatrics, Boston Medical Center, Boston, Massachusetts
78. Thumb Sucking

W. Thomas Boyce, MD

Professor of Epidemiology and Child Development, University of California at Berkeley School of Public Health, Berkeley, California
14. Coping with Stressful Transitions

Robert J. Boyle, MD

Professor of Pediatrics, University of Virginia School of Medicine, Charlottesville, Virginia; Attending Neonatologist, Department of Pediatrics, University of Virginia Health System, Charlottesville, Virginia
61. Prematurity: Primary Care Follow-up

T. Berry Brazelton, MD

Professor Emeritus of Pediatrics, Harvard Medical School, Boston, Massachusetts; Child Development Unit, Children's Hospital, Boston, Massachusetts
4. Touchpoints of Anticipatory Guidance in the First Three Years

Margaret J. Briggs-Gowan, PhD

Associate Research Scientist, Department of Epidemiology and Public Health, Yale University School of Medicine, New Haven, Connecticut
12. Screening for Social and Emotional Delays in Early Childhood

Robert B. Brooks, PhD

Assistant Clinical Professor of Psychology, Department of Psychiatry, Harvard Medical School, Boston, Massachusetts; Consultant, Department of Psychology, McLean Hospital, Belmont, Massachusetts
66. Self-Esteem and Resilience

John C. Carey, MD

Professor of Pediatrics, University of Utah School of Medicine, Salt Lake City, Utah; Chief, Division of Genetics, University of Utah Health Sciences Center, Salt Lake City, Utah
37. The Dysmorphic Child

Elizabeth B. Caronna, MD

Associate Professor of Pediatrics, Boston University School of Medicine, Boston, Massachusetts; Directors, Pediatric Assessment of Communication Clinic, Boston Medical Center, Boston, Massachusetts
26. Autism

Alice S. Carter, PhD

Professor of Psychology, University of Massachusetts at Boston, Boston, Massachusetts
12. Screening for Social and Emotional Delays in Early Childhood

Jonathan M. Cheek, PhD

Professor of Psychology, Wellesley College, Wellesley, Massachusetts
70. Shyness

Edward R. Christophersen, MD

Professor of Pediatrics, University of Missouri at Kansas City School of Medicine, Kansas City, Missouri; Staff Psychologist, Developmental and Behavioral Sciences Section, Children's Mercy Hospital, Kansas City, Missouri
13. Behavioral Management: Theory and Practice

William Lord Coleman, MD

Professor of Pediatrics, University of North Carolina at Chapel Hill School of Medicine, Chapel Hill, North Carolina; Staff Member, Department of Pediatrics, Center for Development and Learning, Chapel Hill, North Carolina
8. Family Systems

Eve R. Colson, MD

Assistant Professor of Pediatrics, Yale University School of Medicine, New Haven, Connecticut; Director, Well Newborn Nursery, Yale-New Haven Hospital, New Haven, Connecticut
46. The Gifted Child

James Coplan, MD

Clinical Associate Professor of Pediatrics, University of Pennsylvania School of Medicine, Philadelphia, Pennsylvania; Director, Leadership Education in Neurodevelopmental Disabilities, Children's Hospital, Philadelphia, Pennsylvania
49. Language Delays
Appendix C. Early Language Milestone Scale

David L. Coulter, MD

Associate Professor of Neurology, Harvard Medical School, Boston, Massachusetts; Assistant in Neurology, Children's Hospital, Boston, Massachusetts
53. Mental Retardation: Diagnostic Evaluation

Howard Dubowitz, MD, MS

Professor of Pediatrics, University of Maryland School of Medicine, Baltimore, Maryland; Chief, Division of Child Protection, University of Maryland Hospital, Baltimore, Maryland
55. Neglect

Paul H. Dworkin, MD

Chair and Professor of Pediatrics, University of Connecticut School of Medicine, Farmington, Connecticut; Physician-in-Chief, Connecticut Children's Medical Center, Hartford, Connecticut
63. School Failure

Margorie Engel, MBA, PhD

President and CEO, Stepfamily Association of America, Lincoln, Nebraska
96. Stepfamilies

Ilgi Ozturk Ertem, MD

Associate Professor of Pediatrics, Ankara University School of Medicine, Cebeci, Ankara, Turkey
17. Early Child Development in Developing Countries
51. Masturbation

Brian W. C. Forsyth, MB, ChB, FRCP(c)

Associate Professor of Pediatrics, Yale University School of Medicine, New Haven, Connecticut; Director, Pediatric Primary Care Center, Yale New Haven Hospital, New Haven, Connecticut
99. Vulnerable Children

Deborah A. Frank, MD

Professor of Pediatrics, Boston University School of Medicine, Boston, Massachusetts; Director, Grow Clinic, Boston Medical Center, Boston, Massachusetts
40. Failure to Thrive

Frances Page Glascoe, PhD

Adjunct Professor of Pediatrics, Vanderbilt University School of Medicine, Nashville, Tennessee
11. Developmental Screening

Joseph M. Gonzalez-Heydrich, MD,

Assistant Professor, Harvard Medical School, Boston, Massachusetts; Medical Director, Outpatient Services, Department of Psychiatry, Children's Hospital, Boston, Massachusetts
19. Psychopharmacology

Linda M. Grant, MD, MPH

Associate Professor of Pediatrics, Boston University School of Medicine, Boston, Massachusetts; Staff, Department of Pediatrics, Boston Medical Center, Boston, Massachusetts
68. Sex and the Adolescent

Ross W. Greene, PhD

Associate Professor in Psychology, Department of Psychiatry, Harvard Medical School, Boston, Massachusetts; Director, CPS Institute, Massachusetts General Hospital, Boston, Massachusetts
21. The Aggressive, Explosive Child

Stanley Greenspan, PhD

Clinical Professor of Psychiatry, Behavioral Sciences, and Pediatrics at George Washington University Medical School, Washington, DC
Appendix F. Socioemotional Development of Infants and Children: Themes and Behaviors

Jessie R. Groothius, MD

Vice President, Clinical Affairs, Hollis-Eden Pharmaceuticals, San Diego, California
98. Twins

Betsy McAlister Groves, LICSW

Assistant Professor of Pediatrics, Boston University School of Medicine, Boston, Massachusetts; Director, Child Witness to Violence, Boston Medical Center, Boston, Massachusetts
84. Witness to Violence

Angela S. Guarda, MD

Assistant Professor of Psychiatry, Johns Hopkins University School of Medicine, Baltimore, Maryland; Director, Eating Disorders Program, Johns Hopkins Hospital, Baltimore, Maryland
22. Anorexia Nervosa and Bulimia

Barry Guitar, PhD

Professor of Communication Sciences, University of Vermont, Burlington, Vermont
73. Stuttering

Randi Jenssen Hagerman, MD

Tsakoponlos-Vismara Professor of Pediatrics, University of California at Davis School of Medicine, Davis, California; Medical Director, MIND Institute, Sacramento, California
43. Fragile X Syndrome

Lawrence D. Hammer, MD

Professor of Pediatrics, Stanford University School of Medicine, Palo Alto, California; Medical Director, Ambulatory Care Center, Lucile Packard Children's Hospital, Palo Alto, California
57. Obesity

Alexander H. Hoon, Jr, MD, MPH

Associate Professor of Pediatrics, Johns Hopkins University School of Medicine, Baltimore, Maryland; Director, Phelps Center for Cerebral Palsy and Motor Disorders, Kennedy Krieger Institute, Baltimore, Maryland
32. Cerebral Palsy

Barbara J. Howard, MD	Assistant Professor of Pediatrics, Johns Hopkins University School of Medicine, Baltimore, Maryland *15. Managing Behavior* *29. Biting Others*
Carol Lee Hubbard, MD, MPH, PhD	Clinical Assistant Professor of Pediatrics, University of Vermont College of Medicine, Burlington, Vermont; Director, Division of Developmental-Behavioral Pediatrics, Maine Medical Center, Falmouth, Maine *8. Family Systems*
Laura A. Jana, MD, FAAP	Pediatrician, Physicians Clinic, Inc., Methodist Health System, Omaha, Nebraska *87. Child Care*
Michael S. Jellinek, MD	Professor of Psychiatry and Pediatrics, Harvard Medical School, Boston, Massachusetts; Chief, Child Psychiatry Services, Massachusetts General Hospital, Boston, Massachusetts; President, Newton Wellesley Hospital, Newton, Massachusetts *35. Depression*
Carole Jenny, MD, MBD	Professor of Pediatrics, Brown University School of Medicine, Providence, Rhode Island *58. Physical Abuse* *69. Sexual Abuse*
Alain Joffe, MD, MPH	Associate Professor of Pediatrics, Johns Hopkins University School of Medicine, Baltimore, Maryland; Director, Student Health and Wellness Center, Johns Hopkins Hospital, Baltimore, Maryland *22. Anorexia Nervosa and Bulimia*
Margot Kaplan-Sanoff, EdD	Associate Professor of Pediatrics, Boston University School of Medicine, Boston, Massachusetts; Director, Sharing Books with Babies, Division of Behavioral and Developmental Pediatrics, Boston Medical Center, Boston, Massachusetts *89. Divorce*
Theodore A. Kastner, MD, MS	Associate Professor of Clinical Pediatrics, University of Medicine and Dentistry of New Jersey, Newark, New Jersey; Attending Physician, Department of Pediatrics, Mountainside Hospital, Montclair, New Jersey *52. Mental Retardation: Behavioral Problems*

John R. Knight, MD

Assistant Professor of Pediatrics, Harvard Medical School, Boston, Massachusetts; Director, Center for Adolescent Substance Abuse Research, Children's Hospital, Boston, Massachusetts
74. Substance Abuse in Adolescence

Perri E. Klass, MD

Assistant Professor of Pediatrics, Boston University School of Medicine, Boston, Massachusetts; Medical Director and President, Reach Out and Read National Center, Somerville, Massachusetts
7. Promoting Early Literacy

Barbara Korsch, MD

Professor of Pediatrics, University of Southern California Keck School of Medicine, Los Angeles, California; Attending Pediatrician, Children's Hospital of Los Angeles, Los Angeles, California
1. Talking with Parents
5. Difficult Encounters with Parents

John M. Leventhal, MD

Professor of Pediatrics, Child Study Center, Yale University School of Medicine, New Haven, Connecticut; Attending Physician, Department of Pediatrics,Yale-New Haven Hospital, New Haven, Connecticut
51. Masturbation

Melvin D. Levine, MD

Professor of Pediatrics, University of North Carolina at Chapel Hill School of Medicine, Chapel Hill, North Carolina; Director, Center for Development and Learning, Chapel Hill, North Carolina
81. Unpopular Children

Melvin Lewis, MBBS, FRCPsych, DCH

Professor Emeritus of Child Psychiatry and Pediatrics, Yale University School of Medicine, New Haven, Connecticut; Attending Physician, Child Psychiatry and Pediatrics, Yale-New Haven Hospital, New Haven, Connecticut
90. Dying Children

Yi Hui Liu, MD, MPH

Fellow in Developmental and Behavioral Pediatrics, University of California at San Diego School of Medicine, San Diego, California; Children's Hospital of San Diego, San Diego, California
2. Talking with Children

Julie Lumeng, MD

Research Investigator, Center for Human Growth and Development, University of Michigan, Ann Arbor, Michigan; Clinical Instructor, Department of Pediatrics and Communicable Diseases, University of Michigan, Ann Arbor, Michigan
59. Picky Eating

Deborah Madansky, MD

Executive Director/Medical Director, CARE Children's Counseling Center, Santa Rosa Medical Center, Santa Rosa, California
69. Sexual Abuse

Bruce J. Masek, PhD

Associate Professor of Psychology, Harvard Medical School, Boston, Massachusetts; Clinical Director, Child and Adolescent Psychiatry, Massachusetts General Hospital, Boston, Massachusetts
23. Anxiety Disorders

Rebecca J. McCauley, PhD, CCC-SLP

Professor of Communication Sciences, University of Vermont, Burlington, Vermont
72. Speech-Sound Disorders

Barbara A. Morse, PhD

Assistant Research Professor of Psychiatry, Boston University School of Medicine, Boston, Massachusetts; Program Director, Fetal Alcohol Education Program, Concord, Massachusetts
42. Fetal Alcohol Syndrome

Michael E. Msall, MD

Professor of Pediatrics, University of Chicago Pritzker School of Medicine, Chicago, Illinois; Chief of Developmental and Behavioral Pediatrics, Comer Children's and La Rabida Children's Hospitals, Chicago, Illinois
83. Visual Impairment

Robert Needlman, MD

Associate Professor of Pediatrics, Case Western Reserve University School of Medicine, Cleveland, Ohio; Attending Pediatrician, MetroHealth Medical Center, Cleveland, Ohio
76. Temper Tantrums
94. Sibling Rivalry

Karen Norberg, MD

Assistant Professor of Psychiatry, Boston University School of Medicine, Boston, Massachusetts; Attending Psychiatrist, Boston City Hospital, Boston, Massachusetts
75. Suicide

Karen N. Olness, MD

Professor of Pediatrics, Family Medicine, and International Health, Case Western Reserve University, Cleveland, Ohio; Director of International Child Health, Rainbow Babies and Children's Hospital, Cleveland, Ohio
18. Self-Regulation Therapy

Judith A. Owens, MD, MPH

Associate Professor of Pediatrics, Brown University School of Medicine, Providence, Rhode Island; Director, Pediatric Sleep Disorders Clinic, Hasbro Children's Hospital, Providence, Rhode Island
71. Sleep Problems

Lee M. Pachter, DO

Professor of Pediatrics and Anthropology, University of Connecticut School of Medicine, Farmington, Connecticut; Senior Attending Physician, Department of Pediatrics, Saint Francis Hospital and Medical Center, Hartford, Connecticut
88. Cultural Competence

Frederick B. Palmer, MD

Shainberg Professor of Pediatrics, University of Tennessee Health Sciences Center, Memphis, Tennessee; Director, Boling Center for Developmental Disabilities, Memphis, Tennessee
32. Cerebral Palsy

Steven Parker, MD

Associate Professor of Pediatrics, Boston University School of Medicine, Boston, Massachusetts; Director, Division of Developmental and Behavioral Pediatrics, Boston Medical Center, Boston, Massachusetts
3. Teachable Moments in Primary Care
25. Attention Deficit Hyperactivity Disorder
34. Colic
80. Toilet Training

Ellen C. Perrin, MA, MD

Professor of Pediatrics, Tufts University School of Medicine, Boston, Massachusetts; Director, Division of Developmental-Behavioral Pediatrics, The Floating Hospital for Children, New England Medical Center, Boston, Massachusetts
10. Behavioral Screening
33. Chronic Conditions
45. Gender Identity Issues
92. Gay and Lesbian Parents

Siegfried M. Pueschel, MD, PhD, JD, MPH

Professor of Pediatrics, Brown University School of Medicine, Providence, Rhode Island; Director, Child Development Center, Rhode Island Hospital, Providence, Rhode Island
36. Down Syndrome

Leonard A. Rappaport, MD, MS

Mary Deming Scott Associate Professor of Pediatrics, Harvard Medical School, Boston, Massachusetts; Director, Developmental Medicine Center and Associate Chief, Division of General Pediatrics, Children's Hospital, Boston, Massachusetts
20. Recurrent Abdominal Pain
38. Encopresis
39. Enuresis

Gary Remafedi, MD, MPH

Professor of Pediatrics, University of Minnesota, Minneapolis, Minnesota; Director, Youth AIDS Project, University of Minnesota Health Sciences Center, Minneapolis, Minnesota
44. Gay, Lesbian, and Bisexual Youth

Nancy J. Roizen, MD

Professor of Pediatrics, SUNY Upstate Medical University, Syracuse, New York; vice Chair of Pediatrics, University Hospital, Syracuse, New York
85. Adoption

Adrian D. Sandler, MD

Clinical Associate Professor of Pediatrics, University of North Carolina at Chapel Hill School of Medicine, Chapel Hill, North Carolina; Medical Director, Olson Huff Center, Mission Children's Hospital, Asheville, North Carolina
79. Tics and Tourette Syndrome

Nerissa B. San Luis, MD

Fellow in Developmental-Behavioral Pediatrics, University of California at San Diego School of Medicine, San Diego, California; Children's Hospital San Diego, San Diego, California
50. Lying, Cheating, & Stealing

Celine A. Saulnier, MD

NAAR Fellow in Child Psychology, Child Study Center, Yale University School of Medicine, New Haven, Connecticut
24. Asperger Syndrome

Glenn Saxe, MD

Chairman of Child and Adolescent Psychiatry, Boston University School of Medicine, Boston, Massachusetts; Chairman, Department of Child and Adolescent Psychiatry, Boston Medical Center, Boston, Massachusetts
60. Posttraumatic Stress Disorder (PTSD) in Children

Neil L. Schechter, MD

Professor and Head of Division of Developmental and Behavioral Pediatrics, University of Connecticut School of Medicine, Farmington, Connecticut; Director, Pain Relief Program/Developmental Pediatrics, Saint Francis Hospital/Connecticut Children's Medical Center, Hartford, Connecticut
16. Pain
46. The Gifted Child

Barton D. Schmitt, MD

Professor of Pediatrics, University of Colorado School of Medicine, Denver, Colorado; Director, General Pediatric Consultative Services, The Children's Hospital, Denver, Colorado
62. School Avoidance

David J. Schonfeld, MD

Associate Professor of Pediatrics, Child Study Center, Yale University School of Medicine, New Haven, Connecticut; Co-Chair, Decedent Affairs Program, Yale-New Haven Hospital, New Haven, Connecticut
90. Dying Children

Alison D. Schonwald, MD

Instructor in Pediatrics, Harvard Medical School, Boston, Massachusetts; Assistant in Medicine, Division of General Pediatrics, Children's Hospital, Boston, Massachusetts
19. Psychopharmacology
38. Encopresis
39. Enuresis

C. Wayne Sells, MD, MPH

Associate Professor of Pediatrics and Director, Division of Adolescent Health, Oregon Health and Science University, Portland, Oregon; Division Chief, Adolescent Health, Doernbecher Children's Hospital, Portland, Oregon
44. Gay, Lesbian, & Bisexual Youth

Prachi Edlagan Shah, MD

Clinical Instructor of Pediatrics, Boston University School of Medicine, Boston, Massachusetts; Boston Medical Center, Boston, Massachusetts
93. Screening for Maternal Depression

Jack P. Shonkoff, MD

Dean, The Heller School for Social Policy and Management, Brandeis University, Waltham, Massachusetts; Associate, Children's Hospital, Boston, Massachusetts
6. Helping Families Deal with Bad News

Benjamin S. Siegel, MD

Professor of Pediatrics and Psychiatry, Boston University School of Medicine, Boston, Massachusetts; Pediatrician, Boston Medical Center, Boston, Massachusetts
86. Bereavement and Loss

Joshua D. Sparrow, MD

Assistant Professor of Psychiatry, Harvard Medical School, Boston, Massachusetts; Special Initiatives Director, Brazelton Touchpoints Center, Children's Hospital, Boston, Massachusetts
4. Touchpoints of Anticipatory Guidance in the First Three Years

Terry Stancin, PhD

Professor of Pediatrics, Psychiatry, and Psychology, Case Western Reserve University, Cleveland, Ohio; Head, Pediatric Psychology, MetroHealth Medical Center, Cleveland, Ohio
10. Behavioral Screening

Martin T. Stein, MD

Professor of Pediatrics, University of California at San Diego School of Medicine, San Diego, California; Director of Developmental-Behavioral Pediatrics, Children's Hospital, San Diego, California
2. Talking with Children
47. Headaches
50. Lying, Cheating, & Stealing

Naomi Steiner, MD

Developmental and Behavioral Pediatrician, Tufts-New England Medical Center, Boston, Massachusetts
65. Selective Mutism

Victor C. Strasburger, MD

Professor of Pediatrics, University of New Mexico School of Medicine, Albuquerque, New Mexico; Chief, Division of Adolescent Medicine, University of New Mexico Hospital, Albuquerque, New Mexico
97. Television

Peter G. Stringham, MD, MS

Assistant Clinical Professor of Pediatrics, Boston University School of Medicine, Boston, Massachusetts; Department of Pediatrics and Adolescent Medicine, East Boston Neighborhood Health Center, East Boston, Massachusetts
82. Violent Youth

Margaret A. Swank, PhD

Clinical Fellow in Psychology, Department of Psychiatry, Harvard Medical School, Boston, Massachusetts; Massachusetts General Hospital, Boston, Massachusetts
23. Anxiety Disorders

Moira Szilagyi, MD, PhD

Assistant Professor of Pediatrics, University of Rochester School of Medicine, Rochester, New York; Medical Director, Foster Care Pediatrics, Monroe County Department of Public Health, Rochester, New York
91. Foster Care

Lane Tanner, MD

Clinical Professor of Pediatrics, University of California at San Francisco School of Medicine, San Francisco, California; Associate Director, Division of Developmental and Behavioral Pediatrics, Children's Hospital and Research Center at Oakland, Oakland, California
95. Single Parents

Maria Trozzi, MEd

Assistant Professor of Pediatrics, Boston University School of Medicine, Boston, Massachusetts; Director of the Good Grief Program, Boston Medical Center, Boston, Massachusetts
86. Bereavement and Loss

Stanley Turecki, MD

Attending Psychiatrist, Lenox Hill Hospital, New York, New York
77. Tempermentally Difficult Children

Douglas L. Vanderbilt, MD

Instructor in Pediatrics, Boston University School of Medicine, Boston, Massachusetts; Fellow in Developmental and Behavioral Pediatrics, Boston Medical Center, Boston, Massachusetts
31. Bullying

John S. Visher, MD

Lecturer Emeritus in Psychiatry, Stanford University School of Medicine, Stanford, California; Former President, American College of Psychiatrists, Berkeley, California
96. Stepfamilies

Fred R. Volkmar, MD

Professor of Pediatrics, Child Study Center, Yale University School of Medicine, New Haven, Connecticut; Attending Physician, Child Psychiatry and Pediatrics, Yale-New Haven Hospital, New Haven, Connecticut
24. Asperger Syndrome

Kevin K. Walsh, PhD

Director of Quality Management and Research, Developmental Disabilities Health Alliance, Inc., Clementon, New Jersey
52. Mental Retardation: Behavioral Problems

Lyn Weiner, MPH

Associate Professor of Public Health, Boston University School of Medicine, Boston, Massachusetts; Executive Director, Fetal Alcohol Education Program, Boston University School of Medicine, Brookline, Massachusetts
42. Fetal Alcohol Syndrome

Karen E. Wills, PhD, ABPP

Pediatric Neuropsychologist, Psychological Services, Children's Hospitals and Clinics, Minneapolis, Minnesota
48. Hearing Impairment

Laurel M. Wills, MD

Assistant Professor of Pediatrics, University of Minnesota School of Medicine, Minneapolis, Minnesota; Director, Developmental Pediatric Clinic, Hennepin County Medical Center, Minneapolis, Minnesota
48. Hearing Impairment

Janet Wozniak, MD

Assistant Professor of Psychiatry, Harvard Medical School, Boston, Massachusetts; Director, Pediatric Bipolar Disorder Research Program, Child and Adolescent Psychiatry, Massachusetts General Hospital, Boston, Massachusetts
28. Bipolar Disorder in Children

Yvette E. Yatchmink, MD, PhD

Assistant Professor of Pediatrics, Brown University School of Medicine, Providence, Rhode Island; Developmental-Behavioral Pediatrician, Child Development Center, Rhode Island Hospital, Providence, Rhode Island
6. *Helping Families Deal with Bad News*

Barry Zuckerman, MD

Joel and Barbara Alpert Professor of Pediatrics, Boston University School of Medicine, Boston, Massachusetts; Chief, Department of Pediatrics, Boston City Hospital, Boston, Massachusetts
3. *Teachable Moments in Primary Care*
9. *Promoting Parental Self-Understanding*
30. *Breath Holding*
56. *Nightmares and Night Terrors*

Pamela M. Zuckerman, MD

Associate Clinical Professor, Boston University School of Medicine, Boston, Massachusetts; Private Practice, Brookline, Massachusetts
9. *Promoting Parental Self-Understanding*

Behavioral and developmental issues play a role in almost every pediatric encounter and are often among the most challenging diagnostic and therapeutic dilemmas facing the pediatric primary care clinician. Busy practices, significant time constraints, inadequate training, reluctance to delve into all but purely "medical" problems, and a lack of scientifically validated solutions—all result in the neglect of such issues by many clinicians.

Behavioral and Developmental Pediatrics: A Handbook for Primary Care evolved from our work as primary care clinicians and as educators in developmental and behavioral pediatrics for practitioners. We have learned that primary care clinicians are most effective when they can form therapeutic alliances with children and families; sensitively elicit information; understand the psychological, biological, and social roots of problems; and have ready concrete, practical, and effective treatment strategies.

This book is intended to strengthen these skills in primary care clinicians— pediatricians, family practitioners, nurse practitioners, physicians' assistants, pediatric nurses, and others who care for children. Chapters are written by experts in the field and provide the key information needed to effectively address specific problems. This book is *not* meant to provide encyclopedic, exhaustive information. Rather, we have asked experts to *distill* their experience and the extant scientific literature into a concise, user-friendly format that can be easily understood and applied by the busy clinician. For those desiring more extensive information, a bibliography at the end of each chapter refers to additional key articles or chapters.

Part I discusses the fundamentals of behavioral and developmental pediatrics. It is designed to enable the clinician to create a therapeutic atmosphere in primary care and covers such topics as forming a therapeutic alliance, interviewing, diagnosis, and management. This information informs and enriches the subsequent sections and adds depth and sophistication to the clinician's skills.

Parts II and III address issue-specific developmental and behavioral problems. Each chapter is presented in a similar format to enhance accessibility. Most chapters provide sample questions to facilitate the history-taking process by modeling sensitive ways to elicit the information. The descriptions of the problems are intended to provide sufficient information to allow the clinician to explain the relevant issues to parents and children in a way that demystifies the problem and enhances families' ability to deal with it. Additionally, we have provided useful developmental and behavioral questionnaires and screening instruments in the appendixes for the interested clinician.

We hope this book will help to promote excellence in the management of behavioral and developmental problems during primary care visits and enhance the clinician's satisfaction in addressing such issues. As the pace of social change has quickened, so too have threats to children's behavioral and developmental well-being multiplied in frequency and severity. It is often the health care provider who is in the best position to help families and children deal with these threats. As we approach the twenty-first century, it is clear that pediatric clinicians must become more efficient, sophisticated, and clever in addressing behavioral and developmental issues if families and children are to be well served. We hope *Behavioral and Developmental Pediatrics* will contribute to the achievement of that end.

We thank Margaret Stanhope-Lavoye and Jeanne McCarthy for their invaluable help in the preparation of this manuscript. Their attention to detail, organizational skills, support, and timely responsiveness at crunch time are greatly appreciated.

S.P. B.Z.

Preface

Developmental and Behavioral Pediatrics (DBP) has undergone spectacular growth since the publication of the 1st edition of *Developmental and Behavioral Pediatrics: A Handbook for Primary Care:*

- The field of Developmental and Behavioral Pediatrics (DBP) was granted status as an official subspecialty of Pediatrics.
- Qualified pediatricians have, for the first time, been awarded official subspecialty designation as DBP specialists.
- The Pediatric Residency Review Committee (RRC) has mandated that all Pediatric Residency Training programs must devote at least two months to DBP training to maintain accreditation.

At the same time, most pediatric primary care providers have expanded the DBP services they provide to families. Rather than referring a child with ADHD to a specialist, for example, most pediatric clinicians are now comfortable with its diagnosis and treatment in the majority of cases. Likewise, awareness and suspicion (if not diagnosis) of Autistic Spectrum Disorder in primary care has become more the rule than the exception. Many more clinicians are now willing to serve as a "medical home" for children with disabilities. And the issues that families face (let alone how we define "family") are ever changing, challenging the pediatric clinician to expand his/her repertoire of therapeutic interventions to address the newest "new morbidity".

As in the first edition, this Handbook is meant to further the integration of DBP into primary care and to enhance the efforts in this area of the busy primary care clinician. Towards this goal, we have added many new topics and updated all of the original chapters. We hope it will serve as a succinct, accurate, up-to-date and practical reference, the starting point from which the interested clinician can find immediate support, timely information, and wise counsel.

SP
BZ
MA

The Fundamentals of Developmental and Behavioral Pediatrics

1 Talking with Parents

Barbara Korsch

I. **Description.** The therapeutic alliance is achieved in large measure during the interview. Rapport building, engaging the patient, eliciting psychosocial and personal aspects of the patient's experiences, supporting the parents in their roles as parents, including the child, grandparent, and other significant others—all of these are essential to establish a therapeutic relationship.

   In many communities today, the clinician is faced with cultural and language barriers that complicate the interview. There are no easy solutions for this problem. For language problems, a skilled professional interpreter (preferably not a family member) is the only desirable approach. In the presence of an interpreter, it is essential that the physician maintain eye contact with the patient, continue to address the patient and family directly, and not discuss problems with the interpreter instead of the patient or caretaker (avoid saying "tell her that" or "ask him what"). Cultural sensitivities pose unique challenges to effective healthcare and require the clinician to emphasize all the skills for assessing an individual patient's perceptions, value systems, and health beliefs, especially when offering advice and counsel.

   Although there are no techniques that work for all patients or all clinicians, there are some basics that virtually always strengthen the therapeutic alliance (Table 1-1).

II. **Optimal communication with parents.**

   A. **Listening.** Letting the parent know that you are listening is basic. Body language—sitting down, looking at the parent, leaning forward, showing appropriate concern—is effective in conveying a listening attitude and does not require extra time in the interview. Responding to nonverbal expressions of parent affect is also essential. For example, if the mother's face falls when the clinician suggests the use of a pacifier for a colicky baby, the responsive clinician needs to inquire, "You do not seem to like that idea. Is there any special reason why you do not want your baby to use the pacifier?" He or she may find out that the mother had difficulty in weaning her first-born from the pacifier or that she finds pacifiers disgusting. When screening, behavioral checklists have been used (see Appendices A and B); the parental responses can provide the topics for discussion.

   B. **Facilitating the dialogue.** The parent's story should be facilitated by appropriate empathetic responses, such as, "Tell me more about that" or "I can see that it did not work out so well for you," or "That must be hard for you." The clinician should avoid interruptions, subject changes, and judgmental comments and not prematurely pursue other diagnostic hypotheses, which can derail the parent's narrative. Attentive listening during the opening of an interview promotes communication and rarely takes more than a couple of minutes. Yet it has also been shown that, on average, physicians interrupt the patients within 18 seconds. The reason is conflicting agendas: patients want to tell their story, and clinicians want to pursue their decision making. There are other strategies to facilitate a diagnosis:

   C. **Elicit the reasons for the parent's concerns early in the interview.** "What worried you especially when you brought John in to see us today? Why did that worry you?"

   D. **Elicit the parent's expectations for the visit and acknowledge them.** "What had you hoped we might be able to do for your child today? What would you like to have us explain to you today?" These inquiries may reveal unrealistic expectations for specific therapies or magical cures. At other times, such questions make the clinician's job simple; it may be that all the family wants is reassurance. Once the parent's expectations have been acknowledged, the clinician, the parents, and the child can set an agenda for the visit, which synthesizes the parent's concerns and biomedical issues. It is only after this opening—after listening attentively to the parent—that the clinician can afford to pursue his or her line of questions and fact finding. The first phase of the interaction has taken care of urgent concerns, relaxed the parent, and made

Table 1-1 How to enhance the therapeutic alliance

Process steps	Sample comments
Greet	
Introduce self	
Set agenda jointly	
Listen	
Allow pauses	
Maintain eye contact	
Facilitate	"Tell me more about that."
Do not judge	
Do not interrupt	
Elicit and acknowledge parent's concern	"What are you hoping we'll do for her today?"
	"You thought the high fever might bring on a seizure?"
Elicit and acknowledge parent's expectations	"What are you hoping we'll do for her today?"
Involve the child	"What has this been like for you?"
	"Do you understand why you are here?"
Be family centered	
Guide (not dominate) discourse	
Elicit the parent's solutions	"What have you tried so far?"
	"What would you like to try at this time?"
Make treatment decisions jointly	"Do you think you'll be able to give him the medicine 4 times a day?"
Make closure and agenda setting explicit	

her or him realize that the clinician is interested. The parent will now be a better historian and partner in the task-oriented portion of the interview.

    E. Guide but do not dominate the discourse. General questions allow parents to broach subjects of interest to them. For child health supervision visits, clinicians can use simple questions: "How are things going?", "What are some new things the baby is doing?", "How do things work out at bedtime?", "What is the hardest part of taking care of him now?", "What is most enjoyable about taking care of him?", "Is the baby's father (or mother) able to give you any help?" Open-ended, non-judgmental questions are essential for this phase of the interview.

    F. Use common courtesy. All the amenities of nonmedical human interaction must also be observed. Even clinicians who usually have good manners will, in the task-oriented medical encounter, omit greetings, introductions, and courtesies (such as knocking on the door before entering the examining room or explaining the reasons for keeping someone waiting). These courtesies should include a few appropriate remarks acknowledging the parent as a person, such as, "You sure have your hands full today," to the parent who comes with several children and all the attending paraphernalia, or, "I bet you are impatient with us for having kept you waiting so long. I had to deal with an emergency upstairs."

  III. Talking with the child. Early in the visit, an appropriate approach must be made to the child; this is especially important when the social distance between practitioner and family is great or when communication is difficult because of the parent's anxiety, suspicion, or hostility. The awareness of a mutual interest in helping the child creates a bond between parent and clinician. Throughout the interview, in spite of the necessary record keeping, the practitioner must maintain eye contact with the child and parent and watch for nonverbal signs of distress or disagreement or of reassurance and relief.

  IV. Dealing with acute illnesses. During an acute illness, the interview must be focused. As the parent tells the story of the illness, the practitioner can facilitate responsively: "So the fever has been high for almost 3 days now··· What are some of the other things you have noticed?···. How did you handle that?···. How did that work out?···. What about feeding?···. Sleep?···. Any other changes?"

    • If the parents have used home remedies, it is essential not to make judgmental statements. If the treatment was harmless and the parent feels it was effective (even when the practitioner would not have chosen it), it is best to support the parent's approach.

    • If a parent has attempted an intervention that is potentially harmful (e.g., giving aspirin for a viral infection), the clinician should not use this moment to give alarming warnings (e.g., about Reye's syndrome). Yet the family needs to be informed. Our approach is: "I am glad she is feeling better, but I need to give you some new information. Aspirin has been around a long time, and it has provided relief for many patients. However, we have learned that aspirin can have side effects that involve severe liver damage and can be very serious, although rare. Your baby is obviously fine, but I feel strongly that, from now on, you should avoid aspirin and use acetaminophen instead."

- After the episode is over and the parent is less likely to be overwhelmed by guilt and anxieties, more complete and forceful information can be given. Alternatives and additional treatments can be suggested without undermining the parent's self-confidence and self-esteem.
- To avoid embarrassment and fractures of the clinician–parent alliance, at all times the clinician should ask, "How have you handled that? What have you been doing or giving her so far?", before launching into medical advice. Whenever possible, the parent's own solution should be supported. When developing other approaches, it is best to involve the parent. For example: "Has anyone suggested to you that it is time to give up the bottle feeding? Have you yourself contemplated making a change? How ready are you to make the necessary changes?" Before giving what seems to be appropriate advice, the clinician must assess the families' readiness to change, their conviction that change is necessary, and their confidence that they can, indeed, change. A therapeutic plan has to be a joint venture; rarely should it be imposed without parental input.

V. **Redirecting the interview.** The clinician needs to keep control of the interview, even while being supportive and accepting. When the discussion gets off track, the clinician needs to redirect the discourse—for instance, "We must sit down and discuss that on another occasion after he is over this illness," or "There is some other information I need right now so we can decide about the treatment for this illness." If the parent makes an unreasonable request, such as, "You will give him a shot of penicillin today, won't you?", the clinician can back off and state, "I do not know whether that will be necessary today. We will talk about that after I have examined your son."

VI. **Counseling and reassurance.** Advising and counseling the patient and family can be a continuing process. Some concerns may be addressed at the first mention. For example, if the mother says, "He still wakes up once in the night and calls for me," the clinician may reassure promptly that this is not unusual at his age: "He misses you in the dark alone in his bedroom. Just comfort him, but do not start a night bottle again." Other concerns may best be allayed during the physical examination: "The arches of the foot normally do not develop before the child has been weight bearing for a while." Other topics require a discussion at the end of the visit or even at another scheduled conference time: "I can see you are having real difficulty in setting limits for his behavior at this time. We need to take some time to see what we can work out to help him accept your discipline and to make your life a little easier."

VII. **Closure.**
- **A.** Summarize the relevant points the parent has raised and information he or she has given toward the end of the encounter.
- **B.** Offer other educational materials, such as handouts, and individualize them by underlining certain specific issues or relating them to the parent's concerns.
- **C.** Invite questions from caregivers, family, and child. Even when there is no time for full responses, they can be included in jointly setting the agenda for subsequent visits and follow-up healthcare.

BIBLIOGRAPHY

Beckman H, Frankel R. The effect of physician behavior on the collection of data. *Ann Intern Med* 101:692–696, 1984.

Korsch B, Harding C. *The Intelligent Patient's Guide to the Doctor-Patient Relationship.* New York: Oxford University Press, 1997.

Korsch BM, Aley EF. Pediatric interviewing techniques. *Cur Prob Pediat* 3:33–42, 1973.

Roter D, Hall J. *Doctors Talking With Patients; Patients Talking With Doctors.* Westport, CT: Auburn House, 1997.

Stewart M, Roter D (eds). *Communicating with Medical Patients.* Newbury Park, CA: Sage Productions, Inc. 1989.

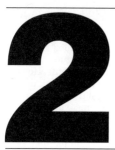

Talking with Children

Yi Hui Liu
Martin T. Stein

I. **Goals.**
   A. **Pediatric clinicians acknowledge the significance of nurturing an independent and trusting relationship with the child.** As a child's primary care provider, the pediatric provider has the unique opportunity to develop such a bond over time. Even brief encounters with children can benefit from the skills required to sustain a longitudinal relationship.
   B. **The child should feel recognized and valued as an equal partner and active participant in their care.** This enhances the child's self-esteem as he or she learns about and develops responsibility for his or her own health and helps the child to view the pediatric provider not only as a source of treatment but also as a source of guidance and support. The child should recognize the pediatric clinician as *his or hers*, not the parents'. These experiences mold the child's self-view and may contribute to his or her response to health and illness in adulthood.
   C. **The establishment of a therapeutic alliance with the child allows the clinician to ascertain important information about the child and the child's environment.** This information includes the child's strengths, stressors, and developmental status. At the same time, the pediatric clinician is able to assess language, speech, and auditory functioning.
   D. **By sensitively communicating with the child, the pediatric clinician models for parents the art of listening to and respecting the views of their child from as early as infancy.**
II. **Creating the environment: promoting effective communication.**
   A. **The reception area.** A child-friendly environment conveys to the child that this place is for children. If possible, provide separate areas for different ages with age-appropriate décor and materials. Toys, a fish tank, books, a drawing board, room to crawl and walk, child-sized furniture, children's drawings, and children's pictures—all impart a welcoming environment. Paper and crayons allow the child to draw pictures which may be used to facilitate conversation or to illustrate the child's perception of self, family, or situation.
   B. **The exam/interview room.** Toys, books, drawing materials, child-sized furniture, and child-friendly décor are once again useful in making the child feel at ease. A quiet, appealing, and private environment encourages the child to interact with the pediatric clinician. There should be no barriers (such as a large desk) between the pediatric clinician and child, and the pediatric clinician should be positioned at the child's eye level.
   C. **The greeting.** When appropriate, speak to the child first. This promotes the message that the child is the patient. Approach the child in a calm and friendly manner and ask him or her what he or she would like to be called. Commenting on a toy or book that has been brought or clothes that are worn can be a pleasant icebreaker.
III. **Communication tools.**
   A. **Open-ended questions.** Start with open-ended questions to allow the child to express her or his thoughts and concerns for the visit. Further questions may elicit the child's personal and culturally influenced perception of the situation, helping the pediatric clinician to understand the child's frame of reference. Targeted questions may follow open-ended questions to generate additional, specific information. Members of some cultures will not respond to or be comfortable with an open-ended question if they are expecting the physician to act in a more directive manner.
   B. **Pauses and silence.** Allowing the child time to organize thoughts or regain composure and then to express feelings without pressure shows the child respect and concern.
   C. **Reflection (repetition).** If the child makes a puzzling or significant comment, repeat the key words or phrases back in a neutral tone to encourage him or her to clarify or elaborate further.
   D. **Empathy.** Acknowledge and respond to the child's feelings to convey warmth and sympathy. Listen for the message behind the words.

E. **Active listening.** Provide undivided attention and facilitate the conversation through open-ended questions, silences, and repetition to communicate to the child respect and concern. Both body language (leaning forward, eye contact) and verbal expressions (e.g., "tell me more") can convey support and interest, allowing the child to feel comfortable in expressing feelings and thoughts and, thus, to more fully participate in the visit.

F. **Tracking.** Allow the child to set the interview's style, pace, and language.

G. **Summarizing.** After explaining the assessment and plan to the child, review the major points; avoid using medical jargon. Asking the child to summarize what has been said will ensure that the information has been understood. It is helpful to make the recommendations practical and concrete.

IV. **Communication techniques for different age groups.**
  A. **General Techniques.**
   1. Engage the child early in the visit with talk, play, or other activities to lessen anxiety. Be mindful of the child's temperament and approach the child accordingly.
   2. Use age-appropriate words and eye contact. Children younger than 2 years, for example, may find eye contact to be threatening. They gain comfort from watching their parents respond to the pediatric clinician in a friendly manner. In addition, questions about "when" and "why" may not be useful in young children who do not yet understand time and causality.
   3. Start with casual questions about familiar and comfortable subjects in an encouraging manner before moving on to more difficult ones. Talk about a child's interests (sports, music), family, friends, or school to develop a rapport. Use special interests as an opener for subsequent visits.
   4. Approach difficult questions in a nonjudgmental and matter-of-fact manner. Indirect statements and questions can be effective in opening discussions about potentially sensitive areas (bullying, fears, school failure, drug use, sex, suicide risk, family conflicts). Starting the discussion about children in general, followed by acquaintances, and then the child, is less threatening. For example, "Some kids tell me that they have a tough time with other kids at school. Do you know anyone with this problem? What has been your experience?"
   5. Humor can dispel anxieties and make the visit enjoyable at all age levels.
   6. The TEACHER method (trust, elicit, agenda, control, health plan, explain, rehearse) (Table 2-1) can enhance communication with children and their parents.
  B. **Communicating with children less than 6 months.**
   1. Developmental stage: Symbiotic. The infant and primary caregiver have a strong attachment. The child is not significantly fearful of strangers.
   2. At this age, the pediatric clinician can model for the parent appropriate ways of speaking to and encouraging language development in babies.
  C. **Communicating with children 6–36 months.**
   1. Developmental stage: Separation—individuation. The child often has stranger awareness and may cling to parents as he or she gradually loosens early attachment and develops a sense of autonomy.

Table 2-1 TEACHER: A method for enhancing communication with pediatric patients and their parents

T	Trust	Build trust and rapport with the child by asking nonthreatening questions not related to illness
E	Elicit	Elicit information from parent(s) and child regarding parental fears and concerns and the child's understanding of the reason for the visit
A	Agenda	Set an agenda early in the visit to help ensure that the parents' concerns are addressed
C	Control	Help the child feel control over the visit (e.g., knowing what will and will not happen) to help decrease fear and increase cooperation
H	Health plan	Establish a health plan with child and parent to meet the child's needs and limitations
E	Explain	Explain the health plan to the child in a way he or she can understand
R	Rehearse	Have the child rehearse the health plan as a way of assessing comprehension; reinforce the child's jobs in relation to healthcare; explore any potential problems in the plan with the child and parent

From Bernzweigt J, Pantell R, Lewis CC. Talking with Children. In Parker S, Zuckerman B, (eds). *Behavioral and Developmental Pediatrics*. New York: Little, Brown & Co. 1995, p. 7

      2. The child should be allowed to stay close to the parent (sitting on parent's lap) for reassurance.

      3. Avoid direct, prolonged eye contact with the child younger than 2 years, as this may be perceived as threatening.

      4. Approach this child gently and gradually. Watch body language to judge acceptance. Wait until he or she is willing to leave his or her parent's lap.

      5. Use play (peek-a-boo, keys, flash light, or toy) to capture the child's attention and ease anxiety.

      6. Prepare the child for physical contact. Imitation with the parent or a doll or stuffed animal will ease the child's anxiety during the physical examination and any procedures.

  D. Communicating with children 3–6 years.

      1. Developmental stage: Preschool age—age of initiative. The child has increasing language skills and engages in fantasy play. The child's understanding of illness is mediated by magical thinking.

      2. Use simple language. Expressive and receptive language skills starting at age 3 years allow the pediatric clinician to begin use of the communication techniques described above to elicit the child's concerns and thoughts. Remember, a child's receptive language is more advanced than his or her expressive language.

      3. Encourage the child to ask questions.

      4. Engage the child by explaining procedures and allowing him to participate in the examination. Offer choices when possible and talk to him about his health care.

      5. As these children enter school age, some time alone with the pediatric clinician can further the development of an independent relationship.

  E. Communicating with children 6–12 years.

      1. Developmental stage: School age—age of industry. The child has improved cognitive skills and has developed the ability to understand cause and effect. Concrete thinking characterizes younger school-age children, whereas the ability to generalize and begin to understand causes of illness occurs in older preadolescents.

      2. School-age children enjoy talking about family, friends, school, and other facets of their lives. Their interests and strengths are easily determined.

      3. Explanation of procedures, assessments, and plans becomes important and helpful in eliciting the preadolescent's cooperation.

      4. Spend some time alone with the school-age child to determine any further concerns and to continue to foster a relationship with the child.

  F. Communicating with Adolescents.

      1. Developmental stage: Age of identity. The adolescent is focused on changing body features and is developing abstract reasoning. He or she is able to understand the general principles of illness and recovery.

      2. Interview the adolescent separate from the parent to respect growing independence, to recognize individuality, and to cultivate the therapeutic alliance.

      3. Elicit and address the adolescent's concerns.

      4. Emphasize and clarify confidentiality issues, as adolescents may withhold information that they believe will be relayed to their parents. Obtain the adolescent's permission to share information or discuss certain issues with others.

      5. Do not pressure the adolescent to talk. Be patient and respect the adolescent's privacy. It is better to revisit difficult topics on a later date after trust has been gained.

      6. Address difficult topics (drugs, sex, depression, anxiety, eating disorders) in a nonjudgmental manner after a rapport has been developed. Indirect questions and statements, as well as asking first about the experience of the adolescent's friends, are helpful.

      7. Talking about "stress" may be easier than asking directly about depression and anxiety. This is less threatening since stress is perceived as a normal part of life.

      8. Always be truthful.

      9. Acknowledge that the adolescent is responsible for personal healthcare and advocate for the adolescent with parents.

V. Clinical pearls and pitfalls.

  A. Cultural sensitivity.

      1. Respecting a child and family's cultural values, beliefs, and attitudes is essential in facilitating communication and cooperation. Ask about cultural interpretations of medical and social issues. "What do you call this problem? What do you think caused it? How do you treat it? What do you expect the treatment to do?"

      2. Knowledge about cultures is useful in avoiding unintentional distress. For example, Southeast Asians will show respect to a physician by avoiding direct eye contact.

Being overly complimentary about a child may elicit fears in the Hmong, who feel this may bring unwanted attention from malevolent spirits.
B. Nonverbal communication. Body language (posture, facial expressions) and quality and tone of speech are important clues to the psychological state of a child. With clinical practice, nonverbal clues may provide crucial information about the veracity or full disclosure of information by a child or adolescent and receptivity to the provider's assessment and advice.
C. The parent–child interaction. Assess parent–child interactions that may provide insights to attachment, parenting style, and parenting skills. Model appropriate use of language, soothing behaviors, and discipline techniques when a teachable moment presents.
D. Procedures. Developmentally appropriate explanations of procedures (e.g., immunizations, venapuncture, operations) are critical, and rehearsal of the sequence of events helps to ease a child's anxieties. The parent's presence during a procedure usually lessens the stress to the child; separation should generally be avoided. Be truthful if a procedure will cause any pain. Offer choices to the child if possible (which arm to draw blood from, what color cast they would like).
E. Illness and hospitalization.
  1. Anticipatory guidance about diagnostic/therapeutic procedures and an elective hospitalization helps both child and parent. A preschool child's "magical" thinking, a school-age child's concrete thinking, and an older school-age child's emerging ability to understand causality moderates their response to illness and the clinician's language and content of information.
  2. Hospitalization is associated with a sudden environmental change and loss of independence. Provide the child with a description of the hospital environment and the procedures encountered.
F. Common pitfalls.
  1. Communicating only with parents. When the pediatric clinician communicates primarily with the parents, an opportunity to uncover important information and to nurture an independent relationship with the child may be missed. As a preventive measure, start an encounter by greeting the child; the implied message is that the child is the patient.
  2. Simultaneously examining and interviewing. This technique does not allow the physician to establish eye contact, communicate effectively, or promote a trusting relationship with the child.

BIBLIOGRAPHY

For Parents

Brazelton TB.Your Child's Doctor. In Brazelton TB. *Touchpoints: Your Child's Emotional and Behavioral Development*. Reading, MA: Perseus Publishing, 1992, pp. 451–461.

For Professionals

American Academy of Pediatrics. *Guidelines for Health Supervision III*. Elk Grove Village, IL: American Academy of Pediatrics, 2002.
Beresin EV.The Doctor-patient relationship in pediatrics. In Kaye DL, Montgomery ME, Munson SW. *Child and Adolescent Mental Health*. Philadelphia: Lippincott Williams & Wilkins, 2002.
Coleman WL.The interview. In Levine MD, Carey WB, Crocker AC. *Developmental-Behavioral Pediatrics*. Philadelphia: W.B. Saunders Company, 1999.
Stein MT.The development-based office: doing more with each visit. In Dixon SD, Stein MT. *Encounters with Children: Pediatric Behavior and Development*. St. Louis: Mosby, 2000, pp. 46–65.
Stein MT:Encounters with Illness: Opportunity for Health Promotion. In Dixon SD, Stein MT. *Encounters with Children: Pediatric Behavior and Development*. St. Louis: Mosby, 2000, pp. 524–545.
Taylor L, Willies-Jacobo L. The culturally competent pediatrician: Respecting ethnicity in your practice. *Contemporary Pediatrics* 20:83, 2003.

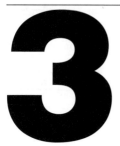

Teachable Moments in Primary Care

Barry Zuckerman
Steven Parker

I. Description. Teachable Moments (TM) represent a strategy to help pediatric clinicians provide effective education for parents within the time constraints of a typical office visit. TM uses the basic assessments of the pediatric visit—history taking, physical examinations, and developmental surveillance—as interventions by exploiting the educational opportunities they present. The strategy of teachable moments is to use the clinician–parent interactions in the office as a compelling, shared experience that furthers parents' insights into their child and enhances their sense of competence as a parent. Using everyday questions and experiences in the office as a shared context for discussion as the visit progresses is an efficient way to address such issues without appreciably lengthening the visit.

The goals of teachable moments are to:
- Enhance parents' understanding of the child's needs
- Promote "goodness of fit" between parent and child
- Model constructive interactions with the child
- Improve the relationship between the pediatric clinician and the parent

A. Using behavior in the office as a teachable moment.

1. Discussions of the infant's or child's behavior in the office provide a fruitful context for teachable moments. Newly developed skills and behaviors may challenge the equilibrium between parent and child. Frequently a specific behavior that parents find disturbing—e.g., mouthing toys at 6 months of age, throwing blocks or food at 8 months, refusing to lie down to be diapered at 10 months, irrepressible exploration at 18 months, playing with the penis at 3 years—is developmentally normal and expectable. Parents' concerns about these issues create a special opportunity to promote parental understanding of health and development.

   a. Concerns new parents bring to pediatric visits in the first months of a child's life provide a wealth of teachable moments. Table 3-1 offers examples of common teachable moments during infancy. The infant's behavior creates a special opportunity to promote parental understanding and support. For example, if the infant cries inconsolably during the visit or is difficult to read, the clinician can explore how parents feel and empathize with their frustration at not being able to calm the baby. The goal of this teachable moment is to blend information about development with the message that the parents are "experts" on their baby.

2. When a child's behavior in the office provides a teachable moment, it is up to the clinician to capitalize on it. During these teachable moments, one might "read" the child's behavior or temperament together with the parents, and offer constructive interpretations of its significance. The clinician should then ask parents how they feel about the behavior or use their own reactions to explore parental concerns. If the clinician finds the child's behavior exasperating, chances are so do the parents.

3. If useable behaviors do not occur spontaneously, the clinician may employ routine strategies to engage the child and discuss the implications for behavior and development (Table 3-2). Parents observe with interest as the pediatric clinician engages the child in activities—e.g., handing the child a toy or a book, rolling a ball back and forth, listening to the heart or looking into the ears—that demonstrate a particular behavioral or temperamental quality or developmental skill.

   a. In some cases a pediatric clinician can direct his comments to the child rather than to the parents: "You like seeing the pictures of babies in the books, don't you?" as you show parents that even 6-month-olds get excited about books. If this serves to encourage parents to start sharing books with babies, the first step in learning to read has been taken. When children push the clinicians hand away as he attempts to listen to the heart, the clinician can talk about other behaviors in which the child is "uncooperative".

4. By observing and commenting on the child's behavior, the pediatric clinician encourages the parents to step back and speculate about its meaning. Unrealistic expecta-

Table 3-1 Eliciting teachable moments

Birth to 4 months of age

Maneuver	Comment
Rock a fussy newborn in your arms and speak softly to console him. Hold a drowsy newborn in a vertical position on your shoulder to bring him to an alert state.	Whether or not your tactics work, explain what you are trying to do and draw the parents' attention to the infant's reactions. If their baby is unresponsive or difficult to arouse or console, they may be feeling rejected. By showing them that this is difficult for you too, you help them understand they are not to blame. Explaining about temperament as an inherent characteristic can encourage them to try new approaches to arousing and consoling their child.
Draw parents' attention to the reciprocal interaction you see going on between mother and 2- to 3-month-old as they take turns smiling and cooing at each other.	Tell parents that this playful exchange shows normal emotional development (baby's smiling, happy face), the beginning of language (vowel sounds, ahs and coos), and cognitive ability (taking turns).
Smile at the 3- or 4-month-old and try to get the baby to smile back; then ask the parents to try.	Point out that parents got a quicker, bigger smile. Explain that while infants at this age smile at everyone, they smile more readily and more fully at the people they feel closest to. This can lead to a discussion of who else gets big smiles (grandparents, the babysitter) and help prepare parents for the next stage when baby's general friendliness will be replaced by stranger anxiety.

tions, which can contribute to parental frustration and lead to child abuse or neglect, can be gently corrected. If parents' reactions are negative, the clinician can reframe the child's behavior in a more positive light. The more mobile 12–18 month can be described as "exuberant" or "exploratory" rather than "disobedient". The child who is "uncooperative" with the physical exam is really "asserting his independence".

a. For example, parents describe how the child throws his food off the high chair tray, making a mess for the parents to clean. They often respond by controlling the feeding and not allowing the child to feed himself. The clinician can join with the parents around how messy babies can be. They can reframe the throwing behavior, explaining how shaking and throwing are the infant's way of exploring objects to discover what they can do. This can easily be demonstrated by giving the child a toy in the office and watching him bang, shake, and throw it. The clinician can create a teachable moment by narrating the child's actions, reframing them as acts of exploration rather than as deliberate attempts to make a mess. The clinician can explain how seemingly unimportant tasks, like using a pincer grasp to pick up a Cheerio, are important windows into a baby's development and learning.

b. Another example of reframing behavior involves stranger anxiety. Many children are visibly upset by the 12–15 month visit because of their heightened stranger and separation anxiety. They may express this anxiety by actively refusing to cooperate with the exam and by protesting when the pediatric clinician tries to examine them. This behavior, often embarrassing to parents, can be used as a teachable moment to discuss stranger anxiety, its developmental function, and to explore its ramifications for the families. Parents are usually relieved to understand why it is a developmental inevitability for their baby to become wary of strangers and actively and loudly resist separation. They are also pleased to learn that these behaviors are linked to cognitive growth in object permanence.

c. The **18-24 month period** is marked by struggles over control, by limit testing, and by the toddler's ability to get herself into serious trouble as he climbs too high or runs away too quickly from a parent. The physical exam and immunizations usually produce enough negative responses from the toddler to bring these issues

Table 3-2 Teachable moments: exploring the world

With each maneuver, comment on the child's interest, attention, and excitement. Point out that these attributes will serve the child well in future learning situations.

Teachable moments 6-12 months

Maneuver	Comment
1. Put a Cheerio in front of the baby within reach. Tell parents to observe how the baby tries to get it.	At 6 months, the baby will use her or his thumb and all her or his fingers in an uncoordinated, raking movement. Explain to parents that babies at this age don't have the fine motor coordination to pick up a small object. Tell them to keep watching. At 9 months, when her or his nervous system is more mature, he or she will pick up a Cheerio with a pincer movement of the thumb and forefinger and put it into her or his mouth. Point out that a baby who can do this with a Cheerio can pick up other small objects as well, not all of them edible or safe. Warn about keeping small objects out of reach.
2. Give the child a toy car, about 2 inches long.	What the baby does with the car will change over time. At 5 to 6 months, he or she will probably put it in his or her mouth. Tell parents that mouthing is the first stage in a sequence of learning about the nature of objects. By 7 to 8 months, they can expect him or her to be into throwing and banging, and at 9 months he will inspect the car intently, turning it over and over in his or her hand and feeling its contours. Each stage yields more information about the car's properties than the one before. At about 1 year of age, he or she will show his or her understanding of the toy's function by running its wheels along the floor.
3. Hide a favorite object under a cloth while the baby is watching.	When the infant takes the cloth away, discuss how this demonstrates their beginning understanding of object permanence. The knowledge that objects continue to exist even when the baby can't see them adds to his or her knowledge that the world has some consistency and dependability to it. Infants are beginning to have a mental representation of the object which explains why they can search and find the hidden toy now when they could not do it at 6 months of age. Compare this ability to understand object permanence with person permanence Discuss how separation anxiety and protest when the mother leaves the room demonstrates that the baby now has a mental symbol of the mother and the discrepancy between that symbol and her not being there evokes crying and protest in an attempt to get the mother to return.
4. Engage the child in reaching for a pen which is extended to him.	The pediatric clinician can again demonstrate improved visual-motor functioning. The infant will shape his fingers midway through the reach, depending on the placement of the pen. This again is a reflection of neuro-maturational development and greater efficiency of the visual-motor process

(continued)

Table 3-2 Teachable moments: exploring the world *(continued)*

12 months (1 year) of age

Maneuver	Comment
1. Again offer the extended pen to the child.	Starting at about 12 months of age stranger anxiety prevents the child from reaching toward a stranger.
2. Give the baby a pop-up toy or busy-box to play with.	Discuss the strategies that the child uses to figure out how to get the toy to perform. The baby who uses a variety of schemes like banging, shaking, and poking has developed more ways to use objects and to extract meaning from objects. This broadens his or her cognitive understanding of how the world works. Relate these exploratory schemes for discovering causality to the classic complaint of most parents that 1-year-olds are "into everything." Emphasize that while this can be annoying to parents and cause for safety concerns, it is the toddler's way of learning about the objects in his or her environment. Discuss ways to amuse busy toddlers while the parents cook, eat, and go about their normal routines.
3. The child's autonomy and stranger anxiety can be seen when the child tries to fend off the physical examination.	This presents an opportunity to discuss with parents the child's temperament, level of persistence and intensity, and autonomy regarding everyday activities

15 months of age

Maneuver	Comment
1. In many cases the pediatric clinician need not do anything to provoke an example of the child's growing autonomy. Most children scream as soon as they get into the room with strangers.	The pediatric clinician can model *how* by slowly approaching the child using his or her voice as a distraction technique. If that approach is unsuccessful, the pediatric clinician can point to his or her own frustration and how other family members or friends who see the child infrequently may feel rejected by the child.
2. Place a string toy just out of reach of the child with the string near his hand.	Note the baby's efforts to get the toy. Discuss the use of the string as an extension of the hand and how at this stage the child must still actively try out each solution to solve the problem. Soon he or she will begin to think about how to get things that are out of reach, but now he or she still needs to actively experiment to figure out how to achieve his or her goals. This is an example of means–ends relations. The toddler has to separate the means (grasping) from the ends (to get) by inserting another operation (pulling the string to get the toy).
3. Give the child a toy telephone and see if he or she can demonstrate functional use by putting the phone to his or her ear. Ask him or her to let a doll talk on the phone.	Discuss the child's ability to represent the use of a toy phone on a doll. This stage of cognitive development signals the beginning of symbolic representation, when the child can use one object to represent another object that is not present. Children at this age can demonstrate the functional use of cars, dolls, and care giving activities like feeding, and can imitate housework like vacuuming and washing dishes.

(continued)

Table 3-2 Teachable moments: exploring the world *(continued)*

18 months of age

Maneuver	Comment
1. Give the child a container and blocks.	Note the seemingly endless delight that toddlers have in dumping and filling. There is a sense of satisfaction and fulfillment to the activity. There is also a cognitive component. Toddlers are learning about the properties of objects in space, about completing a task (when the bucket is full), and about a parent's reaction to the toddler's goal of filling and dumping. This also gives the pediatric clinician the opportunity to talk about throwing objects and offer suggestions for how to handle limit setting with young toddlers.

24 months (2 years) of age

Maneuver	Comment
1. Give the child a simple two- or three-piece puzzle to work.	Talk about the child's attempts at problem solving. Does he or she try to bang the pieces into place? Does he or she examine each one first? This activity also offers the opportunity to talk about the child's persistence and frustration level. Point out how highly persistent children can excel at sticking with a task until they get it and can focus for long periods of time. Also note how persistent children are when they want an object that they can't have. Similarly, children who are easily frustrated by new tasks are easier to distract. Use the opportunity to view persistence in children as having both a positive and negative impact on parent–child relations. Ask the parent to help the child complete the task. Comment on "joint attention," ways to support problem solving, and following the child's lead in play.

30 months of age

Maneuver	Comment
1. Demonstrate the child's receptive language skills by asking the child to complete two and three step commands using symbolic representation. For example, using a doll, bottle, and tissue, ask the child to feed the baby or pose the question "The baby's hungry, what should we do? Put the baby to sleep?" The same activity can be done with fitting toy people into a toy car.	Watching their child perform these tasks correctly can be particularly important for parents who are worried about their child's language development. Demonstrating the sophistication with which the child can follow directions often calms the fears of a parent who is worried about a child who is not talking as well as his or her age mates. It also tells a lot about a child's ability to use symbols as a means for organizing and understanding his or her world. This can also be an indicator of expressive language issues depending on how great the skew.

Pretend play also tells a lot about a child's ability to use symbols as a means for organizing and understanding his or her world.
Many children who are within the normal range for expressive and receptive language may show different abilities for each skill. However, a wide gap between expressive and receptive language abilities may indicate a language delay. |

36 months (3 years) of age

Maneuver	Comment
1. Use a ball to introduce simple games.	While playing ballgames with the child, point out the child's ability to take turns, understand reciprocity, keep the ball within the physical limits set by the game (between your legs and his), and kick it forward.

Adapted from Zuckerman B, et al. *Contemporary Pediatrics.* Dec. 1997.

to the surface. Since clinician and parent have both observed these behaviors, they create yet another teachable moment, giving the clinician insight into how the parents understand the behavior and how they respond to it. It is important at moments like these to

- *Empathize* with the parents. They need assurance that their child's behavior is normal, as is their frustration and embarrassment or anger at their child
- *Explain* that a toddler's autonomy struggles often feel like the child is "refusing to listen"
- *Model* verbal and behavioral strategies to help the child cope with the experience of being in the office, e.g., demonstrating for the parents the importance of setting safe limits for the child while trying to avoid unnecessary power struggles regarding parental control
- *Help* the child feel like he has mastered a stressful situation by commenting on her or his attempts at control: "I know it was hard for you, but you did a good job when I looked in your ears." Instead of the child feeling like a failure and the parents feeling embarrassed or angry or both, the family can feel that you understood and accepted their reactions and that you still like their child and respect their parenting efforts

B. **Using history taking as a teachable moment.**
1. **Evocative questions** during history taking, especially in the first year of life, can create special teachable moments. Such questions might include asking about the parents' own upbringing, the "ghosts in the nursery" that influence their child-rearing practices and their feelings about themselves as parents. Eliciting a family history of depression and alcoholism may help parents understand the impact of these factors on their parenting and their fears about their child's (and their own) vulnerability to these or other mental health problems.
2. Questions about the **child's behavior and development** give parents a chance to discuss concerns in these areas. Especially useful in the early years are questions about the child's temperamental characteristics, developmental milestones, behavioral and family issues, and how the mother and father feel about these issues.
3. A dialog about **parental disagreements** is another example of a potential teachable moment during history taking. Asking how a family handles anger or resolves disputes often leads to a discussion of these issues and their impact on child behavior and development. The clinician might say that children benefit when they see their parents come to a peaceful conclusion after an argument, or point out that conflicts are an opportunity to teach children about frustration, anger, and disagreements without fear of the loss of love.
4. Clinical judgment is always required to distinguish when it is appropriate to expand, and when to narrow, the content of the discussion. Also, it is helpful to remember that while some parents find it helpful to discuss their feelings, others experience personal questions as intrusive. Sensing when not to intrude on the parents' privacy is as important as knowing what, how, and when to probe.
5. Finally, clinicians should be aware that teachable moments also occur when children who are old enough to understand are asked directly about their health and behavior. Asking 3-year-olds whether they brush their teeth or eat their vegetables, conveys the message that they have a responsibility to take good care of their bodies. The opportunity should not be missed.

C. **Using the physical examination as a teachable moment.**
1. The physical examination provides the pediatric clinician with a window into the child's behavior and development. One can comment how *this* child at *this* age responds to the examination, compared to another child of the same age. As the pediatric clinician performs the examination, he or she should narrate a running commentary about the findings: "Heart sounds great—good, strong heart! Lungs are clear . . . No sign of bronchitis. Ears have a little bit of fluid—do you think he is hearing okay?" This running narrative serves, first and foremost, to reassure mothers and fathers that their child is healthy. In this regard, one should avoid ambiguous statements such as: "Well, he doesn't sound too bad or I can't find anything wrong." Such equivocation does little to reassure and may set the anxious parent's mind racing.
2. The examination also serves as a natural springboard to elicit more information or concerns from the observing parent. Neutral, nonjudgmental comments about the child's behavior (e.g., "He certainly is a busy guy, isn't he?") may trigger a host of parental concerns, elicited all the more easily by focusing ostensibly on the child's physical examination and not the parental feelings.
3. Finally, the physical examination is a wonderful opportunity for the pediatric clinician

to reframe the child's behavior in order to enhance the parent–child interactions. One's demeanor toward the child serves as a model for the parent. Certainly, the physical examination must be approached with respect for the child and sensitivity to issues of power and control. For example, the obstreperous toddler who resists examination offers the opportunity to discuss the child's attempts at autonomy, individuation, and his understandable desire to maintain control of his body. The child who cries but then consoles himself sets the stage for a discussion of his coping skills.

BIBLIOGRAPHY

For Clinicians

Parker S, Zuckerman B. Therapeutic aspects of the assessment process. In Meisels S, Shonkoff J (eds) *Handbook of Early Childhood Intervention.* New York: Cambridge University Press, 1990, pp. 350–371.
Zuckerman B, Parker S. Teachable moments: Assessment as Intervention. *Contemporary Pediatrics* Dec 1997. Available at: http://www.contpeds.com/be_core/content/journals/k/data/1997/1200/kca041.html
Zuckerman B. Family history: A special opportunity for psychosocial intervention. *Pediatrics* 87: 740, 1991

4

Touchpoints of Anticipatory Guidance in the First Three Years

T. Berry Brazelton
Joshua Sparrow

I. **Description of Touchpoints**™.

  A. **Touchpoints are the periods in the first years of life when children's developmental spurts predictably result in disruption of the family system.** Developmental progress is often preceded in the infant and child by a transient (and inexplicable) period of behavioral disorganization and distress. The succession of Touchpoints in a child's development is like a map that can be identified and anticipated by both parents and pediatric providers.

  1. Thirteen touchpoints have been noted in the first 3 years, beginning in pregnancy. They are centered on care giving themes that matter to parents (e.g., feeding, discipline), rather than traditional milestones. The child's negotiation of these Touchpoints can be seen as a source of satisfaction and encouragement, as well as a source of stress, for the family system. Foreknowledge of these Touchpoints and strategies for dealing with them can help reduce negative interactions that might otherwise throw the child's development off course and result in problems in the areas of sleep, feeding, toilet training, among others.

  2. Touchpoints may occur somewhat later in **premature** infants, but they will be even more important as opportunities for supporting anxious parents.

  3. Atypically developing children's Touchpoints may in some instances occur at different times or have different features from those of typically developing children. It is preferable to carefully observe, understand, and respect each child's behavior for evidence of developmental disorganization and reorganization rather than to make unhelpful comparative judgments.

  B. **The guiding principles of the Touchpoints model.** Professionals can use these principles as a framework for each encounter with families during a child's first 3 years (Table 4-1).

  1. Several guiding assumptions about parents form the core of Touchpoints' practice with families (Table 4-2) . Perhaps the most important one for the clinician to keep in mind is that *parents are the experts on their child's behavior.* Together, professionals and parents can discover themes that recur and strategies to negotiate upcoming challenges.

     • For example, for 4-month-olds, providers can predict a burst in cognitive awareness of the environment. The baby will be difficult to feed. He will stop eating to look around and to listen to every stimulus in the environment. To parents' dismay, he will begin to awaken again at night. His awareness of his surroundings will be enhanced by a burst in visual development. Yet, when parents understand the disorganization as reflected in these behaviors as a natural precursor to the rapid and exciting development that follows, they will not need to feel as if it represents failure.

     • From the Touchpoints framework, the guidance that professionals can give parents is supportive rather than prescriptive. Anticipatory guidance is not delivery of '"expert advice", but a dialogue, a shared discussion about how parents will feel and react in the face of predictable challenges to come. This is, in part, based on how they have dealt with related issues in the past.

  2. Parents find it reassuring that bursts and regressions in development are to be expected. This represents a shift in thinking for parents who, without this information, would often misunderstand their child's behavior as pathological and question their own caregiving efficacy. In the face of their children's behavioral regressions, they wonder what they are doing wrong. Sharing these Touchpoints preventively helps parents feel more confident in themselves and in their child.

  C. **A paradigm shift.** In order to fulfill this opportunity to use the spurts in the baby's development and the vulnerability they stir up in parents to establish and deepen their relationships with families, a provider must make a difficult paradigm shift (Fig. 4-1).

  1. Healthcare professionals are trained to look for the failures and defects in the child

Table 4-1 The guiding principles of the Touchpoints model

Value and understand the relationship between you and the parent
Use the behavior of the child as your language
Value passion wherever you find it
Focus on the parent–child relationship
Look for opportunities to support mastery
Recognize the beliefs and biases that you bring to the interaction
Be willing to discuss matters that go beyond your traditional role

Table 4-2 Touchpoints parent assumptions

The parent is the expert on his/her child
All parents have strengths
All parents want to do well by their child
All parents have something critical to share at each developmental stage
All parents have ambivalent feelings
Parenting is a process built on trial and error

and parents. Unfortunately, these do not endear us to the parents of our patients. They sense our search for their failures. If we can change to a **model of observing and valuing their successes,** as opposed to a top-down, agenda (guidelines)-driven model, we can engage parents in a collaborative rather than a prescriptive relationship. Parents are aware and grateful for such a change. When we focus on their strengths, they are far more likely to share with us their vulnerabilities.

   a. Though this paradigm shift is easy for many professionals to endorse, it is more difficult for them to alter their interactions with families accordingly. We are too well trained in our medical search for impairments that we can "fix", such that it can be difficult to acknowledge parents' expertise and look for opportunities to support their mastery. As a result of our focus on their problems, we leave parents wary and defensive. When we can join them in a collaborative approach, they let down defenses and become available to develop an effective and satisfying working relationship with us.

  2. A systems model is a valuable way to think of how clinicians can be most effective (Fig. 4-2). Systems theory assumes that **each member of the system is in balance**

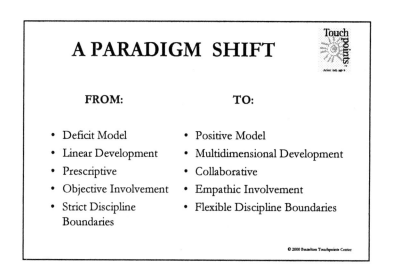

Figure 4-1. A paradigm shift.

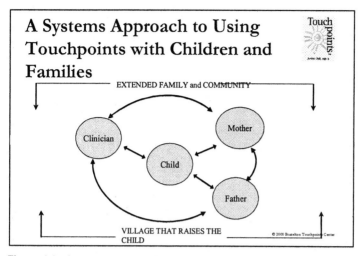

Figure 4-2. A systems approach to using Touchpoints with children and families.

with each other member. If there is a stress on the system, each member must adjust to the stress. As a result, stress can be an opportunity for learning.

If a provider wants the system to learn to succeed, he or she must **become an equal member of the system**. As a member, the professional must learn to understand and value the culture, the ethnicity, the religion, and the belief systems of the other members. Understanding a different culture is a lesson in humility, for the more we learn, the more we realize there is much that escapes us. Such a stance, which empowers the families we work with to transform us, is a far cry from the medical training of talking down to and of giving instructions to patients.

- In order to effect this change the clinician should greet a family with an initial observation of the infant or child's behavior. Initially, the provider can observe evidence of temperament and stage of development, and share these behaviors with parents.
- Other meaningful behaviors to be shared with parents are those that offer evidence

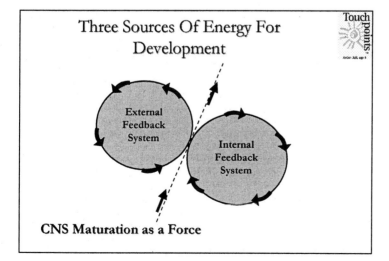

Figure 4-3. Three sources of energy for development.

of a child's own satisfaction in a new accomplishment. When a child strives to succeed at a developmental task, he registers his success with the behavior of "I did it", as the inner feedback cycle closes. The inner feedback cycle (Fig. 4-3), which is registered in the child's behavior as he makes an effort to succeed, is a powerful observation to share with parents. This cycle, coupled with the parent's efforts (as represented by the external feedback cycle), fuel the processes of development driven by the maturation of the central nervous system. Parents can be encouraged by the provider to observe these two cycles and to revel in them, if they don't already.

- Child behaviors that are meaningful for providers to share with parents emphasize the child's strengths and the parents' major contributions to the child's development. These shared observations can serve as an introduction to the relational approach of provider–parent visits. Parents drop their defenses and are more likely to become available to history taking and sharing concerns with the provider. Each visit then becomes more valuable in fostering a working relationship between parents and provider, as parents come to trust that, along with their strengths, their vulnerabilities will be respected and valued.

3. The trust of parents is also more readily won when providers demonstrate their understanding of and sensitivity to the predictable developmental needs of their child. For example, when the clinician respects a 9-month-old's stranger anxiety, he or she has shown their capacity to care for a child more powerfully than by simply saying "I care". The clinician should not be too intrusive by trying immediately to engage the infant. Rather, the clinician should engage the infant in response to the infant's signals of readiness and interest.

4. A Touchpoint provides an opportunity for deepening the mutual relationship between provider and parent. Each one is dependent on the predictable stresses of a child's developmental surges and is matched by the parent's passionate desire to do well by the child. Each of these stresses represents an opportunity. As we join the parents in their urge to foster the child's optimal development, each contact becomes rewarding to them as well as to us as providers.

BIBLIOGRAPHY

Brazelton TB. *Touchpoints: Emotional and Behavioral Development.* Reading, MA: Addison-Wesley, 1992.

Brazelton TB. Soapbox: How to help parents of young children: the Touchpoints Model. *Clinical Child Psychology and Psychiatry* 3(3):481–483, 1998.

Brazelton TB, Sparrow JD. *Touchpoints: 3-6.* Cambridge, MA: Perseus, 2001.

Websites for Professionals

www.touchpoints.org

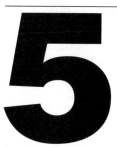

Difficult Encounters with Parents

Barbara Korsch

I. **Description of the problem.** No honest clinician in pediatrics can claim to love all patients all of the time or to communicate well with everyone who appears in the practice. There are certain names on the day's schedule that make the practitioner's heart sink and feel fatigued in advance.

II. **Factors in difficult encounters.** The situations that trigger negative emotions are not the same for every practitioner. It is of fundamental importance for each practitioner to develop awareness and insight into his or her own individual sensitivities and idiosyncrasies in order to minimize counterproductive encounters and to develop strategies for assuring his or her own well-being.

   A. **The clinician–parent relationship.** It is too easy to blame the parent: "The mother was a poor historian" or "She was ignorant, opinionated, and uncooperative." Unflattering labels are often used to take the onus and the blame off the clinician. If it were entirely the parent's "fault" that the medical encounter was difficult, there would be no way of mending the relationship. It is more productive for the clinician to realize that a ruptured relationship usually involves both sides. Knowledge, critical self-awareness, and an explicit focus of interest on the communication process and where it went wrong are helpful in this regard.

   B. **Ambiguity.** Clinicians are trained to solve problems and finish tasks. They want diseases that can be named (labeling is one approach to mastery) and symptoms that can be cured. Yet patients' problems often defy simple solutions. A common reason for difficult encounters lies in the clinician's (or parents') discomfort with this ambiguity. Patients with symptoms that do not point to a known disease entity are annoying and frustrating.

   C. **The overanxious parent.** In pediatrics, the parent who recites the child's complaints in an overanxious and overemotional manner is judged the equivalent of the hypochondriac in adult practice. He or she is equally unpopular and frequently given short shrift, although sympathetic listening to the concerns might reveal significant issues underlying the emotionality. Concluding that "it's the parent who is the problem" and not the child, too often does not lead to problem recognition, empathy, and sympathetic treatment.

   D. **Slow treatment response.** Just as clinicians thrive on the instant gratification of a patient's getting well quickly, so too are they annoyed by patients who do not respond to treatment. Blaming the patient for a poor response to treatment (even unconsciously) impedes the collaboration with the family. The practitioner needs to join the family and patient in facing their common disappointments: "I know you had hoped to see him better by now. So did I. But we will have to be patient a little longer. We do know we are on the right track".

   E. **Clinician limitations.** All clinicians encounter certain issues, which lead them to communicate less effectively, because of special sensitivities. There may be something in the parent's personality or in the presenting illness of the child that touches a sensitive nerve in the clinician. This often leads to over identification, which interferes with accurate empathy. It is crucial that the physician develop enough awareness of these special vulnerabilities so that they do not interfere with optimal patient care"—physician know thyself".

      1. A frequent barrier to effective communication lies in the clinician's difficulty in accepting his or her own limitations. A parent who "shops" for medical care; who quotes other authorities ("When the child next door had the same thing, the doctor gave him penicillin and he was fine the next day"); who reads independently and forms strong opinions ("I read on the Internet that new medicine A is really more effective"); who challenges directly ("How many children have you raised doctor?" or "How many kids with this condition have you treated?" or "How long have you been in practice?")-these are all unpopular parents. The reason, often, is that the

health professional needs to feel that parents will accept *only his or her* authority. The idea that a parent might inquire elsewhere, quote information or misinformation from the Internet, and that there are other valid (and sometimes better) ideas may seem unacceptable. But such paternalism is unjustified in all respects, especially in a therapeutic alliance between clinician and patient-family.

2. Failure to accept personal limitations in knowledge and competence may lead the practitioner to perceive patients as difficult. A simple, "You know, I have not really seen this particular combination of signs and symptoms before. I would like you to see Dr. X who has more experience in this line," may be an effective approach that relieves clinician stress and parental anxiety.

F. **Cultural differences.** The clinician's lack of knowledge about cultural factors that may provoke certain kinds of patient symptoms or behavior can also lead to irritation and impatience. For instance, resistance on the part of certain Latino families to have their daughter's perineum inspected might be interpreted as ignorance and resistance. The informed clinician understands that the mother's reluctance is not a personal reaction but is based on the cultural belief that privacy must be protected in young girls at all costs. There are also differences in cultures of medical care and it is increasingly important for the clinician to assess the families' ideas concerning complementary or alternative medical practices and to include these in the joint decision making.

1. Cultural sensitivities pose special challenges in our Western culture. We take pride in our nonpatronizing approaches, with patients and physicians working as partners, and on maximum information sharing and joint decision making. There are problems in applying this approach with all patients in all situations. Yet even in our community there are instances where patients do not wish to be informed and desire their physicians to make important decisions for them.

2. In many other societies, communication about health and illness is handled much less openly. This is true within families where relatives protect family members from information, and also applies in the clinician–patient relationship. Being informed about fatal illness and bad prognosis may be considered harmful to the patient. These patients' belief systems need to be explored and respected by the physician, even when his own preferences are different. Over time an agreement may be achieved, but the relationship and trust can be damaged by insensitive insistence that our approach be used.

3. Decision making is especially difficult for those patients who have been taught not to challenge their doctors or to ask questions. They may suffer when pressured to decide, for fear or angering the doctor, and also because they do not have the necessary knowledge.

4. Another cultural barrier with which everyone is struggling has to do with language, and as the population gets more heterogeneous increased skills in using interpreters and overcoming language barriers will be needed.

G. **Ambiguous boundaries.** Some parents are unwilling to assume any responsibility, thus putting everything onto the clinician's shoulders" (Can you tell my daughter to stand up straight or she'll make her back crooked"? or "Oh! doctor, tell me what to do! You've got to help me"!) Having once become trapped in such a situation, the clinician will subsequently have to deal with a parent who continues to act helpless and expects him or her to solve every problem. This is a no-win situation with inevitable disappointment for the family. Instead, the clinician needs to support and mobilize the parents' resources and to help the family take ownership of their problems. Recognizing and setting clear boundaries about what the clinician is (and is not) able to do and establishing reasonable expectations for parent–patient responsibility is one of the essential principles of avoiding counterproductive clinician–parent communication.

H. **Judgmental attitudes.** Besides the need for power, authority, success, and the wish to please, other attributes of the clinician constrain open communication. Some clinicians do not like fat children; others overreact to lack of cleanliness. Ways of dressing, sexual orientation, or mannerisms may trigger emotional reactions in clinicians of which they are not even aware.

I. **Overidentification.** Certain diagnoses (such as, developmental disability, leukemia, blindness) may arouse feelings based on the clinician's personal experiences that negatively color the encounter. Overidentification, which is also a lack of boundary setting, is as counterproductive to the therapeutic alliance as is a lack of empathy.

J. **Systems problems.** Another barrier to good clinician–patient relationships lies in systems problems: lack of time; difficulty in obtaining relevant data; excess waiting time for families, which angers them before they even begin the encounter; pressures imposed by quality control and utilization review committees; fear of litigation; and the many other irritants in the healthcare system. When clinicians themselves feel abused by the system and helpless to overcome certain obstacles to optimal care, they are likely to transfer their frustrations to colleagues, families, and patients. Acknowledgment of the pressures for all involved and allowing mutual expression of frustration will often clear the air and lead to better cooperation (e.g., "I can understand that it annoys you that you are not seeing the same doctor today. It is difficult for me too because we could work things out better if I had all the information at hand. In the meantime, let's do the best we can").

K. Time constraints. Especially in busy practices, patients who take a lot of time are very irritating. Clearly, there are patients who suffer from such extreme psychosocial or emotional problems that they do not fit into the constraints of regular medical practice. Patients who arrive without appointments, bring in two children, or ask for advice for other family members need to be redirected with appropriate boundaries and limit setting. It will save the clinician time and frustration to learn to detect the truly pathologic personalities as early as possible so their care can be appropriately shared with mental health professionals or outside community agencies.

Instances of this type, however, are far less frequent than are those in which extra time is needed due to ineffective communication and the failure to recognize communication breakdown. When in the course of an encounter the clinician feels annoyed and impatient, repeating the same message with the sense that it is not getting across (e.g., "What you need is just a regular bedtime routine" to a mother who is struggling to survive in a chaotic and overwhelming family situation), he or she needs to consider: What is going wrong? Why am I angry? Why does this parent act so aggressively? Is there another approach I could try? What can I learn from this difficult encounter that could help this family or parent?

III. Dealing with difficult encounters.

A. Address the problem. Acknowledging that it is the *encounter* and not the parent that is difficult is the most important step. A number of techniques can be helpful.

  1. Confront the parent: "You seem angry. Can you tell more about why?"

  2. Acknowledge the difficulty: "I am having a problem here. I feel we are talking at cross-purposes. Let's see whether we can get off to a better start. What I really need to hear from you right now is …."

  3. Use the common concern over the child: "Let's watch him walk together. Perhaps we'll observe the things that concern you about him, and then we can discuss plans".

  4. Offer a concrete sign of wanting to help. For instance, if a parent is anxious about a sibling who will be getting out of school, allowing her to call a neighbor on the office telephone may turn things around. An extra diaper from the office supply or a quarter for the parking meter may make the point that the clinician does indeed want to help.

B. Expand the system. After setting boundaries for what can appropriately be dealt with, it may be time to expand the system.

  1. Include other family members: "Could you get your husband to come in or telephone me so we can include his ideas in our planning?"

  2. Call on other members of the healthcare team, depending on the urgency and the main focus of the problem.

  3. Look to the community-not necessarily to a health professional but perhaps to the family's clergy or other religious adviser. Sometimes the grandparent becomes a key figure.

C. Give it time. Many things cannot be dealt with on a single visit, and if the task cannot be completed to the parent's or the clinician's satisfaction, both will be frustrated. But if the clinician is able to deal at least partially with the problem and can explicitly defer some of the other concerns to a later occasion, harmony can be restored toward the end of the visit. Solutions may also be more likely after a certain amount of reflection and time has passed. Frequently the parents who annoy the clinician the most are those who require the most prompt follow-up.

BIBLIOGRAPHY

Korsch BM. Do you know these patients? High risk pediatric encounters. *Pediatr Rev* 10:100–105, 1988.

Korsch BM, Gozzi EK, Francis V. Gaps in doctor-patient communication. I. Doctor-patient interaction and patient satisfaction. *Pediatrics* 42:855–871, 1968.

Miller R, Rollnick S. *Motivational Interviewing.* New York: The Guilford Press, 1991.

Prochaska JO, DiClemente CC. Transtheoretical therapy: Toward a more integrative model of change. *Psychotherapy* 20:161–173, 1982.

Quill TE. Recognizing and adjusting to barriers in doctor-patient communication. *Ann Intern Med* 111:51–57, 1989.

6 Helping Families Deal with Bad News

Jack P. Shonkoff
Yvette E. Yatchmink

I. **Issues in delivering bad news.** Conveying difficult information—the diagnosis of a serious chronic illness, a significant developmental disability, or a fatal disease—is one of the most intellectually and emotionally challenging responsibilities a clinician faces. Helping families understand and come to terms with such knowledge can be a rewarding professional and personal experience.

  A. **The clinician–patient relationship.** The clinical challenge of sharing difficult information can be understood best within the broader context of the health care provider-patient relationship. Three essential features of that relationship are particularly critical.

   1. All interactions must be open, honest, and built on a firm foundation of trust. The practitioner must be comfortable with sharing all that he or she knows; the family must have confidence that nothing is withheld.

   2. All interactions must reflect a genuine sense of caring. The need for professional objectivity and rational thinking should never be confused with the destructiveness of emotional detachment.

   3. Supportive relationships cannot be developed instantaneously. They must be nurtured and allowed to evolve over time.

  B. **Individual variations.** Studies of the process that individuals experience as they attempt to cope with stressful knowledge have postulated various stages of adaptation. Such models typically describe a sequential experience of shock, resistance, or denial, followed by sadness or anger, and ultimate accommodation and adaptation. Such frameworks can provide a general understanding of the process of adjustment to bad news, but individual differences among people must guide clinical behavior. Skilled clinicians are sensitive to such variation and have the intellectual and emotional flexibility to respond constructively. It is equally important, however, for practitioners to be aware of the extent to which their own individual values, personalities, and intellectual styles can affect their clinical approaches to difficult interactions with patients.

  C. **Self-awareness.** No clinician can deal with the communication of bad news in a helpful manner before confronting his or her own feelings. Each professional must be aware of his or her own attitude toward chronic illnesses, significant disabling conditions, and the threat of death, and should be able to separate these feelings from those of the patient. Second, clinicians should have insight into their own tolerance for ambiguity and uncertainty, an issue that is embedded in much of the content of the bad news. Finally, all healthcare providers must be able to deal comfortably with a number of affective and cognitive boundaries. These include the capacity to share painful, intimate feelings in a way that is comforting and not burdensome for families and to acknowledge the limits of one's clinical powers without feeling personally responsible for the existence of the problem. As a skill that can be taught and refined with experience, the ability to share threatening or unpleasant information incorporates both the science and the art of clinical medicine.

II. **The process of delivering bad news.** Although the process of sharing difficult information cannot be programmed and must retain a significant degree of flexibility to meet individual needs and circumstances, the following framework may serve as a general clinical guide.

  A. **Tell the family as soon as possible.** Studies of parents' reactions to hearing bad news about their child have demonstrated that most families would prefer to be told as soon as the healthcare provider suspects that there is a problem. Sensitive clinicians must feel comfortable sharing available information, even if it is incomplete and uncertain.

  B. **Arrange for a private setting.** Difficult information should be shared in an environment that provides protection and security. A quiet setting that is free of distractions or interruptions will afford an opportunity for reflection and the provision of meaningful support. Bad news should never be transmitted over the telephone, in a hallway or crowded waiting room, or when strangers are present. Everyone involved should be seated. It must be clear that the family has the clinician's undivided attention.

C. **Ensure that key people are present.** Every effort should be made to ensure that both parents are present when difficult information about their child is conveyed. When appropriate, other important people (e.g., grandparents) may be present, at the discretion of the parents. The inclusion of more than one person provides an additional source of support and relieves one family member of the responsibility of transmitting information and answering questions for the others. If it is not possible to have all key people present when difficult information is first shared, a prompt follow-up visit should be offered.

D. **Personalize the discussion.** It is important for families to believe that the clinician who is sharing difficult news knows them and their child. Always refer to the child by name and acknowledge specifically his personal characteristics (both positive and worrisome).

E. **Get to the point.** Before sitting down with the family, the practitioner should identify the most important message to convey. When multiple issues are to be addressed, it is essential that the core message relate closely to the primary concerns that have prompted medical intervention. Recognizing the possibility that traumatic news may result in a self-protective "tuning out," the most salient information should be delivered at the beginning. Prior to initiating the conversation, the clinician might ask himself or herself: "What is the most important message for this family to understand?" Such information should then be provided briefly, directly, and sensitively.

F. **Stop, look, and listen.** Once the central message has been conveyed, the clinician should stop and wait for a reaction. The critical clinical challenge at this point is to assess the cognitive and emotional dimensions of the parents' verbal and nonverbal reactions. The experienced clinician will be prepared with an agenda for further discussion but will look to the family for guidance on the direction of the dialogue. A professional who is anxious has a tendency to talk too much at the beginning. Under such circumstances, it is particularly important to exert the self-discipline required to be brief, to stop, to listen, and to wait for guidance from the family on where to go next.

G. **Invite affect.** Multiple studies of parents' reactions to the experience of receiving bad news have underscored the importance of having an opportunity to discuss feelings. Because families vary dramatically in the extent to which they feel comfortable sharing their inner feelings, it is important that the clinician invite affective responses. Simple comments, such as, "How do you feel about what I have just shared with you?" or "I know that this is difficult to hear" send a signal that discussing feelings is part of the parent–professional relationship. The clinician should be prepared to allow and support a range of emotions, including tears, anger, and withdrawal. By conveying a sense of caring, kindness, and compassion and by remaining supportive whatever the realities, the sensitive healthcare provider offers a broad range of options that parents will pursue according to their own individual needs.

H. **Answer questions.** Sufficient time should be allocated for parents to ask questions. Some respond with a barrage of specific inquiries; others may ask very little beyond "Why did this happen?" or "What can we do?" All questions must be answered directly and openly. When the answer is unclear, it is particularly important to distinguish between responses to questions that cannot be answered because of the limitations of the clinician's knowledge (e.g., "I don't know the answer to that question, but I will help you find out") and responses to questions that are essentially unanswerable (e.g., "It is *difficult to say what your child will be like 5 years from now*"). In the latter case, it is helpful to explain why the question cannot be answered and to discuss the process by which the healthcare provider and family together can try to reach a greater understanding, if not a definitive conclusion. It also may be useful during this part of the interaction to raise and answer questions that the parents do not identify (e.g., if the child's problem is in any way their fault), as well as to offer future opportunities to answer further questions after the information has been assimilated.

I. **Titrate the message.** One of the most important goals of the process of sharing bad news is to reach some closure (at least for this session) on a well-informed and balanced understanding of the child's problem. Some parents may react to the initial information with a sense of despondency and hopelessness. Others may seem not to hear the gravity of the situation. A skilled and sensitive clinician will listen to the parents and make a judgment about whether their assimilation of the information is overly pessimistic or excessively optimistic. In the former case, it is important to underscore a sense of hopefulness with specific examples of potential positive outcomes (e.g., "Your child will always continue to gain new skills"). In the latter case, it may be necessary to acknowledge the grounds for optimism but gently remind the family about the concerns and their probable sequelae (e.g., "Your child will always need special help in school"). As the clinician watches and listens to the parents, it is useful to ask oneself whether the family's perceptions are reasonably balanced, given the seriousness of the child's problem. No family should leave this session without any sense of hope.

   J. Discuss next steps. The session should end with a concrete discussion regarding specific plans for further referrals, evaluations, and arrangements for appropriate therapeutic, educational, and supportive services. There should be no ambiguity with respect to the division of responsibilities between parent and professional regarding subsequent management and care. Individual differences are important to acknowledge. Some parents may want as much additional information as possible, others very little. Requests for second opinions should be honored and facilitated, and not interpreted as threatening. Follow-up plans should be negotiated collaboratively, and areas of agreement should be clear before the session is ended.

   K. Check whether the message has been heard. As the meeting is terminated, it is important for the clinician to determine whether the family has heard and understood all of the important content. A useful technique is to ask the parents whether someone is waiting to hear about the results of this meeting. The clinician can then ask the parents what they will say and invite them to practice their response. This provides a useful opportunity to hear what the parents have retained from the discussion and to offer constructive assistance in "completing the story."

BIBLIOGRAPHY

Cuddigan M, Hanson MB. *Growing Pains-Helping Children Deal with Everyday Problems Through Reading.* Bethesda, MD: Association for the Care of Children's Health, 1988.

Drotar D, et al. The adaptation of parents to the birth of an infant with a congenital malformation: A hypothetical model. *Pediatrics* 56:710–717, 1975.

Krahn GL, Hallum A, Klime C. Are there good ways to give "bad news"? *Pediatrics* 91:578–582, 1993.

Myers BA. The informing interview: Enabling parents to "hear" and cope with bad news. *Am J Dis Child* 137:572–577, 1983.

Nursey AD, Rohde JR, Farmer RDT. Ways of telling new parents about their child and his or her mental handicap: A comparison of doctors' and parents' views. *J Ment Def Res* 35:48–57, 1991.

Promoting Early Literacy

Perri Klass

I. **Description of the problem.** Children who grow up without being read to and with little exposure to books and to printed language during the first 5 years of life are at a greatly increased risk for reading failure and general school failure. They are likely to reach the age of school entry with poorer language skills, poorer school readiness, and poorer motivation. They may be unskilled in handling books, lacking positive associations with the printed word or with books as sources of pleasure and information. Children who are not able to develop reading skills on grade level in first grade are at increased risk for ongoing reading challenges and subsequent risk of school failure.

II. **Epidemiology.** Approximately one-third of U.S. children enter school without the requisite language preparation to learn to read on schedule. When reading skills are tested in the fourth grade, approximately one-third of the children in the United States cannot read on grade level. Low socioeconomic status and poor parental literacy skills significantly increase children's risk.

A. **Etiology/contributing factors.** There are many reasons why children may not be read to or may grow up in print-poor environments.
   - Parents who were not themselves read to as children may not understand the importance of reading aloud especially to very young children.
   - Parents who have poor literacy skills may not be in the habit of using written language (newspapers, magazines, books, written messages) to convey or receive information.
   - Adults who struggled in school, or who still struggle with written language, may look on reading aloud as a difficult task, or a reminder of failure and defeat.
   - Families may be under significant time stress, lack resources to buy books, or live in areas where appropriate children's books are not easily available.
   - Non–English-speaking parents may not have books available in their languages, may be intimidated by books in English, or may deliberately refrain from reading (or even speaking) to their children in their native language in the hope that the children will grow up speaking English.
   - Parents who are themselves educated may not be directly caring for their own young children, or may feel unsure about what books and reading techniques are suitable for infants and toddlers.

III. **Which families need literacy promotion?** Literacy promotion in pediatric primary care should be offered to all families, regardless of socioeconomic status and parents' educational level. Special attention should be paid to families whose economic circumstances or educational background place their children at additional risk, to parents who have not completed high school, to parents whose English language skills are limited, to adolescent parents, and to families under extreme social and/or financial stress. Despite these warnings, it should still be kept in mind that literacy promotion should take place on a highly positive note, since it offers a tool with which parents can help their children learn and achieve, and also an experience which both parent and child are likely to enjoy.

A. **History.** Ask about the child's language skills, and ask parents if they are already reading to their young children, and ask them what books their children enjoy, or what they enjoy doing with books. Ask about whether books are already incorporated into the routine of the child's day. Ask if anyone in the family has a library card.

B. **Identifying families at risk.** It is important to try and identify parents who may be at increased risk, and may need extra help because they themselves have limited literacy skills. The children of these parents are at risk for reading difficulties and school problems, but these families may also be at additional health risk because of the parent's limited ability to understand other written materials, including prescriptions, handouts, and pamphlets. Asking about parental literacy level may feel uncomfortable and intrusive for many professionals, and it may be easiest to ask for objective information (i.e., how far a parent went in school) as a routine part of patient intake. One study has shown that the number of children's books in the home can be a good indicator of parental literacy level, with parents who claim less than ten children's books in the home more likely to perform poorly on a test of health literacy.

IV. **Management: literacy promotion in primary care.**
  A. **A model for effective literacy promotion.** Reach Out and Read (ROR) was founded in 1988 by pediatric clinicians and early childhood educators. ROR advocates a three-component model of literacy promotion in pediatric primary care.
   1. Primary care providers are trained to counsel parents about books and reading aloud at the health supervision visit.
   2. Providers give each child a new, age-appropriate children's book at every health supervision visit from 6 to 60 months, so that the child acquires a home library of 9 to 10 books by school entry age.
   3. Volunteers in the waiting room read aloud to children and thereby model reading-aloud techniques for parents.
      In multiple published studies, ROR has been shown to result in significantly higher rates of parents reading to children, significantly more positive attitudes towards books and reading on the part of parents and children, and significantly improved receptive and expressive language skills in children as young as 18 months.
  B. **Anticipatory guidance.** Anticipatory guidance offered to parents around literacy should be:
   1. Brief and age-appropriate.
      a. Parents need to understand what to expect from young children with respect to books and reading (e.g., that it is normal for a 6-month-old immediately to put a board book in his mouth, or that a 2-year-old may not sit still for an entire story).
      b. Encourage age-appropriate dialogue, as in asking a toddler to name a picture or asking a 4-year-old to tell you what he thinks will happen next.
   2. Linked to other issues of behavior and development discussed in the health supervision visit.
      a. Discuss reading at bedtime in the context of discussing sleep issues and bedtime routines.
      b. Offer suggestions for how to incorporate books into other aspects of the child's routines.
      c. Encourage parents who are looking at daycare and preschool programs to look for situations where books are available and reading aloud is built into the schedule.
      d. When talking about television watching and young children, offer reading aloud as an alternative entertainment.
      e. Discuss the importance of reading aloud in the context of language exposure and acquisition for infants and toddlers.
      f. Discuss the relationship of reading aloud and school readiness with preschoolers.
   3. Positive and reinforcing for the parents.
      a. Give parents positive feedback if they are already reading.
      b. Emphasize the importance of the parent's voice to the child.
      c. Encourage physical contact between parent and child, cuddling, "face time," all of which will make the books and reading more desirable and important to a young child.
      d. Present reading with the child as something that should be fun; acknowledge the parent's wish to see the child learn and succeed.
  C. **Using books in the exam room.**
   1. If books are available to be given to the child at the visit
      • Bring the book in early in the visit
      • Offer the book to the child and observe the child's behavior with the book while you speak with the parent
      • Use the book as part of your developmental assessment of the child
  D. **Choosing age-appropriate books for children.**
   1. For **6–12 months of age**, choose small board books, with pictures of faces and only a few words per page.
   2. For **1–2 years of age**, choose board books with pictures of familiar objects, family life, animals; choose simple stories, books with rhyme and repetition.
   3. Many **2-year-olds** can handle paper pages, and enjoy books with more complex stories; rhyme and repetition remain important.
   4. For **3–5 years of age**, it is often helpful to offer the child a choice of books. Fantasy

stories are popular, as are funny stories and family stories; also consider alphabet books and counting books.

E. Books as developmental assessment tools.

   1. Observe fine motor development as child handles book, looking for pincer grasp in turning pages and pointing with one finger (at 9 months of age), for increasing skill in handling paper pages (by 2 years of age).

   2. Assess speech and language as child responds to book; infants should vocalize, 1- to 2-year-olds should label with single words, older children may be asked to name objects or colors.

   3. Discuss child's language with parents in the context of the book: by 15 to 18 months, children begin filling in words at the ends of familiar sentences; by 2 years, they can "read" familiar books to themselves or their stuffed animals.

   4. Assess parent–child interaction, and whether parent is able to pick up child's cues, answer child's questions, respond to child's interests.

V. Clinical pearls and pitfalls.

   • Be sure to have the book in the room during the visit, and not to use it as a "give-away" (like a sticker or a lollipop) at the end of the visit.

   • Model simple book-reading strategies in the exam room—pointing at pictures and naming them with infants and toddlers ("That's a baby, that's the baby's nose!"), asking more complicated questions with older children ("What do you think will happen if he gives that cookie to the mouse?").

   • Compliment parents when children take pleasure in the books, or manifest book-handling skills ("He (or she) really seems to like books-that's because you read to him (or her) at home.")

   • If there are any concerns about the parent's own literacy skills, encourage the parent to enjoy the book with the child without emphasizing the word "read," by talking about looking at books together, naming the pictures, telling a story.

   • Be prepared to offer referrals to adult and/or family literacy programs to parents who express a desire to improve their own literacy skills.

   • With non–English-speaking families, it is of course very helpful to have books available in the appropriate language; but when this is not possible, parents should be encouraged to look at pictures and discuss books with their children, even when they cannot read the words.

   • Older siblings can be encouraged to read aloud to younger children.

   • Don't let this become a drill, or a way of pressuring children to read early-reading aloud should be about enjoying books together. Older children will certainly begin to pick up information about print and letters, and parents can encourage this, but hearing a story should not be a test!

   • Help parents understand the link between a younger child who enjoys being read to—in part, because it means parental attention-and an older child who likes books and feels eager and ready to learn to read.

BIBLIOGRAPHY

For Parents

Web Sites

http://www.drspock.com/topic/0,1504,432,00.html
http://www.bankstreet.edu/literacyguide/main.html

Books

Lipson ER. *The New York Times Parent's Guide to the Best Books for Children* (3rd ed). New York: Three Rivers Press, 2000.

National Research Council. *Starting Out Right: A Guide to Promoting Children's Reading Success.* Washington, DC: National Academy Press, 1999.

Trelease J. *The Read-Aloud Handbook* (5th ed). New York: Penguin, 2001.

For Professionals

High PC, LaGasse L, Becker S, Ahlgren I, Gardner A. Literacy promotion in primary care pediatrics: can we make a difference? *Pediatrics* 104:927–934, 2000.

Mendelsohn AL, Mogilner LN, Dreyer BP, et al. The impact of a clinic-based literacy intervention on language development in inner-city preschool children. *Pediatrics* 107:130–134, 2001.

National Research Council. *Preventing Reading Difficulties in Young Children.* Washington, DC: National Academy Press, 1998.
Needlman R, Klass P, Zuckerman B. Reach out and get your patients to read. *Contemporary Pediatrics* 19:xxx–xxx, 2002.

Web Sites

www.reachoutandread.org

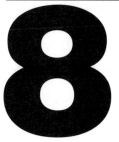

Family Systems

Carol Hubbard
William Lord Coleman

I. **Description of the issue.** Family function has a huge impact on the physical and mental health of family members. Children's behavioral issues, for example, can disrupt the family balance and make parents feel frustrated or powerless; and parental challenges, such as depression, can profoundly affect children's behavior, mood, and even physical health. Almost any behavioral, emotional, or physical complaint in a child may be a manifestation of underlying distress in the family system. The pediatric clinician is uniquely poised to provide family guidance, often being the only healthcare professional in regular contact with the family during the early years of a child's life.

II. **Family assessment.**
   A. **How family issues present.** Table 8-1 describes particular clues or "red flags" that raise the suspicion of underlying family stress.
   B. **Shifting the focus from the child to the family unit.** Techniques that can help to explore a problem within a family context include
      1. Showing empathy for parents by acknowledging the impact of the child's problem on the family": This must be a challenge for you all to deal with as a family. How are you handling it?" An opportunity for such a comment can occur when parents use the term "we" to refer to the people affected by the child's issues.
      2. Asking directly "Who are all the people who are affected by your child's health or behavior problem?"
      3. Soliciting family members' opinions about the source of the difficulties, "What do you think is going on?" and inviting them to work together as a team with you to address the problem.
   C. **Gathering family information.** Information gathering can sometimes jump start the therapeutic process toward better family functioning by encouraging family members to think about the issues involved. History taking also provides an opportunity for the clinician to comment on a family's strengths and past efforts to address problems. Key areas to consider are found in Table 8-2.
      Further techniques for gathering family data include
      1. Eliciting family narratives. Family stories or narratives develop over time to explain past behavior, events, or illness, and are shaped by family members' perceptions and selective memories of past events. Subsequent events are often interpreted in light of the pre-existing story, and may perpetuate the problem. A child, for example, may be labeled "bad" or the "black sheep of the family," and much of their behavior interpreted with that bias. The clinician can listen for such themes, and guide family members to remember other details (exceptions to the dominant narrative) that might support a different "story," one with a more positive slant.
      2. Asking circular questions. This powerful technique involves asking one family member about the perceptions of another. Examples include asking a child "How do you think your mother feels when you and your sister argue?" or asking a parent "What does your spouse think about your son's illness?" Circular questions can be used with several family members present to encourage dialogue and understanding of each other's points of view, or with one person at a time to learn more about their relationships with other family members.
      3. Screening tools. A number of questionnaires are available to be used by the clinician during an interview or completed by parents to assist in assessing topics such as family function, parental depression, and social support, including the Child and Family Evaluation (CAFE), the Family APGAR, and the Pediatric Symptom Checklist.
      4. Construction of a genogram to diagram family structure, mental health, and psychosocial issues is often an illuminating exercise for parents and clinicians.
      5. Family drawings. The child and other family members can be asked to "Draw your family doing something". The drawings can then be reviewed and compared. Alter-

Table 8-1 "Red Flags" for potential family factors in a child's presentation

1. An ambiguous chief complaint or reason for the visit
2. Recurrent, multiple, or chronic complaints without an obvious medical explanation
3. Lack of improvement of symptoms with standard therapy
4. Sudden unexplained changes in a child's behavior or health
5. Unusual parental concern or anxiety about a child
6. Concerning parental behavior and affect (anger, hopelessness) in the office
7. Obvious conflict or estrangement between family members
8. A major family transition or crisis

natively, family members can be asked to collaborate and do a drawing together. Both approaches can provide much information about family structure and dynamics.

   6. Positive feedback. Liberal use of compliments and positive feedback can remind the family of previous success, reinforce positive behaviors, and instill hope. A *positive reframe* of a negative perception may serve to change the family narrative in a way that facilitates problem resolution.

III. Meeting with the family. There are times when it is useful to gather the family together, in order to learn more about a child's issues, to provide them with information (for example about a new diagnosis), or to brainstorm about a problem. Simply letting parents know that they are welcome to bring significant family members or support-givers to the child's

Table 8-2 Areas to consider when assessing family function

Family structure and relationships	Who is considered part of the family?
	Strength of the parents relationship?
	Sibling relationships?
	Who is in charge and makes decisions ("the Executive")?
	Who provides emotional support?
	Appropriateness of boundaries between the members and generations
Family/parenting style	Cohesive versus disengaged and distant?
	Adaptable versus rigid?
	How is affection demonstrated?
Communication style	Can difficult subjects be discussed?
Sources of stress on the family	Internal or external stressors?
	Recent crises or transitions: deaths, births, children leaving home, divorce, illness in family members, substance abuse, domestic violence? Is the home perceived as a safe place?
Background	Ethnicity and culture
	Religion
	Education level
	Parent's upbringing and families of origin (and how their own parenting has been shaped by their experiences)
Environment factors	Socioeconomic level
	Employment
	Neighborhood
	School
	Peer relationships
	Community agency involvement
	Sources of support outside the family

Table 8-3 Steps in convening a family meeting

1. **Contact the family to arrange the meeting**. Have them write down their questions in advance. Encourage participation of the affected members, especially "the Executive."
2. **Before the meeting, formulate your thoughts, questions, and hypotheses about what family factors may be contributing to the problem.**
3. **Find a place to meet with adequate seating for all participants** (a conference room or after-hours waiting room).
4. **Greeting and seating:** Perform introductions and explain the purpose of the meeting.
5. **Social or warm-up time:** If appropriate, ask demographic information about each person (e.g., their connection with the group). Identify the authority figures or spokespersons. Try to match your communication style (e.g., warm, reserved, joking) to the family.
6. **Problem identification/information sharing:** Briefly introduce the issues to be discussed. Then ask each person to describe the problem. Encourage them to be specific, and to describe behavior and feelings. Direct communication between members is facilitated and blaming discouraged. Attempts are made to engage all members.
7. **Goal definition:** Past attempts at solutions are discussed, emphasizing successes. Be positive and encouraging about the group's strengths and the possibility of progress. Assist the family in defining what they would like to see change. Goals should be specific, positive, and realistic.
8. **Homework assignment:** Suggest specific, small, achievable tasks to be done by individual family members before the next meeting to move the group closer to the goal.

appointments can lead to opportunities for group discussion. A family meeting is more effective if the affected family members are present, particularly the family "Executive" or decision maker. A meeting may allow the clinician to meet previously "hidden" but important members. It can be informative to ask which family members are not present, and what they would think about the topics being discussed. A positive, supportive tone, with emphasis on past successes the family may have had in addressing the problem can help motivate family members to work together. The meeting is likely to be most productive if focused on goals and problem solving rather than lengthy descriptions of the problem. A suggested format for a family interview is given in Table 8-3.

  IV. **When to refer.** Referral to a mental health professional is appropriate when the pediatric clinician's work with a family has not ameliorated the problems or when family issues are uncovered that are outside the clinician's ability or comfort level (for example substance abuse or domestic violence). Other factors to consider in deciding on referral include the severity and acuity of the problem, and any associated protective or risk factors.

BIBLIOGRAPHY

Allmond BW, Tanner JL. *The Family is the Patient (2nd ed)*. Philadelphia: Lippincott Williams & Wilkins, 1999.

Coleman WL. *Family-Focused Behavioral Pediatrics: Clinical Techniques for Primary Care*. Philadelphia: Lippincott Williams & Wilkins, 2001.

Coleman WL, Howard BJ. Family-focused behavioral pediatrics. *Pediatr Rev;* 16:448–455, 1995.

McDaniel S, Campbell TL, Seaburn DB. *Family-Oriented Primary Care*. New York: Springer-Verlag, 1990.

9

Promoting Parental Self-Understanding

Barry Zuckerman
Pamela M. Zuckerman

I. **Description of the problem.** Adults are challenged by novel tasks when they first become parents and they often experience concerns, anxieties, and fears. New parents must also address previously unexplored values and attitudes now brought to the fore by the birth of their baby. New day-to-day activities and routines, new problems needing solutions, and normal struggles and uncertainties can elicit heightened emotional responses from parents.

Mundane and minor matters can elicit worry (e.g., parents' great anxiety when their infant has not had a bowel movement in 2 days). More serious and threatening experiences also cause internal upset (e.g., a mother's feelings of exhaustion and being literally consumed by her ever-hungry new infant; a father's dismay at his wife's physical and at times emotional unavailability as she completely focuses on the new infant).

In addition to these universal early experiences, parents know that ahead of them are the even more challenging tasks and risks of child rearing.
- How will they protect the child from their own occasional frustration, anger, or irritability?
- How will they avoid being overindulgent and also set limits that are not too harsh or arbitrary?
- How will they balance providing praise appropriately and correcting unwanted behaviors effectively without being either too strict or overly permissive?

II. **Process of self-understanding.** The pediatric clinician input around child development information and child rearing strategies is often inadequate to help parents negotiate the myriad feelings and the complex tasks involved in successful parenting. What parents really need to be successful is to develop understanding and insight into their own past, especially their relationship to their own parents, and to also understand their own patterns of behavior. Self-understanding for parents develops over time through review of their past upbringing through remembering, retelling, reflecting on and perhaps reinterpreting past events. This process is catalyzed and assisted through ongoing conversations with spouse, relatives, friends, and other parents and professionals.

Without adequate self-understanding, problems can arise for parents when experiences, attitudes, and fears arising from their own upbringing, cause them to respond inconsistently or behave inappropriately toward their child. And when parents do direct excessive anger, withdrawal, sarcasm, harsh criticism, or rigid orders toward their child, it can be upsetting, confusing and ultimately damaging for the child. In order to short-circuit inappropriate responses to their child, parents need to be aware of the origins of their attitudes and behaviors. Again, this is achieved through reflection and self-exploration.

Pediatric clinicians can foster self-understanding in parents by asking key questions at critical times and then listening to the answer. Questions that are particularly important address parents' attitudes and values, especially as they relate to their own childhood and how their parents raised them. Growing up in a family that's overly strict or harsh or lacks emotional warmth can program children to recreate the same family style when they become parents. But when parents have reviewed their own upbringing thoughtfully, have considered which aspects were positive and which were not, and have decided how they would like to raise their own children, research shows they are much less likely to repeat maladaptive patterns learned in the past.

A. **Questions for self-understanding.** There are a number of simple, straightforward questions that pediatricians can ask that will help parents begin to look at their own personal stories and make connections between their current experiences being a parent now and their past experiences as a child growing up.

General themes to be addressed include experiences of love, nurturing, separation, care when distressed, times of feeling threatened, and experiences of loss. Other related topics, which may also be helpful, include experiences of being disciplined, the presence of siblings, and changes in the relationship with the parents during adolescence and adulthood. Parents can be relieved when they gain insight into the connections between

Table 9-1 Questions for parental self-reflection

These questions can be asked over the course of many visits over many years.

Do you plan to raise your child like your mother and father raised you? What was your parents' philosophy in raising children? What was it about it that you liked? What was it about it that you didn't like?

How did you get along with your parents? How did the relationship evolve throughout your youth and up until the present time?

How did your relationship with your mother and father differ and how were they similar? Can you describe three characteristics of your childhood relationship to each of your parents? Why did you choose these adjectives? Are there ways in which you try to be like, or try not to be like, either of your parents?

Do you recall your earliest separations from your parents? What was it like? Did you ever have prolonged separations from your parents?

What kind of discipline do your parent use? Did your mother or father differ? What impact did that have on your childhood, and how do you feel it affects your role as a parent now?

Did you ever feel rejected or threatened by your parents? Were there other experiences you had that felt overwhelming or traumatizing in your life, during childhood or beyond? Do any of these experiences still feel very much alive? Do they continue to influence your life?

Did anyone significant in your life die during your childhood or later in life? What was that like for you at the time, and how does that loss affect you now?

How did your parents communicate with you when you were happy and excited? Did they join with you in your enthusiasm? When you were distressed or unhappy as a child, what would happen? Did your father and mother respond differently to you during these emotional times? How?

Was there anyone else besides your parents in your childhood who took care of you? What was that relationship like for you? What happened to those individuals? What is it like for you when you let others take care of your child now?

If you had difficult times during your childhood, were there positive relationships in or outside of your home that you could depend on during those times? How do you feel those connections benefited you then, and how might they help you now?

How have your childhood experiences influenced your relationships with others as an adult? How has your childhood shaped the ways in which you relate to your children?

Adapted from Siegel DJ, Kaetzel M. *Parenting from the inside out.* New York: Putnam Books, 2003.

difficult events in their past and unexpected eruptions in their present life with their children. When these connections are made and parents gain insight into some of the underpinnings of their own behavior, parents are often then able to let go of some struggles or rigidity they are involved in with their children.

The pediatric clinician can begin with gentle questions (see Table 9-1) to open the door, to invite parents to remember, to retell and to rethink the emotional meanings of their past lives in context with their new role as a mother or a father. Because the pediatric clinician is a trusted professional the parents can tolerate and respond thoughtfully to these personal questions. The pediatric clinician need not ask all these questions at one visit and should consider this as an ongoing conversation that may vary in need and intensity at different stages in the child's development or parents' life circumstances.

By bringing up these questions in the first year of life, the pediatric clinician can use information obtained as a base to further elicit parents' feelings and reflections when normal parent–child difficulties arise. The longitudinal and trusting relationship is a special advantage that pediatricians have over mental health professionals when a problem arises. It potentially promotes timely, effective resolution before a problem progresses.

Asking these or related questions needs to be accompanied by a little time to listen to a parent's responses. Pediatric clinicians don't have to listen indefinitely or hear it all at once, nor do they have to respond with explanations or advice immediately. If necessary, the appropriate "referral" is to a spouse, friends, or selected family members. The professional can say something like, "It sounds like you have many memories and feelings. I would encourage you to talk to your spouse, sister, friends about them to give you insight into what you want to do and don't do as a parent."

Outside the pediatric office setting the issues can be explored in greater depth and complexity in the parents' circle of friends and family, and with other therapeutic professionals if appropriate or desired. Spouses and friends can assist parents in continuing the process of insightful exploration, "making sense" of a parent's personal history with supportive, empathic, emotionally directed conversations.

Both science and clinical experience tell us that parents' self-understanding can greatly enhance their ability to be good parents and to foster their children's optimal development. The pediatric clinician's role is to raise the issues and support the process of parental self-understanding through reflection and discussion with others. A continuity of care setting allows questions and the unfolding answers and their clarification and import to occur over time.

BIBLIOGRAPHY

For Parents

Siegel DJ, Hartzel M. *Parenting from the inside out.* New York: Penguin Putnam, 2003.

For Professionals

Fraiberg S, Adelson E, Shapiro V. The Nursery. *J Am Acad Child Psychiatry* 14:387–421, 1975.
Mav M. Attachment: overview with implications for clinical work. In: Goldberg S, Muir R, Kerr J, eds. *Attachment theory: social, developmental, and clinical perspectives* Hillsdale, NJ: Analytic Press, 407–474, 1995.
Zuckerman B, Zuckerman P, Siegel DJ. Beyond giving information: promoting parental self understanding. *Contemporary Pediatrics,* in press.

Behavioral Screening

Terry Stancin
Ellen C. Perrin

I. **Description of the problem.** Behavioral and emotional problems have been shown to be common in children, yet they are often unrecognized and untreated. Studies in primary care settings have shown that close to 25% of children have *significant* behavioral problems, yet pediatric clinicians fail to identify many of them and refer successfully only a minority of children to mental health professionals for further evaluation and treatment. The use of standardized instruments and other systematic procedures have been shown to increase identification of child behavior problems in primary care settings. Unfortunately, routine systematic behavioral screening is not widespread in pediatric practice. Screening should be done within the context of a clinical evaluation that combines information from a thorough history, direct observation, physical examination, and diagnostic tests. A screening procedure should be psychometrically sound, acceptable to parents, accurate, cost effective, and fit into the practice setting.

Most of the screening methods for behavioral problems rely on parent report, often via questionnaire or rating scales. Some providers may prefer to tailor non-standardized screening procedures to the needs of their practice. Standardized rating scales allow comparisons to normative standards, analogous to showing parents a child's weight on a standardized growth chart. Most can be administered in advance of clinical encounters and scored easily by clerical staff, and thus are efficient and inexpensive methods for collecting information. Rating scales also can be an excellent way to collect and compare the opinions of multiple observers, especially teachers.

II. **Selection and utilization of behavioral screening instruments.**

A. **Selection of screening methods depends on the particular goals of screening but should take into consideration the following factors**
   - Ages of the children to be screened
   - Informants (parent, teacher, child)
   - Characteristics of available screening tools (sensitivity, specificity, acceptability, efficiency, and cost)
   - Impact of procedures on practice (e.g., training and supervision of staff responsible for implementation and maintenance of screening procedures)
   - Reimbursement issues
   - Procedures for further evaluation and interventions of children who screen positive
   - Mental health resources available
   - Possible adverse consequences to screening

   Table 1 contains a list of some behavioral screening instruments that have been recommended for use in pediatric settings. Comparative studies have not been conducted to allow a recommendation of any one method over the others.

B. **Incorporating behavioral instruments into practice.**
   1. Short "first stage" screening measures are appropriate to administer routinely to all children in a setting, such as the pediatric clinician's waiting room. First stage measures focus on broad concerns such as general psychosocial dysfunction, disruptive behavior, or family functioning and can be completed and scored in less than 10 minutes. An example of this is the Pediatric Symptom Checklist (PSC).
   2. A longer, "second stage" screening instrument may follow positive results of a first stage screening or whenever a clinician has identified a problem, in order to obtain more detailed information about the nature and severity of behavioral concerns. These instruments, such as the Child Behavior Checklist (CBCL) and the Behavioral Assessment Scale for Children (BASC), tend to be multidimensional in focus and have normative standards by which to evaluate severity of problems.

C. **Cautions regarding the use of standardized questionnaires.**
   - Interpretation of results must take into account the fact that any caregiver's perceptions are subject to biases. Procedures that rely on parent report may yield false

Table 10-1 Selected behavioral screening instruments

Title of instrument	Screening focus	Informant	Ages (years)	Time (minutes)	Comments
1st Stage Screening					
Pediatric Symptom Checklist (PSC) http://psc.partners.org	General psychological functioning	Parent	4–16	<5	Specifically designed for use in pediatric settings to screen for psychosocial dysfunction. Cutoffs, but no standard scores. Can be downloaded and used free of charge. Acceptable psychometrics.
Parent Guides to Pediatric Visits www.aap.org	General developmental and behavioral concerns	Parent	0–21	10	Easily administered by staff in office area. Parent and child self-identify concerns for discussion with primary care pediatrician. Can be downloaded and used free of charge. Psychometrics not available.
Brief Infant-Toddler Social-Emotional Assessment Scale (BITSEA) Email: ITSEA@yale.edu	Emotional competencies and problems of infants and toddlers	Parent	1–4	15	Developmentally and clinically sensitive. Obtain free from test developers. Acceptable psychometrics.
Parents' Evaluation of Developmental Status (PEDS) www.pedstest.com	Developmental and behavioral concerns	Parent	0–8	5	Questions prompt parents to observe and describe concerns. Acceptable psychometrics.
Eyberg Child Behavior Inventory (ECBI) www.parinc.com	Disruptive behavior problems	Parent	2–16	5	Easy to administer and score; disruptive problems only. Acceptable psychometrics.
Family Psychosocial Screening http://www.pedstest.com/links/resources.html	Family psychosocial risk factors	Parent	All	<15	Can be used as clinic intake form. Free in public domain. Acceptable psychometrics.
McMaster Family Assessment Device (FAD), General Functioning Subscale Email: Familyresearch@lifespan.org	Global family functioning	Parent	4–16	5	Brief and sensitive measure of global family functioning. Provides limited information on specific concerns unless entire 60-item test is given. Acceptable psychometrics.

(continued)

Table 10-1 Selected behavioral screening instruments (*continued*)

Title of instrument	Screening focus	Informant	Ages (years)	Time (minutes)	Comments
2nd Stage Screening Child Behavior Checklists (CBCL, TRF, C-TRF, YSR) http://ASEBA.uvm.edu	Multi-dimensional behavioral screening and assessment	Parent, teacher and child self-report formats	1.5–Adult	20	Broad-based measure of pathology. Provides a profile of internalizing and externalizing problems. Standard T-scores provide norm-based comparisons by age and gender, with DSM-compatible scales. Spanish versions available. Computer scoring or Internet administration recommended. Acceptable psychometrics.
Behavior Assessment System for Children (BASC) www.agsnet.com	Multi-dimensional behavioral screening and assessment	Parent, teacher and child self-report formats	2–18	20	Broad-based measure of pathology. Provides a profile of internalizing and externalizing problems, other problems (atypicality, withdrawal); and adaptive skills. Standard T-scores provide norm-based comparisons by age and gender. Validity check included. Norms available by age and gender. Computer scoring recommended. Acceptable psychometrics.
Infant-Toddler Social-Emotional Assessment Scale (ITSEA) Email: ITSEA@yale.edu	Emotional competencies and problems of infants and toddlers	Parent	1–4	40	Extension of BITSEA. Developmentally and clinically sensitive. Obtain free from test developers. Acceptable psychometrics.

Portions adapted from: Perrin E, Stancin T. A continuing dilemma: whether and how to screen for concerns about children's behavior in primary care settings. *Pediatrics in Review* 23: 264–282, 2002; and from Stancin T, Aylward GP. Screening instruments: behavioral and developmental. In Ollendick T, Schroeder C (eds). *Encyclopedia of Pediatric and Child Psychology*. New York: Kluwer Academic/Plenum, 2003;574–577.
Test author references available at most test websites.

negative results when the parent does not perceive behaviors as problematic. Use of multiple informants is ideal.
- Screening procedures carry costs for implementation (e.g., purchase of materials, implementation costs, scoring, subsequent care).
- New administrative demands are placed on office staff to administer questionnaires properly. Training, supervision, and expertise are necessary to ensure proper scoring and valid interpretation of results. To properly interpret results, the provider must be familiar with and understand the meaning of a test's psychometric properties and norms.
- Screening is intended to identify those in need of further evaluation and assessment, not to provide a diagnosis. Because of the complexities described above, pediatric providers should seek consultation from a knowledgeable pediatric psychologist when selecting and incorporating formal rating scales into practice.

D. **Beyond Screening.** Most pediatric providers will benefit from help with the *management* of children with behavioral problems even more than with their identification. *Screening for any condition presupposes a system in place for following up appropriately when a problem is identified.* Communication between mental health professionals and primary care pediatricians is often cumbersome and frequently inadequate. Therefore, a collaborative relationship with one or more mental health professionals in the community is advisable. New models of collaborative care and improved payment mechanisms are urgently needed to create a fully responsive system for regular and comprehensive child health supervision and care.

BIBLIOGRAPHY

Eisert DC, Sturner RA, Mabe PA. Questionnaires in behavioral pediatrics: Guidelines for selection and use. *J Dev Behav Pediatr* 12:42–50, 1991.
Perrin EC. Ethical questions about screening. *J Dev Behav Pediatr* 19:350–352, 1998.
Perrin E, Stancin T. A continuing dilemma: Whether and how to screen for concerns about children's behavior in primary care settings. *Pediatrics in Review* 23:264–282, 2002.
Stancin T, Aylward GP. Screening instruments: behavioral and developmental. In: Ollendick T, Schroeder C (eds). *Encyclopedia of Pediatric and Child Psychology*. New York: Kluwer Academic/Plenum, 2003;

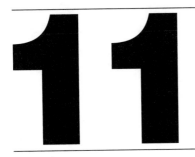

Developmental Screening

Frances Page Glascoe

I. **The problem of underdetection.** Most children with developmental and behavioral problems have subtle symptoms that are not readily apparent in the absence of measurement. Because few medical professionals use standardized screening tests routinely, **70% to 80% of children with disabilities are not detected prior to school entrance**, vital opportunities for early intervention are missed.

II. **Pitfalls.** Developmental checklists, such as those incorporated into patient encounter forms, appear to be a major contributor to underdetection of disabilities in pediatric settings. All lack validated scoring criteria and many include items that are far too easy for the age levels given. Checklists lack any proof of accuracy. Similarly, the subtle and emerging nature of developmental problems, the gradual adverse impact of psychosocial risk factors, and dearth of dysmorphology and physical symptomotology in children with disabilities, illustrate the problems of clinical observation in detecting those with disorders and delays.

III. **Pearls.** The optimal tools for identifying developmental and behavioral problems in primary care are those that:
- Have proven levels of accuracy (at least 70% to 80% of children with and without problems should be detected correctly).
- Rely on information from parents. Parent-based screens take little time to administer (because parents can complete them in waiting or exam rooms) and are easy to use because pediatric clinicians need not elicit skills directly from children who may be fearful, uncooperative, sick, or asleep. Parents, regardless of their level of education or parenting experience, are equally able to provide predictive information about their children. For non-English speaking parents, some screens are published in multiple languages.

IV. **Tools.** Several good quality measures relying on information from parents are presented in Table 11-1. Two additional screens involving direct elicitation of children's skills are also included in the recognition that some clinicians prefer this approach.

One of the measures listed in Table 11-1, Parents' Evaluation of Developmental Status (PEDS) is particularly suitable for pediatric offices because it:
- Capitalizes on typical aspects of a pediatric encounter-asking parents about their concerns-while using questions proven to be effective.
- Takes about two minutes to score.
- Offers decision support on when to refer and where, when to counsel families, when to screen further (or refer for additional screening), when to watchfully wait, versus reassure and continue to monitor developmental and behavioral progress. Completed Response and longitudinal Interpretation forms are presented in Figures 11-1 and 11-2. The Score form (not shown) is printed on the back of the Interpretation form and illustrates the concerns predictive of developmental problems according to children's ages and the American Academy of Pediatrics' well visit schedule—thus providing documentation for chart audits.
- Improves parent satisfaction with health care.
- Reduces parents' frustration with child-rearing and promotes use of positive disciplinary techniques (e.g., time-out versus spanking).
- Appears to reduce "oh by the way" concerns, shorten visit length, improve provider confidence in decision-making, and enhance patient flow.

V. **Making it work in primary care.** There are many approaches to organizing pediatric settings so that developmental and behavioral problems can be easily detected and addressed while maintaining patient flow and office efficiency. Table 11-2 is a list of such methods. *(Text continues on page 50)*

Table 11-1 Screening tools

Developmental screens relying on information from parents	Age range	Description	Scoring	Accuracy	Time frame and costs
Parents' Evaluations of Developmental Status (PEDS) (1997) Ellsworth & Vandermeer Press, Ltd. P.O. Box 68164 Nashville, TN 37206 Phone: 615-226-4460; fax: 615-227-0411 www.pedstest.com ($30.00)	Birth–9 years	10 questions eliciting parents' concerns in English, Spanish, Vietnamese, and Chinese. Written at the 5th grade level. Determines when to refer, provide a second screen, provide patient education, or monitor development, behavior/emotional, and academic progress	Identifies children as low, moderate, or high risk for various kinds of disabilities and delays	Sensitivity 74%–79% and specificity 70%–80% across age levels	About 2 minutes (if interview needed) Materials ~$.31 Admin. ~$.88 Total ~$1.19
Infant Development Inventory (1992) Behavior Science Systems P.O. Box 580274 Minneapolis, MN 55458 Phone: 612-929-6220 ($11.00)	3–18 months	Presents parents with a grid with very brief descriptions of 60 skills sorted by developmental domains. Parents mark each as tasks children can, can't yet, or are beginning to do, and these are then compared to a age cutoffs. The 300-item Child Development Inventory may be useful in subspecialty clinics and produces a range of scores	A single cutoff tied to 1.5 standard Deviations below the mean	Sensitivity in detecting children with difficulties is excellent (>75% across studies) and specificity in correctly detecting normally developing children is good (70% across studies).	About 10 minutes (if interview needed) Materials ~$.40 Admin. ~$3.40 Total ~$3.80
Ages and Stages Questionnaire (formerly Infant Monitoring System) (1994) Paul H. Brookes, Publishers P.O. Box 10624, Baltimore, MD 21285 Phone: 800-638-3775. ($190) www.pbrookes.com	4–60 months	Parents indicate children's developmental skills on 25–35 items (4–5 pages) using a different form for each well visit. Reading level varies across items from 3rd to 12th grade. Can be used in mass mail-outs for child-find programs. In English, Spanish, French	Single pass/fail score	Sensitivity 70%–90% at all ages except the 4-month level; specificity 76%–91%	About 15 minutes (if interview needed) Materials ~$.40 Admin. ~$4.20 Total ~$4.60

(continued)

Table 11-1 Screening tools

Developmental screens relying on information from parents	Age range	Description	Scoring	Accuracy	Time frame and costs
BEHAVIORAL/EMOTIONAL SCREENS RELYING ON INFORMATION FROM PARENTS					
Eyberg Child Behavior Inventory/Sutter-Eyberg Student Behavior Inventory Psychological Assessment Resources P.O. Box 998 Odessa FL: 33556 Phone: 800-331-8378 ($120.00) www.parinc.com	2–16 years	The ECBI/SESBI consists of 36–38 short statements of common behavior problems. More than 16 suggests the referrals for behavioral interventions. Fewer than 16 enables the measure to function as a problems list for planning in-office counseling and selecting handouts. The tools are helpful in monitoring behavioral progress	Single refer/ nonrefer score for externalizing problems (conduct, attention, aggression, etc.)	Sensitivity 80%, specificity 86% to disruptive behavior problems	About 7 minutes (if interview needed) Materials ~$.30 Admin. ~$2.38 Total ~$2.68
Pediatric Symptom Checklist Jellinek MS, Murphy JM, Robinson J, et al. Pediatric Symptom Checklist: Screening school age children for academic and psychosocial dysfunction. *Journal of Pediatrics* 112:201–209, 1988 (the test is included in the article; also can be freely downloaded at http:// psc.partners.org or with factor scores at www.pedstest.com	4–16 years	35 short statements of problem behaviors including both externalizing (conduct) and internalizing (depression, anxiety, adjustment, etc.) Ratings of never, sometimes, or often are assigned a value of 0, 1, or 2. Scores totaling 28 or more suggest referrals. Factor scores identify attentional, internalizing, and externalizing problems. Factor scoring is available for download at: http://www.pedstest.com/links/ resources.html	Single refer/ nonrefer score	All but one study showed high sensitivity (80%–95%) but somewhat scattered specificity (68%–100%)	About 7 minutes (if interview needed) Materials ~$.10 Admin. ~$2.38 Total ~$2.48
Parents' Evaluations of Developmental Status (PEDS) (1997) Ellsworth & Vandermeer Press, Ltd. P.O. Box 68164 Nashville, TN 37206 Phone: 615-226-4460; fax: 615-227-0411 www.pedstest.com ($30.00)	Birth–9 years	10 questions eliciting parents' concerns in English, Spanish, Vietnamese, and Chinese. Written at the 5th grade level. Determines when to refer, provide a second screen, provide patient education, or monitor development, behavior/ emotional, and academic progress	Identifies children as low, moderate, or high risk for various kinds of disabilities and delays	Sensitivity 74%–79% and specificity 70%–80% across age levels	About 2 minutes (if interview needed) Materials ~$.31 Admin. ~$.88 Total ~$1.19

(continued)

Table 11-1 Screening tools (continued)

Developmental screens relying on information from parents	Age range	Description	Scoring	Accuracy	Time frame and costs
Ages & Stages Questionnaires: Social-Emotional (ASQ:SE) Paul H. Brookes, Publishers P.O. Box 10624, Baltimore, MD 21285 Phone: 800-638-3775 ($125) www.pbrookes.com	6–60 months	Designed to supplement the ASQ, the ASQ:SE consists of 30-item forms (4–5 pages long) for each of 8 visits between 6 and 60 months. Items focus on self-regulation, compliance, communication, adaptive functioning, autonomy, affect, and interaction with people	Single cutoff score indicating when a referral is needed	Sensitivity 71%–85%; specificity from 90%–98%	10–15 minutes (if interview needed) Materials ~$.40 Admin. ~$4.20 Total ~$4.40
FAMILY SCREENS					
Family Psychosocial Screening Kemper KJ, Kelleher KJ. Family psychosocial screening: instruments and techniques. *Ambulatory Child Health* 4:325–339,1996. (the measures are included in the article) and downloadable at www.pedstest.com	Screen for parents and best used along with the above screens	A two-page clinic intake form that identifies psychosocial risk factors associated with developmental problems including: a 4-item measure of parental history of physical abuse as a child; a 6-item measure of parental substance abuse; and a 3-item measure of maternal depression.	Refer/nonrefer scores for each risk factor. Also has guides to referring and resource lists.	All studies showed sensitivity and specificity to larger inventories >90%	About 15 minutes (if interview needed) Materials ~$.20 Admin. ~$4.20 Total ~$4.40
DEVELOPMENTAL SCREENS RELYING ON ELICITING SKILLS DIRECTLY FROM CHILDREN					
Brigance Screens (1985) Curriculum Associates, Inc. 153 Rangeway Road, N. Billerica, MA, 01862 Phone: 800-225-0248 ($501.00) www.curriculumassociates.com	0–90 months	9 separate forms, one for each 12-month age range. Taps speech-language, motor, readiness and general knowledge at younger ages and also reading and math at older ages. Uses direct elicitation and observation. In the 0–2 year age range, can be administered by parent report	Cutoff, quotients, percentiles, age equivalent scores in various domains and overall.	Sensitivity and specificity to giftedness and to developmental and academic problems are 70%–82% across ages	10–15 minutes Materials ~$1.53 Admin. ~$10.15 Total ~$11.68

(continued)

Table 11-1 Screening tools (continued)

Developmental screens relying on information from parents	Age range	Description	Scoring	Accuracy	Time frame and costs
Battelle Developmental Inventory Screening Test (BDIST) (1984). Riverside Publishing Company 8420 Bryn Mawr Ave, Chicago, IL 60631 Phone: 800-767-8378 $143.00+$339 if materials kit is purchased but test stimuli can be obtained for about $50 by shopping at discount department stores www.riverpub.com	12–96 months	Items use a combination of direct assessment, observation, and parental interview. The receptive language subtest may serve as a brief prescreen. Difficult to administer and takes 15 minutes for younger children and 35 for older ones. Well standardized ard validated. Instructional videos and scoring software are available. English only	Age equivalents (somewhat deflated), cutoffs at 1.0, 1.5, and 2.0 standard deviations below the mean	Sensitivity and specificy are 70%–80% across ages	15–35 minutes Materials ~$.40 Admin. ~$20.15 Total ~$20.55
Bayley Infant Neurodevelomental Screen (BINS) (1995) The Psychological Corporation 555 Academic Court, San Antonio, TX 78204 Phone: 800-228-0752 ($265) www.psychcorp.com	3–24 months	Uses 10–13 directly elicited items per 3–6 month age range assess neurological processes (reflexes, and tone); neurodevelopmental skills (movement, and symmetry) and developmental accomplishments (object permanence, imitation, and language)	Categorizes performance into low, moderate or high risk via cut scores. Provides subtest cut scores for each domain	Specificity and sensitivity are 75%–86% across ages	10–15 minutes Materials ~$.30 Admin. ~$10.15 Total ~$10.45
Denver Developmental screening test (DDST II)	0–6 years				

(continued)

Table 11-1 Screening tools

Developmental screens relying on information from parents	Age range	Description	Scoring	Accuracy	Time frame and costs
ACADEMIC SCREENS					
Pediatric Symptom Checklist Jellinek MS, Murphy JM, Robinson J, et al. Pediatric Symptom Checklist: Screening school age children for academic and psychosocial dysfunction. *Journal of Pediatrics* 112:201–209, 1988 (the test is included in the article); also can be freely downloaded at http://www.dbpeds.org/handouts or with factor scores at www.pedstest.com	4–16 years	35 short statements of problem behaviors including both externalizing (conduct) and internalizing (depression, anxiety, adjustment, etc.) Ratings of never, sometimes, or often are assigned a value of 0, 1, or 2. Scores totaling 28 or more suggest referrals. Factor scores identify attentional, internalizing and externalizing problems. Single item on school difficulties predictive of academic dysfunction	Single refer/ nonrefer score, error analysis needed to identify school dysfunction	All but one study showed high sensitivity (80%–95%) but somewhat scattered specificity (68%–100%).	About 7 minutes (if interview needed) Materials ~$.10 Admin. ~$2.38 Total ~$2.48
Safety Word Inventory and Literacy Screener (SWILS) Glascoe FP. Clinical Pediatrics (in press). Items courtesy of Curriculum Associates, Inc. The SWILS can be freely downloaded at: www.pedstest.com	6–14	Children are asked to read 29 common safety words (e.g., High Voltage, Wait, Poison) aloud. The number of correctly read words is compared to a cutoff score. Results predict performance in math, written language, and a range of reading skills. Test content may serve as a springboard to injury prevention counseling	Single cutoff score indicating the need for a referral	Sensitivity and specificity 78%–84% across all ages	About 7 minutes (if interview needed) Materials ~$.30 Admin. ~$2.38 Total ~$2.68

This chart lists measures that meet standards for screening test accuracy, meaning that they correctly identify at least 70% of children with disabilities while also correctly identifying at least 70% of children without disabilities. All included measures were standardized on national samples and validated against a range of measures. Not included are measures (such as the Denver-II) that fail to meet standards (limited standardization, absent validation, and no proof of accuracy) or measures of single developmental domains (e.g., just language or motor). The first column provides publication information and the cost of purchasing a specimen set. The Description column provides information on alternative ways (if available) to administer measures (e.g., waiting rooms). The Accuracy column shows the percentage of patients with and without problems identified correctly. The Time Frame/Costs column shows the costs of materials per visit along with the costs of professional time (using an average salary of $50 per hour) needed to administer each measure. For parent report tools, administration time reflects not only scoring of test results, but also the relationship between each test's reading level and the percentage of parents with less than a high school education (who may or may not be able to complete measures in waiting rooms due to literacy problems and will need interview administrations).
Updated from Glascoe FP. *Collaborating with Parents.* Nashville, TN: Ellsworth & Vandermeer Press, Ltd, 1998.

Table 11-2 Organizing pediatric offices for developmental/behavioral promotion and detection

1. Ask parents to complete parent-report instruments while in waiting or exam rooms.
2. To avoid incomplete, incorrect, or non-returned parent report screens, ask parents if they would like to complete the measure or on their own or have someone go through it with them. Almost all poor readers will select the latter.
3. Considering mailing parent-report tests in advance of well visits so that physicians need only score and interpret during the visit. This is often improves the quality of parent report because families may sufficient time to respond more thoughtfully. Advance mailings are also helpful with families whose English is limited because they can usually find someone in the community to help translate items.
4. Set up a return visit devoted to screening when developmental concerns are raised unexpectedly toward the end of an encounter. A similar alternative is to have office staff call families after an encounter and administer a screen over the telephone.
5. Train office staff to administer, score, and even interpret screening tests.
6. Many low-income families do not readily seek well-child care and so miss opportunities for screening, anticipatory guidance, developmental promotion, etc. For these families, use return visits to screen development and behavior. This can be facilitated by sending them home from a sick visit with forms to bring with them to the return visit.
7. Pool resources with partners so that the practice can hire a developmental specialist to administer screening tests (and perhaps provide parent counseling, run parent training groups, assist with group well-child visits, diagnostic evaluations and referrals).
8. Recruit education majors or train volunteers to administer screening tests on a periodic basis (e.g., set a regular screening day in your office).
9. Maintain a current list of telephone numbers for local service providers (e.g., speech-language centers, school psychologists, mental health centers, private psychologists and psychiatrists, parent training classes, etc.) The availability of brochures describing services may promote parental follow-through on referral suggestions.
10. Encourage professionals involved in hospital-based care (e.g., child-life workers) to screen patients.
11. Collaborate with local service providers (e.g., day care centers, Head Starts, public health clinics, department of human services workers, etc.) to establish community-wide child-find programs that use valid, accurate screening instruments.
12. Keep parent information sheets handy. Many clinics keep them in plastic binders (so that originals are not lost). When an issue arises, retrieve the original handout, copy it, read it on the way back to the exam room (in order to refresh on the contents) and then go through the highlights with parents.
13. Use screens as designed, adhering to standard wording, scoring, and decision-making. Violating test standardization decreases validity and increases the likelihood of underdetection.
14. It is possible that experienced pediatric clinicians memorize test items and internalize norms. This may lead them to rely heavily on clinical judgement. Since human reasoning is not infallible and judgement can drift over time, professionals should test their decisions at least periodically by comparing them to the results of standardized screening tests. This should help keep clinical skills honed and provide an appropriate model for less experienced professionals such as residents and medical students.

Adapted from Glascoe FP. *Collaborating with Parents.* Nashville, TN: Ellsworth & Vandermeer Press, Ltd, 1998.

Child's Name Billy Morris

PEDS INTERPRETATION FORM

Specific Decisions

0–3 mos. counseled re: colic

4–5 mos. happy baby, happy mom, gave info on promoting sleep

6–11 mos. no concerns gave info babyproofing house

12–14 mos. concerns about delayed walking, gave info on wide age range

15–17 mos. no concerns re: poor response to no. Disc. limits of memory, child-proofing house

18–23 mos. no concerned re: sufficient caloric intake. Growth rate normal

2 yrs. progressing well, no concerns. Gave info on tantrums and positive discipline

3 yrs. Sent home with PDI to return 4/28
4/28: passed; counseled mo re: SEL, return w

4–4½ yrs.

4½–6 yrs.

6–7 yrs.

7–8 yrs.

Path A: Two or more significant concerns?
Yes? → Two or more concerns about self-help, social, school, or receptive language skills?
Yes? → Refer for audiological and speech-language testing. Use professional judgment to decide if referrals are also needed for social work, occupational/physical therapy, mental health services, etc.
No? → Refer for intellectual and educational evaluations. Use professional judgment to decide if speech-language, audiological, or other evaluations are also needed.

Path B: One significant concern?
Yes? → Screen or refer for screening.
If screen is passed, counsel in areas of concern and watch vigilantly.
If screen is failed, refer for testing in area(s) of difficulty.

Path C: Nonsignificant concerns?
Yes? → Counsel in areas of difficulty and follow up in several weeks.
If unsuccessful, screen for emotional/behavioral problems and refer as indicated. Otherwise refer for parent training, behavioral intervention, etc.

Path D: Parental difficulties communicating?
Yes? → Foreign language a barrier?
No? → Use a second screen that directly elicits children's skills or refer for screening elsewhere.
Yes? → Use foreign language versions, send PEDS home in preparation for a second visit; seek a translator, or refer for screening elsewhere.

Path E: No concerns?
Yes? → Elicit concerns at next checkpoint.
No? → Use PEDS between checkpoints (e.g. sick- or return-visit).

Figure 11-1. PEDS Interpretation Form.

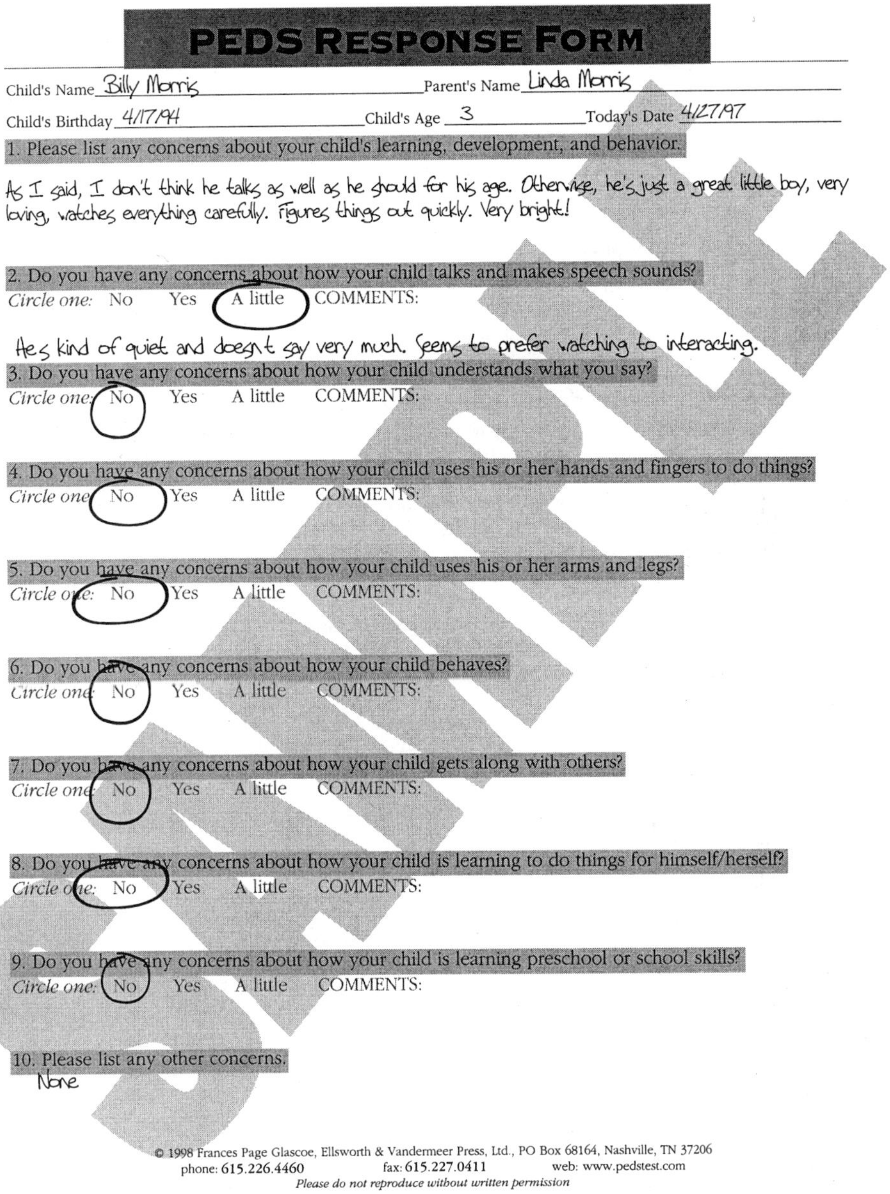

PEDS RESPONSE FORM

Child's Name _Billy Morris_   Parent's Name _Linda Morris_

Child's Birthday _4/17/94_   Child's Age _3_   Today's Date _4/27/97_

1. Please list any concerns about your child's learning, development, and behavior.

As I said, I don't think he talks as well as he should for his age. Otherwise, he's just a great little boy, very loving, watches everything carefully. Figures things out quickly. Very bright!

2. Do you have any concerns about how your child talks and makes speech sounds?
Circle one: No   Yes   (A little)   COMMENTS:

He's kind of quiet and doesn't say very much. Seems to prefer watching to interacting.

3. Do you have any concerns about how your child understands what you say?
Circle one: (No)   Yes   A little   COMMENTS:

4. Do you have any concerns about how your child uses his or her hands and fingers to do things?
Circle one: (No)   Yes   A little   COMMENTS:

5. Do you have any concerns about how your child uses his or her arms and legs?
Circle one: (No)   Yes   A little   COMMENTS:

6. Do you have any concerns about how your child behaves?
Circle one: (No)   Yes   A little   COMMENTS:

7. Do you have any concerns about how your child gets along with others?
Circle one: (No)   Yes   A little   COMMENTS:

8. Do you have any concerns about how your child is learning to do things for himself/herself?
Circle one: (No)   Yes   A little   COMMENTS:

9. Do you have any concerns about how your child is learning preschool or school skills?
Circle one: (No)   Yes   A little   COMMENTS:

10. Please list any other concerns.
None

© 1998 Frances Page Glascoe, Ellsworth & Vandermeer Press, Ltd., PO Box 68164, Nashville, TN 37206
phone: 615.226.4460   fax: 615.227.0411   web: www.pedstest.com
Please do not reproduce without written permission

Figure 11-2. PEDS Response Form.

BIBLIOGRAPHY

For Parents

Patient Education

Schmitt BD, Jacobs JT, Fletcher J. (eds). *Instructions for Pediatric Patients (2nd ed)*. Philadelphia: Saunders, 1999.
Wyckoff, Unell. *Discipline Without Shouting or Spanking: Practical Solutions to the Most Common Preschool Behavior*. Minnetonka, MN: Meadowbrook Press, 2001.

Guidance on a range of topics and downloadable handouts from the following Websites

www.kidshealth.org [Nemours Foundation]
www.kidsgrowth.com
www.teengrowth.com

Referral and Disability Resources

www.dbpeds.org The American Academy of Pediatrics' Section on Developmental and Behavioral Pediatrics Home Page has a Website with information on typical and atypical child development and an excellent e-mail discussion list offering continuing medical education credit.
www.eparent.com Exceptional Parent, P.O. Box 3000, Dept. EP, Denville NJ 07834, 1-800-562-1973. Published monthly, this journal also produces an annual resource issue that lists Websites, phone numbers, and addresses of organizations devoted to specific disabilities and conditions, parent-to-parent programs, mental health resources, parent training and information services, etc.
www.nectas.org National Early Childhood Technical Assistance System has a Websites listing all the coordinators for 0-3 and preschool programs, state by state. These individuals have complete lists of early intervention programs. The site provides phone numbers, e-mail, and street addresses.
www.irsc.org Internet Resources for Special Children. Links to National Institutes of Health and other government clearinghouses, disability specific foundations, etc.
www.firstsigns.org First Signs includes information on early detection and treatment of autism.

For Professionals

Meisels SJ, Shonkoff JP (eds). *Handbook of Early Childhood Intervention (2nd ed)*. Cambridge: Cambridge University Press, 2000.
Wolraich ML (ed). *Disorders of Development and Learning: A Practical Guide to Assessment and Management (3rd ed)*. Chicago: Mosby-Year Book, Inc., 2002.
American Academy of Pediatrics. Committee on Children with Disabilities. Developmental surveillance and screening of infants and young children. *Pediatrics* 108:192–196, 2001. Available at: http://www.aap.org/policy/re0062.html

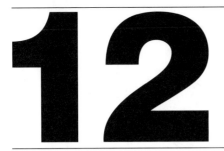

Screening for Social and Emotional Delays in Early Childhood

Margaret J. Briggs-Gowan
Alice S. Carter

I. **Introduction.** Across all ages of childhood, as many as 1 in 5 children are estimated to have mental health problems. However, the majority of children with such difficulties do not receive mental health services. Lack of attention likely prolongs and exacerbates children's difficulties and contributes to increased parent and family stress. Whereas for older children, schools are a primary setting for identification, pediatric clinicians are often relied upon to identify and make referrals for young children's social and emotional behavioral problems. Although some concerned parents do not share their concerns with any professional, those who do consult a professional about a social and emotional behavioral problem are most likely to turn to their pediatric provider. Yet, pediatric clinicians must balance the task of identifying mental health problems with competing medical and developmental demands that are inherent to the well-child visit. Achieving this balance is further complicated by shortened visits under managed care. To address such barriers to early identification of children with social and emotional behavioral problems, the American Academy of Pediatrics has recommended that pediatric clinicians routinely screen for these mental health problems.

II. **Goal of screening.** The general goal of screening is to identify children who may be experiencing delays or difficulties in a particular developmental domain (e.g., language, cognition, social emotional), with the expectation that additional follow-up will be needed to determine the specific nature of the problem and whether any intervention or referral is warranted. In some cases, the practitioner may choose to employ a two stage screening in which a brief screener is followed by a longer measure that provides a more in depth assessment of the child's difficulties and will help in referral or treatment planning.

III. **Choice of screening tool.** The age of the child will influence the choice of an appropriate screener. For school-age children, screening for social and emotional behavioral problems is generally sufficient, as cognitive delays are likely to be identified through the school system. Screening tools for school-age children have existed for quite some time and are well-validated and reliable.

- **Pediatric Symptom Checklist** (**PSC**) (Jellinek et al., 1988), which addresses social and emotional behavioral problems. When a child is in the "at-risk" range on a screener, such as the PSC, follow-up with a clinical interview or lengthier measure is useful to obtain more detailed information about the specific nature of the child's difficulties and the contexts in which the difficulties are apparent.
- **Behavior Assessment Scale for Children Parent Rating Scales** (**BASC-P**) (Reynolds & Kamphaus, 1992) for 6- to 11-year-olds is a more lengthy measure (138 items) which includes assessment of both problems and competencies.
- **Conners' Rating Scale-Revised** (**CRS-R**) (Conners, 1997) an 80-item problem behavior checklist for ages 3 to 17 years.
- **Child Behavior Checklist** (**CBCL**) (Achenbach, 2001) for ages 6 to 18 years is a 113-item checklist.

Each of these measures has parent, youth, and teacher versions that allow one to obtain information from multiple perspectives. An advantage of the BASC is that it assesses social-emotional skills, as well as emotional/behavioral problems.

For young children, it is important to screen for developmental delays in addition to social and emotional behavioral problems, as the former may increase risk for social and emotional problems, and social and emotional competencies are not expected to exceed a child's developmental level. Screening for delays is particularly important in early childhood because, unlike older children, some infants and toddlers have limited contact with formal childcare or preschool settings and are therefore less likely to come into contact with professionals who recognize developmental delays. It is also important to note that, in contrast to findings for older children, parental concern about a young child does not appear to be an accurate predictor of social, emotional, and behavioral problems. Recent work indicates that, although worry about their child does appear to motivate parents to discuss concerns with their pediatric clinician, many parents who report high levels of

Table 12-1 Social-emotional/behavioral problem screeners for early childhood

	Ages and stages questionnaires social-emotional (ASQ-SE)	Brief infant-toddler social & emotional assessment (BITSEA)	Devereux early childhood assessment (DECA)	Eyberg child behavior inventory	Ages and stages questionnaires (ASQ)	Brigance screens – infant and toddler screen
Age range	6–60 months	12–36 months	2–5 years	2½–11 years	4 months–5 years	0–23 months (older version goes to 90 mo)
Respondent	Parent or caregiver	Parent or caregiver	Parent or caregiver	Parent	Parent or caregiver	Administered by paraprofessional
Number of items	19–33 items	42 items	37 items	36 items	30 items	83–85 items
Completion time	10–15 minutes	5–7 minutes	10 minutes	5 minutes	10–20 minutes	10 minutes
Validity as screener	Acceptable	Acceptable	Not adequate	Acceptable	Acceptable	Acceptable
Problem areas assessed	Social-emotional behavioral	Internalizing Externalizing Dysregulation	10 problem behaviors	Conduct Aggression Inattention	None	None
Competence or social skills assessed	Social-emotional competencies	Social-emotional competencies	Initiative Self-control Attachment	None	Personal-social	Self-help Social-emotional skills
Autism Spectrum Behaviors	Yes	Yes	None	None	None	None
Developmental domains	None	None	None	None	Commun. Gross motor Fine motor Problem solving	Fine motor Gross motor Receptive language Expressive language
Scores	Problem	Problem Competence	Problem Competence	Problem	Developmental delay	Developmental delay

Four screeners that focus on social-emotional issues in early childhood are presented as well as two that focus on developmental delay.

ASQ-SE: Squires J, Bricker D, Twombly E. *Ages & Stages Questionnaires: Social-Emotional: A parent completed, child-monitoring system for social-emotional behaviors.* Baltimore, MD: Paul H. Brookes Publishing, 2002.

BITSEA: Briggs-Gowan MJ, Carter AS, Irwin J, Wachtel K, Cicchetti D. The Brief Infant-Toddler Social and Emotional Assessment: Screening for social-emotional problems and delays in competence. *Journal of Pediatric Psychology* 29:143-155, 2004.

Eyberg: Eyberg S. The Eyberg Child Behavior Inventory. *Journal of Clinical Child Psychology* 9:22-28, 1980.

DECA: LeBuffe PA, Naglieri JA. The Devereux Early Childhood Assessment (DECA): A measure of within-child protective factors in preschool children. Devereux: Institute of Clinical Training and Research, 2003. Available at: http://www.devereuxearlychildhood.com (accessed June 10, 2003).

Brigance: Brigance AH, Glascoe FP. *Brigance Infant and Toddler Screen.* North Billerica, MA: Curriculum Associates, Inc., 2002.

ASQ: Bricker D, Squires J. *The Ages & Stages Questionnaires: A parent-completed, child monitoring system, second edition.* Baltimore, MD: Paul H. Brooks Publishing, 1999.

emotional/behavioral problems do not report worry about their child. These findings highlight the importance of inquiring about specific child behaviors, as parents of young children may have difficulty determining when difficult child behavior crosses the boundary between normal and atypical.

The number of screening tools available for early childhood has grown in recent years. Four screeners that focus on social-emotional issues in early childhood are presented in Table 12-1. A parent with a 6th grade reading level can complete each of the social-emotional screeners independently in less than 10 minutes. These screeners have been translated into Spanish and other languages. Many have caregiver/teacher versions that allow one to gather information about the child's behavior in different contexts, such as childcare. The BITSEA and the ASQ-SE are the most comprehensive in scope, addressing both social and emotional behavioral problems and delays in competencies. As many of these tools were developed recently, research concerning their validity is still emerging. Nonetheless, the BITSEA, ASQ-SE and Eyberg have shown acceptable validity in detecting children with elevated social, emotional, and behavioral problems. In addition, the BITSEA has demonstrated sensitivity in identifying children with Autism Spectrum disorders. As with older children, it may be beneficial to follow at-risk screening results with more lengthy measures.
- **Infant-Toddler Social & Emotional Assessment (ITSEA)** (Carter et al., 2003) designed for 12 to 48 months of age, offers a comprehensive profile of social and emotional behavioral problems and competencies.
- **Behavior Assessment Scale for Children (BASC-2½-5)** (Reynolds and Kamphaus, 1992) for 2½- to 5-year-olds also measures problem behaviors and social-emotional skills.
- **Child Behavior Checklist (CBCL/1.5-5)** (Achenbach and Rescorla, 2000) assesses emotional and behavioral problems.

IV. **Cultural issues.** Although many of the developers of these tools strove to take ethnicity or culture into consideration during measurement development, these tools have not been normed within specific cultural groups. There is increasing evidence that parents from different cultures may expect particular child behaviors or skills to emerge at different points in development. Therefore, it is important to discuss "problem" responses with the parent to determine whether the specific behavior is considered to be atypical or unusual in the family's cultural group.

V. **Clinical pearls.**
- At a time when pediatric clinicians face increased demands to address the physical, developmental, and mental health needs of their patients, it is critical to advance methodologies that can facilitate the identification and management of children with social, emotional, and behavioral problems.
- Screening tools offer a time and cost effective means of detecting children who may be experiencing social, emotional, and behavioral problems that warrant additional follow-up. However, it is equally critical to develop methodologies for addressing the mental health problems that are identified through screening, for example, by developing intervention approaches that can be provided within the pediatric setting and by improving linkages between pediatrics and existing mental healthcare systems.

BIBLIOGRAPHY

American Academy of Pediatrics. Committee on Children with Disabilities. Developmental surveillance and screening of infants and young children. *Pediatrics* 108:192–196, 2001.

Briggs-Gowan MJ, Carter AS, Skuban EM, Horwitz SM. Prevalence of social-emotional and behavioral problems in a community sample of 1- and 2-year-old children. *Journal of the American Academy of Child & Adolescent Psychiatry* 40, 811–819, 2001.

Glascoe FP. Early detection of developmental and behavioral problems. *Pediatric Review* 21, 272–280, 2000.

U.S. Public Health Service. *Report of the Surgeon General's Conference on Children's Mental Health: A National Action Agenda.* Washington, DC: Department of Health and Human Services, 2000.

Screening Tools

Achenbach T. *The Child Behavior Checklist for Ages 6 to 18.* Burlington: University of Vermont, 2001.

Achenbach T, Rescorla L. *Manual for the ASEBA Preschool Forms and Profiles.* Burlington: University of Vermont, 2000.

Bricker D, Squires J. *The Ages & Stages Questionnaires: A parent-completed, child monitoring system, second edition.* Baltimore, MD: Paul H. Brooks Publishing, 1999.

Brigance AH, Glascoe FP. *Brigance Infant and Toddler Screen.* North Billerica, MA: Curriculum Associates, Inc., 2002.

Briggs-Gowan MJ, Carter AS, Irwin J, Wachtel K, Cicchetti D. The Brief Infant-Toddler Social and Emotional Assessment: Screening for social-emotional problems and delays in competence. *Journal of Pediatric Psychology* 29:143–155, 2004.

Carter AS, Briggs-Gowan MJ, Jones SM, Little TD. The Infant-Toddler Social and Emotional Assessment (ITSEA): Factor structure, reliability, and validity. *Journal of Abnormal Child Psychology* 31:495–514, 2003.

Conners CK. Conners' Rating Scales-Revised (CRS-R), 1997. Available at: http://www.mhs.com/onlineCat/product.asp?productID = CRS-R; accessed December 14, 2003.)

Eyberg S. The Eyberg Child Behavior Inventory. *Journal of Clinical Child Psychology* 9:22–28, 1980.

Jellinek MS, Murphy JM, Robinson J, et al. Pediatric Symptom Checklist: screening school-age children for psychosocial dysfunction. *Journal of Pediatrics* 112:201–209, 1988.

LeBuffe PA, Naglieri JA. *The Devereux Early Childhood Assessment (DECA): A measure of within-child protective factors in preschool children.* Devereux: Institute of Clinical Training and Research, 2003. Available at: http://www.devereuxearlychildhood (accessed June 10, 2003).

Reynolds CR, Kamphaus RW. *BASC: Parent Rating Scales, 6-11.* Circle Pines, MN: American Guidance Service, Inc., 1992.

Squires J, Bricker D, Twombly E. Ages & Stages Questionnaires: Social-Emotional: A parent completed, child-monitoring system for social-emotional behaviors. Baltimore, MD: Paul H. Brookes Publishing, 2002.

13

Behavioral Management: Theory and Practice

Edward R. Christophersen

Traditional behavioral management techniques can be very useful to the primary care clinician. This chapter describes the concepts and techniques that parents can routinely use in interacting with their children.

I. **Techniques to teach or improve behaviors.**
   A. **Time-In and verbal praise.**
      1. *Time-In* refers to the way parents interact with their children when they do not necessarily deserve praise but when their behavior is acceptable. Parents should be encouraged and educated to provide their children with frequent, brief, nonverbal, physical contact whenever their child is not engaging in a behavior the parents consider unacceptable or offensive. They do not have to wait for "good behavior."
      2. *Verbal praise* is used only when a child has done something "good." The best time to use verbal praise is during natural breaks in an activity. For example, when a child is coloring, the parent should provide lots of brief; nonverbal, physical contact (time-in); simple physical contact, without any praise, is much less likely to distract a child. When the child has finished coloring or stops coloring to show it to a parent, verbal praise is appropriate.

         Advantages. Time-in and verbal praise encourage children to continue to engage in acceptable behaviors. These techniques take no additional parent time and do not distract children.
   B. **Incidental learning.** Children learn behaviors by being around individuals who engage in those behaviors naturally. This is called *incidental learning.* For example, if both parents smoke cigarettes, their child is significantly more likely to become a smoker than if neither parent smokes. A surprising number and variety of children's behaviors appear to have been learned incidentally, including language, gestures, and anger management strategies.

      Advantages and disadvantages. Incidental learning can be achieved without any additional effort on the part of the parents. They need only be aware that such learning occurs naturally and be cognizant of incidental learning during the time they spend with their children. The negative side is that children also learn behaviors the parents never intended for them to learn (e.g., swearing).
   C. **Modeling.**
      1. Two basic modeling techniques exist: live and videotape. Most modeling procedures work best if the model is approximately the same age as the target child. For example, a 6-year-old boy who has previously had his teeth cleaned by a dentist and who behaved appropriately during the procedure could be observed live or on videotape while being examined. A second child who observes the dental procedures being performed on this model can learn both what to expect of dental procedures and how to react to those procedures.

         Advantages and disadvantages. Children are more likely to believe what they see a peer doing than what their parents *tell* them, particularly if the two messages are contradictory (e.g., one a verbal message that the child should relax, and the other the anxiety that a child feels in the dental chair). However, modeling can teach maladaptive behaviors as well as adaptive behaviors. For example, if a child is observing a peer model in the dentist's office and the peer model becomes very upset, the target child will probably have a more difficult time when it is his turn for the procedure.
   D. **Reinforcement.** No other topic in the behavioral literature has been more misunderstood than reinforcement. An item or activity can be said to have reinforcing properties for an individual child if and only if that child has previously worked in order to obtain access to that item or activity.
      1. *Choosing rewards.* Under the right circumstances, reinforcement, by definition, will work with virtually any age group and with many different behaviors. However, no item or activity can be accurately described as a reinforcer unless and until it has

produced a change in behavior. For example, although candy is reinforcing for the vast majority of children, it cannot be referred to as a reinforcer until it has been demonstrated that the child will either work to obtain the candy or stop a behavior that prevents him from receiving it.

Principles of reinforcement, or the manner in which the reinforcer is made accessible to a child, are extremely important:

a. **Small rewards offered frequently are better than large rewards offered infrequently.** A physical hug offered several times during a household chore will usually be more effective than a big reward at the end of the chore. Small rewards during the chore and a reward at the end will also work nicely.

b. **Repetition, with feedback, enhances a child's learning.** A child will learn more from performing the same task repeatedly, with help from his parent, than from performing it once. While parents will often expect their child to perform a task correctly the first time, the child will actually learn the task better if he has many opportunities to practice. For example, a child who helps one of his parents do the laundry several times each week for two years will probably be able to do the laundry for the rest of his life.

c. Children learn more quickly and retain the learning better if they are **relaxed while they are learning.** While children can be very frustrating, the parent who becomes angry or impatient only exacerbates the situation. Similarly, an upset child does not learn as rapidly or as permanently as a calm child.

d. **Warnings only make children worse.** While parents have a natural tendency to warn their children, it is far more effective to discipline the child for not performing the task and then give the child another opportunity to do it, rather than frequent warnings that the tasks must be done.

e. **A behavior must already be learned before it can be reinforced.** If the child doesn't know how to perform the expected behavior, offering a reward, in lieu of teaching the child how to perform the behavior, is ineffective.

Advantages and disadvantages. Reinforcing items and activities frequently can become part of normal, everyday life without substantial planning on the parents' part. Reinforcing items and activities may sometimes be inadvertent. For example, when a parent picks up a child who has been crying in bed after bedtime, the parent may be reinforcing that child for crying.

Additionally, the child's behavior may return to its prereinforcement level as soon as the reinforcers are no longer available. For example, in research on the use of reinforcers for automobile seatbelt use, many children stopped wearing their seatbelts as soon as the reinforcers were no longer available. Procedures that have been shown to be successful in maintaining desired behaviors after reinforcement ceases include gradually making the reinforcer available less often (e.g., on the average, every second behavior is reinforced, then every third behavior, then every fourth behavior). Once a behavior becomes habitual, the individual will engage in it whether it is reinforced or not.

E. **Conditioned reinforcers.** Many items and activities that have no intrinsic reinforcing properties can take on reinforcing properties. Money, for example, is not usually a reinforcer to a small child. When the child learns what he can purchase with money, it begins to take on reinforcing properties. As another example, to a distressed child in the middle of the night, even the sound of the bedroom door opening can take on reinforcing properties, as the child associates the sound of the door opening with receiving attention from a caregiver.

Advantages. Conditioned reinforcers are usually more readily available than the actual reinforcer, and most children work just as hard for a conditioned reinforcer as they will for the actual one. Conditioned reinforcers, such as money, also have the advantage that they can be traded for a wide variety of items or activities as the child's tastes and preferences change.

F. **The token economy.** Conditioned reinforcers work best if there is a consistent method of exchange. In the case of money, the exchange system is already in place, and the money becomes a "token" of what can be purchased. Entire "token economies" have been devised as treatment programs for children from age 4 years to adulthood. The term token economy refers to the organized manner in which tokens are gained and lost, as well as what can be purchased with them. The success or failure of a token economy depends almost entirely on how it is implemented and on how many reinforcing activities are realistically available to the individual who must earn, lose, and spend tokens. The mere use of tokens does not make a token economy.

Token economies are most effective when they are used as motivational sys-

tems to encourage children to engage in socially appropriate behaviors. Three different types of token economies are widely used with common behavioral problems:

1. A **simple exchange system** provides a means of keeping track of the child's appropriate and inappropriate behaviors. A list of behaviors can be taped to the door of the refrigerator. As the child completes assigned or volunteered tasks or chores, he marks these on the "positive side" of the exchange chart. Similarly, as the child engages in inappropriate behaviors, he marks these on the "negative side." When the child wants a special privilege or activity, there must be more positive marks than negative marks to "afford" the special privilege. The simple exchange system is appropriate for children age 5–12 years.

2. Under **chip systems**, the child earns a token, such as a poker chip, for positive behaviors. Each time poker chips are earned, the parent acknowledges the child's appropriate behavior while offering chips. The child is then expected to take the chips from the parent's hand, look the parent in the eye, and say, "thank you." In this way, the child not only receives the tokens for the appropriate behavior but also practices appropriate social behaviors. Similarly, when the child engages in a behavior that loses chips, he is expected to hand the chips to the parent politely and may receive one chip back for "taking the fine so nicely." The chip system is useful for ages 3–7 years.

3. The **point system** is similar to the chip system but can be much more sophisticated. Points can be used to motivate children and teenagers to practice the behaviors they are lacking, such as taking feedback well and sharing their feelings appropriately. Each time they engage in these types of behaviors, they earn points that can be used to purchase items and activities they want. The point system is useful for children ages 6–16 years.

G. Fading. Fading refers to changing something gradually instead of abruptly changing it. For example:

- Instead of taking away a toddler's bottle, a cup can be available with milk in it while the bottle is gradually diluted from 100% milk to 90% milk:10% water, then 80% milk:20% water, and so on, until the toddler is drinking pure water from the bottle and pure milk from the cup.
- Raising training wheels on a bicycle 1/8 in. every 2 weeks until they are about 3 inches off the ground and no longer necessary.
- Changing a child's bedtime 15 minutes each night at daylight savings time instead of abruptly changing it the entire hour in one night.
- Teaching a child how to swallow pills by starting out with very small cake sprinkles to wash down with a favorite beverage, then moving to slightly larger pieces of candy. Typically using 6 to 8 steps (sizes) is very effective.

Advantages and disadvantages. Fading often helps to avoid confrontations with a child. It can be used to accomplish something without incident that otherwise may have been difficult to accomplish. The disadvantage of fading is that parents have to spend more time than they would if their child could abruptly make the desired changes.

II. Procedures to decrease or discourage behaviors.

A. Time-In and time-out. Probably the most often recommended disciplinary technique is time-out. As initially used, time-out was actually referred to as "time-out from positive reinforcement." Over the past two decades or so the term has been shortened to time-out, and, in doing so, the idea of removing a pleasant interaction has been ignored or forgotten. Time-in and time-out are effective from less than age 1 year to early adolescence. But, in absence of good "time-in," there really is no such thing as "time-out."

The following variables have the most impact on the effectiveness of time-out;

- It must be presented immediately after an inappropriate behavior.
- It must he presented every time the inappropriate behavior occurs.
- The time-out must remove or make unavailable an otherwise pleasant state of affairs (i.e., time-in).
- The time-out should not be considered "over" or "finished" until the child has quieted down.
- All warnings about using time-out should be carried out.
- The child should be completely ignored during the time-out, regardless of how outrageous the behavior might become. One study demonstrated that time-out becomes more effective when the time-in is "enriched" (more fun, more enjoyable) and becomes less effective when the time-in is "impoverished."

Advantages. Time-in and time-out provide parents with an effective alternative to nagging, yelling, or spanking. Their consistent use also encourages children to develop self-quieting skills (a child's ability to calm himself without the assistance of a parent). It encourages these skills because the parents are modeling the ability to cope with an unpleasant situation and because the child is learning how to cope with feelings he experiences when they do not like something their parents have done.

B. Extinction. Extinction is defined as the withdrawal of all attention after a child engages in undesirable behaviors. The most common example of extinction is letting a child cry at bedtime instead of paying attention to the whining, fussing, or screaming. When used properly, extinction involves completely ignoring a child's behaviors and protests.

A major problem with using extinction is an initial sharp increase in the child's inappropriate behavior, called an *extinction burst*. For example, when a child is ignored during a temper tantrum or when whining at bedtime, these behaviors usually increase at first, perhaps discouraging the parents from continuing the extinction procedure. If the parents continue with the extinction procedure, however, the change in the child's behavior will usually be forthcoming.

Although extinction procedures are often successful, parents may not be able to tolerate the technique. Several modifications have been made to make extinction techniques more acceptable to parents. For example, the day correction of bedtime problems technique involves teaching the parents to use extinction for whining and fussing during the day. The parents then gain confidence in their ability to use it properly and the child learns that the parents will follow through with the use of extinction once they start it. Only after the parents and the child are familiar with the use of extinction during the day are the parents encouraged to use it at bedtime. The day correction technique is actually more effective than using extinction only at bedtime.

Advantages and disadvantages. Extinction procedures have been effective with many different childhood problems. The time necessary to educate parents on the use of these procedures is reasonable, given the constraints of primary care practices. The main disadvantage is the extinction burst and the parents' inability to tolerate their child's initial distress at being ignored.

C. Planned Ignoring. The parents gradually ignore their child's behavior more and more (as opposed to introducing complete extinction abruptly). Planned ignoring may result in less of an extinction burst, but it takes longer to be effective.

D. Spanking. With spanking, caregivers can vent their own frustration at the same time they are discouraging a child from engaging in the behavior that resulted in the spanking. Additionally, spanking will often produce an immediate decrease in the child's behavior.

Advantages and disadvantages. Spanking can teach a child that hitting is acceptable. The child, after being spanked, is likely to avoid or try to escape from the caregiver who administered the spanking. Spanking can also result in other discipline methods losing their effectiveness. Thus, a child who is frequently spanked at home is less likely to be responsive to the use of extinction at daycare. Since time-in and time-out can produce virtually the same effects as spanking but without the side effects, spanking does not need to be the first alternative that professionals recommend for parents.

E. Job grounding. A form of grounding whereby the child has control over how long the grounding is in effect. When a child has broken a major rule (e.g., gone to a shopping center by bike without telling parents), he is "grounded". The child loses all privileges (including television, telephone, having a friend over, playing with games, snacks and desserts) until he has completed one job properly. The jobs, which can each be written on a 3x5 card, should be agreed upon by both parent and child during a quiet, peaceful time. The child, upon being grounded, is asked to pick from a stack of cards that are held face down by the parent. Once the job is chosen, the child is restricted from most activities until the job is completed. The parents are instructed to refrain from nagging, prodding, and reminding. As soon as the child has completed the job (most jobs should take only 5–10 minutes to complete and be tasks that the child has done many times before), he is "off grounding." Job grounding differs from traditional time-based grounding in that the child determines how long the grounding lasts and, under most circumstances, the child has the option of getting the job done without missing valued social activities.

Advantages and disadvantages. Job grounding is usually effective, it lets the child practice a job that he probably did not want to do in the first place, and it gives him the opportunity to avoid losing a valued activity. The disadvantage is that if the child has no planned activities, he may stall on completing the job until some external motivation is present.

F. Habit reversal. Habit reversal procedures were developed for use with habit disorders. Habit-reversal training requires a level of cognition not reached before a mental age of about 4–5 years.

1. Components of habit reversal:
   - **Increase your child's awareness of the habit on a daily basis**
   - Keeping track of how often the habit occurs is the only way that you and your child can tell when progress is being made.
   - On a daily basis, have your child look in a mirror while performing the habit on purpose.
   - Help your child to become aware of how their body moves and what muscles are being used when they perform the habit.
   - Have your child identify each time they engage in the habit by either raising their hand when the habit occurs, or by stating, "that was one," when the habit occurs.
   - If you see the habit occur but your child does not appear to be aware that it occurred, use a prearranged gesture or expression to help make them aware.
   - Self-monitoring: Your child can record each occurrence of the habit on a 3x5 card.
   - **Competing response should be practiced daily**
   - Have your child practice their competing response in the mirror. This helps your child become comfortable with the response and assures them that the competing response is not noticeable socially. For example, a child who is pulling their hair can practice holding their thumbs on the waist of their pants or skirt.
   - Encourage your child to use the competing response when they feel the urge to engage in the habit or in situations where the child has a history of engaging in the habit.
   - Encourage your child to use the competing response for 1 minute following the occurrence of the habit.
   - **Stress anxiety reduction procedures** (all should be practiced daily)
   - Progressive muscle relaxation training
   - Visual imagery
   - Breathing exercises
2. Parent Involvement
   - **Feedback.** Work with your child to increase awareness of their habit by helping them identify the habit when it occurs.
   - **Support and Encouragement** Encourage your child to use their competing response and praise them when they do so. Praise any noted decrease in rates of their habits.
   - Remember, although many children and adolescents will notice a decrease in their habit within a couple of days, the greatest change from using these habit reversal procedures occurs during the second and third month. Don't quit practicing after only a couple of days or weeks.

   Advantages and disadvantages. Habit reversal training is effective and has no physical side effects. The overall reduction in habit disorders and tics is also far greater with this technique than with medication. The disadvantage is the time it takes to teach and monitor, as well as the time it takes to reduce the habit disorder (usually days).

G. **Positive practice** is the procedure of having a child practice an appropriate behavior after each inappropriate behavior. For example, when a previously toilet trained child wets his pants, he is required to practice "going to the bathroom" 10 times; five times from the place where the accident was discovered and five times from such alternative sites as the front yard, the back yard, the kitchen, and the bedroom. When used correctly, with no nagging or unpleasant behavior on the care givers part, positive practice can produce dramatic results.

Advantages and disadvantages. Positive practice gives a child a lot of opportunities to practice appropriate behaviors. This technique is typically effective quickly. The disadvantages include the length of time necessary to implement the practice, as well as the fact that the practice should be done immediately after the inappropriate behavior, which is not always convenient.

H. **Practice, Praise, Point Out and Prompt.** Several of these procedures can be combined into a very effective teaching tool. For example, when a child's interrupting is a problem, they can be taught an alternative to interrupting. Encourage the parent to practice having their child gently place their hand on the parent's forearm and the parent 'o immediately place their hand on the child's hand and ask them what they want. This should be practiced daily with a reward from practicing. The parent should "point out" to their child when they wait instead of interrupting, or when a character in a book is seen to be waiting. The parent can also "prompt" their child to place their hand, for example, on Daddy's arm when they want to get his attention. This strategy combines incidental learning, modeling, reinforcement, and praise.

III. General remarks and conclusions.

- Although the term "behavior management" frequently has been used to refer to coercive action taken in an effort to discourage a child from engaging in inappropriate behavior, many positive alternatives are available. Generally, the emphasis should be on teaching children appropriate behaviors, rather than concentrating on reducing inappropriate behaviors.
- The single most important consideration in implementing such behavior management strategies is taking a history that can help to identify precisely what strategy should be offered to the caregiver and how to offer that strategy. The primary care provider now has a variety of behavior management strategies available for dealing with situations encountered in the provision of care to normal children with minor behavior problems.
- As with many of the "medical interventions" offered to parents from the primary care provider, the use of written handouts summarizing the treatment recommendations can be very helpful to the parent who is trying to follow their providers recommendations.

BIBLIOGRAPHY

For Parents

Christophersen ER. *Little People: Guidelines for Commonsense Child Rearing (4th ed.),* Shawnee Mission, KS: Overland Press, 1998.
Christophersen ER, Mortweet SL. *Parenting that Works: Building Skills that Last a Lifetime.* Washington, DC: American Psychological Association, 2003.
Schmitt BD. *Your Child's Health (2nd ed).* New York: Bantam Books, 1991.

Web Sites

http://www.patienteducation.com/products/pediatric/
http://www.disciplinehelp.com/instruct/default.htm

For Professionals

Christophersen ER: *Pediatric Compliance: A Guide for the Primary Care Physician.* New York: Plenum, 1994.
Christophersen ER, Mortweet SL.*Treatments that work with children: Empirically supported strategies for managing childhood problems.* Washington, DC: American Psychological Association, 2001.
Mortweet SL, Christophersen ER. Coping skills for the angry/impatient/clamorous child: A home and office practicum. *Contemporary Pediatrics,* 2004, 21(6), 43–55
Schmitt BD (ed). *Pediatric Advisor.* Inglewood CO: Clinical Reference Systems. Computer software, 2003.

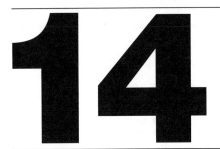

Coping with Stressful Transitions

W. Thomas Boyce

The primary care clinician is often the principal source of assistance for a family or a child during periods of stressful transitions. As such, he or she is especially well placed to offer advice, construct effective interventions, and provide encouragement and empathic care during critical moments in a family's life course. It is precisely during such moments that patients and families may find themselves unusually receptive to the words, reflections, and concerns of a caring professional. What may seem at first an insurmountable difficulty can become, under the guidance of the primary care provider, an occasion for growth and renewal. Stressful transitions may become turning points in a child's life and, through an alchemy of crisis, the pain of a seemingly catastrophic event can be memorably transformed into a moment at which life was indelibly changed for the better.

I. **Types of childhood transitions.** A childhood transition is a period of swift, challenging change that may alter a child's experiences of self, life circumstances, or future possibilities and expectations. Childhood is a period of rapid and dramatic developmental change and is filled with transitional events, ranging from the birth of a sibling or starting school to the death of a beloved grandparent or a parental divorce. Such transitions can be regarded as normative or nonnormative, biological or psychosocial, and "on-time or off-time" events.

   A. **Normative and nonnormative transitions.** Normative events (e.g., entering kindergarten) are those experienced by most children under ordinary conditions growing up in the Western world. Nonnormative transitions (e.g., the death of a parent) are those that represent unexpected deviations from the normal, anticipated sequence of life events. Events deemed as nonnormative within a given society may be regarded as normative in other social or cultural circumstances. Divorce, for example, has become so prevalent in North American society that it could arguably be viewed as a nearly normative stressor for many children. Normative transitional events may be planned, as in a family's move to a new home, or unplanned, as in the changes in a family's economic condition that typically follow the loss of a parent's job.

   B. **Biological and psychosocial transitions.** Transitions in childhood can attend both biological and psychosocial changes. The onset of puberty is an example of a transition with biological origins, but it is also a transition with social and psychological consequences. The endocrine processes in early adolescence that set into motion a cascade of intricately interconnected changes ultimately transform the individual's reproductive capacity, self-identity, relationships with peers, and social role within the context of the family and community. On the other hand, religious rites of passage (such as a bar mitzvah or confirmation) are transitions that constitute points of psychosocial demarcation in the young person's emergence into the adult world.

   C. **On-time and off-time transitions.** On-time or off-time transitions depend on the timing of the event in relationship to personal and societal expectations. Pregnancy, for example, is a fundamentally different event in the life of a married 23-year-old woman than it is in the life of a 13-year-old. While the onset of puberty in a 14-year-old boy may be an occasion for celebration or relief, the same event may be bewildering and distressing to an 8-year-old boy. The meaning and adaptive significance of a transition depends in part on whether its timing conforms to cultural and biological norms regarding its location within life-course development.

II. **Factors defining stressful transitions.**

   A. **Manifestations of stress.** Not all transitions in childhood *are* stressful but many are accompanied by the behaviors and expressions of emotion that signal a child's efforts to overcome and adapt to stress. Transitions are capable of invoking a child's neuroendocrine stress response systems. Starting preschool or kindergarten, for example, has been shown to activate the hypothalamic-pituitary-adrenocortical axis, resulting in measurable elevations in the cortisol levels found in both blood and saliva and alterations in immune and cardiovascular function. Stressful transitions therefore appear capable of changing not only the child's behavior and emotional experience but may also set in motion physiologic processes that may be plausibly linked to the development of disease.

B. Aspects of stressful transitions.

1. **Adaptation to new situations.** Transitions are, by definition, processes that expose the child to novelty and challenge. A move to a new home, for example, is an event that brings with it the challenges of new neighborhoods and communities, new friends, new schools, and new patterns of living. Although the novelties inherent in such transitions can be invigorating and growth promoting, they often require the simultaneous processes of reorientation, reintegration, and re-exploration of the surrounding physical and social landscapes. Each of these processes can result in the experiences and feelings of emotional stress.

2. **Exacerbation of existing problems.** Transitions can create stress by exacerbating or inflaming previously existing problems. A young girl who is struggling with the new academic demands of middle school may find herself overwhelmed by such demands at the time of menarche and its associated biological changes. A 4-year-old who is experiencing difficulty self-regulating his aggressive impulses in preschool may feel (and be) out of control following the birth of a sibling. Points of transition carry with them a tendency to uncover, accentuate, or bring into focus struggles in the psychological life of the child.

3. **Coping with changed relationships.** A family systems perspective on child development teaches that major changes in the life of any family member can be expected to alter systematically each of the relationships that comprise the family unit. With events such as divorce, these changes in relationships are glaringly self-evident. Even more subtle transitions, such as a grandparent's coming to live with the family, will be reliably accompanied by shifts and disequilibria in the various relationships among siblings and parents.

4. **Beginnings and endings.** Transitions may be experienced as stressful by virtue of their capacity either to open up or to close down the opportunities available to the child or family. When a child begins kindergarten, a landmark is passed in the relationship of child and parents. This child has begun a journey that will end almost certainly in eventual parting from the family that conceived, loved, and raised him. While school may open new visions of possibilities and promise, school also signals—for both the child and parents—the end of something: the final, nonnegotiable conclusion of life as a "little girl or boy."

III. Management. While some changes and transitions may be eagerly anticipated, others will be painful, saddening, or even frightening. At such times, a clinician can be of great assistance to the family by offering professional advice, suggesting practical interventions for the family to pursue, and providing small packages of wisdom about the transition and its likely effects.

A. Parents should be taught or reminded of the powerful effects created by their simple **presence and encouragement in their children's lives.** Within the typically hurried pace of a contemporary family's existence, it is easy to forget that one of the greatest and most lasting expressions of a parent's love—beyond the gifts of protection, security, and provision for physical needs—is the gift of time. The cultural myth of "quality time"—so much a part of the late–twentieth-century's parenting lexicon—should be debunked. Parents should be encouraged to be near and available to their children for as much time as possible, particularly during periods of significant transition. The economic requirements of modern life put undeniable constraints on the amount of time many parents can spend with their children. Nonetheless, even single, working parents can be encouraged to put aside the 30–40 minutes it takes to talk to their children about the day or play a family game.

Parents often underestimate the efficacy of simple encouragement, but there is no question that the support and love of a parent can do more than almost anything else to sustain children through times of difficulty and change. In both words and behavior, parents should be encouraged to convey to their children the message: "This is a difficult time for you and for our family. But I know that better times are ahead, and I know that you, and we, can move through it together."

B. It may be helpful for parents to make special efforts to uphold and adhere to **family rituals and routines** during times of transition. For children at all developmental stages, clinging to the enduring, predictable aspects of day-to-day life may be especially helpful during periods of overwhelming change. Parents may know this already, having observed the tenacity and persistence with which children follow routine. Events as mundane as eating dinner together each night, reading together as a family, or taking a daily walk may take on special significance for children during times of upheaval in their family's life.

C. Families may find that it is helpful to children, when possible, to **reduce the rate of environmental changes**. Stress research suggests that it is usually not the isolated stressor that is deleterious to children's health and well being, but rather the cumulative effects of multiple stressors over a relatively brief period of time. A proliferation of such stressors is likely to occur, for example, during a divorce, when the painful loss of a parent's presence is attended by a wide variety of other changes, such as the selling of the family home, residential moves to new communities and schools, the loss of peer relationships, and the alterations in routine that accompany change in a parent's employment status. When possible, parents should consider slowing the rapidity with which such changes occur, allowing children to spread their adaptive efforts over a longer span of time.

D. **Fantasy and play** are natural, effective means of coping for young children in difficult transitions. Most children instinctively use imaginative play to process and work through the emotionally conflictive aspects of a transitional event. Parents may support these adaptive efforts by allowing children sufficient time for play, by engaging them in imaginative games and conversations about the event, by encouraging the use of art and drawing, and, most important, by not stifling or discouraging their playing through troubling or difficult aspects of their experiences. It has been noted, for example, that among children living in war-torn areas of the world, those children able to "play war" are more likely to show adaptive strengths and sustain positive developmental outcomes.

E. Clinicians and parents should share with children the **personal coping strategies** that have helped them to lighten the difficulties they have encountered during major life transitions. Adaptive hints—such as approaching transitions a single day at a time or dividing the task into smaller steps of graded intensity—may provide substantial benefits to children who have attained sufficient cognitive development to understand such concepts. Among latency-age and older children, parents can teach the importance of pacing oneself by allowing adequate time during periods of stress for sleep, relaxation, and play. With adolescents and young adults, parents and clinicians can encourage the displacement of emotional distress onto physical activities, such as vigorous exercise and competitive athletics.

F. Parents should be encouraged to provide for their children, as a preventive measure for later stressful experiences, opportunities for the **development of competence and mastery**. Parents often fail to place meaningful responsibilities in the hands of children, thereby disallowing the discovery of their own competencies and talents. Even preschool children can be given meaningful household tasks that support the collective life of the family. Responsibilities of increasing difficulty and significance can be progressively shared as children grow. Taken together over the span of years, these opportunities for the production of meaningful work can support the development of a child's sense of mastery and personal confidence in facing the vicissitudes of life.

Parents may also need, at times, to foster the development of mastery by gently urging children into situations that tax or stretch their abilities. An extremely shy or inhibited child, for example, may need to be quietly but persistently encouraged to join a soccer team in order to discover his innate athletic abilities. Through such experiences of bearing responsibility and engaging in controlled risk taking, children become increasingly aware of their internal strengths and their adaptive capabilities.

BIBLIOGRAPHY

Boyce WT. Life events and crises. In Green M, Haggerty RJ (eds), *Ambulatory Pediatrics* (4th ed), Philadelphia: Saunders, 1990.

Haggerty RJ, Garmezy N, Rutter M, Sherrod LR. *Stress, Risk, and Resilience in Children and Adolescents: Processes, Mechanisms, and Intervention.* Cambridge: Cambridge University Press, 1993.

Rutter M. Pathways from childhood to adult life. *J Child Psychol Psychiatry* 30(1):23–51, 1989.

Shonkoff JP, Jarman FC, Kohlenberg TM. Family transitions, crises, and adaptations. *Cur Probl Pediatr* 17(9):507–553, 1987.

Websites

American Academy of Pediatrics. Information for Community Physicians Caring for Children. Available at: http://www.aap.org/moc/aapresponse.htm

Death of a Child in the ED Policy Statement. Available at:http://aappolicy.aappublications.org/cgi/content/full/pediatrics%3b110/4/839

For Parents

Garmezy N, Rutter M. *Stress, Coping and Development in Children.* New York, NY: Johns Hopkins University, 1988.
Haggerty R. *Stress Risk and Resilience in Children and Adolescents: Process, Mechanisms and Intervention.* New York, NY: Cambridge University Press, 1996.

15

Managing Behavior

Barbara Howard

I. **Description of the problem.** Behavioral and emotional issues comprise an estimated 25%–50% of all pediatric problems raised by parents. Pediatric primary care clinicians are in an ideal position to deal with such concerns: they are well known to the family, generally respected, viewed as supportive by both parent and child, and already know much about the child and the family. Additionally, the office setting is seen as friendly, nonstigmatizing territory.

II. **Identifying problems.**
A. **Open-ended questions.** The first requirement for addressing behavioral problems is their identification. This is not always easy since children rarely ask for help and the parents may not realize that the clinician has either the interest or the expertise to help. Discussing behavior and development at each visit, using screening questionnaires, and educating oneself to have practical advice will all encourage parents to discuss psychosocial concerns. Open-ended questions (ones that cannot be answered by Yes or No), such as "How are things going?" allow the parent and child to express their own agenda for the visit. In other families, the clinician may need to ask specifically about *behavior at home, at school, or in day care*. Another approach that broadens the agenda is to ask routinely, "What is the hardest part of taking care of a X-month old?"

B. **Observations in the office.** Observations of behavior in the office and waiting room can be revealing. Toys in the medical bag or examination room are an invaluable way to observe the child's behavior and development (as well as to enhance the enjoyment of the visit). These observations can then be used to start the discussion (e.g., "I noticed that he is very active. How is that for you at home?"). Such comments should be asked in a nonjudgmental way so that the parents' response can reveal if they view the behavior as problematic. The clinician's own feelings and intuitions about the child and family should be compared with parental and child reports and used to raise questions or to formulate clinical hypotheses about the child's behavior.

C. **Screening questionnaires.** Questionnaires can be a valuable time saver and tool for identifying behavioral problems and adding to office documentation. This method is discussed in Chapter 10.

III. **Managing behavioral problems.**
A. **Addressing the problem.** The first step to successful problem resolution occurs during the initial discussion in defining the problem. After initial open-ended questions, it is crucial to elicit details about the onset and attempted solutions, as well as times when the problem wasn't present to look for relevant causal factors. A survey of the areas of daily functioning (including bedtime, meals, toileting, peer interaction, separation abilities, family relationships and school adjustment) are all needed to detect patterns that suggest areas of weakness or dysfunctional management.

It is important for the clinician to summarize the parent's (or his or her own) concerns to demonstrate that their worries have been heard. The problem should be discussed nonjudgmentally and reframed in a positive light and in terms of new specific desired behaviors rather than the ending of a behavior (e.g., "You would like him to listen to instructions [rather than to not act up]"). The initial discussion should set the stage for treatment by **clarifying the problem, setting a positive tone, engaging other family members by determining how it affects them and not blaming or insulting the child (who may be listening)**.

The next step is to convey some **hope and confidence** that a solution is possible and design "homework" that addresses a relevant goal for behavior change. It is important to guide family members in selecting homework tasks that apply to the family dynamic that seems causative, include tasks for each family member that are doable and measurable, and are of a scope that is not overwhelming but also not trivial. Additional diagnostic information comes from seeing how the family acted on this advice when they come for a follow-up.

B. Levels of intervention in primary care. There are different levels of behavior management suitable for different practitioners depending on their amount of interest, skill, and time available for this work.

1. **Education.** The simplest level of behavioral intervention is caregiver education. This usually entails informing the family about what the behavior means to the child, what behavior is normal for age, how temperament may be involved, and how behaviors may be reinforced, for example by attention. This level of intervention should also include teaching families how to set up the environment to reduce the child's frustration and stress and how the caregivers should model how to manage emotions themselves e.g. through self control, verbalizing feelings, or walking away.

2. **Advice.** The second level of intervention involves all of the above plus giving specific advice for the problem behavior. Obtaining details about a specific incident's Antecedents (what happened before the problem behavior, the Behavior itself (what the child did), and the Consequences (for the child and the parent) is essential and will generally reveal the patterns of family interaction. Often children act up at times when they are being asked to make a transition to a new activity. When this is a factor parents may need coaching on how to anticipate these scenarios and how to verbalize about, praise and give marks or points for even small improvements in emotion control or flexibility.

3. **Dealing with underlying issues.** Higher-level interventions involve dealing with underlying issues in the child, adult, family interaction or the environment. To successfully work on this level the clinician needs to understand and make hypotheses based on a transactional model that takes into account mutual influences among these factors.

    a. **Child issues.** Child issues that result in frustration such as functional weaknesses in motor skills, language, emotional regulation or attentional control may need further evaluation. Treatment for weaknesses can be advised including special school placement, adopting bypass strategies, therapy for strengthening skills, reducing demands and medication.

    The behavior itself or the situations eliciting the problem may have meaning to the child that must be addressed directly or symbolically. Clinicians may efficiently hypothesize these meanings based on an understanding of developmental stages and commonly associated family issues, for example sibling jealousy that emerges when infants begin to crawl and get into the other's toys. Other ways of determining the meaning of a behavior include asking directly, "What does it make you think when he does that?" or telling the child or family "Any kid who... (e.g., wonders if a divorce is his fault might act up to see if his parents still care)" while watching the person's emotions. Sometimes the meaning can be inferred from a reaction to "homework" that addresses the issue e.g. infantilizing activities during special time for the child who seems to act up due to seeking more nurturance.

    There are common patterns of family dynamics associated with child behavior problems at different ages. For example, young children may be out of control when a laissez-faire style has resulted from a reaction against a parent's own history of being punished harshly as a child. Child sleep problems may result when there is marital discord causing ambivalence about the parents sleeping together. Biting may occur when parents can't agree on whether or not to use corporal punishment. School underachievement may occur when a sibling is glorified for academics. Promiscuity may signal incest or sexual abuse. Substance abuse may result from depression. After gathering data for a hypothesis about meaning the clinician shares this with the child and/or family and works to both help the family members clarify and communicate the truth and establish new adaptive ways of interacting that are no longer based on reactions to these issues but fill the needs of all parties.

    b. **Parent issues.** It may become clear after simple advice has failed that interfering parent issues need to be addressed such as the parent viewing the child as special or vulnerable, inability to tolerate angry emotions from the child due to their own past exposure to violence, inability to prevent interfering with the other parent's management, covert satisfaction in a child's misbehavior, or lack of energy or motivation to do the hard work of behavior management.

    Eliciting past experiences that are reawakened during child management is often the key. Engaging cooperation from all relevant adults for their own motivation is always helpful and may be essential. When the adult understands how their own issue in affecting the child's behavior they are better able to change their interaction patterns. Writing down the costs and benefits to maintaining the interaction patterns is a useful intervention. Further individual work or therapy for the adult may also be needed.

    c. Interactional issues . A parent with reasonable overall parenting skills may still be susceptible to maladaptive practices with an individual child. This may be due to a mismatch in temperament with the child, an unreasonable expectation given this child's attributes, or a change in circumstances or energy for providing adequate attention to the child's positive behaviors. Education and clarification may be sufficient but providing alternative nurturers for the child is sometimes the only solution.

    d. Environmental issues . It is not unusual for a child's behavior to be due to outside conditions especially with the current culture of extensive time in childcare. Toxins, poor quality care by others, models or stress from observing dysfunctional adult behaviors should all be considered when kindly, reasonable parents are unable to resolve child behavior in a previously well adjusted child. The mediating factors may also be sleep debt, hunger, sibling or peer influence or abuse. These factors often occur in combination with the above so that all need to be addressed.

C. Special "problem visits." Once a problem has been identified, one or more visits of longer duration than usual are generally needed. To arrange an effective "problem visit," the vitally important people in the child's life should be invited to attend if possible. Boyfriends, distant cousins, and babysitters, for example, may be crucial to the solution of the problem. If a key person refuses to attend, a personal telephone call by the clinician that seeks his or her opinion and stresses this person's importance to the child can change a recalcitrant attitude.

    1. Visit duration. Frequently, a longer (e.g., one-half to 1 hour) problem visit can be scheduled at the beginning or the end of the workday, when no sick children are waiting to be seen and telephone calls can be postponed. (It is often advantageous to schedule the problem visit at the beginning of the day, when energy is high). Sometimes the most delicate or powerful issue is not raised until the last moments of the visit in a "parting shot." Such important statements at the end of the hour need to be acknowledged with appropriate empathy, recorded in the chart, and promised as first agenda items at the next visit (which may need to be scheduled sooner, depending on the information revealed).

        Another problem occurs when families or key family members arrive late for an appointment. This may be an important statement of that person's ambivalence about the issues being discussed. The emotional difficulty can be acknowledged directly and with empathy, but the visit should be kept on schedule.

    2. Space considerations. Many offices lack an examining room large enough to seat all the family members. A conference room or even the waiting room may better serve and can be private enough before or after regular office hours.

    3. Documentation of the visit. Since details of the session are critical to understanding and managing the problem and documenting complexity for billing, the clinician should leave adequate time to write down the salient aspects of the visit. Note taking is possible during the session for some clinicians, but should be interrupted when it interferes with the therapeutic alliance with the family and patient.

    4. Billing for the visit. It is important that the extended problem visit be adequately billed with a higher level of care usually based on time spent. Patients should be informed of the fee *before* the first extended visit. Offering to accept payment over time may decrease the burden of the extra fee for some families. Third-party reimbursement may be available depending on the diagnosis, the clinician's experience and training, and state insurance regulations. Clinicians generally cannot refer their own patients to themselves and record the visit as a consultation. Experience suggests that most patients *are* willing to pay for counseling if they are able. Many of the barriers to adequate billing are in the mind of the clinician, who is insecure about whether she or he really has something valuable to offer.

D. Expanding counseling skills. Books, journals, lectures, videotapes of master therapists, workshops, courses, and fellowships in behavior and development, child psychiatry, or family therapy are available to help clinicians strengthen their behavioral counseling skills. The ultimate method, however, is through experience. For example, working as cotherapists with a more experienced clinician in the session with the family is a very valuable format. Case discussions with another clinician or in a group provides support and insight into the family's and clinician's emotional reactions, as well as input into the content and process of management. This process is called *supervision* and can be either direct (another professional attends the counseling session or observes through a one-way mirror) or indirect (the other professional reviews cases later from audiotape, videotape, verbatim process notes, standard notes, or recall, and makes suggestions to be incorporated into future patient visits). The Bureau of Maternal and Child Health has funded a number of Collaborative Office Rounds demonstration projects to provide such case discussion for groups of 8 to10 practicing pediatric clinicians or such groups can be gotten together with an agreement to pay the supervisor for their time.

E. **Communicating with schools.** Some behavioral problems are situationally specific and occur only in school or day care. In such cases it is useful to obtain an objective description of the problem from the school. Have parents sign a note of consent for two-way communication at the first visit that can be faxed to the other relevant sites. A behavioral questionnaire can be sent to the teacher or a written note requested. Ideally, direct telephone contact between clinician and teacher is the most revealing. (It is easiest to reach teachers at 7:30 A.M. or noon.) Teachers are generally very grateful for the clinician's interest and can be extremely helpful in providing more information about the family and the child. A single clinician visit to a school to meet one child's teachers, principal, and guidance counselors can facilitate communication for years to come about many children.

F. **Making effective referrals.** One of the most important (and underrated) skills of the primary care clinician lies in making effective referrals. An estimated 68% of mental health referrals made for children are unsuccessful because the family has been poorly prepared, the referral is ill timed, the family has negative perceptions of mental health professionals, or there is a poor fit between the specialist's therapeutic style and the family's or child's expectations.

1. **Help the family to identify their distress.** The first steps in making an effective referral are to ensure that each member of the family feels that his or her voice has been heard and to identify the distress that will motivate the family and child to accept counseling. It is always better for a clinician to refer the family for a problem that bothers *them,* even if it is not the one that appears primary to the clinician (e.g., a referral for the child's truancy rather than the father's alcoholism). The therapist taking on the case may need to do further work before the family is able to face the central issue.

2. **Discuss issues in a constructive way.** Behavioral and family issues should be discussed in nonjudgmental terms, citing strengths and using issues from the family's current (rather than past) situation to suggest further work. In the case of a separation from an abusive spouse, for example, one might say, "It took so much courage to make this break that I can see that you really want what is best for your son. Now you can focus on improving your relationship with him and seeing him as a different kind of male from your ex-husband."

3. **Find the appropriate referral.** The next step in making an effective referral is to identify an appropriate consultant for the family. The clinician should inquire about the family's past experiences with counseling and demystify the process of counseling (e.g., by pointing out that therapy is just like the talking that has been going on in the exploratory sessions).

   It is helpful to have ready the names and telephone numbers of several therapists who are available and have interest and skills in the type of problem at hand. This takes some preparation in getting to know the counseling style of a cadre of therapists: for example, what kinds of cases they prefer; whether they practice cognitive behavioral therapy, family therapy or psychodynamic therapy; and whether they offer groups. Determine their fees and accepted insurance.

   Consider a face-to-face meeting with a therapist. It allows some basis for discussing the therapist with a family and will facilitate future communications between physician and therapist. The clinician should provide the family and patient with details about the therapists so that they can make an informed choice. The gender of the therapist is not usually central to the success of treatment, although some family members may have a strong preference, which should be respected. The relationship of the family with this professional is vital to the treatment, so they should be actively involved in the initial referral. Additionally, they should be told that they can always change counselors, should the need arise. This is important so that their problems do not go unresolved simply because of an initial mismatch.

4. **Follow-up.** Finally, it is important for the family to know that the primary care clinician will stay involved and will continue to manage other problems as before. This reassures them that they are not being rejected, especially if they have revealed information about themselves that could be perceived as undesirable. The clinician should be clear in defining exactly what problems will be handled by which profes-

sional, and stay in touch with the referral therapist in order to assist or back up the therapist's plans and to facilitate ongoing communication with the family.

G. Alternative counseling strategies in the office.

   1. Groups for families. Group sessions for a number of families concerning common behavioral problems (e.g., temper tantrums, toilet training, discipline issues, choosing a day care provider, teenage risk-taking behaviors) can be an effective way to address those issues and to provide parents with a support system of other parents in similar circumstances. Other groups can be made available for parents of children with a specific problem, such as attention deficit hyperactivity disorder, oppositional defiant disorder, mental retardation, or substance abuse. Local branches of national diagnosis specific organizations may already offer these or will arrange them when sufficient interest is shown. It has been shown that noncategorical groups, e.g., for parents of children with a variety of chronic illnesses, can be as effective as diagnosis specific groups. One-time sessions may be arranged to deal with crises, such as a suicide, disaster, abuse in a local day care center, or death of a public figure. For families, the existence of others with similar problems can be a tremendous relief in itself.

   These groups can be led by a primary care clinician in the practice or by an outside consultant, or co-led by both. They may be offered in the office or elsewhere, sponsored by the practice, or simply made known to patients in the practice. It is important to remember that the needs of the individual child or family are frequently not entirely met by these groups, so the leaders must carefully monitor the participants and ensure that supplemental support, guidance, or management is available if needed.

   2. Group checkups. There are some advantages to offering health supervision visits in groups. By seeing eight 6-month-old babies together over 1 hour, the clinician can spend much more time providing teaching, anticipatory guidance, and discussion of behavioral issues. It is important to also offer some private time for each family, however, as there may be issues that are not appropriate for the group to hear.

   3. Call hour. Many offices have a designated call-in hour for health and behavior questions conducted by either the physician or an experienced nurse or nurse practitioner. While telephone consultations have obvious major disadvantages, when supervised carefully they can be part of a spectrum of office services for dealing with behavioral problems and help motivate families for behavior counseling if the call line information alone does not suffice.

   4. Housing other professional disciplines within the practice. Many practices are choosing to provide offices for specialists from other disciplines to deal with specific behavioral and emotional problems. In private practices, the specialist may receive the space free, share in the costs and income of the group, set lower fees for patients from the practice, be paid a salary by the group, or be a totally independent contractor renting space and billing independently. The practice benefits by having a known, trusted, and readily available person to whom to refer their patients. The entire practice can be strengthened by the comprehensive care that ends up being delivered within its walls.

BIBLIOGRAPHY

Allmond BW, Tanner JL with Gofman HF. *The Family Is the Patient.* Baltimore: Williams & Wilkins, 1999.

Coleman WL.Family-focused pediatrics: Solution-oriented techniques for behavioral problems. *Contemp Ped* 14:121–134, 1997.

Coleman WL, Howard BJ. Family Focused Behavioral Pediatrics: Clinical Techniques for Primary Care. *Ped in Review* 16:448–455, 1995.

Coleman WL, Taylor EH (eds), Family-Focused Pediatrics: Issues, Challenges, and Clinical Methods, *Ped Clin N Am* 42:1–239, 1995.

McDaniel S, Campbell TL, Seaburn DB. *Family-Oriented Primary Care: A Manual for Medical Providers.* New York: Springer-Verlag, 1990.

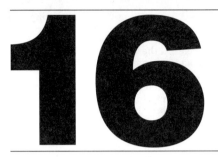

Pain

Neil L. Schechter

I. **Definition and background.** Pain is defined by the International Association for the Study of Pain as "an unpleasant sensory and emotional experience associated with actual or potential tissue damage or described in terms of such damage." This definition implies that pain has two components—a neurophysiologically determined sensation that results from stimulation of nociceptors and the interpretation of that stimulus which is impacted by a host of personality, cognitive, and emotional factors. These may magnify or dampen the amount of pain and suffering that the stimulus causes the individual. Current understanding of pain, therefore, implies that there is no set amount of pain allowable for a given injury or illness because of enormous individual variation and experience that accounts for varying interpretations of that symptom. This section will focus on acute pain; chronic pain problems such as headache and recurrent abdominal pain are reviewed elsewhere in this volume.

Historically, pain has been significantly undertreated in children for a variety of complex reasons. Difficulties with pain assessment in children, social attitudes, and ethical and financial constraints on research diminished interest and allowed for the persistence of myths ("infants do not feel pain") that denigrated the importance of treatment. There has been an outpouring of research in the last 10 years, however, and it is now clearly established that by the end of the second trimester, fetuses have in place the anatomical and chemical capabilities to experience discomfort. Preterm and newborn infants may, in fact, be hyperalgesic because they have the same number of nociceptors in a smaller surface area and because they lack descending modulation of pain through psychological means.

Inadequate pain management may in fact, have short and long term negative consequences. Untreated pain may be responsible for worsening the child's clinical condition and has been implicated as a contributing cause of IVH (intraventricular hemorrhage) in newborns. Inadequately addressed pain in young and school-age children with illness causes unnecessary suffering and worries about procedure pain during routine health supervision. For many children with chronic conditions, inadequately treated procedure pain is the worst part of their illness, often worse than the disease itself and creates anxiety about subsequent medical encounters.

II. **Diagnosis.** Adequate assessment is the cornerstone of pain treatment. An individual's self-report of his/her discomfort is the gold standard for assessment. In adults and children over the age of 8, the visual analogue scale that quantifies pain intensity from 0–10 is traditionally used. Because of developmental immaturity in children age 3 to 8 years, modification of the visual analogue scale is necessary. Color scales, cartoon faces, manipulatives such as poker chips representing pieces of hurt, and photographs of children in discomfort have all been used as modified visual analogue scales. For children under 3 years, physiologic parameters (increased heart rate, increased respiratory rate, decreased SaO_2) and behavioral measures such as facial expression, body position, and crying have all been used as nonspecific indicators of pain. Attempts have been made to cluster together these parameters into clinically-usable scales (examples of these include the CHEOPS, OBSS, OPS, and NIPS).

III. **Treatment.**
   A. **General principles.** The primary goal of treatment is to make the child as comfortable as possible, recognizing that it may not be possible to eliminate all discomfort and that there is often a balance between pain relief and the side effects associated with analgesics. A number of general principles have emerged, however.
   1. It should be generally assumed that whatever hurts an adult will hurt a child and appropriate pain relief should be planned.
   2. A preventative approach is key. Where pain is predictable, it makes much more sense to prevent pain from occurring than to ablate it once it has occurred. This suggests that around-the-clock dosing as compared to PRN dosing is preferable.
   3. Pharmacologic, cognitive-behavioral, and physical approaches should be considered.

4. As often as possible, nonnoxious routes of administration should be used, avoiding intramuscular, rectal or intranasal routes if possible.
5. Needle sticks are extremely troubling for children and wherever possible, local anesthetics should be used when needle sticks are necessary.

B. **Behavioral/cognitive/physical approaches.** These nonpharmacologic approaches vary, depending on the type of pain and the age of the child. In situations where limited pain may be magnified anxiety, they may be the only approach necessary. In general, however, they are used in conjunction with pharmacologic approaches.
   1. **Parental presence.** Parental presence during painful procedures and parental involvement in treatment decisions often has a significant impact on pain the child experiences. During procedures, parents can function as a "coach," stroking, soothing, or talking to the child. They can be instructed in age-appropriate pain relieving techniques. In general, when parents can be included in treatment decisions, they feel less anxious and less helpless and their security is often transmitted to the child and pain is reduced.
   2. **Preparation.** Knowledge about the pain and its expected time course also reduces anxiety about it, which has the effect of decreasing pain. Discussion about illness and procedures clearly improves coping. Preparation for procedures should include a description of how the child will feel as well as a more detailed description of what will happen.
   3. **Visual imagery/distraction/hypnosis.** These techniques help a child cope with painful illnesses or painful procedures by focusing their attention away from their discomfort. Approaches in this category include breathing techniques, blowing on pinwheels, blowing bubbles, being told stories, reading books, and imagining a more pleasant, desirable place. Hypnosis actively involves the child in a fantasy and uses suggestion to reframe the experience.
   4. **Physical approaches.** Massage, heat, cold, pressure and vibration in the form of transcutaneous electrical nerve stimulation all work by flooding the nervous system with nonnoxious stimuli, therefore decreasing the impact of the painful stimulus.

C. **Pharmacologic approaches.** A number of categories of pharmacologic agents are helpful in pain relief. They may have direct pain-relieving properties, anxiety-reducing properties, or potentiate analgesia.
   1. **Local anesthetics.** A number of local anesthetics are presently available which should be used during pain associated with needle insertion or other painful procedures involving the skin.
      - **EMLA**, a topically administered combination of lidocaine and prilocaine, is extremely effective for venous cannulation, phlebotomy, and reservoir access, and has some efficacy on the pain associated with intramuscular injections as well. EMLA requires approximately 1 hour to work, and provides 2–4 mm of anesthesia.
      - Another topical formulation of lidocaine is **ElaMax** which is 4% lidocaine encapsulated by liposomes which allow for transdermal delivery. It is available without prescription and in theory works in approximately one half-hour.
      - One additional topical anesthetic is **amethocaine** (4% tetracaine cream), which is equivalent to EMLA but works more rapidly and is a vasodilator, not constrictor. It is not yet available in the United States.
      - **Lidocaine** can also be injected or administered by iontophoresis. Lidocaine burns when injected, but this burning is decreased if Lidocaine is buffered 9–1 with sodium bicarbonate. Iontophoretic lidocaine takes only 10 minutes to work, and achieves anesthesia to 8–10 mm. Administration by this approach is uncomfortable for some children, however.
      - Topical refrigerants or **vapocoolant sprays** produce immediate anesthesia for a few seconds and therefore may reduce injection or immunization pain.
   2. **Acetaminophen and NSAIDs (see Table 16-1).** These categories of drugs act peripherally and inhibit cyclooxygenase, which has a role in prostoglandin synthesis. All of the drugs in this category have a "ceiling" effect, beyond which no further analgesia is achieved.
      - **Acetaminophen**, the most commonly used drug in this category, provides analgesia but has no anti-inflammatory effect.
      - Unfortunately, all available over-the-counter **NSAIDs** which have antiinflammatory activity, also have associated bleeding and gastrointestinal side effects. These agents are preferable to acetaminophen for pain associated with inflammation such as pain associated with otitis media, pharyngitis, and muscular aches.
      - A new category of drugs, the **COX-2 inhibitors**, is now available which appear

Table 16-1 Dosing data for NSAIDs

Drug	Usual adult dose	Usual pediatric dose	Comments
Oral NSAIDs			
Acetaminophen (paracetamol)	650–1000 mg q 4 hr	10–20 mg/kg q 4 hr	Acetaminophen lacks the peripheral antiinflammatory activity of other NSAIDs
Ibuprofen	400–600 mg q 4–6 hr	6–10 mg/kg q 6–8 hr	Available as several brand names and as generic; also available as oral suspension
Naproxen	500 mg initial dose followed by 250 mg q 6–8 hr	5 mg/kg q 12 hr	Also available as oral liquid
Rofecoxib	25 mg q 24 hr	0.6 mg/kg	COX-2 inhibitor may cause less bleeding and gastritis

to provide analgesia and anti-inflammatory effects with reduced bleeding and gastrointestinal problems.

3. **Opioids (See Table 16-2).** Opioids are the drugs of choice for moderate to severe pain.
   - The "weaker opioids," **codeine and oxycodone**, are available in fixed drug preparations as well as in long-acting preparations (Tylenol #3, Percocet, Tylox).
   - For more severe pain, **morphine** remains the drug of choice. It can be administered through a number of routes and its pharmacokinetics are well-established in children. These agents can be used safely in children but should be used with caution in a carefully monitored setting in infants.
   - For severe pain that persists, **long acting opioids** (MSContin, OxyContin, Kadian) are now available but should only be prescribed for severe chronic pain, not acute unstable pain.
   - A short-acting opioid should be always be prescribed simultaneously for breakthrough pain. There are known side effects predictable side effects associated with these drugs, such as constipation, respiratory depression and itching, which should be anticipated.
   - Although diversion and abuse of these drugs for illicit purposes exists, concerns about addiction, which have hampered the legitimate medical use of these drugs in the past, are essentially negligible.
4. **Sedative-hypnotics.** Drugs in this category include the short-acting benzodiazepine, midazolam, which is often used in conjunction with an opioid during painful procedures and provides amnesia as well as anxiolysis and chloral hydrate. These agents are often used for procedures which require cooperation but are not associated with pain such as MRIs and CT scans.
5. **Adjunctive drugs.** Drugs in this category include anticonvulsants, such as carbamazepine and gabapentin, which have efficacy against the pain of nerve injury, neuropathic pain, which is often opioid-resistant, and tricyclic antidepressants, such as amitryptiline which are also efficacious against neuropathic pain and helps with insomnia.

IV. **Summary.** Most acute pain problems are treatable using relatively simple, safe approaches. A small percent of cases will require regional or other anesthetic approaches. A systematic approach to assessment is the cornerstone of adequate treatment, as, unless pain is documented, it cannot be adequately treated nor can the success of interventions be monitored. Pharmacologic and behavioral approaches are both very successful in children and both should be incorporated in any comprehensive plan for pain relief.

Table 16-2 Dosing data for opioid analgesics

Drug	Equianalgesic parenteral dose	Equianalgesic oral dose	Recommended adult dose[1] parenteral	Recommended adult dose[2] oral	Recommended pediatric dose parenteral	Recommended pediatric dose oral
Morphine	10 mg	30 mg	10 mg q 3–4 hr	30 mg q 3– hr	0.1 mg/kg. q 3-4 hr	0.3 mg/kg. q 3–4 hr
Codeine	130 mg	200 mg	Not recommended	30–60 mg q 4 hr	Not recommended	0.5-1 mg/kg. q 3–4 hr
Hydromophone	1.5 mg	7.5 mg	1 mg q 3–4 hr	2–4 mg q 3–4 hr	0.02 mg/kg. q 3–4 hr	0.04-.08 mg/kg. q 3–4 hr
Oxycodone	Not available	30 mg	Not available	5–10 mg q 3–4 hr	Not available	0.2 mg/kg. q 3–4 hr
Methadone	10 mg	20 mg	5–8 mg q 4 hr	5–10 mg 3–4 hr	0.1 mg/kg. q 6–8 hr	0.1–0.2 mg/kg. q 6–8 hr
Meperidine[3](pethidine)	100 mg	300 mg	50–75 mg q 3 hr	100–150 mg q 2–3 hr	0.8–1 mg/kg. q 2–3 hr	2–3 mg/kg. q 3–4 hr

1. Doses refer to children older than 6 months.
2. Greater than 50 kg
3. Meperidine should be avoided if other opioids are available. With long-term use, its metabolite may cause seizures.

BIBLIOGRAPHY

Books

Acute Pain Management Guideline Panel. *Acute Pain Management: Operative or Medical Procedures and Trauma: Clinical Practice Guideline. AHCPR Pub, No, 92-0032.* Rockville, MD: Agencyfor Health Care Policy and Research, Public Health Service, U.S. Department of Health and Human Services, 1992.
Schechter NL, Berde CB, Yaster M.*Pain in Infants, Children, and Adolescents (2nd ed).* Philadelphia: Lippincott Williams & Wilkins, 2003.
Yaster M, Krane E, Kaplan R, Cote C, Lappe D.*Pediatric Pain Management and Sedation Handbook.* St. Louis: Mosby, 1997.

Organizations

International Association for the Study of Pain 909 NE 43rd St., Suite 306 Seattle, WA 98105-6020 www.iasp-pain.org Society that focuses on pain management and research; has frequent meetings and a special interest group on pediatric pain.
Society for Developmental and Behavioral Pediatrics 17000 Commerce Parkway, Suite C Mt. Laurel, NJ 08054 www.sdbp.org Yearly hypnosis training seminar that often focuses on pain management prior to annual meetings.

Websites

Pediatric pain Website available at: www.dal.ca/~pedpain Dalhousie University supports a superb website that serves as a clearinghouse of pediatric pain information for children, families, and clinicians. They also sponsor a listserve on pediatric pain for clinicians.

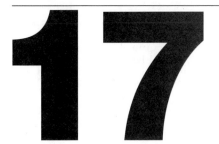

Early Childhood Development in Developing Countries

Ilgi Ozturk Ertem

I. Description of the problem.

A. The majority of the world's children live in developing countries. Although prevention of childhood mortality remains the focus in the developing world, many countries are looking to promote early childhood development via healthcare delivery systems within the context of the following universal principles:

- **Optimal development is the basic right of the child.** The adoption of the United Nations Convention of the Rights of the Child by many countries has brought increased awareness that regardless of where a child may live in the world, an environment that promotes his/her full developmental potential is a basic right of the child.
- **Development during early childhood has implications across the life span.** The quality of relationships in early life shape the child's developing brain. Furthermore, there is evidence that as the health and development of young children is optimized, so is the health, well being and performance of the overall population.
- **Links between physical health and psychosocial development are better understood.** The biomedical model that has dominated the approach to healthcare delivery in developing countries has limited attention to psychosocial and developmental issues. Recent research emphasizes that causes of poor health (e.g., malnutrition) also affect development and that causes of poor development (e.g., unresponsive caring environments) also impact on health. International organizations such as the World Health Organization (WHO) and the United Nations Children's Fund (UNICEF) appreciate that when healthcare delivery includes a developmental context, there are beneficial effects on survival, physical health, and development.
- **The healthcare system is often the only existing infrastructure reaching young children.** Research in western countries has shown that child development can be supported during pediatric healthcare encounters. Healthcare encounters may be the only opportunity available for professionals in developing countries to positively influence caregivers of young children.

B. Risks to early childhood development are multiple in developing countries. It is often impossible to separate biological and psychosocial risks, as they almost invariably coexist and impact on health and development. Poverty, lack of education, unemployment, malnutrition, chronic illness including HIV/AIDS, and deficiencies in family planning often place parents at risk for "unprepared" parenting. Rates of consanguineous marriages and genetic conditions associated with developmental disabilities may be high. Standard prenatal care may not be accessible and both neonatal and maternal mortality and morbidity from unattended delivery, birth trauma, infection and low birth weight is high. Malnutrition is prevalent. Iron deficiency anemia coexists with malnutrition, but may be prevalent in otherwise well nourished children. Chronic illness, particularly infections further impede growth and development.

- **Little information on child development may reach families.** Young children may not be regarded as receptive to interaction and may not be given opportunities for exploration and play. Gender inequalities may place women at higher risk for difficulties in caring for themselves and their young children.
- **Maternal depression** in developing countries is at least as prevalent and has all the consequences that are present for Western children. Furthermore, recent research has shown that in developing countries, young children of depressed mothers have higher mortality and morbidity rates than children of mothers who are not depressed.
- With displacement due to war or move into urban life, **the support of extended family may be lost.** As women increasingly join the work force without appropriate childcare facilities, young children may be left in the care of aging grandparents, or other children. Problems also exist within healthcare systems in developing countries.
- There are far **fewer encounters with healthcare providers**, and these are typically not for well child are visits, but during acute illness.

- **Healthcare professionals may not be equipped with information on developmental or psychosocial issues**, mental health professionals may be very few in number and multi- disciplinary teams may not exist. The support to the development of young children may be regarded as a luxury that is not relevant to health care.
C. **Strengths that foster resilience during early childhood in developing countries.** Strengths and resilience co-exist even in most deprived populations. As risks to optimal development differ within populations, reasons for resilience may also differ.
   - The primary role of the mother in caring for her young child, the slow pace of daily life,the presence of fathers and extended family and the "whole village" that circle and nurture the child may be important protective factors for a young child's development.
   - Substance abuse by women, a major risk in Western populations is less common in the developing world. Healthcare professionals are often highly regarded in the community.
   - Systems that western countries spend large funds to install, for example, home visiting for the delivery of primary care, healthcare stations that are regarded as part of communities, may be already in place in developing countries.
D. **Strategies to promote early childhood development.** The promotion of early childhood development does not require expensive equipment, or expensive and lengthy training programs. When existing strengths within local resources are identified, the challenge then becomes how to increase motivation to also place emphasis on promoting early childhood development:
   - **Develop locally owned, sustainable interventions.** Interventions resembling episodic relief work do little to ameliorate problems in the long run. The magnitude of problems and strengths within communities must be understood to ensure a match between interventions and what the population needs, can achieve and can sustain. It is by building local capacity that a sustainable approach can be developed. Academic centers can be supported to transmit knowledge flow from other countries, develop culturally appropriate and innovative interventions, and test their effectiveness.
   - **Assess theoretical construct.** Culturally appropriate interventions that reflect "state of the art" teachings on child development are needed. Early childhood development may be a new concept in the developing world and may be dominated by outdated theories and models. This may result in the removal of children physically or conceptually from the context of their relationships and environments when attempting to promote their development. Focusing on the neuro-developmental milestones of the child, child centered screening, procedures and interventions that do not foster relationships with caregivers are not likely to provide benefit. Practices based on such beliefs and models need to be identified and changed.
   - Current theories that place **caregiver–child interactions at the center of promoting child development,** interventions that enable relationships and partnerships with caretakers, that allow non-threatening, supportive environments within healthcare delivery, and interventions that regard young children as active participants in the process would be most effective.
   - **Adopt a comprehensive approach.** As risks to development are multiple, so must interventions be comprehensive. It will not be enough to simply enhance the play of malnourished children with untreated infections. Similarly it will not be a sufficient boost to development if these children are only fed and given treatment. All components of health and psychosocial care must be taken into account together.
   - **Assess and increase motivation and training of healthcare staff.** The backgrounds of healthcare staff should be assessed. Is up to date information on child development a part of pre-service or in-service training? What are the knowledge, skills and attitudes of clinicians related to the promotion of child development? How can they be motivated to take on yet another and new agenda?
   - **Identify minimum standards.** When identified in each community and setting, key elements that promote child development may prove to be easy to institute, inexpensive and cost-effective. For example in hospital settings: children and adults may be hospitalized separately, caregiver accompaniment of children can be permitted at all times, home made toys can be provided, a trained healthcare worker can be designated to promote child development.
   - **Support continuity of care.** Whereas continuity of care is often feasible, its importance may not have received as much emphasis in other countries as in the United States. Receiving health care from one provider works to promote child development in two directions: it enhances families' experience through better health worker–family

communication and it enhances health workers' experience through opportunities for natural observations of child and family development.

- **Adopt an opportunistic approach.** All opportunities should be used. Incorporating the promotion of child development into community programs, family planning, safe motherhood, obstetric care, delivery, postpartum care, immunizations, nutrition counseling, ill child ambulatory care and hospitalizations are examples of opportunistic approaches.
- **Involve men as well as women.** The role of fathers, extended family, male leaders in community, and policy makers should not be overlooked and may have more impact than recognized in the Western world.
- **Attend urgently to specific problems.** Children affected by war, displacement, the HIV/AIDS pandemic, natural disasters, developmental disorders, orphanage care, abuse, neglect and exploitation deserve specific attention and comprehensive care throughout the world.
- **Work for peace and equality throughout the world.** In all of our efforts to better child health and development we must remember that these depend most on peace and equal distribution of resources.

II. **Examples of interventions.**
   A. **Care for Development Intervention** (CDI) developed by the World Health Organization Department of Child and Adolescent Health and Development, uses the window of opportunity that arises when the child with an acute illness is brought into the healthcare system. The CDI is a standardized interview which assesses how the caretaker plays with and communicates with the child. Observations and intervention strategies offered to parents during the interview include: listening to caregivers and giving specific praise and positive reinforcement; observing for positive interactions between infants and caregivers during the healthcare visit; using basic home made toys to facilitate interactions; pointing out the responses of the infant and the role of the caregiver in eliciting these responses; and providing ideas for age appropriate stimulation. Healthcare workers then explore with the child's caretaker the potential for such interactions in the home, discuss obstacles that caretakers may face in providing care to help the child develop, and ways he can overcome these obstacles. The intervention can be delivered anywhere and adds approximately 10 minutes to the health visit. The training period is approximately 1.5 days. Training materials, comprising of workbooks and videotape for the facilitator and trainees have been tested in the field. This intervention has a "vector" that can carry it across the world. It can be attached to the WHO Integrated Management of Childhood Illness (IMCI) model so that it can be implemented worldwide in countries that may wish to take up this model.
   B. **Comprehensive training of primary healthcare professionals to promote early childhood development.**
   An example from Turkey. As a joint initiative of The Turkish Ministry of Health, UNICEF-Turkey, a 5-day in-service training program for healthcare professionals (general practitioners, home visiting nurses and midwives) was developed. The topics of the training include: child development starting from pregnancy to preschool years, risks to optimal development, ways to decrease risks, preventing developmental delay, common psychosocial problems, techniques for developmental follow-up and supporting families, early identification of children with developmental delay and their rights, community resources available for early intervention and rehabilitation, and child abuse and neglect. The training methods used are interactive, experiential and problem based. Materials comprise of a book with chapters on each topic, a compact disk with a total of 400 slides, video recordings of children and parents and case scenarios. The program has started and is intended to go to scale in Turkey. We find that the topic of early childhood development for primary healthcare professionals has an enchanting effect. When introduced in a form that is appropriate to the context of their ongoing work, healthcare professionals are highly motivated to take on as their mission the promotion of early childhood development.

BIBLIOGRAPHY

The Global Directory of Early Childhood Projects. http://www.worldbank.org/children.
Keating D, Hertzman C (eds). *Developmental health and the wealth of nations: Social, biological and educational dynamics.* New York: The Guilford Press, 2000

Myers, R. *The Twelve Who Survive: Strengthening Programmes of Early Child Development in the Third World.* London: Routledge, 1991.

Olness K. Effects on brain development leading to cognitive impairment: a worldwide epidemic. *J Dev Behav Pediatr* 24:120–130, 2003

Richter LM. Poverty, underdevelopment and infant mental health. *J Paediatr Child Health* 39: 243–248, 2003.

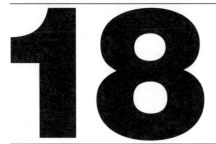

Self-Regulation Therapy

Karen Olness

I. **Description of the issue.** Training in self–self-regulation can prove useful for health professionals and for the children and adolescents they serve. Ongoing studies are comparing the cost-effectiveness and societal impact of self–self-regulation training methods with other treatments. For example, training in self-hypnosis prevents migraine episodes in children, and this may reduce the enormous morbidity associated with adult migraine. Early training in self-regulation may extinguish negative conditioned physiologic responses, such as tachycardia, and thereby avoid more complex adult problems. Perhaps most importantly, such training provides a sense of coping ability and mastery in children. The average child learns quickly, and initial training requires only a few office visits.
   A. **Definitions**
      1. **Cyberphysiology** is the process of governing or controlling one's own physiologic responses.
      2. **Biofeedback** is a strategy of cyberphysiology that provides visual or auditory evidence of physiologic changes. A bathroom scale and a blood pressure monitor, for example, are biofeedback devices. Machines designed to provide feedback of autonomic responses (e.g., galvanic skin resistance, peripheral temperature, heart rate, pulse rate variability, and electromyographic responses) have been used therapeutically.
      3. **Hypnotherapy** is a strategy of cyberphysiology that refers to focusing attention on specific mental images for therapeutic purposes. It often, but not always, involves relaxation. Children, for example, may be physically active when practicing self-hypnosis. All hypnosis is, in fact, self-hypnosis. When those who teach self-hypnosis choose methods consistent with a patient's interests, learning styles, and imagery preferences, it is likely that any motivated person can learn self-hypnosis.
II. **Self-regulation in pediatric care.**
   A. **Applications.** The child health professional may recommend training in a cyberphysiologic strategy as primary or adjunct treatment for a number of problems (Table 18-1). Numerous clinical reports and prospective controlled studies have documented the efficacy of self-regulation in general categories of pain management, chronic illness, habits, and individual performance. In general, training in self-hypnosis is a suitable adjunct to reducing pain, anxiety, nausea, vomiting, and other symptoms associated with chronic disease. There is also evidence that children with chronic problems who learn skills in self-regulation will retain and use these skills as adults.
   B. **Principles of self-regulation treatment.**
      1. Assess the **presenting problem** to rule out biologic causes that may require other types of treatment.
      2. Assess the interest of the child and his or her **willingness to practice self-regulation techniques.** If the problem is primarily of concern to the parent and not the child, the child may not wish to invest the requisite time.
      3. Determine the **child's interest, likes, dislikes, fears, and learning patterns** in order to choose an approach that is likely to be appealing and practical. For example, a 10-year-old boy who likes computer games may be highly motivated by relaxation training associated with computer feedback of his peripheral temperature and galvanic skin resistance.
      4. Because self-regulation is the job of the child, not the parents, **teach the child without the presence of parents,** although they may be present during the initial part of the interview. It is important to say, in the presence of both child and parent, "Your mother is not allowed to remind you to practice. On the way home you can discuss a way to remind yourself to practice, for example, a sign on your bedroom door."
      5. Be certain the child **understands something about the mechanism of the problem.** This can be achieved by simple drawings and concrete language (e.g., diagramming the urinary tract or a pain pathway).

Table 18-1 Applications of self-regulation in pediatrics

Pain Management
   Acute (procedures in office or emergency room)
   Chronic (sickle cell disease, hemophilia, recurrent headaches, etc.)
Habit problems
   Thumb sucking
   Hair pulling
   Simple tics
   Enuresis
   Habit cough
Reduction of anxiety in chronic conditions
   Malignancies
   Hemophilia
   Sickle cell disease
   Lupus erythematosus
   Tourette syndrome
   Diabetes
   Cyclic Vomiting
Improved performance
   Sports
   Drama
   Music
   Exams
Control of conditions involving autonomic dysregulation
   Raynaud's phenomenon
   Reflex sympathetic dystrophy
   Dyshydrosis
   Conditioned hyperventilation
   Conditioned dysphagia
Prevention
   Migraine
   Anxiety
Other
   Insomnia
   Parasomnias
   Warts
   Dysfluencies
   Conditioned hives
   Fears (e.g., flying)
   Eating problems

6. Emphasize your **role as a coach or a teacher.** You are not forcing the child to practice; you only coach him or her to do so. The child decides if and when he or she will do it.

7. Communicate in a way that increases the **child's sense of coping and mastery.** For example, say to a child who is in an isolation room after a bone marrow transplant, "You've done very well in your biofeedback practice. You can decide whether to practice in the morning or afternoon and when you're ready, you can show your mom how you do it."

8. Help the child **predict how life would be different is she or he no longer had the problem.** What would be different? What is the desired outcome? A child with no mental picture of the benefits may not be ready for the self-regulation intervention.

9. Plan, with the child, some **system to record progress,** such as a calendar or sticker chart. It is important to record not only symptoms and their severity but also the frequency of practice.

C. Self-regulation training.

1. **Imagery.** Self-regulation involves directing a child's imagination to focus his attention, at which time the child can give herself or himself instructions to regulate or control a sensation, physiologic function, or action. The mental imagery may be visual, auditory, kinesthetic, or olfactory. The teacher or coach suggests imaginary involvement that is appealing and asks the child to focus on this until she or he is

ready to accept suggestions related to the problem. The child can indicate readiness by lifting a "yes" finger, nodding, or saying, "I'm ready." For example, a child can imagine riding a bicycle to a favorite place and take all the time she or he needs to arrive there. Most children enjoy being offered such control and, after a few minutes, signal their arrival at the special place.

2. **Control.** Giving a child some control in a training session is not only therapeutically sound but also aids in determining if she or he is interested in resolving a habit or performance problem. If the child does not reach the special place on the imaginary bicycle, for example, this may be evidence that she or he is not motivated to change or has not understood what is being taught (or perhaps does not like bike riding). The use of "canned" instructions removes the child's ability to choose and is therefore contraindicated.

3. **Therapeutic suggestions** should be consistent with the child's wishes and previous explanations. The health professional and child should have agreed on the purpose of the visit and should be very clear about what the child wishes to achieve. Suggestions to a child to awaken herself or himself to get out of bed and go to the bathroom will seem strange to the child if they have not been previously discussed. Suggestions should be concrete and refer to language used in earlier explanations and drawings—for example, "When you're ready, you can tell your bladder to send a message to your brain to wake you up when the bladder is full. Tell your brain to wake you up completely and send a message to your legs to get out of bed and walk to the toilet."

4. **Access to the child health professional.** Because parents should not be reinforcers, the child must be able to ask the teacher about the practice, when necessary. Ordinary a follow-up review visit should take place within 10 days. Subsequently, a telephone or email follow-up may be appropriate.

5. **Early training for children with chronic diseases.** It is more efficient and effective to train young children with chronic diseases (such as hemophilia or sickle cell disease) in self-regulation soon after the diagnosis. Children who have developed conditioned anxiety, nausea, and other symptoms associated with procedures can also benefit from self-regulation training, but in general, much more training time is required.

D. **Anticipatory guidance.** Clinicians may choose to include teaching self-regulation in their anticipatory guidance. For example, preschoolers may be encouraged to tell stories during physical examinations. They can be asked, "Where would you like to be?" If the child responds, "At the playground" or "Playing on the swings, " the clinician says,

Table 18-2 Organizations providing training in hypnotherapy

American Society of Clinical Hypnosis
140 North Bloomingdale Road
Bloomingdale, IL 60108-1017
Phone: (630-) 980-4740
www.asch.net

Association for Applied Psychophysiology and Biofeedback
10200 West 44th Avenue, #304
Wheat Ridge, CO 80033-2840
Phone: (303- 422-8436

Society for Behavioral Pediatrics
17000 Commerce Parkway Ste. C
Mount Laurel, NJ 08054
Phone: 856-439-0500
Email: sdbp@ahint.com

Society for Clinical and Experimental Hypnosis
Washington State University
PO Box 642114
Pullman, WA 99164-2114
Phone: (509-) 335-7504
Email: sceh@wsu.edu

"Good. Pretend you're there right now. Tell me about it." This type of interaction can be repeated and becomes useful if painful procedures are required at some later time. For younger children who must undergo procedures, nurses, clinic assistants, and parents can be instructed in holding techniques that give a child a sense of control (e.g., sitting upright on a nurse's lap). A supply of pop-up books, headphones, tapes of appropriate music or stories, or bubbles provide excellent distracters that mitigate the distress of procedures. Simply asking a child to pretend he is blowing out a birthday candle will make it easier for him to tolerate a procedure.

Regardless of whether the child health professional decides to study this area in formal workshops, he or she can practice using language in a way that is encouraging and inspires confidence. For example, during a visit for a minor injury, the clinician may say, "When you go home, what's the first thing you will do?" or "Your blood looks strong and healthy." These simple messages reiterate that a positive outcome is expected and engender, hopefully, a self-fulfilling prophecy.

III. **Training for the professional.** The most practical training is a beginning pediatric hypnotherapy course sponsored by the Society of Behavioral Pediatrics or the Society for Clinical and Experimental Hypnosis. These 3-day workshops are organized for those who work with children and adolescents. Other venues are listed in Table 18-2.

BIBLIOGRAPHY

For Parents

Coleman D, Gurin J (eds). *Mind Body Medicine Consumer Reports*. Yonkers, NY: Consumer Reports Books, 1993.
No Fears, No Tears Canadian Cancer Society No Fears, No Tears 13 Years Later Canadian Cancer Society, 955 West Broadway, Vancouver BC. V5Z 3X8, Canada. www.fanlight.com.

For Professionals

Kohen DP, Olness K. Hypnotherapy with children. In Rhue J, Lynn S, Kirsch I (eds), *Handbook of Clinical Hypnosis*. Washington, DC: American Psychological Association, 1993.
Olness K, Kohen DP. *Hypnosis and Hypnotherapy for Children (3rd ed)*. New York: Guilford, 1996.
Sugarman, L. Training Video: Imaginative Medicine: Hypnosis in Pediatric Practice, 880 Westfall Road, Suite E, Rochester, NY 14618-3906.

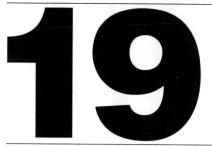

Psychopharmacology

Alison Schonwald
Joseph Gonzalez-Heydrich

I. **Description of the Problem.** The use of psychopharmacologic agents in children most commonly occurs in the treatment of attention deficit hyperactivity disorder ADHD/impulse control problems, mood and anxiety symptoms, and psychosis. While many studies demonstrate highly effective and safe treatment of pediatric (ADHD), data for efficacy with other symptom complexes is less compelling. With childhood depression and anxiety, for example, serotonergic antidepressants have rarely shown more than 60% response rate (compared to a 45% response to placebos). Because of the lack of research on children, most use of medications for non–ADHD symptoms remains "off label." At the same time, pediatric primary care providers are being increasingly asked to prescribe and manage psychotropic medication beyond stimulants for their patients. This demand is likely to increase as more and safer medications become available. Each pediatric provider will then need to decide his level of comfort (or lack thereof) in participating as a member of the mental health team around the management of psychoactive medications.

II. **Epidemiology**
   - Mental health disorders may affect up to 20% of U.S. children and adolescents
   - ADHD affects 3%–7% of U.S. children
   - Depression affects up to 3% of children and 8% of adolescents
   - Up to 15% under age 18 years suffer from anxiety disorders
   - Several studies have reported that over 80% of children who have early-onset bipolar disorder will meet full criteria for ADHD. By some estimates, bipolar disorder (manic-depressive illness) affects close to 1 million children and adolescents in the United States at any given time.

III. **Deciding to treat with medication.** Determining that a child's presentation indicates the need for psychopharmacology requires
   - Identification of target symptoms
   - Degree to which they are causing functional impairment
   - Informed consent

   These decisions can be complicated by difficulties in clearly diagnosing the pediatric population, as well as concerns about potential long-term effects of psychotropics on brain development. Children with depression, anxiety, severe aggression, or psychotic thinking should work with a therapist, who can help identify contributing stressors, and teach the child strategies to better cope with tension, worries, fears, and negative thoughts. For many, however, individual psychotherapy will be augmented by psychopharmacological intervention.

IV. **History: Key clinical questions**
   - "What are your greatest concerns at this time? How impairing are these behaviors or feelings?" Medication may be helpful to the child whose depression, anxiety, or aggression prevents adequate learning, participation in the classroom, or social success. Setting realistic expectations to improve sleep, brighten affect, or improve school behavior comes from clear discussion of what the problems are and how the medication will help.
   - "What interventions or medications have been tried in the past?" Confirming that therapeutic and behavioral support has been appropriately offered is often the first step. Positive and negative responses to different medications and doses might inform the decision of what medications to consider or avoid.

V. **Treatment** Dosing in children is often not established. While taking the adult dose and dividing by 75 yields an approximate mg/kg/day dosing target, this will often underestimate the dose required. It is important to consult the package insert and the clinical trial literature for more specific dosing guidelines. When dosing guidelines for psychiatric indications are not available, there may be some guidance from the dosing for other indications.
   A. **Selective serotonin reuptake inhibitors (SSRIs)** SSRIs are often chosen to treat depression and anxiety in children and adolescents (Table 19-1). This group of medications requires no laboratory monitoring, and most come in liquid and pill forms. Side effects are usually minimal; however, there is a substantial risk of manic activation and a

Table 19-1 Selective serotonin reuptake inhibitors (SSRIs)

Brand name (generic name)	Age and approved indications	Off-label clinical indications	Metabolism	Preparation	Start dose per day	Target dose per day
Prozac® (**fluoxetine**)	≥7 yr: OCD, depression	Anxiety	IID6, IIIA3–4, IIC19	10, 20, 40 mg 20 mg/5 mL	2.5–10 mg	2.5–40 mg c 10–80 mg a
Zoloft® (**sertraline**)	≥6 yr: OCD	Depression, anxiety	Weak IID6, IIC19	25, 50, 100 mg 20 mg/mL	12.5–50 mg	25–200 mg
Luvox® (**fluvoxamine**)	≥8 yr: OCD	Depression, anxiety	IA2, IIIA3–4, IIC19	25, 50, 100 mg	12.5–25 mg	25–300 mg
Paxil® (**paroxetine**)	Not approved in kids; not recommended for depression under 18 yr	Anxiety	IID6	10, 20, 30, 40 mg 10 mg/5 mL	5–10 mg	10–60 mg
Celexa® (**citalopram**)	Not approved in kids	Depression, anxiety	Weak IID6	10, 20, 40 mg 10 mg/5 mL	5–10 mg	10–60 mg
Lexapro® (**escitalopram**)	Not approved in kids	Depression, anxiety	Weak IID6	10, 20 mg 5 mg/5 mL	1.25–5 mg	2.5–20 mg

c, child; a, adolescent; OCD, obsessive compulsive disorder

Table 19-2 Atypical antidepressants

Brand name (generic name)	Age and approved pediatric indications	Off-label clinical indications	Metabolism	Preparation	Start dose per day	Target dose per day
Buspar® (buspirone)	Over 18 yr	Anxiety, depression	IIIa4	5, 10, 15, 30 mg	2.5 mg	20–60 mg divided tid
Anafranil® (clomipramine)	Over 10 yr for OCD	ADHD	IId6, Ia2, IIa4/5	10, 25, 50 mg	25 mg	Up to 200 mg (2–5 mg/kg)
Norpramin® (desipramine)	Over 18 yr	ADHD, chronic pain	IId6	10, 25, 50, 75, 100 mg	10–25 mg	100–200 mg (2–5 mg/kg)
Desyrel® (trazodone)	Over 18 yr	Sedation, anxiety	IIIa4/5	50, 100, 150, 300 mg	25 mg	25–150 mg qhs
Effexor® (venlafaxine)	Over 18 yr; not recommended for depression under 18 yr	Depression, anxiety, ADHD	IId6, IIIa4	25, 37.5, 50, 75 100 mg tabs; 37.5, 75, 150 mg XR	37.5 mg XR	37.5 –225 mg XR
Tofranil® (imipramine)	Childhood enuresis in chidren over 5 yr	ADHD	IId6,IIe9, 11c18/19, IIa4/5	10, 25, 50, 75 mg tabs	10–25 mg	75 mg
Pamelor® (nortriptyline)	Over 18 yr	ADHD	IId6	10,25 mg caps	10–25 mg	0.5–4mg/kg, plasma level 50–175 ng/mL
Remeron® (mirtazapine)	Over 18 yr	Insomnia, depression, anxiety, weight loss	IId6, Ia4, 3a4	15, 30, 45 mg	15 mg qhs	15–45 mg
Serzone® (nefazodone)	Over 18 yr	Depression, insomnia, anxiety	IIIa4/5	100, 150, 200, 250 mg	50 mg bid	300 mg under 12 yr old
Wellbutrin® (bupropion)	Over 18 yr	Depression, ADHD	IIb6, IIIa4	75, 100 mg regular; 100, 150, 200 mg SR; 150, 300 mg XL	50 mg SR	50–200 SR bid, 150–450 XL qd

OCD, obsessive compulsive disorder; ADHD, attention deficit hyperactivity disorder

Table 19-3 Atypical antidepressant side effects

Generic medication	Notable side effects	Management considerations
Nefazodone	Liver toxicity, dry mouth, sedation; may be less activating than SSRIs	Labs: consider LFTs, following may not prevent serious injury
Clomipramine and all tricyclics	Increases PR, QRS, QTc; tremor, sedation, dry mouth, constipation, blurry vision, dizzy	Monitor vital signs, plasma levels and EKG; do not provide more than 1 week supply to patients at risk for overdose
Bupropion	Weight loss, tics, activation, lower seizure threshold	Avoid in patients with bulimia, uncontrolled seizures, risk for seizures
Mirtazapine	Sedation, increased appetite, rare agranulocytosis	Use for insomnia and poor appetite, consider monitoring CBC
Trazodone	Sedation, priapism	Use for insomnia
Venlafaxine	Sustained hypertension	Avoid in patients with high BP

SSRIs, selective scrotin reuptake inhibitors; PR, QTc, corrected QT; LFTs, liver function tests; CBC, complete blood count; BP, blood pressure.

slight increase in the risk of suicidal ideation which families must closely monitor. The SSRIs are not as toxic in overdose as tricyclic antidepressants. SSRIs generally require several weeks to reach full efficacy, and should be weaned over weeks to minimize withdrawal symptoms. Cytochrome P450 interactions are common with fluoxetine, fluvoxamine, and paroxetine. Common medications with which they can interact include dextromethorphan, theophylline, phenytoin, tricyclic antidepressants, and atomoxetine.

   B. **Atypical antidepressants.** Several antidepressants that work via mechanisms other than selective serotonin reuptake inhibition are also widely used, though none are approved in the pediatric population (Table 19-2). Unlike selective serotonin reuptake inhibitors, several atypical antidepressants have side effect profiles that must be carefully considered when prescribing (Table 19-3).

   C. **Antiepileptics and mood stabilizers.** This group of medications has played an increasing role in treating childhood bipolar and impulse/aggression disorders. They are often well-tolerated, but may require combined pharmacotherapy and sometimes blood tests for monitoring (Table 19-4). Many interact with commonly used medications, such as antidepressants (Table 19-5).

   D. **Atypical neuroleptics.** With less risk for extrapyramidal side effects than the first generation of antipsychotics, atypical neuroleptics are used with increasing frequency in children with psychosis, bipolar and disruptive behavior disorders, tic disorders and autism (Table 19-6). However, they can have significant short- and long-term side effects, and there remains modest data indicating efficacy and safety. Risperidone, olanzapine, and quetiapine are linked to weight gain, and possibly to diabetes and hyperglycemia. EKG changes are seen most prominently with ziprasidone, and prolactin elevation most prominently with risperidone. Further studies are necessary for better risk-benefit decisions, and so present monitoring recommendations are controversial and highly varied. Clozaril has significant risk of agranulocytosis, and is associated with seizures and myocarditis; it is rarely prescribed for children. Atypical neuroleptics often interact with antidepressants and antiepileptics.

VI. **Clinical pearls and pitfalls**
   - "Start Low, Go Slow": Start at the lowest possible dose and increase slowly. Children may respond to a lower dose of medication than an adult needs, and may have more side effects as the dose increases.
   - Consider the rest of the picture: If the medication "stops working" or seems to have new side effects, ask if there are other contributors to the child's presentation, such as classroom changes, stressors at home, concomitant illness, new medications, or puberty.
   - Choose medications with side effects in mind: For children who have trouble sleeping you may opt for a sedating drug, while in overweight children you may avoid medications that tend to cause weight gain.
   - Read the newspapers and the journals: Pediatric psychopharmacology is a hot topic in the media, where parents often learn both valid and invalid information. New medications and new potential side effects of older medications are often well publicized, so keep on top of the field to provide top care.

Table 19-4 Antiepileptics and mood stabilizers

Brand name (generic)	Age and approved pediatric indications	Off-label clinical indications	Metabolism	Preparation	Start dose per day	Target dose per day or plasma Level
Depakote (valproate)	Manic episode, epilepsy in children over 10 yr	Mixed mania, behavioral disorders, prophylaxis of major depression	Glucorinidation, mitochondrial oxidation	125 mg sprinkles; 125, 250, 500 mg tabs; 250, 500 mg ER	10–15 mg/kg divided tid, or qd with ER	Plasma level 50–125 mcg/mL
Lithium (lithium carbonate)	Bipolar disorder in children 12 yr and older	Explosive or extreme aggression, Major depression with predictors of bipolar disorder	100% bioavailablility, mostly excreted by kidneys	150, 300, 600 mg caps, 300 mg slow release caps, 450 mg controlled release caps 8 mEq/5 mL, 16 mEq/mL	Dose by weight	Plasma level 0.6–1.2 meq/L
Klonopin (clonazepam)	Panic disorder over 18 yr, seizure disorders in children	Anxiety with insomnia	IIIa	0.5, 1, 2 mg tabs; 0.125, 0.25, 0.5, 1, 2 mg wafers	0.01–0.03 mg/kg divided bid–tid	0.02 to 0.2 mg/kg
Lamictal (lamotrigine)	Adjunct for partial seizures in children, bipolar disorder in adults	Mood stabilization, depression	Glucorinidation	25, 100, 150, 200 mg tabs; 2,5,25 mg chewable	Dosing depends on weight, age, and concomitant medications	Consult package insert for titration schedules
Neurontin (gabapentin)	Adjunct for partial seizures in children over 3 yr	Anxiety, posttraumatic stress disorder	Not metabolized	100, 300, 400 mg caps; 600, 800 mg tabs; 250 mg/5 mL solution	100–300 mg divided tid	400–2400 mg divided tid
Tegretol (carbamazepine)	Childhood epilepsy	Mania, intermittent explosive disorder, rage	IIIa4	Multiple: tabs, solution, chewable, XR	7–10 mg/kg	Plasma level 8–12 mcg/mL
Topomax (topiramate)	Partial onset seizures, or primary generalized tonic-clonic seizures and Lennox-Gastaut syndrome in children over 2 yr	Mood stabilization	Not extensively metabolized	25, 100, 200 mg tabs; 15, 25 mg sprinkles	1–3 mg/kg or 25–50 mg/day	5–9 mg/kg up to 200–400 mg
Trileptal (oxcarbazepine)	Childhood epilepsy	Mania, intermittent explosive disorder, rage	Reduced by cytosolic liver enzymes	150, 300, 600 mg tabs; 300 mg/5 mL	8–10 mg/kg, up to 600 mg divided bid	Target dose based on weight

Table 19-5 Side effects of antiepileptics and mood stabilizers

Medication	Side effects	Management considerations
Carbamazepine	Neutropenia, agranulocytosis, hepatitis, rash, sedation	Baseline CBC, LFTs, TSH, EKG and follow-up CBC, LFTs, plasma level
Depakote®	Nausea, vomiting, pancreatitis, hepatitis, weight gain, thrombocytopenia, tremor, rash	Baseline CBC, LFTs, BUN/Cr, EKG, follow up CBC, LFTs, plasma level; take with meals
Lithium®	Weight gain, kidney and thyroid dysfunction; low therapeutic index	Baseline EKG, baseline and follow up thyroid and kidney function, plasma level q 1–3 mo
Neurontin®	Disinhibition in 10%–15%	Few medication interactions, no serum monitoring
Topomax®	Weight loss	May be used to minimize weight gain

CBC, complete blood count; LFTs, liver function tests; TSH, thyroid stimulating hormone; EKG, electrocardiograph; BUN/Cr, blood urea nitrogen/creatinine.

Table 19-6 Atypical neuroleptics

Brand name (generic)	Age and approved pediatric indications	Off-label clinical indications	Metabolism	Preparation	Start dose per day	Target dose per day
Abilify® (**aripiprazole**)	Schizophrenia in adults	Psychosis, manic and aggressive symptoms	IId6, IIIa4	5, 10, 15, 20, 30 mg	2.5–5 mg	10–30 mg for adults
Clozaril® (**clozapine**)	Treatment resistant schizophrenia in adults	Severe psychosis not responsive to other neuroleptics	Ia2, IId6, IIIa4	25, 100 mg tabs	12.5 mg	50–900 mg divided bid–tid
Geodon® (**ziprasidone**)	Schizophrenia in adults	Psychosis, manic and aggressive symptoms	IIIa4, Ia2	20, 40, 60, 80 mg tabs	20 mg bid	1–3 mg/kg up to 160 mg divided bid
Risperdal® (**risperidone**)	Schizophrenia in adults	Psychosis, manic and aggressive symptoms	IId6	0.25, 0.5, 1,2,3,4 mg tabs; 1 mg/mL	0.25 mg bid	0.5–6 mg divided bid–tid
Seroquel® (**quetiapine**)	Schizophrenia in adults	Psychosis, manic and aggressive symptoms	IIIa4	25, 100, 200, 300 mg tabs	25 mg	25–500 mg divided bid
Zyprexa® (**olanzapine**)	Schizophrenia and bipolar disorder in adults	Psychosis, manic and aggressive symptoms	Ia2, IIIa4	2.5, 5, 7.5, 10, 15, 20 mg tabs	2.5 mg	5–20 mg divided qd–tid

BIBLIOGRAPHY

For Parents

Wilens, TE. *Straight Talk about Psychiatric Medications for Kids.* New York, NY: Guilford Press, 2002.
Dr. King, Clinical Instructor in Pediatrics, Harvard Medical School. http://drkingsoffice.com/GS_psychopharm.htmL

For Professionals

Bostic JQ, Prince J, Frazier J, DeJong S, Wilens TE. "Pediatric Psychopharmacology Update." Available at: http://www.psychiatrictimes.com/p030988.htmL
Kutcher SP, Fletcher J (eds). *Child & Adolescent Psychopharmacology.* Philadelphia: WB Saunders Company, 1997.
Perry P, Kuperman S [Original authors]; Perry P, Kuperman S, Lund BC [Latest revisers]."Pediatric Psychopharmacology: Depression." Available at: http://www.vh.org/adult/provider/psychiatry/CPS/40.htmL

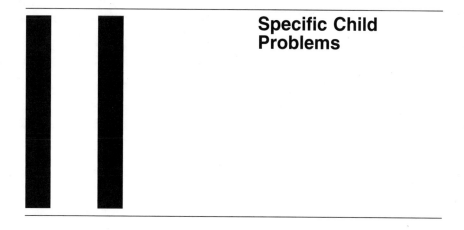

Specific Child Problems

20 Recurrent Abdominal Pain

Leonard Rappaport

I. **Description of the problem.** Recurrent abdominal pain (RAP) is defined as repeated paroxysms of abdominal pain occurring at least once a month, lasting for at least 3 months, with intervening asymptomatic periods. Each episode is severe enough to interfere with normal activities.

   A. **Epidemiology.**
   - Recurrent abdominal pain occurs in approximately **one in seven children** aged 5–12 years. It is one of the most prevalent of childhood symptoms brought to the attention of primary care clinicians.
   - There is a **slight female predominance**.
   - Prevalence is **unrelated to social class, birth, or family size**.

   B. **Etiology.** Three factors, in varying combinations, have been implicated in RAP. For all factors, a family that is overinvolved with the pain symptoms may exacerbate the pain complaint.
      1. **Clear-cut organic pathology.** While the list of possible etiologies is legion, **only 10% of children presenting with recurrent abdominal pain have an identifiable organic etiology.**
      2. **Psychogenic pain.** This is often secondary to a combination of temperament, stress, family, and adjustment factors.
      3. **Physiological pain.** This pain is generated intra-abdominally as a result of normal physiologic processes (termed dysfunctional RAP). This category is subdivided into those with recognizable causes (e.g., imbalance between a stressor and a normal physiologic variant, such as lactose intolerance) and those with nonspecific RAP (no organic etiology can be identified).

II. **Making the diagnosis.**

   A. **Signs and symptoms.** In RAP, the abdominal pain is typically periumbilical, lasts 30–60 minutes, and occurs during the day (rarely awakening the child from sleep). The child will often appear pale and diaphoretic. Alterations from this pattern have been associated with a higher incidence of organic pathology and have been termed red flags> (Table 20-1).

   B. **Differential diagnosis.** While recurrent abdominal pain can be caused by almost any pediatric disease process, most studies have shown that 33%–50% of the identified pathology can be found in the genitourinary tract.

   C. **History: Key clinical questions.**
      1. *"When did the abdominal pain begin? How often does it occur? Where does it hurt?"* Have the child locate the area by pointing with one finger.
      2. *"Are there associated symptoms when the pain occurs?"* For example, is there fever, vomiting, dizziness, or other pain locations?
      3. *"Does the child have regular bowel movements?"* A significant cause of recurrent abdominal pain is constipation.
      4. *"Has there been weight loss?"*
      5. [To both parent and child] *"What do you think causes the pain? How upset does your child become and how much does it interfere with his activity? What is your response?"* It is important to know how the family views this problem. Does it remind them of some bad occurrence in their family (e.g., a child with unrecognized appendicitis or a tumor)? Is the family fixated on the abdominal pain? Is the family rewarding the child for having the pain, and has it become "the currency" of interaction in the family?
      6. *"How is this pain interfering with your child's life?"* It is important to establish whether the pain has been associated with a global withdrawal from school, family, and social interaction. This behavior has been termed the extended syndrome of RAP, in which the pain becomes the focus of the child's life.
      7. *"What do you think causes the pain? Is there anything you can do to get rid of the*

Table 20-1 Red flags: signs and symptoms

Pain farther away from the umbilicus
Fever
Weight loss
Blood in stools (guaiac positive)
Pain awakening the child at night
Anemia
Dysuria
Elevated erythrocyte sedimentation rate (ESR)

pain?" It is essential to know just how important the pain is to the child. Often, for example, a child can say that the pain is mild but that everyone is worried about it.

  D. **Behavioral observations.** The clinician should observe the parents' interactions with the child. How upset do they appear over the pain symptom, and is the child acting at an age-appropriate developmental level? Do the parents allow the child to answer the questions?

  E. **Physical examination.** A complete physical examination, including a neurologic and rectal examination, is essential. Any area not examined at this time should be clearly noted so it can be examined in the future.

  F. **Laboratory evaluation.** If the history and physical examination suggest a specific etiology, appropriate tests should be ordered. Otherwise, the initial laboratory evaluation should be quite limited(Table 20-2).

III. **Management.**

  A. **Primary goals.** The primary goals in managing RAP are to identify and treat organic disease appropriately, lessen pain whenever possible, and decrease the impact of the abdominal pain symptom in the child's life. These goals are accomplished by a thorough initial examination and the institution of an explicit management and treatment plan with the family at the initial visit.

  B. **Initial treatment strategies.**

    1. **Explanation.** On the day of the initial evaluation, the clinician should explain that only 10% of children will have an identifiable organic etiology for their pain and that some children will continue to have abdominal pain several years after the initial presentation. The clinician should explain that the objective of the initial visits is to find organic disease, if present, and to manage the symptoms with available interventions.

    2. **Trial of fiber.** The initial history, physical examination, and laboratory screening are usually negative in recurrent abdominal pain. In most cases, management of the pain complex becomes the major issue. While there have been many suggested treatments for RAP, only one placebo-controlled trial has yielded positive results. This trial utilized fiber in a dosage of 5 g/day (in a fiber cookie). The group receiving this intervention had a significant decrease in abdominal pain during the study period. Therefore a trial of fiber would seem appropriate for most children with RAP.

    3. **Biofeedback** . There have been several well done trials of biofeedback in the treatment of recurrent abdominal pain that show that simple biofeedback method can be taught to children that lessens the frequency of pain episodes.

Table 20-2 Initial workup

Complete physical examination including
   Rectal examination (including stool guaiac)
   Examination of spine
   Neurologic examination
Initial laboratory examination
   Urinalysis (culture in females)
   CBC and erythrocyte sedimentation rate (ESR)
   Stool for ova and parasites (or *Giardia* antigen) in geographic areas where *Giardia* is common
   Lactose breath test (if suggested by history and physical)
   Abdominal ultrasound (if suggested by history and physical)

4. **Parents' role.** It is important to outline the red-flag symptoms for parents, those the clinician should hear about immediately, should they occur (Table 20-1). This should include an explanation of the extended syndrome of recurrent abdominal pain, which includes social withdrawal.

C. **Back-up strategies.** Since the pain of RAP often persists even after a fiber intervention, it is essential for the clinician to remain vigilant for an etiologic cause and not to be discouraged. Care, rather than cure, is often the approach that must be taken at this time. Failure to find a cause or rid the child of the pain is disappointing to all parties, but the clinician should continue to focus energy on limiting the impact of the pain just as he or she does when coping with other chronic conditions for which there is no cure.

IV. **Clinical pearls and pitfalls.**
- There is no substitute for a complete and thorough initial history and physical examination. Unnecessary laboratory and radiologic tests often lead parents to believe that there is an organic etiology for the abdominal pain. Under such circumstances, a negative workup can lead to unnecessary repeat evaluations, which can be quite traumatic for the child.
- Stay in touch. It is helpful to see a child with RAP on a monthly or bimonthly visit to monitor the pain symptom. Show the parents that you are not ignoring the pain, and reassure the child that you will be monitoring the pain.
- Rectal examinations are more easily done with the child lying on the back facing you in a modified lithotomy position. You then tell the child to bear down as though they are going to have a bowel movement while the rectal examination is completed. In this way the child can look at you while you talk and can be distracted from whatever discomfort may be caused by the examination. Additionally, you can clearly see any discomfort the child is experiencing. Having the child face away from you on the examining table, as is often done, can be frightening to the child and provides no additional data.
- Explain to the child that abdominal pain is common in children their age and that the pain does not mean that there is something wrong. Often children are secretly afraid that something truly bad is occurring to them.
- If a family is uncomfortable with your evaluation of their child's abdominal pain, do not discourage a second opinion. It is often helpful to have a specialist in mind whom you feel has a reasonable approach to the care of children with RAP.
- When you note the onset of the extended syndrome, it is time to refer the child to a mental health professional who has an expertise in the management of chronic disease and pain symptoms.
- It is important for parents to understand that the pain is a product of physiological and psychological stressors—not one or the other in most cases.

BIBLIOGRAPHY

Crushell D, Rowland M, Doherty M, Gormally S, Harty S, Bourke B, Drumm B. Importance of parental conceptual model of illness in severe recurrent abdominal pain. *Pediatrics* 112: 1368–1372, 2003.

Frazer CH, Rappaport LA. Recurrent pains. In: Levine MD, et al. *Developmental Behavioral Pediatrics.* Philadelphia: Saunders, 1999.

Humphreys PA, Gevirtz RN. Treatment of recurrent abdominal pain: components analysis of four treatment protocols. *J Pediatr Gastroenterol Nutr* 31(1):47–51, 2000.

Rappaport L, Leichtner A. Recurrent abdominal pain. In: Schechter N, et al. *Pain in Infants, Children, and Adolescents (2nd ed).* Baltimore: Williams & Wilkins, 2002.

Zeiter DK, Hyams JS. Recurrent abdominal pain in children. *Pediatr Clin North Am* 49(1):53–71, 2002.

For Parents

Websites

University of Michigan Health System http://www.med.umich.edu/1libr/pa/pa_abdopain_hhg.htm

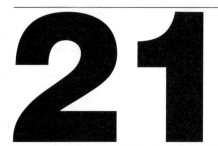

21

The Aggressive, Explosive Child

Ross W. Greene
J. Stuart Ablon

I. **Description of the Problem.** Oppositional-defiant disorder (ODD) refers to a recurrent childhood pattern of developmentally inappropriate levels of negativistic, defiant, disobedient, and hostile behaviors toward authority figures. Specific behaviors associated with ODD include temper outbursts; persistent stubbornness; resistance to directions; unwillingness to compromise, give in, or negotiate with adults or peers; deliberate or persistent testing of limits; and verbal (and minor physical) aggression. These behaviors are almost always present in the home and with individuals the child knows well, and often occur simultaneously with low self-esteem, mood lability, low frustration tolerance, and swearing.

A. **Epidemiology.** Prevalence rates range from 2%–16%. While the data that exist suggest a male predominance in ODD, data regarding age, social class, and ethnicity are not established.

B. **Comorbidity.**

1. **Conduct disorder.** Until recently, ODD has received limited research attention, perhaps due to its relatively recent introduction into the diagnostic nomenclature and because it was viewed merely as an early variant of conduct disorder (CD). However, it is now known that approximately two-thirds of children diagnosed with ODD do not subsequently develop CD. ODD youths—with and without CD—have been found to have significantly elevated rates of other comorbid disorders, significant social impairment, and family dysfunction.

2. **ADHD.** Many of the comorbid psychiatric disorders with ODD share core compromised skills in emotion regulation, problem-solving, frustration tolerance, and adaptation. For example, there is a well-established overlap and developmental continuity between ODD and attention deficit hyperactivity disorder (ADHD), a diagnosis often applied to children compromised in the skills of self-regulation, deficient in higher-order problem-solving, and unable to adjust behavior to fit shifting environmental demands. Approximately 65% of children diagnosed with ADHD have comorbid ODD, and over 80% of children diagnosed with ODD have comorbid ADHD.

3. **Mood and anxiety disorders.** The overlap between ODD and mood and anxiety disorders is also increasingly documented. Researchers have shown extremely high rates of ODD in children diagnosed with depression and bipolar disorder. In recent studies, nearly 70% of children diagnosed with severe major depression and 85% of children diagnosed with bipolar disorder were also diagnosed with ODD. Meaningful rates of anxiety disorders have also been found in youths with ODD: in one recent study, over 60% of youths diagnosed with ODD had a comorbid anxiety disorder and 45% of youths diagnosed with an anxiety disorder had comorbid ODD.

4. **Language disorders.** Language development is also crucial to the evolution of problem-solving, emotion regulation, frustration tolerance, and adaptability. Recent data indicate that over 20% of youths diagnosed with ODD have a comorbid language processing disorder, and that 55% of youths with language processing disorders are also diagnosed with ODD.

C. **Contributing factors.**

1. There is some evidence to suggest that **genetic factors** may contribute to the development of ODD. Recent data provide evidence that both ODD and CD are familial, albeit with stronger association in CD than in ODD. The reciprocal nature of interactions between parents and their difficult offspring likely contribute to familial aggregation whether genes are involved or not.

2. From a transactional perspective, oppositional behavior would be viewed as only *one of many possible manifestations of adult–child incompatibility*, in which the characteristics of one interaction partner (the child) are poorly matched to the characteristics of the second interaction partner (e.g., the parent or teacher), thereby contributing to disadvantageous behavior in both partners which, over time, contrib-

utes to more durable patterns of incompatibility. Such a conceptualization has important implications for the process and goals of treatment, because interventions aimed at reducing children's oppositional behavior must take into account the transactional processes (incompatibilities between child and adult characteristics) giving rise to such behavior. Therefore, effective treatment typically requires the active involvement of child and adult.

   3. Research on noncompliance in children has historically overemphasized *adult* characteristics. Significantly greater attention is now being paid to *child* characteristics, with a specific emphasis on **emotion regulation**, **frustration tolerance**, **adaptation**, and **problem-solving skills**. The skill of compliance—defined as the capacity to defer or delay one's own goals in response to the imposed goals or standards of an authority figure—can be considered one of many developmental expressions of a young child's evolving capacities in these domains.

   When compliance is viewed both as a complex skill and as a critical milestone on the trajectory of emerging self-regulation and affective modulation, then *non*compliance (i.e., oppositional behavior) can be conceptualized as one of many potential byproducts of what might best be described as a "compromised trajectory" in these domains.

II. **Making the diagnosis.** In addition to the diagnostic features listed at the beginning of the chapter, assessment of context is helpful. A *situational analysis* provides indispensible information about the child, adult, and environmental characteristics contributing to oppositional transactions and the incompatibility that gives rise to such transactions.

   A. **History: Key clinical questions.**
      1. Who (e.g., mother, father, peer, soccer coach) is the child interacting with when oppositional episodes occur? How are the combined characteristics of interaction partners related to incompatibility?
      2. What task precipitates oppositional behavior and how is it understood in terms of incompatibility?
      3. Where do oppositional episodes occur (school, home, playground)? How is this understood in terms of compatibility?

   The following questions apply to the child and his interaction partners:
      1. What were they like regarding temperament, trauma history, and family history? Has previous medical or nonmedical treatment been tried?
      2. Were these prior treatments effective, and for how long?

   Given the other prior discussion regarding factors contributing to the development of oppositional behavior, formal assessment by a neuropsychologist or similar psychometrician is invaluable (in both child and adult interaction partners) in the following domains: *general cognitive skills* (provides a backdrop for general level of expectations and a basis for judging relative strengths and limitations); *executive functions* and *language processing skills*; *social skills*, and *problem solving skills*.

III. **Management.**
   A. **Initial management.** The pediatric clinician frequently helps parents with young children who have temper tantrums (see chapters on temper tantrums and managing behavior) and other challenging behavioral problems. However, given that the lines between "developmentally appropriate" temper tantrums and oppositional behavior are increasingly blurred, parental reports of behavior problems in children increasingly signal the need for competent assessment and treatment, neither of which is easily provided during a medical visit.

   B. **Criteria for referral.** Referral to a psychologist or other mental health professional should occur when behaviors associated with these tantrums are causing significant and escalating conflict in child's and family's life (whether or not it is believed that the diagnostic criteria for ODD are met), and/or if parent requests a referral because of their inability to deal with such behaviors regardless of their intensity or frequency. The assessment approach and treatment description in this chapter allows the primary care clinician to clarify for parents and physician the context and potential precipitant of explosive behavior and approach to treatment.

   C. **Interventions aimed at reducing children's oppositional behavior** must take into account the transactional processes (incompatibilities between child and adult characteristics) giving rise to such behavior. Effective treatment requires the active involvement of child *and* adult to address and resolve issues related to their incompatibility.
      1. **Parent training (PT) and behavioral family therapy** focus primarily on altering patterns of parental discipline that contribute to the development of oppositional behavior and problematic parent–child exchanges. Skills typically taught to parents in such models include positive attending; use of appropriate commands; contingent

attention and reinforcement; and use of a time-out procedure. In general, research has documented the efficacy of these procedures.

2. **Collaborative problem solving (CPS)** . Adults are helped to conceptualize oppositional behavior as the byproduct of a "learning disability" in the domains of emotion regulation, frustration tolerance, problem-solving, and/or flexibility. This cognitive-behavioral approach helps adults respond to oppositional behavior in a less personalized, less reactive, and more empathic manner, and is crucial to helping adults understand the necessity for a specialized approach to intervention that emphasizes remediation of these cognitive issues. The specific goals of the CPS approach are to help adults.

  a. To understand the specific adult and child characteristics contributing to the development of a child's oppositional behavior

  b. To become cognizant of three basic strategies for handling unmet expectations, including (1) imposition of adult will, (2) collaborative problem-solving, and (3) removing the expectation

  c. To recognize the impact of each of these three approaches on parent–child interactions; to become proficient, along with their children, at collaborative problem-solving as a means of resolving disagreements and defusing potentially conflictual situations so as to reduce oppositional episodes and improve parent–child compatibility.

BIBLIOGRAPHY

For Parents

Books

Greene RW. *The Explosive Child: A New Approach for Understanding and Helping Easily Frustrated, "Chronically Inflexible" Children (2nd ed)*. New York: Harper Collins, 2001.
Waugh LD. *Tired of Yelling: Teaching Our Children to Resolve Conflict*. Marietta, GA: Longstreet, 1999.

Websites

Parents and Teachers of Explosive Kids (PTEK), a web-based support group. www.explosivekids.org
Center for Collaborative Problem Solving, provides resources for those interested in learning more about the CPS model. www.ccps.info
Federation of Families for Children's Mental Health, provides resources and information for children with mental health needs and their families. www.ffcmh.org

For Professionals

Greene RW, Ablon JS.*Collaborative Problem Solving: Cognitive Theory and Treatment of Oppositional Defiant Disorder*. New York: Guilford Press.

22 Anorexia Nervosa and Bulimia

Angela S. Guarda
Alain Joffe

I. **Description of the problem.** Anorexia nervosa and bulimia are clinical syndromes belonging to a spectrum of conditions best understood as **disorders of dieting behavior**. The two key characteristics common to both diagnoses are (1) **a morbid fear of fatness coupled with** (2) **a disturbance in eating habits** concerned with the consumption or disposal of ingested calories. These behaviors include: restricting intake, binge eating, excessive exercise, self-induced vomiting and/or laxative/diuretic/diet pill abuse. The main distinction between anorexia nervosa and bulimia is ultimately based on weight, with anorexia being defined by underweight.
- Patients with **anorexia nervosa** have a body weight that is at least 15% below ideal body weight or fail to gain the amount of weight normally expected during the pubertal growth spurt. The term anorexia nervosa is a misnomer, since it implies lack of appetite that is not a symptom of this condition. Although patients may deny hunger in their attempts to rationalize their dieting behavior, they are constantly preoccupied with thoughts about food and weight.
  - Amenorrhea is also a prominent finding, although the applicability of this criterion to younger adolescents who may have not yet achieved menarche or who normally have irregular periods is problematic.
  - Besides restricting calories and exercising excessively, a subset of anorectics also binge and may vomit or abuse laxatives and diuretics. This purging anorectic subgroup tends to have a worse prognosis.
- All patients with **bulimia nervosa** engage in binge eating, characterized by the ingestion over a 2-hour period of an amount of food that is distinctly greater than the amount most individuals would consume under similar circumstances.
  - These binge eating episodes are accompanied by feelings of guilt and lack of control.
  - Patients with bulimia nervosa are further subdivided according to whether or not they purge in an attempt to prevent weight gain. Purging behaviors include self-induced vomiting or use of laxatives, diuretics or enemas. Nonpurging bulimics alternate periods of bingeing with severe dietary restriction and or excessive exercise.

A. **Epidemiology.**
1. It is estimated that up to 1% of young females may have anorexia nervosa. Adolescent onset between the ages of 12–18 is found in 50% of cases.
2. Approximately 3% of late adolescent and young adult females meet psychiatric diagnostic criteria for bulimia nervosa, with age of onset (approximately 18) being slightly older than that for anorexia. A brief period of anorexia nervosa often precedes the onset of bulimia and bingeing behavior.
3. Males account for 10% of individuals with eating disorders.
4. Both disorders are seen among all racial and ethnic groups. The belief that anorexia nervosa and bulimia are disorders of Caucasian women of high socioeconomic status is proving to be in part a reflection of patterns of referral for treatment.

B. **Genetics.**
1. The concordance rate for anorexia nervosa among monozygotic twins is 55% (vs 7% for dizygotic pairs), suggesting a strong genetic contribution to this syndrome. First degree relatives of probands are 8 times more likely to develop anorexia than are first degree relatives of healthy controls.
2. The concordance rate for monozygotic twins with bulimia (22.9%) is higher than that for dizygotic pairs (8.7%).

C. **Etiology.** There is no single cause for an eating disorder. Factors that may predispose, precipitate or sustain an eating disorder are
1. **Sociocultural.** Our society places a high premium on being thin, especially for women. Thinness is often equated, implicitly or explicitly, with success, attractiveness, and self-control. Not surprisingly, women in professions in which thinness is prized, such as models or ballet dancers, have very high rates of eating disorders.

2. **Physiologic.** During female puberty, there is a widening of the hips and increased deposition of adipose tissue. These normal changes run counter to pervasive sociocultural pressures for thinness that target female adolescents. This may lead to a preoccupation with weight and dissatisfaction with one's emerging body shape.

    a. Patients with anorexia nervosa and/or bulimia nervosa have been shown to have multiple metabolic, hormonal, and neurotransmitter abnormalities. However, most of the abnormalities result from starvation or from the purging behaviors associated with eating disorders, thereby precluding a straightforward cause and effect relationship from being established. Nonetheless, some of these abnormalities e.g. delayed gastric emptying or preoccupation with food secondary to starvation, are believed to help sustain the disordered eating behaviors.

3. **Developmental.** Predisposing adolescents to the development of eating disorders are such temperamental or personality factors as being introverted, perfectionist, self-critical, or eager to please. Patients who primarily restrict calories tend to be risk-avoidant. In contrast, those who binge and purge may be self-injurious or display impulsive behaviors such as substance abuse, sexual promiscuity, and shop-lifting.

    a. Adolescence is a time of great physiological, psychological, and sociocultural change. Adapting to a markedly changed body, developing a personal and sexual identity and separation from parents are all-important developmental tasks. At this time, adolescents who are otherwise vulnerable to the development of an eating disorder, are particularly sensitive to comments about being "too fat" and to media images that portray thinness as the ideal of beauty, sexual attractiveness, and self-control.

4. **Familial.** Families of bulimics are characterized as hostile and chaotic whereas those of anorectics have often been noted to be over enmeshed and rigid. However, recent research suggests that some characteristics associated with families of eating disorder patients are also typical of families of chronically ill children, suggesting that these patterns of interaction are a consequence rather than a cause of the illness.

II. **Making the diagnosis.**

A. **Signs and symptoms.** Young women rarely disclose an eating disorder to their primary care clinician. Just as anorectics deny hunger as they pursue the ideal body shape, so too will they ignore or cover up various manifestations of their illness. For example, they may wear bulky clothing in an attempt to hide their weight loss. Similarly, patients with bulimia will be quite secretive about their bingeing behavior (which occurs alone) and about vomiting or their use of laxatives or diuretics to minimize weight gain. Hence, the clinician must maintain a high index of suspicion and gently but firmly pursue the diagnosis when symptoms suggest or are consistent with an eating disorder. The signs and symptoms associated with eating disorders are highlighted in Table 22-1. What is apparent on physical examination is a function of whether the patient is starving herself to the point of being significantly underweight and/or whether she uses purging techniques to control her weight. Girls who develop anorexia nervosa at the onset of or early in puberty will present with failure to gain the weight normally expected with physical maturation or with delayed onset of secondary sexual characteristics or primary amenorrhea.

B. **Differential diagnosis.** In developing a differential diagnosis, clinicians should remember that patients with illnesses whose signs and symptoms are similar to anorexia nervosa and bulimia generally indicate discomfort with these manifestations and do not have a persistent and overriding concern with body shape and weight. While they may be initially pleased with a limited amount of unexpected weight loss, they become alarmed as their weight continues to fall. They do not exclusively limit fat and calories and concerns about weight and body shape do not preoccupy them to the exclusion of all else. Diseases that can mimic these disorders are listed in Table 22-2. A thorough history that addresses all aspects of an adolescent's life (HEADSS: Homelife, Education, Activities/Affect, Drug use and Sexuality/sexual behaviors, Suicidal thoughts/actions), a careful physical examination and perhaps a few screening labs (such as counts for erythrocyte sedimentation rate, occult blood in stool, and thyroid-stimulating hormone) are generally sufficient to exclude these diagnoses.

C. **History: Key clinical questions.** Clinicians should focus their questions in the following areas

- Weight and dietary history
- Extreme concerns about being fat and dissatisfaction with body shape
- Methods used to lose weight or prevent weight gain, including exercise patterns and details of bingeing and purging episodes
- Symptoms of a concomitant affective disorder
- Use of drugs and alcohol

Table 22-1 Signs and symptoms of eating disorders

	Associated with starvation	Associated with purging
General	hyperactivity or lethargy irritability sleep problems dizziness, confusion syncope hypothermia	dizziness, syncope confusion
Skin	subcutaneous fat loss dry, brittle hair or loss of hair lanugo hair on torso or face yellow skin	ulcerations, scars, or calluses on back of hand over knuckles perioral acne
Oral		dental caries enamel erosion or discoloration of teeth (lingual surface) parotid gland hypertrophy
Cardiovascular	hypotension bradycardia	arrhythmias
Gastrointestinal	constipation decreased bowel sounds	epigastric tenderness gastroesophageal reflux abdominal distension ileus
Neuromuscular	muscle weakness/wasting decreased deep tendon reflexes	muscle weakness, paresthesias decreased deep tendon reflexes
Extremities	cold, mottled hands and feet	edema of feet
Genitourinary	thin, pale, dry, atrophic vaginal mucosa; amenorrhea, low libido	
Musculoskeletal	osteopenia/fractures	

Note: Patients who are malnourished and engage in purging behaviors will display signs and symptoms from both columns.

Table 22-2 Differential diagnosis of eating disorders

CNS	Hypothalamic disorders (e.g., brain tumor)
Endocrine	Addison's disease
	Diabetes mellitus
	Hyperthyroidism
Gastrointestinal	Inflammatory bowel disease
	Achalasia
	Malabsorption syndromes
Immunologic	Systemic lupus erythematosus
Gynecologic	Pregnancy
Psychiatric	Depression
	Thought disorders
Miscellaneous	Any detected malignancy
	Drug abuse (e.g., amphetamines, alcohol)

1. *"How do you feel about your current weight? What would you like to weigh?"* Begins to elicit information about fear of fatness and body shape dissatisfaction (e.g., feeling fat or wanting to lose "just a few more pounds" even when the teenager appears emaciated).

2. *"What is the most and least you have ever weighed since puberty began and how old were you at each of those times?"* (For prepubertal girls: "What is the least/most you have weighed in the last few years?") Establishes baseline measurements and reflects degree of weight loss. Updating of growth charts is essential.

3. *"Tell me what you ate for breakfast, lunch, dinner, and snacks yesterday and was this a typical day for you?"* Establishes caloric intake, meal patterns and food preferences and helps indicate distorted thoughts about food or restriction of food repertoire to low-calorie, low-fat choices. Information must be obtained in great detail (e.g., what was on the sandwich, how much of it was eaten).

4. *"Tell me about your exercise routine. How many hours do you spend exercising in the average week? Have you increased the amount of exercise you do lately?"* Patients with eating disorders will often exercise intensely as a way to increase caloric expenditure and/or to compensate for binge eating episodes. Information about the specific types and duration of exercise should be elicited.

5. *"How often do you weigh yourself?"* Frequencies greater than once daily indicate an over-preoccupation with body weight.

6. *"How would you generally describe your mood—happy, sad, down, etc.? How did you feel last year?"* Depression is commonly associated with eating disorders, either as a primary or secondary phenomenon. Screening questions about sleep problems, decreased concentration, fatigue, loss of interest in usual activities, frequent crying and feelings of self-blame, guilt or suicidality should be covered.

7. *"Which of the following have you used to control your weight: laxatives, water pills (diuretics), ipecac, diet pills?"* These represent commonly used weight loss methods. Any positive answers should be followed up with questions about current use and frequency of use.

8. *"How often do you binge eat? Tell me exactly what you ate during your last binge?"* A true binge includes consumption of large quantities of food, often several thousand or more calories. In contrast, some young women mistakenly interpret eating a few cookies or an ice cream sundae as a binge. During a binge episode, food is usually consumed quickly and while alone.

9. *"How do you feel before and after you binge? Are there situations or feelings that trigger binge episodes?"* Binge eating typically is associated with feelings of lack of control, self-deprecating thoughts, and guilt. Binges are often triggered by specific feelings such as being disappointed, feeling criticized, lonely, or bored.

10. *"How often do you vomit after a binge episode? What do you do to make yourself vomit?"* These questions elicit details of the binge/purge cycle. Use of emetics such as ipecac on a chronic basis can lead to life threatening complications (cardiotoxicity).

   D. Behavioral observations. While eliciting the history, it is important to note the patient's general affect and the willingness to answer questions directly. Patients with eating disorders often minimize their symptoms. They typically show little concern for a degree of weight loss that others would find alarming and are ambivalent about entering treatment. The interviewer should note the quality of any interactions between patient and family, such as who answers questions and how family members regard each other. It is often helpful to initially interview the adolescent alone to build rapport and trust.

   E. Physical examination. Key aspects of the physical examination are noted in Table 22-1. Severely anorectic patients with a greater degree of weight loss will display more of these features, especially if they also binge and purge. Conversely, patients with bulimia alone may display few physical findings and be of normal weight or above. Patients must be undressed completely (except for a gown and underpants) in order to accurately assess their physical condition. The external genitalia should also be examined; however, a complete pelvic examination is necessary only for those who are sexually active.

     Tests. Women with severe anorexia nervosa or bulimia will have many abnormal laboratory tests but it is not essential to identify all of them. Table 22-3 includes the most commonly noted abnormalities that can help to confirm or eliminate the diagnosis or identify potentially life threatening conditions. In the presence of the classic syndrome of anorexia nervosa or bulimia with fear of fatness and dieting behavior, an exhaustive diagnostic workup is generally not indicated. Gastrointestinal complaints are common among such patients and almost always remit with treatment.

III. Management.

   A. Primary goals. Restoration of weight is the primary goal in the treatment of patients

Table 22-3 Laboratory values in eating disorders

Hematologic	Anemia (mild)
	Leukopenia
	Thrombocytopenia
Endocrine	Follicle-stimulating hormone/luteinizing hormone:low/low normal
	Thyroxine/thyroid-stimulating hormone: low/low normal
	Elevated cortisol (in starvation)
GI	SGOT/SGPT normal or elevated
	Salivary amylase increased (in vomiting)
Renal	BUN normal or elevated
	Urine pH >7
	Urine specific gravity normal or elevated (may also be very low in anorectic patients who drink excessive water).
Metabolic	Metabolic alkalosis
	Decreased Na^+, K^+, CL^-
	Ca^{++} normal or low
	Mg^{++}, PO_4 PO normal or low
	Increased CO_2
ECG	Low voltage
	Bradycardia
	Depressed T waves
	Prolonged QTc interval

ECG, electrocardiogram; SGOT, serum glutamic-oxaloacetic transaminase; SGPT, serum glutamic-pyruvic transaminase.

with severe anorexia nervosa. Until this goal is achieved, patients may not benefit from other therapeutic modalities as a result of the intense preoccupation with food and weight and of depressive symptoms sustained by their starved state. For patients with bingeing and purging behaviors, normalization of eating behaviors and cognitive behavioral therapy including maintenance of a food log and identification of triggers for bingeing are initial goals. Other goals for patients with eating disorders include

- Education about nutrition based on the food pyramid and eating three regular meals daily
- Improvement in personal and social functioning, improvement in family functioning, correction of medical complications
- Treatment of comorbid psychiatric conditions (e.g., depression, anxiety disorders, drug and alcohol abuse)

B. Treatment. Management of a young woman with an eating disorder depends on a number of factors: the stage of the illness at which the patient is diagnosed; the primary behaviors employed to control weight and their intensity; the clinicians assessment of the family dynamics and the level of support likely to be offered by her family; the presence of a concomitant affective disorder and/or substance abuse problem; and,

Table 22-4 Indications for psychiatric hospitalization

Weight less than 60% of normal weight for height
Continued weight loss or failure to gain weight in anorexia nervosa or to decrease binge-purge behavior in bulimia following 2–3 months of outpatient treatment
Cardiovascular compromise
Cardiac arrhythmias
  bradycardia (slower than 40–50 bpm)
  QTc prolongation (>500 msec)
Postural hypotension with presyncopal symptoms or systolic blood pressure <70 mm Hg
Hypothermia (<36°C)
Significant dehydration
Electrolyte disturbances (e.g., K <2.5 mEq/liter, metabolic alkalosis)
Severe psychiatric symptoms (e.g., comorbid depression or anxiety or substance abuse)
Suicidal ideation or recurrent self-injurious behavior

finally, the skill level of the clinician in working with these patients. In general, younger patients with supportive families and recent onset of the eating disorder without significant comorbidity can be effectively managed by the primary care clinician on an outpatient basis.

The optimal outpatient treatment of most patients occurs with a multidisciplinary treatment team consisting of a pediatric clinician, nutritionist, mental health worker and nurse. More complicated patients, those who fail to gain weight after several weeks of outpatient therapy, or those with a long standing eating disorder will likely require admission to a specialty inpatient treatment program. Immediate hospitalization is necessary if any of the conditions in Table 22-4 are present.

The primary care clinician is ideally suited to serve as coordinator of the treatment process. Often, he or she has a long-standing relationship with the patient and her family and can explain the nature and severity of the illness. The clinician can also assume the role of monitoring weight gain and the potential medical complications of the illness (such as amenorrhea or hypokalemia).

1. **Weight gain.** Patients should be weighed weekly dressed in a gown and underpants only. They should urinate before being weighed. The goal should be a slow, steady gain of 1–2 pounds per week. The target weight should be the 50th percentile for the patient's height and pubertal development. Restoration of menses is a reliable indicator that an appropriate weight threshold has been achieved. Patients usually tolerate an initial caloric intake of 1,500–2,000 kcal/day, with increments of 500 kcal per week until the patient gains at least 1 pound per week. Weight gain usually occurs once the adolescent consumes 3,000–4,000 kcal/day; the last 1,000 kcal may need to be provided in a liquid supplement form, e.g., as three 350 kcal supplements daily between meals. It will be necessary for the clinician or nutritionist to be very specific about what kinds of foods the young woman will need to eat in order to reach her daily caloric requirements. Many young women with eating disorders have developed a list of "forbidden" foods and will need considerable firm, concrete instruction and support in changing their diet. Parents should be instructed to select the menu during the early treatment phase.

2. **Restrictions** on activities and privileges are necessary, both as a means of assuring the safety of an underweight patient and because patients are unlikely to gain weight if permitted to exercise. In most cases, no exercise should be permitted until the goal weight is achieved.

3. **Body image.** Much of the ongoing treatment will revolve around addressing the young woman's concerns about her body shape and fear of fatness. The clinician can review with her what happens to a young woman's body as she matures (e.g., the hips widen) and that these changes do not indicate that the patient is becoming fat. Many young women find it helpful to know that their peers are struggling with the same issues and that our society creates unreasonable expectations for them in terms of defining characteristics for physical attractiveness and success.

4. **Nutrition.** In conjunction with the nutritionist, the role of proper nutrition as critical to appropriate physiologic functioning should be stressed. Since many patients with eating disorders are concerned with athletics, it may be helpful to indicate that optimal performance requires adequate intake of essential nutrients. Many adolescents (and their parents) have inaccurate information about the caloric content of various foods and the appropriate diet for a maturing adolescent. It is important to stress, for example, that a low calcium diet, coupled with a hypoestrogenic state, can lead to osteopenia, which is largely irreversible and that this complication occurs early, often within 6 months of the onset of amenorrhea. Many of the symptoms the patient experiences and finds distressful are due to physiologic alterations secondary to weight loss; clarifying this relationship will lend credence to the team's insistence on weight gain. The importance of choosing foods following the food pyramid guide should be stressed. Some fat should be consumed with each meal and no diet, fat-free, or sugarless products should be eaten until the target weight is achieved.

5. **Purging.** Teenagers may not be aware that self-induced vomiting or regular use of diuretics or laxatives often results in water weight loss rather than true weight loss yet can induce dehydration or a variety of life-threatening complications. The clinician should routinely ask if patients have used or are using any of these products or to what extent they are purging. Hypokalemia (serum K+ < 3.0 mEq/dl) suggests a patient is vomiting at least daily.

6. **Family dynamics** and problems that contribute to the eating disorder must also be assessed. Treatment goals and expectations among team members and the family must be clear to all involved parties so that the patient, family members, and mem-

bers of the treatment team are not pitted one against another. Again, the clinician can play a critical role in coordinating these treatment efforts and assuring that everyone is in agreement with treatment plans. Family therapy is an essential component of the treatment for eating disorders among adolescents and has been shown to be more effective than individual therapy alone.

7. **Medications,** such as the serotonergic reuptake inhibitors, have been found to be helpful in decreasing episodes of bingeing and purging. No medication has been found to be particularly useful in achieving weight gain among anorectics but serotonergic antidepressants are often helpful in patients with comorbid psychiatric disorders. Hormonal treatments to induce or regulate menses have not been demonstrated to be effective in preventing osteoporosis. Refeeding and weight gain will usually result in resumption of menses and halt bone loss.

BIBLIOGRAPHY

For Parents and Patients

Pamphlets

"Eating Disorders" American College Health Association P.O. Box 28937 Baltimore, MD 21240-8937 FAX for orders: 301-843-0159
"Eating Disorders—What? Why?" and "Dieting—What's Normal? What's Not?" ETR Associates 1-800-321-4407 www.etr.org
Eating Disorders Resource Catalogue Gurze Books P.O. Box 2238 Carlsbad, CA 92018 1-800-756-7533 www.gurze.com
"Facts About Eating Disorders and the Search for Solutions" National Institute of Mental Health www.nimh.nih.gov

National Organizations

American Anorexia/Bulimia Association (AABA) 165 West 46th Street, #1108 New York, NY 10036 212-575-6200
National Association of Anorexia Nervosa and Associated Disorders (ANAD) P.O. Box 7 Highland Park, IL 60035 847-831-3438
National Eating Disorders Association (NEDA) 603 Stewart Street, Suite 803 Seattle WA 98101 206-382-3587 www.edap.org

For Professionals

American Psychiatric Association Work Group on Eating Disorders. Practice guideline for the treatment of patients with eating disorders (revision). *American Journal of Psychiatry* 157(1 Suppl):1–39, 2000.
Golden NH, Katzman DK, Kreipe RE, et al.; Society for Adolescent Medicine. Eating disorders in adolescents: position paper of the Society for Adolescent Medicine. *J Adolesc Health* 33(6): 496–503, 2003.
Pederson KJ, Roerig JL, Mitchell JE. Towards the pharmacotherapy of eating disorders. *Expert Opin Pharmacother* 4(10):1659–1678, 2003.
Rome ES, Ammerman S, Rosen DS, et al. Children and adolescents with eating disorders: the state of the art. *Pediatrics* 111(1):98–108, 2003.
Strober M, Freeman R, Morrell W. The long-term course of severe anorexia nervosa in adolescents: survival analysis of recovery, relapse, and outcome predictors over 10-15 years in a prospective study. *Int J Eat Disord* 22:339–360, 1997.
Thompson JK (ed). *Handbook of Eating Disorders and Obesity.* Hoboken, NJ: Wiley, 2003.

23

Anxiety Disorders

Travis R. Adams
Margaret A. Swank
Bruce J. Masek

I. **Description of the problem.** Anxiety disorders are the most common class of psychiatric illness affecting children and adolescents. This chapter will identify and describe factors associated with generalized anxiety disorder (GAD) and separation anxiety disorder (SAD).

   A. *Generalized anxiety disorder* (GAD) refers to a pattern of **excessive anxiety** or worry that is difficult to control, **lasts at least 6 months** and **creates impairment in functioning**. It is accompanied by at least one of the following physiological symptoms: **restlessness, easily fatigued, difficulty concentrating, irritability, muscle tension, and/or sleep disturbance.**

   B. *Separation anxiety disorder* (SAD) is defined by excessive anxiety or worry about being **separated from attachment figures or home, lasting at least 1 month, that causes significant disturbance in important areas of functioning** and is **developmentally inappropriate** (i.e., may be developmentally appropriate from 7 months to 6 years of age).

   C. **Epidemiology.** Anxiety disorders impact approximately 13% of children and adolescents. It is estimated that 33% of children diagnosed with one anxiety disorder will also meet criteria for at least two other anxiety disorders, with depression and attention deficit hyperactivity disorder also being common comorbid conditions. The course of an anxiety is often chronic: 70% of adults diagnosed with an anxiety disorder report that their symptoms developed before adulthood.

      1. **GAD.** The prevalence rate for school-aged children is 3% and increases in adolescence to 10%. GAD has been documented as early as age 4, but the mean age of onset is **between 10–13 years of age**. Gender ratio is approximately equal until adolescence, when it tends to be more common in females. If untreated, GAD is a significant risk factor for future anxiety disorders, major depression, suicide, and psychiatric hospitalization.

      2. **SAD.** The prevalence rate is estimated to be around 4% for school-aged children and young adolescents. SAD is more common in younger children, with a mean age of onset **at 7.5 years**. Gender ratio is approximately equal. There is a higher incidence among low socioeconomic status and single parent families.

   D. **Etiology.**

      1. **Genetic.** Empirical evidence suggests a genetic predisposition for anxiety disorders. Children having at least one biological parent with an anxiety disorder are at a significantly greater risk of developing an anxiety than control groups. As a risk factor, genetics accounts for approximately one-third of the variance. In addition, child twin studies found anxious symptoms had a heritibility estimate of 59%.

      2. **Environmental Factors.** Many parents unintentionally reinforce their child's anxious or insecure behaviors, but it is very difficult to tell whether a nervous parent promotes anxious behavior in their child or an anxious child elicits certain behaviors from their parent. The parental behaviors that have been correlated with the development and maintenance of childhood anxiety include over-involvement, affectionless control, high levels of rejection, and low intimacy. Also, stressful environmental factors such as a death, physical or sexual assault, or even ordinary transitions can lead to the manifestation of an anxiety disorder.

      3. **Temperament.** Behavioral inhibition or a shy temperament style has been most closely associated with anxiety. Behaviorally inhibited children tend to withdraw from new situations and are described as shy and hesitant to go far from their parents. In contrast, children who are characterized as secure and willing to explore the unfamiliar are less likely to be anxious in later life.

II. **Making the diagnosis.**

   A. **Signs and symptoms.**

      1. **GAD.** In general, these children worry excessively about past, current, and future happenings, often without overt evidence or cause for concern. Common worry

themes include academic performance, natural disasters, social life, and physical assault. These children tend to be overly conforming and perfectionist and will seek constant approval and reassurance about their worries.

They may have similar worries to other children their age, but the intensity of these worries tends to be more extreme and as adolescents they are more likely to report disturbing dreams and somatic complaints (especially gastrointestinal symptoms).

2. **SAD.** School refusal is the most common behavior associated with SAD, occurring in 75% of the children. Other symptoms tend to vary according to age and major developmental transitions
   - **Young children (5–8 years):** Refusal to sleep or fall asleep alone is a common manifestation of SAD at this age. Children often report nightmares and fears about harm befalling parents or family members.
   - **Middle children (9–12 years):** Observable distress when separated from parents is common. Children may be physically clingy to parents and follow them from one room to another.
   - **Adolescence (13–16 years):** Somatic complaints such as nausea and headaches and frank expressions of worry and sadness are common when separation from parents or other attachment figures occurs or is anticipated. Older children are likely to have an additional anxiety or depressive disorder.

B. **Differential diagnosis.** Making an accurate diagnosis of an anxiety disorder in a pediatric population can be very difficult. Fears and worries are a common element of childhood and most children have worries that mildly interfere with daily functioning. Also, the constant changes associated with normal childhood development complicate the clinical picture. Clinicians should focus on factors such as **duration, frequency, and intensity of symptoms,** within the context of development.

1. **Anxiety disorders** must also be distinguished from medical conditions that can mimic anxiety, including hypoglycemic episodes, hyperthyroidism, cardiac arrhythmias, caffeinism, pheochromocytoma, seizure disorders, migraine, neurologic disorders, and medication reactions. Reactions to medications should also be ruled out.

2. **GAD.** Although other anxiety disorders are often comorbid conditions with GAD, the worries associated with GAD tend to be more global than the specific fears associated with a simple phobia (fear of a particular object or situation), social phobia (fear of public embarrassment), separation anxiety, or hypocondriasis (fear of illness).

3. **SAD.** With school refusal being the most common symptom of separation anxiety, clinicians should seek to understand the underlying cause of the refusal. Refusal associated with avoidance of the anxiety associated with being away from the home or parent is the hallmark of SAD. School refusal also may occur in an attempt to avoid social contact and fear of embarrassment associated with social phobia. Practical conditions at home that reward school avoidance or at least do not deter school refusal should also be considered.

C. **History: Key clinical questions.** Even with very structured interview formats, there is a low concordance rate between what parents and their children report. In an effort to make an accurate diagnosis, it is recommended that information be obtained from multiple sources, at a minimum from parent and child.

Questions for child (GAD)
1. *"Do you think that you worry more about things than other children your age?"*
2. *"What things do you worry most about?"*
3. *"How do worries interfere with things like going to school, friendships, fun activities, or sleep?"*
4. *"About how long have these worries been bothering you?"*
5. *"What happened that lead you to worry about···?"*

Questions for parent (GAD)
1. *"Would you describe your child as being nervous or a worrier?"*
2. *"Does your child frequently ask for reassurance?"*
3. *"How does your child's nervousness interfere with daily activities like school, friendships, fun activities, or health? How long has it interfered?"*
4. *"What events may be related to your child's nervousness or worries?"*
5. *"Does anyone in the extended family have a history of anxiety or depression?"*

Questions for child (SAD)
1. *"Are you ever afraid that something bad might happen to your mom or dad?"*
2. *"Do you sometimes get nervous when you are alone?"*
3. *"Do you worry about getting lost or kidnapped?"*

Questions for parent (SAD)
1. *"Does your child have any difficulty going falling asleep or sleeping alone?"*
2. *"Does your child cry or have temper tantrums when anticipating being left with others?"*
3. *"Does your child follow you from room to room?"*
4. *"Do your child's worries ever keep them from normal activities including school or other fun activities away from home?"*
5. *"Does your child complain of headaches, stomachaches, or body aches frequently on weekdays, but not on weekends?"*

III. **Management.**
   A. **Clinical approach.** The clinical approach to GAD and SAD depends on the age of the child, severity of symptoms, and the family's motivation for treatment. For younger children (up to 8 years of age), **parent guidance** is typically the first step. For children over 8 years old, parent guidance may be combined with **cognitive-behavioral therapy.** **Medication** is considered when symptoms are severe to the point of interfering with the child's ability to function in school or is significantly disrupting family life.
   1. **Parent guidance.** The goal of this intervention is to provide parents with strategies to manage their child's acute anxiety episodes, identify and shape adaptive coping responses, and insight about when to gently push for independent functioning versus when to back off yet avoid reinforcing anxiety-provoking behavior.
   2. **Cognitive-behavioral therapy.** This is an empirically supported treatment that is focused on teaching the child how to modify negative thought patterns that lead to emotional distress and poor coping. Another component of treatment is to teach the child relaxation techniques and how to use them to modulate excessive arousal and motor hyperactivity. A third component that is often employed is the use of positive reinforcement to shape and strengthen new, adaptive behavior patterns. This approach is most effective when the child presents with some insight into their problem and is motivated to change.
   3. **Medication.** Serotonergic reuptake inhibitors, such as fluoxetine, paroxetine and citalopram, are most often prescribed for severe GAD and SAD because of their relatively favorable safety margin and side-effect profile. Other anti-anxiety agents found to be useful include clonazepam and mirtazapine. Studies of efficacy are lacking.
   B. **School.** It is helpful and often necessary to educate school personnel about these disorders and provide guidance about handling the child's symptoms in the school environment.
   C. **Psychotherapy.** Psychodynamic psychotherapy can be combined with the above interventions to provide a safe and accepting environment for the child to explore feelings and beliefs about self-efficacy and self-worth.
IV. **Clinical pearls and pitfalls.**
   - Externalizing disorders such as ADHD, oppositional-defiant, and bipolar are more easily identifiable than an underlying anxiety disorder such that it may go undiagnosed.
   - Providers should carefully assess for co-morbid conditions with externalizing disorders.
   - When assessing for SAD providers should assess whether the child's somatic complaints tend to occur on weekdays, but not on weekends or other times when parents will be home.
   - SAD may be misdiagnosed in children who live in dangerous neighborhoods who have reasonable fears of leaving home. An assessment of environmental conditions is encouraged.

BIBLIOGRAPHY

For Parents

Books

Dacey JS, Fiore LB. *Your Anxious Child: How Parents and Teachers Can Relieve Anxiety in Children.* San Francisco: Jossey-Bass, 2000.
Manassis K. *Keys to Parenting Your Anxious Child.* New York: Barron's Educational Series Inc., 1996.
Shaw MA. *Your Anxious Child: Raising a Healthy Child in a Frightening World (2nd ed).* Irving, TX: Tapestry Press, 2003.

Websites

Mental Health is a site designed to provide information on mental health to professionals and consumers. www.mentalhealth.com

National Institute of Mental Health is the lead federal agency on research on mental and behavioral disorders. www.nimh.nih.gov

Anxiety Disorders Association of America is a nonprofit organization aimed at informing healthcare professionals and the general public about anxiety. www.adaa.org

For Professionals

Albano AM, Chorpita BF, Barlow DH. Childhood anxiety disorders. In Mash EJ, Barkley RA (eds). *Child Psychopathology (2nd ed)*. New York: The Guilford Press, 2003.

Bernstein GA, Shaw K. Practice parameters for the assessment and treatment of children and adolescents with anxiety disorders. *J Am Acad Child Adolesc Psychiatry* 10(Suppl):69S–84S, 1997.

March JS, Morris TL (eds). *Anxiety Disorders in Children and Adolescents (2nd ed)*. New York: The Guilford Press, 2004.

24

Asperger Syndrome

Celine A. Saulnier
Fred R. Volkmar

I. **Description of the problem.** Asperger syndrome (AS) is a neurodevelopmental disorder characterized by **marked impairments in social interaction** with a **repertoire of restricted interests and activities** as seen in autism, yet *with relatively preserved cognitive and language functioning*. The restricted interests tend to include **intense, unusual, and highly circumscribed interests** that can be all encompassing. Although formal language skills are intact, **conversational skills and pragmatic language are quite idiosyncratic and impaired**. Motor clumsiness is an associated, but not diagnostic feature of AS.

A. **Epidemiology.** The prevalence of Asperger syndrome is about 2–3 cases/10,000. Consistent with higher functioning autism, AS is much more frequent in boys. There is no predilection for any racial, ethnic, or socioeconomic group. In the past, good verbal skills have probably led to the condition being under-recognized and incorrectly diagnosed.

B. **Familial transmission/genetics.** In his original report Hans Asperger (1943) suggested that the disorder tended to run in families. The limited available data support this assumption with perhaps one-third of cases having a close family member with the condition or a significant social disability.

C. **Etiology/contributing factors.** Although a precise etiology has not yet been specified the apparently strong genetic basis and the unusual pattern of development strongly suggest the operation of neurobiological factors in pathogenesis.

II. **Making the diagnosis.**

A. **Diagnostic features.** It has been suggested that the disorder begins during infancy or childhood with clinical features that include

1. **Impaired reciprocal social interaction** (*at least two*).
   - Impaired use of nonverbal behaviors such as social gaze, communicative gestures, body posture, and facial expressions
   - Failure to develop age-appropriate peer relationships
   - Failure to seek others to share enjoyment, interests, and achievements
   - Lack of social and emotional reciprocity

2. **Restricted repertoire of activities and interests** (*at least one*).
   - Unusually intense circumscribed interests that are abnormal in intensity and focus
   - Rigid adherence to nonfunctional routines and rituals
   - Stereotyped repetitive motor mannerisms
   - Preoccupation with parts of objects

3. **Symptoms** cause clinically significant impairment across areas of functioning (e.g., social, educational, occupational, etc.).

4. **No history of delays** in the general development of language, with single words developing by the age of 2 and communicative phrases developing by the age of 3.

5. **No significant delays or impairments** in cognitive functioning, age-appropriate self-help and adaptive behavior skills, and curiosity about the environment.

B. **Clinical features.**

1. **Age of onset.** AS is typically recognized after the age of 3, when atypical social interaction skills and preoccupied interests become evident. If the symptoms are detected prior to the age of three, then the profile of impairments should not meet the criteria for autism or another pervasive developmental disorder (i.e., there should be no delays in the development of formal language).

2. **Language and communication skills.** In AS there should be preservation in the development of formal language skills prior to the age of 3, and language may even appear to be a lifeline for the child early on. However, difficulties will arise as the child matures, particularly in pragmatic language (i.e., in the functional and social use of language). Conversational skills tend to be limited to topics of interest and as a result, communicative exchanges become one-sided and circumstantial. A failure to use and respond to nonverbal cues, such as gestures, body posture, and facial

expressions is also observed. The rate and volume of speech in AS is frequently atypical, which is consistent with autism.

3. **Socialization skills.** The early development of socialization skills in AS may initially appear preserved in that social intent is typically present. Impairments in social interaction become evident when the child attempts to negotiate interactions, as when engaging in conversation. Although the child may be aware of and interested in others, their social exchanges become verbose monologues on their topics of interest without any monitoring of the respective interests of their conversational partner. Thus, there is a lack of social and communicative reciprocity.

4. **Behavioral problems.** Individuals with AS are often accused of conduct problems that tend to result from a lack of social understanding, such as empathy and concern for others. During school years, for example, individuals with AS may engage in inappropriate or atypical behaviors that are perceived as behavior problems when in reality they are consequences of the disorder. Unfortunately, these individuals can then become the victim of rejection and/or ridicule from peers, placing them at risk for developing comorbid conditions such as anxiety and depression.

5. **Cognitive function.** According to the DSM-IV-TR diagnostic criteria, cognitive functioning in AS is at or above age level (i.e., IQ >70). Although this may be the case for generalized IQ scores, the cognitive profiles in AS tend to be highly variable (as in autism), with significant impairments evident in some cognitive abilities. In contrast to individuals with autism whose visual-spatial skills tend to be a relative strength, individuals with AS typically have more facility with verbal information, particularly rote, factually based information. The cognitive profile in AS is often, but not always, indicative of a nonverbal learning disability, where verbal IQ scores are significantly greater than nonverbal IQ scores.

6. **Motor skills.** Individuals with AS have been described as having poor gross motor coordination, which is in contrast to the gross motor agility that is often observed in autism. In addition to motor clumsiness, individuals may also present with fine motor difficulties, including difficulties with fine motor speed and dexterity and grapho-motor weaknesses.

7. **Changes over time.** Although the preservation of skills in the early development of AS suggests that the disorder is a "milder" form of autism, the manifestation of AS over the course of life actually presents numerous challenges. First, because of the preserved cognitive skills and often advanced formal language skills, a child with AS may erroneously be perceived as a "problem child" for acting in inappropriate and maladaptive ways, and their needs may be overlooked and under-addressed. Second, the perseverative interests and social naivete can result in rejection and ridicule from peers. This rejection, coupled with an awareness of not being accepted, places individuals with AS at great risk for developing anxiety and depression, which is often the case beginning in adolescence and young adulthood. This can also be the outcome if an individual with AS does not receive the appropriate social, educational, and vocational supports to successfully navigate through life.

C. **Differential diagnosis.**

1. **Autism,** a pervasive developmental disorder that is marked by impairments in communication that were apparent prior to age 3 in addition to the socialization impairments and restricted interests that are observed in AS.

2. **Schizoid personality disorder,** a pattern of social detachment and restricted range of emotional expression that typically begins in early adulthood and is present across contexts. A qualitative distinction between AS and schizoid personality disorder is that in AS there appears to be an intent for social interaction and distress as a result of failure to engage, whereas in schizoid personality disorder the desire for interaction is not likely present.

3. **Nonverbal learning disability** is a neuropsychological profile marked by well-developed rote verbal abilities in the presence of poor pragmatic language, along with deficits in nonverbal problem solving abilities, visual-spatial–organizational difficulties, and poor arithmetic and grapho-motor skills. Deficits in social perception and judgment are the product of this neuropsychological profile, rather than the hallmark of the disability, as evidenced in pervasive developmental disorders.

4. **Semantic pragmatic language disorder,** a profile of preserved syntactic and phonological skills in the presence of impaired semantic and pragmatic language skills.

D. **History: Key clinical questions.**

1. *"Do you have any concerns regarding your child's socialization and play skills?"* Impairments in socialization are the hallmark features of AS, as in autism and other pervasive developmental disorders.

2. *"Did you have concerns regarding your child's language development before the age of 3?"* Since delays/impairments in the development of language are characteristic of autism, it is essential to inquire about early language development for the purpose of diagnostic differentiation between autism and AS.

3. *"When your child developed speech, did it appear to be formal in nature or precociously verbose?"* Language development in AS is often precocious, yet it can be pedantic or formal in nature (as like "little professors").

4. *"Does your child have any unusual interests or preoccupations with certain topics? If so, to what extent do they interfere with the child's ability to engage in social exchanges?"* Assess the presence of and degree of intrusion of preoccupations.

5. *Are there times when your child simply does not respond to sounds?* Hearing loss and possible seizure activity should always be ruled out.

6. *"Does your child seem to be improving? If so, what appears to be helping?"* What works for one child may not for another, even with the same diagnosis. Treatment plans must always be individualized.

7. *"How are you, your spouse, and other members of your family managing?"* Like autism, AS is a family problem. All members need support.

E. **Physical examination.** There are no characteristic abnormal findings with AS.

F. **Tests and additional evaluations.**

1. **Tests.** No specific medical evaluations are routinely indicated. Specific tests may be indicated based on specifics of the case.

2. **Evaluations.** As in autism, all children with AS should have a detailed evaluation by a developmental and behavioral pediatric clinician, child neurologist, child psychologist or child psychiatrist, and a speech-language pathologist. Evaluation by an occupational or physical therapist will often prove useful as well.

III. **Management.**

A. **Educational/behavioral management.** The educational and therapeutic programming for children with AS should consist of the same intensive and comprehensive intervention developed for individuals with autism, and should be customized to meet the needs of each individual based on his profile of strengths and vulnerabilities. Programs should incorporate a range of intervention strategies to enhance skills across areas, including conversation and social interaction skills, academic functioning, motor control, psychological functioning, adaptive functioning, and behavioral management. Social skills training can range from teaching social scripts and social stories in one-to-one settings, to working with peers, dyads, and small groups to practice and generalize learned strategies. Conversational skills can be improved upon by enhancing awareness of speech volume, tone, and nonverbal gestures, as well as teaching individuals with AS to inquire about the interests of their conversational partner, while restricting their desire to focus on their own topics of interest.

Similar to autism, children with AS tend to learn rote and concrete information with ease, whereas abstract concepts and complex information are more challenging to comprehend. Therefore, applied behavioral analysis techniques that involve breaking down concepts into basic, identifiable parts tend to be successful. Additional academic supports can include strategies to enhance the organization and interpretation of visual material, particularly organizing sequential visual material. When verbal abilities are a relative strength, supplemental verbal and written supports should be provided to enhance comprehension of visual information, which may differ from treatment in autism where the emphasis tends to be on using supplemental visual aids. Furthermore, psychological supports can serve to provide a supportive advocate for the child with AS with whom to problem solve challenging social and academic experiences.

B. **Medications.** In school age children with AS attentional difficulties are often prominent and may respond, at least in part, to stimulant and similar medications. Adolescents appear to be at increased risk for depression. For individuals with depression combined with anxiety, SSRIs (selective serotonin reuptake inhibitors) are often utilized.

C. **Support for families.** Support for the families of individuals with AS can include parent support groups, sibling support groups, family and educational advocates, and respite services.

IV. **Prognosis.** In general the outcome in Asperger syndrome is apparently better than that in higher functioning autism (i.e., autism associated with IQ in the normal range). Many individuals with AS marry and have families; they may be somewhat socially isolated and are often attracted to occupations that minimize socialization requirements.

BIBLIOGRAPHY

For Parents

Organizations

OASIS (Online Asperger Syndrome Information and Support). Web resources for parents on Asperger syndrome and related disorders. www.aspergersyndrome.org

Autism Society of America. Largest nonprofit organization on autism and pervasive developmental disorders. Provides a wealth of written materials, including newsletters, book lists, meeting schedules, and research updates.

Autism Society of America 8601 Georgia Avenue, Suite 503 Silver Spring, MD 20910 Phone: 301-565-0433 Fax: 301-565-0834 www.autism-society.org

Books

Klass P, Costello F. *Quirky Kids: Understanding and Helping Your Child Who Doesn't Fit In: When to Worry and When Not to Worry*. New York: Ballantine Books, 2003.

Ozonoff S, Dawson G, McPartland J. *A Parent's Guide to Asperger Syndrome and High-Functioning Autism*. New York: The Guilford Press, 2002.

Powers M. *Asperger Syndrome and Your Child: A Parent's Guide*. New York: Harper Resource, 2002.

Stewart K. *Helping a Child with Nonverbal Learning Disability or Asperger Syndrome: A Parent's Guide*. Oakland, CA: New Harbinger Publications, Inc., 2002.

For Professionals

Klin A, Volkmar FR, Sparrow SS (eds). *Asperger Syndrome*. New York: The Guilford Press, 2000.

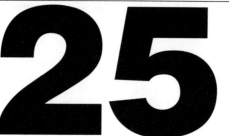

Attention Deficit Hyperactivity Disorder

Steven Parker

I. Description of the problem.

A. Attention deficit hyperactivity disorder (ADHD) is not a simple medical diagnosis. Rather, it is a behavioral syndrome, suspected when a cluster of suggestive behaviors are consistently observed by parents and other caregivers early in the child's life. **In young children** these behaviors cause significant dysfunction in most of the important aspects of the child's experience: challenging relationships with parents and other caregivers, teachers and peers, as well as behavioral and discipline problems in multiple settings, including home, school, and childcare. **In the adolescent and adult,** ADHD may impair job performance, adult relationships, academic achievement, and be associated with increased legal difficulties, motor vehicle accidents, smoking, and substance abuse.

1. **The DSM-IV diagnostic criteria for ADHD are found in Table 25-1.** While meeting these criteria may not be necessary to make a diagnosis in all cases, these criteria represent an excellent list of the symptoms for the pediatric clinician to explore during the diagnostic process.

2. Aside from the "official" behaviors endorsed by the DSM-IV, other issues commonly seen in children with ADHD may be even more important to their social, emotional, and academic well-being. These include

   - **Emotional lability or immaturity** (other children call him "a baby"; when mood swings are extreme, especially with hyperirritable periods, a diagnosis of bipolar disorder may be considered)
   - **Resistance to environmental reinforcement** (much less responsive to positive or negative reinforcement, often rendering behavioral interventions less effective)
   - **Little sense of physical safety** (leading to increased accidents)
   - **Aggressive behaviors** (a major red flag with perhaps the most problematic long-term prognosis, often related to later aggressive behaviors and full-blown conduct disorder if not addressed)
   - **An oppositional stance to the world** (another major red flag, suggesting a suboptimal and negative response of the environment to the behavioral challenges, perhaps presaging a full-blown oppositional defiant disorder if not promptly addressed)
   - **Poor social skills** ("socially tone deaf") and poor peer relations (heartbreakingly few friends),
   - **Low self-esteem** (perhaps the most common damaging long-term outcome of all)

B. Epidemiology.

1. Prevalence studies yield confusing results, depending on the criteria and means for ascertainment. Probably the best estimate is 4%–6% of American school children have ADHD.
   - ADHD has been found worldwide, whenever it has been studied, with rates ranging from 3%–18%.
   - Higher rates are seen in children from low socioeconomic status, but it is unclear whether this represents a true increase or is the result of an environment with fewer resources to ameliorate the challenging behaviors.

2. Male to female ratio had been classically estimated at about 4–6:1. However, recent studies suggest a lower ratio, perhaps as low as 2:1. This is because the diagnostic criteria are oriented to the male presentation (with many externalizing behaviors) and may miss many females (who tend to be diagnosed at a later date, if at all, presenting with subtle attentional challenges in school and difficulties in their social relations).

C. Comorbidity of other diagnoses and ADHD is quite high, although it is often ambiguous whether a second diagnosis has been caused by the ADHD or is cause of behaviors that look like ADHD or coexists as a discrete but interacting true second diagnosis (Table 25-2). More than one of these additional syndromes can be (and often are) identified

Table 25-1 ADHD: DSM-IV criteria

1. Six or more of the following symptoms of inattention have persisted for at least 6 months to a degree that is maladaptive and inconsistent with developmental level:

Inattention
a. Often fails to give close attention to details or makes careless mistakes in schoolwork, work, or other activities
b. Often has difficulty sustaining attention in tasks or play activities
c. Often does not seem to listen when spoken to directly
d. Often does not follow through on instructions and fails to finish schoolwork, chores, or duties in the workplace (not due to oppositional behavior or failure to understand instructions)
e. Often has difficulty organizing tasks and activities
f. Often avoids, dislikes, or is reluctant to engage in tasks that require sustained mental effort (such as homework)
g. Often loses things necessary for tasks or activities (toys, school assignments, pencils, books, or tools)
h. Is often easily distracted by extraneous stimuli
i. Is often forgetful in daily activities

Hyperactivity-impulsivity
2. Six or more of the following symptoms of hyperactivity-impulsivity have persisted for at least 6 months to a degree that is maladaptive and inconsistent with developmental level:

Hyperactivity
a. Often fidgets with hands or feet or squirms in seat
b. Often leaves seat in classroom or in other situations in which remaining seated is expected
c. Often runs about or climbs excessively in situations in which it is inappropriate (in adolescents or adults, may be limited to subjective feelings of restlessness)
d. Often has difficulty playing or engaging in leisure activities quietly
e. Is often "on the go" or often acts as if "driven by a motor"
f. Often talks excessively

Impulsivity
g. Often blurts out answers before questions have been completed
h. Often has difficulty awaiting turn
i. Often interrupts or intrudes on others (such as butting into conversations or games)

A. Some hyperactive, impulsive, or inattentive symptoms that caused impairment were present before age 7 years
B. Some impairment from the symptoms is present in two or more settings (such as in school or work and at home)
C. There must be clear evidence of clinically significant impairment in social, academic, or occupational functioning
D. The symptoms do not occur exclusively during the course of a pervasive developmental disorder, schizophrenia, or another psychotic disorder and are not better accounted for by another mental disorder (such as a mood, anxiety, dissociative, or personality disorder)

Based on type, ADHD may be classified as:
1. Attention deficit/hyperactivity disorder, combined type (if both criteria have been met for the pat 6 months)
2. Attention deficit/hyperactivity disorder, predominately inattentive type (if only criteria for inattention met for the past 6 months)
3. Attention deficit/hyperactivity disorder, predominately hyperactive-impulsive type (if only criteria for hyperactivity-impulsivity met for past 6 months)

American Psychiatric Association, *Diagnostic and Statistical Manual of Mental Disorders* (4th ed). Washington, DC: American Psychiatric Association, 1994.
*For individuals (especially adolescents and adults) who currently have symptoms that no longer meet full criteria, "in partial remission" should be specified.

Table 25-2 Comorbid disorders

Comorbid disorders	% Range of prevalence from several studies
Specific developmental disorders (academic skills disorders, language and speech disorders, motor skills disorder)	20–60
Mild mental retardation	3–10
Oppositional defiant disorder	30–60
Conduct disorder	10–50
Anxiety disorders of childhood or adolescence (separation anxiety disorder, avoidant disorder, overanxious disorder)	10–30
Depressive disorder	5–35 (in adults)
Bipolar disorder	0–10 (15% of adults)
Tic disorders	5–30
Other neurologic disorders	<10
Post-traumatic stress disorder	Unknown

in the same child. Some estimate that comorbid diagnoses are the rule, not the exception, and can be found in 50%–75% of all children with ADHD.

   D. Etiology. ADHD likely has no single invariant cause, but likely represents the final common pathway for a host of neurological and environmental risks.

      1. Genetic factors. The concordance rate of ADHD in identical twins is strikingly high: 0.6-0.8. Additionally, first and second-degree relatives (parents, siblings, and grandparents) of children with ADHD have a much higher incidence of the disorder (20%–25%). Abnormal level protein production by candidate dopamine-related genes (D4, D2, DAT) are being implicated in some. These and other genes are active subjects of intense research.

      2. Medical risks. Intrauterine exposure to maternal smoking and alcohol use increase the risk of ADHD. Premature and low birth weight infants also show a higher prevalence. Increased lead levels, carbon monoxide exposure, and various heavy metals (e.g., cadmium) have been implicated in some cases.

         a. Differences in the brain. Animal studies and the effects of psychoactive medications have led to speculations of altered neurotransmitter profiles and brain function in persons with ADHD. Recent positron emission tomography (PET) and fMRI studies suggest underactivity in parts of the cerebral cortex, especially the frontal lobes, perhaps leading to the challenges in self-regulation described in ADHD. Other areas which have been implicated in studies as having altered function include the cerebellar vermis, cingulated gyrus, frontal-striatal connections, basal ganglia, and brain stem.

            (1) Environmental factors. Environmental issues, such as parental psychopathology and low socioeconomic status, likely play more of a role in exacerbating (or at least not ameliorating) the behaviors of ADHD, rather than as a causal agent. A family environment that includes poor monitoring of behavior and a punitive approach to discipline, for example, may magnify the symptoms of ADHD.

   E. Theories of ADHD. The most popular current theory of ADHD, posited by Russell Barkley, is that ADHD represents **a disorder of "executive function"**. This implies dysfunction in the prefrontal lobes so that the child lacks the ability for *behavioral inhibition or self-regulation* of such executive functions as nonverbal working memory, speech internalization, affect, emotion, motivation, and arousal. Because of this relative inability to inhibit, the child lives pretty much only in the "now" and lacks the ability to modify or delay behavior in view of future consequences.

   F. Prognosis.

      1. Symptoms persist in the majority of young adults and adults, but change in nature (hyperactivity replaced by feelings of restlessness).

      2. Higher incidence of problems are seen, such as antisocial behaviors (about 20%), substance abuse (15%), and other DSM diagnosis (about 35%).

        • However, a recent meta-analysis suggests the incidence of substance abuse in teens is less with those who were treated with stimulant medication.

      3. The majority do well, especially those who were not aggressive or oppositional, who have a high IQ, and come from high socioeconomic backgrounds.

II. Making the diagnosis. There is **no *sine qua non*** for the diagnosis of ADHD. Rather, the pediatric clinician must analyze and integrate the reports of characteristic behaviors by multiple observers, occurring in a variety of different settings, over an extended period of time. These behaviors are described as occurring with greater intensity and frequency than is typical for other children of the same developmental age and, most importantly, **are causing significant problems in the child's functioning and relationships in those settings.**

A. History: Key clinical questions.

1. *"Tell me about the behaviors that concern you? What, exactly does he do? Give me a specific example."* It is important to obtain specific examples to see if the behaviors sound truly more severe than other children at the same developmental level, or if the parent has a low tolerance for a "normal," albeit temperamentally active and intense child.

2. *"Who else is concerned about these behaviors?"* Since children with true ADHD are problematic in most or all settings across time and space, if only the parent is concerned but other significant caregivers or teachers are not, one's index of suspicion should be raised of an etiology other than ADHD.

3. *"When did you first become concerned about these behaviors?"* Often the symptoms have been present for a long time before coming to your attention. Conversely, the abrupt onset of behavioral problems may suggest a stressful trigger and etiology.

4. *"Tell me about his attention span."* Remember that the ability to watch TV or play video games for an extended period does not necessarily connote a good attention span. As these require no input from the child, he may interact without really paying a lot of attention. Instead, ask for examples of *internally mediated attention*, i.e., paying attention to less compelling, more boring activities that require sustained attention to be successful. Ask questions such as: "Is he a daydreamer? Easily distracted? Does he have a hard time completing tasks? Does he have a hard time listening to instructions? Is he a poor listener?"

5. *"Tell me about his activity level."* Some children are obviously extremely active. For others, fidgety and nonpurposeful activity may be more salient than gross motor hyperactivity. Ask: "Does he seem to be in constant motion? Is he fidgety, even when quiet? Does he engage in dangerous activities without a sense of fear? Does he talk a lot?"

6. *"Is he impulsive?"* "Does he often act without thinking? Does he interrupt and butt in on others when they are doing something? Is he often remorseful after an impulsive act, saying, 'I'm sorry, I just couldn't help myself?'"

7. *"Tell me about how he expresses his emotions? Does he seem angry or depressed or anxious or incredibly irritable sometimes?"* The search for another cause (e.g., depression, anxiety, bipolar disorder) or comorbidity begins with the initial history taking.

8. *"Does he get along with other kids? Have many friends?"* Most children with ADHD have poor social relationships, which is a significant cause of unhappiness and low self-esteem.

9. *"Tell me about how he is doing in school or daycare?"* It is important to get a sense of the level of dysfunction and suffering these behaviors may be causing in all-important aspects of his world, including daycare/preschool/school functioning.

10. *"Given all the problems you describe, how do you think they have affected his self-esteem?"* Since enhancing self-esteem may be the pediatric clinician's number one long-term goal, it is helpful to raise the issue early on, especially for parents who have never considered this question before.

11. *"How do you deal with these behaviors? What has worked and what has not?"* Often a child with ADHD has engendered many negative, ineffectual, and punitive responses by his parents. Especially because of their relative lack of response to positive and negative reinforcement, don't be too quick to blame the parents for inadequate limit-setting in a child for whom it requires heroic efforts to set consistent limits and who doesn't respond all that well to them anyway.

12. *"Why do you think these problems are occurring? What do others say is the cause?"* The parents' theories of causation are important to make explicit. Often they have a direct impact on their response (for example, "He's just a bad boy and could behave better if he wanted" can lead to punitive and deprecating interactions). This question can also bring out parental disagreements that can affect later treatment ("His father says he's 'just a boy' and there is no problem, but I'm with him all day and I know better!").

B. Office observations/evaluation.

1. Many children with ADHD can contain themselves in the short time of the visit.

They may be on their best behavior in order not to provoke the powerful pediatric clinician and because the setting is mostly one-on-one with few distractions. Such "good behavior" in the office should not be used to rule out ADHD, which is dependent on his behavior in the usual familiar settings.

2. On the other hand, if a child has many ADHD behaviors in the office, these may help to confirm the diagnosis when otherwise suspected, and perhaps even represents a level of symptomatology that is more pervasive and intense than a child who can contain himself in the office.

3. **Physical examination** is rarely revealing, except insofar as it allows a window into the child's behavior and affect during the exam. Look for any neurologic signs, mild dysmorphic features, signs of autonomic disturbance that might suggest a medical or genetic diagnosis. Assessing for so-called **soft neurological signs** is interesting, but cannot be used to confirm or disconfirm the diagnosis of ADHD.

C. **Diagnostic tests.** Aside from ADHD questionnaire, other testing is rarely indicated unless suggested by the history and physical exam (e.g., lab tests assessing thyroid function, EEG or MRI when unexpected neurological findings are prominent). Computer-based studies of sustained attention (e.g., the "continuous performance task") are neither reliable indicators of the diagnosis nor response to treatment.

1. **Psychological and educational testing** can be illuminating if academic problems are significant to identify a comorbid learning disability or other learning challenge. Some clinicians refer *all* children with ADHD for such testing; others first treat the ADHD and then refer only those children for whom significant academic difficulties persist.

D. **Principles of the diagnostic process once ADHD is suspected.**

1. **Do your homework!** It is rarely sufficient or acceptable to take a suggestive history from a parent, observe the child in the office, and make a definitive diagnosis. The suggestive behaviors must occur in all the child's significant environments.

2. **Obtain a description and seek corroboration of the child's behaviors from caretakers in all settings in which he spends time.** Since interviews with these providers are impractical, use ADHD-specific questionnaires (see Table 25-3). Ask the mother and father and other caregivers in the home to complete questionnaires, as well as all significant outside professionals and caretakers (babysitters, grandparents, teachers, pre-school and Head Start providers, childcare providers).

3. **Review the behavioral descriptions and integrate them with the history and your understanding of the child and family.** Remember these descriptions are not diag-

Table 25-3 ADHD questionnaires

NICHQ Vanderbilt Assessment Scale
Free and downloadable from the **AAP ADHD Toolkit Website** http://www.utmem.edu/
   pediatrics/general/clinical/behavior/aap_adhd_toolkit/

Revised Conner's Questionnaire–Teacher and Parent Rating Scales
Perhaps the best validated and also includes if child meets DSM-IV criteria; is very focused on
   ADHD, with little information on comorbidities (however, is not free). Available through:
Multi-Health Systems, Inc.
P.O. Box 950
North Tonawanda, NY 14120-3003
1-800-456-3003

Behavior Assessment System for Children (BASC)
Longer, but more information on potential comorbid diagnoses (e.g., depression, anxiety). Order
   from:
American Guidance Services (AGS)
4201 Woodland Road
P.O. Box 99
Circle Pines, MN 55014
1-800-328-2560

The ADHD Self-Rating Scale for Girls
Very useful as is specifically targeted for older girls when the diagnosis can be subtle.
http://www.addvance.com/resources/Articles/Checklist.htm

---

nostic. *They merely state whether the behavioral descriptions are consistent with (but not necessarily due to) a diagnosis of ADHD.* Clinical judgment must be carefully applied to sort out such information.

    a. Look for consistency of the reported behaviors and whether they suggest ADHD in all settings. If that is the case, the diagnosis may be more clear-cut.

    b. Look for inconsistencies of the reported behaviors in different settings. Variable descriptions are more problematic to interpret.

- For example, extreme behaviors described at home but not at school may imply stress and/or problematic relationships at home and not true ADHD.
- Conversely, problematic behaviors seen only in school may imply a learning disability, scapegoating, etc. at school, and not true ADHD.
- On the other hand, some parents are quite accepting of their child's inattentive, impulsive behaviors at home or do not challenge the child to exert sustained attention and may downplay those symptoms in a child with true ADHD.

4. Diagnostic certainty is impossible. Especially in situations of problematic environmental characteristics (poor "goodness of fit" with parent or daycare/school, lots of family stress, early adversities in home environment and community, etc.), it can be impossible to gauge if the ADHD-like behaviors are a cause of problematic parental interactions or an effect of environmental adversities.

    a. In such cases, ask yourself a key question: *"How much trouble is this child in? How much dysfunction and suffering in his life are these behaviors causing, regardless of the etiology?"* If the answer is "to a significant degree", then a trial of medications may be warranted despite the diagnostic uncertainty. Conversely, a child who seems to be coping reasonably well in his world may not require such intervention at this time.

5. Be mindful of potential comorbidities. Since ADHD can be associated with learning disabilities, depression, anxiety, posttraumatic stress disorder, developmental disability, an unrecognized genetic syndrome, language delays, etc. (Table 25-2), a diagnosis of ADHD should never shut out the possibility that other challenges may be either causing the behaviors or co-occurring.

6. Discuss with parents your judgment on the diagnosis. It is always helpful to have asked parents to read about ADHD and state whether or not they think their child fits the criteria. The disagreements between clinician and parent can be made explicit and discussed.

    a. If a parent disagrees with your diagnosis, intervention efforts are likely to fail. Rather than try to browbeat them into acceptance, allow them time to learn more and see if things improve. *"We disagree on whether your child has ADHD. But he's your child and you have to make the final decision. Why don't you read some more about it, talk to parents with kids who have ADHD, and let's see if things improve. I think because your child is having such serious problems at school (and at home, with friends, etc.) that we really need to try to help him out. So far nothing has worked well and I'm concerned that, unless we treat him for ADHD, things are only going to get worse. We'll hold for now, but why don't I see you back in a month or so and we can discuss this further."*

    b. It is helpful to explain ADHD to parents with simple metaphors: *"Your child is like a fast car in which the accelerator is stuck down and the brakes don't work very well. One way or another we need to get the brakes to be more effective."*

    c. A diagnosis of ADHD is often helpful because it **takes the onus off the child**: *"I know his behaviors can be exasperating, but mostly he really can't help it. ADHD is caused by differences in the brain, not because he is a 'bad kid' or 'lazy'."* Without the understanding that *biological* factors lead to the child's behavior, his actions are often interpreted as willful and manipulative, and may provoke an angry response, which then aggravates the child's feelings of being misunderstood and picked on.

    d. Explain that ADHD is a **chronic condition**, and is unlikely to go away on its own.

    e. Encourage the parents to read and learn as much as they can in order to best help their child.

III. Management.

    A. Primary goals. The goals of all treatment for ADHD are to enhance the child's successful functioning in the domains that have been impaired and causing distress. These areas almost always include his academic or preschool functioning, family and peer relationships, and self-esteem.

    B. Information for the family.

1. Explain to the family the nature of ADHD and what is known about its treatment, specifically that medication treatment has been demonstrated to be, far and away, the most effective treatment in most children with ADHD.
   a. Have well-chosen handouts for parents at the ready in the office to give to them for later perusal.

C. Medication treatment.

1. **Fundamental rules of ADHD medication treatment** (some of which should also be explained to the parents.)
   - **All decisions are reversible.** Once a decision has been made either to treat or not to treat with medications, it can be changed as circumstances warrant.
   - **Obtain ongoing feedback regarding efficacy and side effects** from the parents and the same caretakers who provided the initial history. This often best done by the provider faxing a brief weekly report (such as the clinical attention profile [CAPS] which can be downloaded for free at: www.dbpeds.org) to the clinician in the initial stages of treatment and then bimonthly once a stable dose is achieved.
   - **If one medication doesn't work, try another.** If a child is a nonresponder to methylphenidate, 80% of the time he will respond to an amphetamine preparation. Likewise amphetamine nonresponders do respond to methylphenidate in 66% of cases.
   - Improvement should be gauged in areas such **as improved academic performance** (volume of work, efficiency, completion, accuracy) as well as **behavior in the classroom, improved self-esteem, decreased disruptive behaviors, improved relationships with parents, siblings, teachers, and peers; and enhanced safety.**
   - In general, one is looking for **a dramatic and clearly beneficial response to the medications.** Reports that maybe there *might* be some subtle or minor changes are not sufficient to view the trial as successful.
   - **Medications are usually the most important, but not the only treatment.** However, the improvement in the child's behavior often greatly enhances attempts at limit-setting, school expectations, etc.
   - **Medications are effective in 70%–80% of children with ADHD.** However the lack of a beneficial response does not necessarily mean the diagnosis is incorrect.
   - **Parental agreement with a medication trial is essential.** Some parents are understandably reluctant to give their child a psychoactive medication. They may have read or heard of frightening side effects and "don't want my child to become a zombie". The clinician should acknowledge and respect such concerns: *"I understand why you are concerned. I am too—I don't want to put a child on medications unless I really think it's necessary and safe to do so, which, in your child's case, I do. First off, if we start this, you will be in **complete control**. If your child is having side effects that worry you or if the meds don't seem to be helping, we'll stop or change the medicine. If it doesn't seem to be helping, we'll stop or change. Just because we start meds, doesn't mean we have to continue them if you or I are unsatisfied with their effects. Second, these medications have been around for a long time and are really very safe. If there are any side effects—and these are usually mild anyway–they go away when the medication is discontinued. Third, there is no question that medications are the most effective way to treat ADHD that we have. So, think about it. I'm not going to start meds unless you give me the okay. If you decide against it now, we can reconsider it in the future if things don't improve for your child. But I suggest giving them a try and seeing how things go."*

2. **Pharmacologic agents.**
   a. **Stimulant medications** remain the first line of medication treatment for ADHD. These include the various preparations of methylphenidate and amphetamines. Table 25-4 contains information concerning their use. All can be effective, but some children may respond to only one. When problems arise with one drug or it is ineffective, another in this group should be tried.
   b. Currently, the second line of ADHD medications, when a stimulant trial proves ineffective due to intolerable side effects or dubious efficacy, is **atomoxetine**, which unlike stimulants is specific noradrenergic reuptake inhibitor. As such, it has no potential for abuse and is unscheduled, with the ability to write for refills.
   c. Third-line medications such as clonidine, guanfacine, buprion are least effective in improving ADHD symptoms and are often used in addition to a stimulant to address aggressive behaviors (clonidine, guanfacine) or depression (buprion).

Table 25-4 Stimulant medication: dosage and techniques of administration*

Pharmacologic Agent	Starting Dose	Maximum Dose	Usual Dosing
First line			
Ritalin	Short acting (3-4 hr)	2 mg/kg/day	tid (lasts 3–4 hr)
Focalin		1 mg/kg/day	bid (lasts 5–6 hr)
Concerta	18 mg q day	2 mg/kg/day	18–72 mg q AM (12 hr duration) (titrated until benefit or side effects occur)
Metadate or Ritalin LA	10–20 mg q AM	2 mg/kg/day	qd (duration 8 hr)
Adderall	(dose is generally ½ 1.5 mg/kg/day of that of methylphenidate 2.5-5 mg)		bid (duration 4-6 hr)
Adderall XR	10 mg qd	1.5 mg/kg/day	qd (duration 8 hr)
Dexedrine	2.5–5 mg qd	1.5 mg/kg/day	bid/tid (duration 4 hr)
Dexedrine	5 mg qd	1.5 mg/kg/day	qd, bid (duration about 6 hr)

Spansules
Second line
Atomoxetine (Strattera) 0.5 mg/kg/day for 2 wk then gradually increase to 1.2-1.4 mg/kg/day (in AM if no drowsiness or HS if there is)

    d. Dosage. In general, a medication is started at the lowest dose and then gradually increased until the optimal response or intolerable side effects are seen. Side effects can usually be minimized by altering the dosage, timing, or form (short- or long-acting) of medication. Table 25-5 lists the common clinical question and side effects and how they can be managed.

- It is best to **start medications or any changes on the weekend** or any time the parents can be the first to witness the effects. They can then be instructed to call the clinician on Monday and relate any benefits or concerns.
- Throughout treatment, **height and weight should be monitored**. Although some children may experience short-term suppression of growth, long-term effects are rarely seen. Even short-term effects can be modified by altering the timing of medication and the time when eating is allowed.
- Once the appropriate dosage is established, it should be reevaluated and adjusted upward as tolerance develops or as the child's growth necessitates a larger dosage.
- The decision to treat only on weekdays or only during the school year is best made in consultation with the parents. **Improved school performance is always a priority**, but when the child's symptoms seem to have a lesser impact on home and peer relationships, weekday use only may be acceptable. However, when the child's relationships at home and with peers is a source of great contention and suffering, taking the medications every day, including holidays and vacations, may be the best option.

    e. Duration of treatment. In general, treatment will need to be continued into and through adolescence (except in the 10%–20% of children with ADHD who may completely "outgrow" the problem). The decision to end treatment can be periodically tested via trials off medication during times of low stress.

   3. Multi-modal treatments. In addition to medication, several psychological and social treatments should be considered).

    a. Parent training in behavioral management. This treatment aims to teach parents how to set limits, provide incentives for appropriate behaviors, and minimize emotionally destructive responses. Training adults (either parents or teachers) in behavioral management skills often requires referral to a specialized program for parents of children with ADHD. For parents, treatment may be done in small groups, which have the advantage of providing support as well as training. The clinician should recognize that the goal of behavioral management therapy is improvement in the environment in which daily living takes place, not to change the child's fundamental nature.

    b. Additional therapies may be needed depending on the circumstances of the family

Table 25-5 Stimulant medication: common clinical questions and side effects and management strategies

Common clinical questions	Management strategies
Short-acting or long-acting?	In general, long-acting preparations (8-12 hr) are preferable, unless the cost is prohibitive or parental preference
Decreased appetite?	Administer medication with or shortly after meals. Offer high calorie foods when hungry
	Encourage eating after school and/or before bedtime
	When severe, institute short periods off medication on weekends
Difficulty falling asleep?	Try a 8 hr, rather than 12 hr preparation. On the other hand, if the child is restless and overactive at bedtime, may try a short-acting PM dose
	Add a mild hypnotic such as an antihistamine or clonidine prior to bedtime
Dazed and/or withdrawn behavior?	Reduce dosage or discontinue medication and try a different class
Gradual return of hyperactive behaviors?	Increase dosage. Be sure is not 'rebound' behavior when blood levels are waning
Gradual onset of symptoms of depression during periods of effective medication dose?	Discontinue medication and try another class. Consider referral for treatment of depression
Development of tics that were not present prior to starting medication?	Discontinue medication and try another class

and the child. Individual psychotherapy for the child with ADHD should be considered in cases of oppositional and aggressive behaviors, as well as to improve self-esteem. There is, however, no evidence that individual psychotherapy improves the child's ability to pay attention or reduces impulsiveness. As the child gets older and becomes more self-aware, however, psychotherapy may facilitate an understanding of how his own behavior affects others. **Family therapy** may be useful for families in which the relationships are stuck in negative responses and for whom the child's behavior has engendered other significant family issues or who need a specific focus in communication skills. **Social skills training** for the child can be helpful in improving peer relationships.

D. **Criteria for referral.** Most primary care clinicians will be involved in two aspects of treatment: (1) explaining the condition to the child and the family and (2) prescribing and following medication. Psychosocial treatments will be given by others, though the clinician should be familiar with each type of treatment and the goals of each treatment strategy. The clinician should develop resources for referral and establish including ongoing communication with those resources. When the child fails to respond to stimulant medication or develops unacceptable side effects or the diagnosis remains ambiguous, referral to a specialist, such as a developmental-behavioral pediatrician or child psychiatrist, is indicated.

BIBLIOGRAPHY

For Parents

A.D.D. Warehouse. A one-stop shopping site with books, videos, and other products to help children with ADHD and their families to understand and manage ADHD problems. Contains an excellent annotated bibliography. A.D.D. Warehouse 300 Northwest 70th Avenue, Suite 102 Plantation FL 33317 1-800-233-9273 http://addwarehouse.com/shopsite_sc/store/html/index.html

CH.A.D.D. (Children with Attention Deficit Disorders). A national organization with local chapters throughout the country. Provides support to families, formation regarding local laws and school policies and an avenue for advocacy. CH.A.D.D. 499 Northwest 70th Avenue, Suite 308 Plantation FL 33317 305-587-3700 www.chadd.org

For Teachers

The Pediatric Development and Behavior Homepages. Helpful information and tips for dealing with ADHD in the classroom. http://www.dbpeds.org/articles/detail.cfm?id = 23

For Professionals

The AAP ADHD Toolkit. Contains very useful, free, downloadable information, handouts for parents, questionnaires, history forms, etc.http://www.utmem.edu/pediatrics/general/clinical/behavior/aap_adhd_toolkit/
These two articles are excellent and available at: http://aappolicy.aappublications.org/practice_guidelines/index.dtl
Clinical Practice Guideline: Diagnosis and Evaluation of the Child With Attention-Deficit/Hyperactivity Disorder. *Pediatrics* 10(5):1158–1170, 19xx.
Clinical Practice Guideline: Treatment of the School-Aged Child With Attention-Deficit/Hyperactivity Disorder. *Pediatrics* 108(4):1033–1044, 19xx.

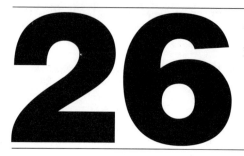

Autism

Elizabeth B. Caronna

I. **Description of the problem.** Autism is a heterogeneous neurodevelopmental disorder. It is defined clinically by characteristic behavioral impairments in
   - Reciprocal social interactions
   - Verbal and nonverbal communication
   - The range of activities or interests

   The DSM-IV-TR uses the umbrella term pervasive developmental disorders (PDD) to include several disorders which appear to have different etiologies, including autistic disorder, Rett's disorder, childhood disintegrative disorder, Asperger sydrome, and pervasive developmental disorder-not otherwise specified (PDD-NOS). Recently there has been increasing use of the term autism spectrum disorder (ASD) as a diagnosis for individuals who show less severe impairment than individuals who meet DSM criteria for autistic disorder. The autism spectrum includes PDD-NOS, atypical autism, high functioning autism, and Asperger syndrome. This shift in nomenclature reflects the broader conceptualization of the disorder to include more individuals with milder symptoms.

   (In this chapter, the term autism is used to denote autistic disorder, PDD-NOS, and ASD. The other PDDs will not be discussed in detail here. Asperger syndrome is addressed in greater detail in another chapter.)

   A. **Epidemiology.** The prevalence of autism is hotly debated. As recently as the 1980s, prevalence estimates were in the range of 0.5–1/1,000. More recent estimates have suggested a rate of ASD (including autistic disorder, PDD-NOS, and Asperger syndrome) as high as 3.4/1,000. The dramatic increase in rate of diagnosed cases may be attributed to several different factors, including changes in diagnostic criteria and the broader definition of ASD, variation in case finding methods, increased public and professional awareness of the disorders leading to earlier diagnosis, availability of behavioral treatment, and a possible true increase in the prevalence.

   Rates of autism are 3–4x higher in males than females. There is no difference based on race, ethnic backgroud, or socioeconomic status.

   B. **Etiology/contributing factors.** Historically, autism was attributed to cold, distant parenting, widely known as the "refrigerator mother theory." The accumulation of evidence that the disorder had a neurological basis (frequency of associated seizures, obvious genetic links, pathological abnormalities in the brain) made psychodynamic theories of etiology untenable. In the majority of cases, the etiology of autism is idiopathic. There are a small number of cases in which there is an underlying metabolic, infectious, or genetic disorder (such as untreated phenylketonuria [PKU], congenital cytomegalovirus [CMV] or rubella, tuberous sclerosis, fragile X syndrome, CHARGE syndrome, neurofibromatosis, and Down syndrome).

   A genetic contribution to ASD is supported by high rates of recurrence of autism in families with one affected child (3%–7% or higher) and twin studies that show up to 60% concordance for autistic disorder and 90% concordance for ASD in monozygotic twins. As expected, lower concordance is seen in dizygotic twins (<3% for autistic disorder and 10%–30% for broader phenotype). Autism is assumed to be a polygenic disorder resulting from gene-environment interactions. Numerous studies have identified various chromosomal "hot spots" in autism including loci on chromosomes 6, 7, 13, 15, 16, 17, and 22. There is a high rate (up to 10%) of fragile X syndrome in individuals with autism. Notwithstanding rampant speculation in the lay press and on the Internet, possible environmental triggers of the disorder in genetically predisposed individuals have not yet been identified.

II. **Making the diagnosis.**
   A. **Signs and symptoms.**
      1. **DSM-IV-TR Criteria for autistic disorder.** The criteria for diagnosis of **autistic disorder** according to DSM-IV-TR are outlined below. The presence of impairment must be judged compared to children of the same developmental level or mental age. The

DSM requires at least six criteria be met from the following three groups of symptoms.

a. **Qualitative impairment of reciprocal social interactions** (*at least two*).
  - Marked impairment in the use of multiple nonverbal behaviors such as eye-to-eye gaze, facial expression, body postures, and gestures to regulate social interaction
  - Failure to develop peer relationships appropriate to developmental level
  - A lack of spontaneous seeking to share enjoyment, interests, or achievements with other people (e.g., by a lack of showing, bringing, or pointing out objects of interest)
  - Lack of social or emotional reciprocity

b. **Qualitative impairments in communication** (*at least one*).
  - Delay in, or total lack of, the development of spoken language (not accompanied by an attempt to compensate through alternative modes of communication such as gestures or mime)
  - In individuals with adequate speech, marked impairment in the ability to initiate or sustain a conversation with others
  - Stereotyped and repetitive use of language or idiosyncratic language
  - Lack of varied, spontaneous make-believe play or social imitative play appropriate to developmental level

c. **Restricted, repetitive, and stereotyped patterns of behavior, interests, and activities** (*at least one*).
  - Encompassing preoccupation with one or more stereotyped and restricted patterns of interest that is abnormal either in intensity or focus
  - Apparently inflexible adherence to specific, nonfunctional routines or rituals
  - Stereotyped and repetitive motor mannerisms (e.g. hand or finger flapping or twisting, or complex whole-body movements)
  - Persistent preoccupation with parts of objects

  In addition, delays must be present in at least one of the core areas (social interaction, social communication, or symbolic/imaginative play) by age 3 years. Though some children with autism demonstrate true regression, it appears that most have atypical features in the first year of life that may not be clinically identified at the time.

2. **DSM-IV-TR: PDD-NOS.** This category is used for severe and pervasive impairment in development of reciprocal social interaction associated with impairment in either verbal or nonverbal communication or with the presence of stereotyped behaviors, interests and activities, but criteria are not met for autistic disorder. This includes atypical autism because of late age of presentation, atypical symptomatology, and/or subthreshold symptomatology.

3. **Clinical features.** Each child on the autism spectrum has a unique presentation with various levels of impairment in each of the three core symptom areas. Common presentations in the often overlapping domains are outlined below.

  a. **Abnormal social interactions.** Deficits specific to autism include lack of joint attention (ability to share interest with another using language, gestures, and eye gaze). Eye contact is usually minimal or fleeting. Children with autism may range from being very withdrawn and appearing unaware of other people, to having variable or odd interactions with others. Despite common misconceptions, they may be quite affectionate with caregivers and have normal attachment to them. They have difficulty establishing friendships with peers, ranging from being aloof to being overly intrusive. They may lack the ability to feel empathy or "put themselves in another's shoes".

  b. **Atypical communication.** Regression of language skills may or may not be present. Children on the spectrum who have meaningful language may demonstrate immediate and delayed echolalia, scripted speech (language heard on videos or in adult conversation), unusual prosody (monotone or singsong quality to speech), pronoun reversal (I/you), and preservative speech. They do not spontaneously use gestures usually acquired by a child's first birthday, including pointing and waving.

  c. **Restricted activities/play.** Children with autism show little imaginative play. Often they engage in repetitive games or routines with toys (lining up, smelling, tapping). They may focus on sensory aspects of objects (spinning fans, flashing lights) or develop fascinations and obsessions with unusual objects (sprinkler systems, picture hooks, manhole covers). They often demand sameness in routines, placement of objects, or other rituals, and may become very agitated with any change. They may engage in repetitive hand or body movement (hand flapping, spinning, rocking) instead of meaningful play.

    d. Rote memory, nonverbal skills. Children with autism may have advanced "splinter skills," such as being able to decode words at a much higher level than expected (hyperlexia), although they rarely have commensurate reading comprehension. They may learn to count into the thousands, say the alphabet backwards, or be able to complete puzzles with the pieces upside down so that no pictures are showing; though they are not able to communicate their wants or needs to their parents.

    e. Sensory sensitivities. Many children appear to be hyper- or hyposensitive to sensory experiences. They may, for example, cover their ears to loud noises, become distressed by textures of food or clothing, or be insensitive to painful stimuli.

    f. Comorbidities. Many children with autism have mental retardation (approximately 50%), although as diagnostic categorization of ASD has broadened, the rates are dropping. Children with mental retardation are more likely to develop seizure disorders as well (approximately 30%). Many have symptoms of hyperactivity and inattention, anxiety, obsessive-compulsive behaviors, self-injurious behaviors, pica, or aggression. Sleep disorders, gastrointestinal and feeding disorders, and allergies are also common.

B. Differential diagnosis.

    1. Global developmental delay/mental retardation. Cognitive abilities may be difficult to assess in young, nonverbal child. Severe cognitive deficits may be associated with some of the repetitive behavioral manifestations of autism.

    2. Developmental language disorder. In the absence of significantly inhibited temperament or anxiety disorder, the child with developmental language disorder alone should demonstrate normal reciprocal social interactions and appropriate play for age.

    3. Hearing impairment. Although not common, it is important to rule out sensory deficits as a cause of language and social delays.

    4. Landau-Kleffner syndrome. Also known as acquired epileptic aphasia, this may cause regression of language and other delays and can be diagnosed by sleep-deprived EEG.

    5. Rett's syndrome. Rett's syndrome is a sporadic X-linked disorder in girls that shares some behavioral features with autism. It is, however, a distinct disorder with a characteristic course including deceleration of head growth, stereotypic hand movements, and dementia. Many cases of Rett's syndrome can be confirmed by genetic testing for the MECP2 gene.

    6. Childhood disintegrative disorder. CDD is much rarer than autism and is notable for apparently normal development followed by regression in at least two (and typically all) of the following areas: language, social skills, adaptive behavior, bowel and bladder control, play, or motor skills.

    7. Severe early deprivation/reactive attachment disorder. Children who have experienced significant abuse and neglect may exhibit some of the symptoms of autism.

    8. Anxiety disorders/obsessive compulsive disorder. There is overlap between these disorders and ASD, although typically children with primary anxiety disorders have joint attention and reciprocal social relations that children with ASD lack.

C. History.

    1. Screening tools. There is an increasing pressure from both parents and professionals for earlier identification of autism so that treatment can begin before the age of 3 years. Various screening tests for autism available for use in primary care may be used as a second level screen if a child demonstrates abnormalities in language or social development. These include the CHAT (Checklist for Autism in Toddlers), the M-CHAT (Modified CHAT), PDDST-II, Stage 1 (PDD Screening Test), and the STAT (Screening Test for Autism in Two Year Olds).

    Children identified as being at risk for autism who "fail" routine screening or surveillance with questions below should be referred to a specialist experienced in evaluating children with autism spectrum disorders (developmental pediatric clinician, neurologist, psychologist, or psychiatrist).

    2. Key clinical questions. When a concern of ASD is raised, the following questions (modified from the CHAT and M-CHAT) are informative.

    1. *"Does your child respond to his name?"* Parents often report that they wonder if their child is deaf since he doesn't respond to voice, although he does turn to other sounds.

    2. *"Does your child prefer to play alone than with others?"*

3. **"Does your child ever use her index finger to point and to show you something? Does your child ever bring a toy over to show you?"** These look at joint attention, which is impaired in autism.

4. **"Does your child [over the age of 18 months] ever pretend when he is playing? (e.g., pretend to talk on the phone or feed a doll)."** Symbolic play is delayed or absent in ASD.

5. Red flags **of development that warrant further evaluation of possible autism**.
- No babbling by 9 months
- No gesturing by 12 months
- No single words by 16 months
- No functional, nonecholalic 2-word phrases by 24 months
- **ANY loss of language or social skills at ANY age**

D. **Physical exam.** Most children with idiopathic autism have unremarkable physical exams. Some have isolated macrocephaly. Most have normal neurologic exams and no motor abnormalities.

E. **Additional evaluations.** The medical workup of ASD should be guided by clues from the history and physical examination.
1. Formal audiologic evaluation and vision testing should be performed on all children.
2. Lead level should be tested if pica or social risk are present.
3. High resolution chromosomes, subtelomeric FISH, and DNA for fragile X if mental retardation present.
4. Repeat newborn screen if not available or performed.
5. Consider EEG if clinical concern of seizures or significant regression (rule out Landau-Kleffner syndrome).
6. Consider MRI if seizures or focal neurologic exam.
7. Consider genetics consultation if dysmorphisms present.
8. Consider metabolic studies if history or physical exam are suggestive.

III. **Management.**
A. **Early, specialized educational/behavioral interventions.** Studies suggest better outcomes in some children who received intensive behavioral services from an early age. The best-studied intervention is applied behavioral analysis (ABA), a very structured, repetitive, and intensive behavioral approach. Coverage of this therapy through IDEA varies nationwide and can be prohibitively expensive. Other commonly used interventions include the "floor time" model which focuses more on engaging young children in social interactions, speech and language therapy (often focusing on sign language and use of picture based systems in addition to spoken language), and occupational therapy, often focusing on sensory integration therapy. A consensus opinion of the National Research Council panel of experts in 2001 recommended 25 hours a week of instruction, for 12 months a year, with a low teacher to student ration (no more than 2:1) utilizing an eclectic approach individualized to the needs of the child, including behavioral interventions, speech and language therapy, occupational therapy, and physical therapy.

B. **Parent education and support.** The diagnosis of ASD can be overwhelming and confusing to families. Parents need guidance in evaluating the quality of information available on the Internet and elsewhere. They require support from providers and community organizations in dealing with the stress caused by living with a child with autism and trying to navigate the process of obtaining services for their child.

C. **Medications.** To date, no medications have been shown to directly treat the core symptoms of autism. However, psychopharmacologic agents can be used as an adjunct to the educational and behavioral interventions. However, children with autism often have idiosyncratic reactions or unacceptable side effects to psychopharmacologic agents, which limit their usefulness. Few placebo-controlled trials have been done in the pediatric population with autism to support the use of these medications, although they are widely prescribed. Below are listed some of the most commonly targeted symptoms and commonly used medications.

1. **Inattention/hyperactivity.** Stimulants often do not have as pronounced an effect as they do in neurotypical children with ADHD. An unintended side effect can be increased perseverative behavior because of improved attention and focus. Clonidine is also commonly utilized but probably has more of a sedative than direct effect on attention. Atomoxetine has had positive effects anecdotally and will undoubtedly be used widely in this population as it has been in typical children with ADHD symptoms.

2. **Aggression and disruptive behavior.** Haloperidol has been shown to effectively reduce aggressive behavior, but the side effects of typical neuroleptics (e.g., tardive

dyskinesia) limit its appeal today. Risperidone has been shown to reduce tantrums, aggression, self-injurious behavior in placebo-controlled trials, although weight gain was a significant side effect. Alpha-adrenergic agents are also commonly used, as are anticonvulsants.

3. **Symptoms of anxiety/OCD.** Selective serotonin reuptake inhibitors (SSRIs) are most commonly used to treat these symptoms.

4. **Sleep disturbances.** Melatonin may be helpful in inducing sleep.

D. **Complementary and alternative medicine.** CAM is frequently used by families of children with autism in addition to more mainstream educational treatments. Providers should ask routinely about their use. Few controlled studies exist in most cases. Some have potentially dangerous side effects, and for many the placebo effect is considerable. Commonly used agents include mega vitamins (especially B6 and magnesium), gluten-free/casein-free diet (widely used), antifungal medications, probiotic agents, secretin, immunotherapy (IVIG), chelation therapy, and DMG (dimethylglycine). Alternative therapies also commonly employed include massage therapy and auditory integration therapy, among others.

Providers should try to help parents evaluate the pros and cons of CAM by exploring the rationale behind the treatment, the evidence for it, the cost, and possible side effects. They should encourage families to keep track of target symptoms that the therapies are supposed to improve to monitor effects on and off the agents.

IV. **Clinical pearls and pitfalls.**
- There is often a significant delay between when parents express concerns about their child's development and when the diagnosis of autism is given. This may result in unnecessary delay of early intervention at the time when it is thought to have greatest impact. Parents' concerns about their child's development should be evaluated seriously and watchful waiting is not always appropriate.
- In the primary care office, providers should be sensitive to the needs of the child with autism by speaking in a quiet voice and not pushing the child beyond his comfort level with eye contact or social interactions.
- Providers should be alert to "hidden" medical conditions that can cause behavioral changes in nonverbal children with autism (dental pain, constipation, etc).

BIBLIOGRAPHY

For Parents

Books

Grandin T. *Thinking in Pictures: and Other Reports from My Life with Autism.* New York: Vintage Books, 1995.

Greenspan S, et al. *The Child with Special Needs.* New York: Perseus Books, 1998. [Outlines the floor time model.]

Maurice C. *Let Me Hear Your Voice: A Family's Triumph over Autism.* New York: Ballantine Books, 1993. [A mother's description of how intensive ABA therapy caused resolution of her children's autistic symptoms. Results are not typical of most children receiving ABA.]

Park C.*The Siege: The First Eight Years of an Autistic Child.* Back Bay Books, reissue 1995. [A mother's description of her child's autism in the "refrigerator mother" era.]

Siegel B. *The World of the Autistic Child: Understanding and Treating Autism Spectrum Disorders.* New York: Oxford University Press, 1996.

Websites

Autism Society of America www.autism-society.org
National Alliance of Autism Research www.naar.org
Has information about a range of treatments, including the TEACCH program www.teacch.com

For Professionals

American Academy of Pediatrics Committee on Children with Disabilities. Technical report: The pediatrician's role in the diagnosis and management of autistic spectrum disorder in children. *Pediatrics* 107:e85, 2001.

First Signs is an organization that has information for parents and professionals about screening. M-CHAT can be downloaded from this site at: www.firstsigns.org

Filipek PA et al. Practice parameter: Screening and diagnosis of autism. *Neurology* 55:468–479, 2000.

National Research Council Committee on Educational Interventions for Children with Autism, Lord C. and McGee J.P. (eds). *Educating Children with Autism.* Washington, DC: National Academy Press, 2001.

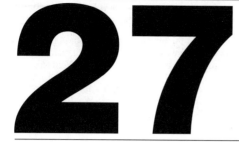

Bad News in the Media

Marilyn Augustyn
Betsy McAllister Groves

I. **Description of the Problem.** Over the last 20 years, media coverage of world events has changed, as has children's exposure to the media.
- In 1965 American children spent 30 hr/week with their parents; in 2002 they spent 17 hr/wk with their parents and 40 hr/wk on average watching TV, using the computer, listening to the radio or CDs, and playing video games.
- TV news coverage may be primarily *episodic* (focused on events) or *thematic* (including attention to trends, data on other conditions, providing context for an event). However, 90% of network crime stories are framed episodically, and it has been hypothesized that this episodic presentation makes the viewer more likely to blame the victim and less likely to think of prevention policies with a public health approach.
- Studies of stories about violence on local news programs suggest that they overemphasize violent crime, distort issues of race, and cultivate fear of urban areas in heavy viewers. Both children and adults who watch a lot of TV come to believe that the world is a far more dangerous place than it really is.

II. **Making the diagnosis.**
   A. **Taking a media history.**
   1. **From parents.** This is particularly important if parents are concerned about how a child may be responding to an event. Key trigger questions include
      - *"Does your child have a TV/computer in his room?"*
      - *"Do you watch TV with your child or know what your child is watching?"*
      - *"Do you monitor Internet or online computer use?"*
      - *"Does your child watch more than 1–2 hours of TV per day?"*
   2. **From the child.** After 4 years of age, children are often good historians about their favorite TV show, what they like to do on the computer, what they understand about current world events, etc.

III. **Advice for families.**
   A. Before parents talk to the child about a potentially distressing event in the media, they should take stock of their own thoughts, beliefs, fears and reactions. Children are great

Table 27-1 Developmental perspectives

Age	Child's understanding	Interventions
Toddlers (2 yr and under)	They will have no understanding apart from the reactions of their caregivers. Their only concern may be how it will impact their world.	Details may frighten them. Shield the child when possible from exposure to the news. Reassure them that their caregivers will keep them safe.
Preschoolers	Their capacity to distinguish real from fantasy is limited. Their main worry will be about their own safety and the safety of their parents.	Keep the TV off and stay close to home during the days surrounding an event. Show your child some things that may help keep him safe like smoke alarms or door locks.
School age children	It's best to start with a question to find out how much your child may know and begin from there. As they have a sense of right and wrong, they are often focused on why an event occurred.	It may be helpful to show the child that people are not powerless in this situation; for example helping the child in an act to aid the situation, donating food to tragedy victims, etc. It is also a prime time to help the child understand how they too deal with anger.

readers of emotional messages and will respond to verbal and nonverbal messages parents send about their own feelings. For some children, parental distress may be more upsetting than the event itself.

B. Maintaining open communication with children about world events is very important. The parents' relationship with the child is the most important ingredient as to how the child will understand the event. Take the child's questions seriously and be prepared to answer the same questions repeatedly.

C. Children communicate their thoughts and worries in both verbal and nonverbal ways. They may draw pictures, use dramatic play or themes to share their feelings. Use these to trigger supportive discussions between parent and child.

D. Limit the child's access to TV, newspapers, and magazines with graphic images of violence.

E. Spend extra time with your children during times of stress. Maintain the daily routine. Predictability and structure are often comforting for children in times of stress.

F. Developmental perspectives. Table 27-1 has suggestions of how to talk to different age children about world events.

BIBLIOGRAPHY

For Parents

Websites

American Academy of Pediatricians http://www.aap.org/family/mediaimpact.htm
Young Media Australia http://www.youngmedia.org.au/mediachildren/
Children Now http://www.childrennow.org/links/links-media.html

For Professionals

AAP Policy Statement on Children, Adolescents and Television. *Pediatrics* 107(2):423–426, 2001.

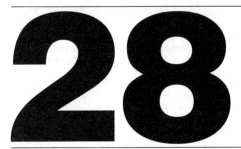

Bipolar Disorder in Children

Janet Wozniak
Joseph Biederman

I. **Description of the problem.** Childhood or pediatric-onset bipolar disorder is now the focus of an increasing number of research studies due to the high degree of disability associated with the symptoms and the suggestion of a higher prevalence than once thought. Up until the mid-1990s, the condition was thought to be so uncommon it was generally not included in the training of child and adolescent psychiatrists or pediatric clinicians and not considered in the differential diagnosis of a moody child. Factors such as symptom overlap with attention deficit hyperactivity disorder (ADHD) and developmentally different presentation from the adult form of bipolar disorder have led to its underdiagnosis in the past.

A. **Epidemiology.** The true epidemiology of childhood bipolar disorder is not known as no definitive epidemiologic studies have addressed the question.
   - One study of adolescents suggests **that 1% are affected, with up to 15% suffering from a subthreshold (but highly disabling) form of bipolar disorder**.
   - Other studies that indirectly address the prevalence of bipolar disorder in youth by examining rates in clinic, depressed and ADHD populations, generally confirm that **1% of children and adolescents are affected**.
   - As research on the pediatric subtype of bipolar disorder increases, new evidence addressing the various subtypes of bipolar disorder present in adults suggests that the **prevalence of bipolar disorder in the adult population may be 4%–5%**, also higher than previously thought.

B. **Etiology/contributing factors.** As in all psychiatric conditions, a complex interplay of environmental influences and genetic factors is responsible for the development of bipolar disorder in adults as well as in children. **There is no evidence that "bad parenting" or traumatic experience is responsible for the dramatic mood swings present in bipolar children** and adolescents. However, **parenting techniques which focus on flexibility and decreased rigidity are gaining acceptance as essential in reducing the frequency and intensity of the rage aspect of bipolar disorder**.
   1. Family studies increasingly implicate the role of genetics as important in the development of bipolar disorder, but a **complex, polygenetic etiology** is more likely than a single gene. Neuroimaging studies implicate the **limbic structures of the brain** as the site of the neurobiologic abnormality.

II. **Making the diagnosis. There is no definitive test for bipolar disorder.** Despite advances in neuro-imaging and in identifying candidate genes, there are currently no biological markers for this disorder. Like other psychiatric disorders, the diagnosis is made clinically, by asking about the specific symptoms in a developmentally appropriate manner. Research studies often use the Young Mania Rating Scale, but this scale was designed for use in adult inpatients and is not as useful in children and adolescents.

A. **Signs and symptoms**. Bipolar disorder is a mood disorder and therefore the diagnosis is anchored by the presence of abnormal mood states that fluctuate between depression and mania. Please see the chapter on depression for information regarding the symptoms of depression.
   1. Mania is characterized by two types of abnormal mood: **euphoric and irritable**. To be diagnosed as having bipolar disorder it is necessary to have had an **episode of mania that lasts 1 week or longer** (hypomania refers to episodes of mania lasting less than a week, but at least 4 days). Most individuals who have episodes of mania also have depression.
   2. **Depression can cycle in an alternating fashion** with mania (a week or more of mania followed by an episode of depression). Some such individuals will then experience an **inter-morbid period of good functioning**, free from abnormal mood states.
   3. Others experience **"mixed" states in which mania and depression occur together**. In such states, an individual may be euphoric for part of a day, rageful/

irritable for another part of the day and depressed/suicidal for another part of the day. **Children and adolescents tend to present with mixed states and complicated cycling patterns** rather than classic episodes of mania alternating with depression. A return to a high functioning, euthymic (even/normal) mood appears to be rare in bipolar youth.

4. **Euphoric states** are characterized by a feeling of being high or hyper, being "on top of the world" or being powerful and able to "accomplish anything".

5. The irritable mood of mania is distinctly different from the irritability associated with depression, ADHD, age appropriate tantrums or "bad days". The **irritability of mania is extreme, persistent, threatening, attacking, and out of control**. Rage episodes can occur with long episodes (20–60 minutes or more) of destructive, out of control and dangerous anger.

6. In addition to abnormal moods, the diagnosis of mania requires at least 3 (or 4 in the absence of euphoria) additional symptoms, often remembered with the mneumonic DIGFAST (**D**istractibility, **I**ncreased activity/energy, **G**randiosity, **F**light of ideas, **A**ctivities with bad outcome, **S**leep decreased, **T**alkativeness).

B. **Differential diagnosis.**

1. With **unipolar depression**. Irritability can characterize both mania and depression. However, the irritability of depression is milder, more complaining/whining/grouchy and is associated with low self-esteem, self-denigrating and self-destructive feelings, joylessness and hopelessness. The **irritability of mania is more severe and dramatic with aggression and explosiveness**.

2. With **ADHD**. Mania and ADHD share the symptoms of distractibility, increased energy or hyperactivity and talkativeness. In addition, ADHD can be associated with irritability and decreased frustration tolerance, although the irritability of ADHD is of lower intensity. Both disorders can be characterized by impulsivity. In general, **the symptoms of mania are much more disabling and of a greater severity than ADHD**. It is important to note that ADHD frequently co-occurs with mania, and both disorders can be present.

C. **History: Key clinical questions.**

1. To **assess overall moodiness**: *"How often (much of each day? How many days out of the week?) and how severe are the child's abnormal mood states? How often do you see age appropriate moods?"*

2. To **assess mania**: *"How common and how severe are angry mood states? How often does grouchy, cranky, whining behavior occur? How common is hitting, kicking, biting, spitting? How common (many times per day, once per day, a few times per week) are rage episodes or explosions? Do rages last a long time (20–60 minutes or more)? Are the rages threatening, aggressive, attacking, or dangerous? How common and how severe are euphoric or goofy/giddy/silly mood states? While all children can be silly, does your child take jokes too far? Does the child alienate others with immature behavior or excessive laughing fits?"*

3. To assess **depression and cycling**: *"How common are depressed, sad, blue or hopeless/joyless mood states? Do these moods occur on the same days as the manic mood states noted above? Do depressed moods occur during weeks or months separate from the manic mood states? Is the child self-destructive, self-abusive, or suicidal?"*

4. To assess **DIGFAST symptoms**

   a. *"Is the child easily distracted from tasks by noise, sights or internal thoughts?"*

   b. *"Does the child have high-energy states with increased motor activity? Is it difficult to calm or slow down the child?"*

   c. *"Is the child grandiose? Does he have inflated sense of self-esteem or does he overestimate his ability to do things? Does the child act or feel stronger/smarter/more powerful than others? Take on big projects? Does the child demonstrate a flagrant disregard for adult authority, acting like the boss? Is the child a braggart or show-off?"*

   d. *"Does the child jump from idea to idea quickly or go off on tangents that are hard to follow when they talk? Does the child complain of "racing thoughts" or thoughts that occur so rapidly they are hard to keep track of?"*

   e. *"Does the child show poor judgment in activities? Is the child reckless? Does the child want to buy or spend money excessively? Is the child sexually inappropriate (e.g., excessive bathroom humor, preoccupation with genitals or sexual matters, excessive or public masturbation, touching others' breasts or private parts, exposing self to others)?"*

   f. *"Does the child function with less sleep than most other children of the same age?*

How many hours less? Has the child ever functioned on no sleep or just a few hours?"

g. *"Is the child talkative? Does the child have pressured speech? Is the child difficult to stop or interrupt?"*

III. Management. While some children may "grow out" of bipolar disorder symptoms (longitudinal studies are underway), bipolar disorder is generally considered to be a chronic, lifelong condition. Longitudinal studies of children suggest a pattern of partial recovery, with frequent relapse.

A. Pharmacotherapy is the mainstay of treatment for bipolar disorder and a combined pharmacotherapy approach (using medications in combination) is typically required. **Mood stabilizing medications** which span various categories are the first-line treatment. Mood stabilizers include **atypical antipsychotics** (risperidone, olanzapine, quetiapine, ziprasidone, aripiprazole), **lithium**, and **certain anticonvulsants** (valproate, carbamazepine, oxycarbazepine, and lamotrigine in older adolescents).

- Clinical trials and clinical experience has suggested that atypical antipsychotics work the fastest and most effectively in youth to control the disabling symptoms of mania as compared to the more traditional agents (lithium and anticonvulsants).
- Pediatric bipolar disorder is difficult to treat and often requires combination therapy using more than one mood stabilizer at a time. Mood stabilizers may control mania, but leave depression untreated, requiring the cautious addition of an antidepressant (cautiously using low doses, as antidepressants can cause worsening of mania).
- Because bipolar disorder is highly comorbid with ADHD and anxiety disorders, medications addressing these conditions are often required. Stimulant medications must be used cautiously as they can exacerbate mania, but frequently improve the functioning of the child who has both mania and ADHD.

B. Other therapies including cognitive behavioral therapy (CBT), dialectical behavioral therapy (DBT), family therapy, group therapy, and individual psychodynamic therapy can all be helpful for various individuals. An approach combining medication treatment with these other therapies tailored to the needs of the individual is generally recommended for the treatment of bipolar disorder

- Helping the bipolar individual develop insight into his condition and to recognize the early signs of relapse aids in treatment.
- Therapy is helpful to ensure medication compliance, which is important in preventing relapse.

C. Psychiatric hospitalization is frequently required in the management of bipolar disorder due to the **dangerous behaviors associated with mania, the suicidality of depression** or **psychosis** associated with either. Many children improve with the containment and structure of hospitalization or residential treatment programs.

D. The presence of comorbid conditions can complicate the management and course of bipolar disorder in youth.

- In bipolar children under age 12, **comorbid ADHD** is almost always present (90% or more).
- In bipolar adolescents, **comorbid ADHD** occurs in 50%–60%.
- **Conduct disorder or antisocial personality disorder** (criminal behaviors) occur in 40% of youth and may or may not improve when the bipolar disorder is treated.
- **Anxiety disorders** are present in 50%–60% of bipolar youth and may be easy to miss, as it may seem counterintuitive to be disinhibited from mania and ADHD, but fearful and inhibited from anxiety simultaneously.
- **Alcohol and drug abuse and addiction** commonly occur in bipolar youth, with adolescent-onset bipolar disorder carrying the greatest risk. Random drug screening is recommended even in youth professing abstinence.

IV. Clinical pearls and pitfalls.

- Pediatric bipolar disorder may be a difficult diagnosis to make because it presents atypically by adult standards with a developmental picture characterized by: 1) more irritability (than euphoria); 2) mixed states and complex cycling; 3) chronicity rather than inter-episode high functioning; and 4) high levels of comorbidity especially with ADHD.
- Parents often feel unfairly blamed by mental health professionals, pediatric clinicians, teachers and family members for "causing" the disorder by not being strict enough or disciplining "bad behavior" effectively. In fact, a gentic etiology is most likely.
- Pediatric bipolar disorder is a neurobiologic disorder affecting thinking, feeling, and behavior in children in a dramatic way. It is characterized by out of control mood swings and frequent episodes of rage, irritability and poor judgment.
- Some children present with different symptoms in different arenas. At certain stages of the disorder and at certain ages, rage and depression may only be evident to those family

members closest to the child and not apparent to teachers, friends, or pediatric clinicians. The reasons for this are unclear, but may relate to the progression of the disorder (most evident to parents initially, later spilling over into other arenas). This feature does not mean that parents are "doing something wrong" and should not discourage parents from seeking professional treatment.

BIBLIOGRAPHY

For Parents

CABF (Child and Adolesent Bipolar Foundation) www.bpkids.org

Greene R. *The Explosive Child: A new approach for understanding and parenting easily frustrated, "chronically inflexible" children.* New York, NY: Harper Collins, 1998.

Papolos D, Papolos J. *The Bipolar Child and reassuring guide to childhood's most misunderstood disorder.* New York, NY: Broadway books, 2002.

For Professionals

Biederman J, Faraone S, Mick E, Wozniak J, Chen L, Ouellette C, Marrs A, Moore P, Garcia J, Mennin D, Lelon E. Attention-deficit hyperactivity disorder and juvenile mania: an overlooked comorbidity? *Journal of American Academy of Child & Adolescent Psychiatry* 35:(8)997–1008, 1996 Aug.

Findling RL, Calabrese JR. Rapid-cycling bipolar disorder in children. *American Journal of Psychiatry* 157:(9)1526–7, 2000 Sep.

Geller B, Craney JL, Bolhofner K, Nickelsburg MJ, Williams M, Zimmerman B. Two-year prospective follow-up of children with a prepubertal and early adolescent bipolar disorder phenotype. *American Journal of Psychiatry* 159:(6)927–33, 2002 Jun.

Wozniak J, Biederman J, Kiely K, Ablon S, Faraone SV, Mundy E, Mennin D. Mania-like symptoms suggestive of childhood onset bipolar disorder in clinically referred children. *Journal of American Academy of Child & Adolescent Psychiatry* 34: 867–876, 1995.

29

Biting Others

Barbara Howard

I. Description of the problem.

A. Epidemiology.

1. Almost all children bite at some time during the first 3 years. For example, 50% of toddlers in childcare are bitten 3 times every year. Bites constitute 6% of injuries to males and 3% to females in daycare.

2. As with most other aggressive behaviors, boys are more likely to bite than girls.

3. Biting is more severe or persistent in children with family dysfunction, where physical punishment is used, or when there is chronic stress.

4. Acceptability or modeling of violence predisposes to aggressive behaviors, such as biting.

B. Contributing factors.

1. **Environmental.** Children are more likely to bite others when they are in social situations beyond their coping abilities. Biting in these situations is usually intended to obtain objects, to gain attention, or to express frustration. It is also a powerful way of acquiring attention from adults. For example, some parents remove the child from the daycare setting for the day after a biting incident. Such *secondary gain* from the environment may prolong the biting phase.

2. **Developmental.** Biting emerges at predictable developmental stages.

   a. The first peak, at the **time of tooth eruption,** is rarely reported as a problem since caregivers interpret it as normal experimentation. Interestingly, breast-fed infants generally learn very quickly not to bite the breast, probably because of their mother's shriek, her affective distress, and the prompt removal of the infant.

   b. The next peak in biting occurs around **8–12** months when infants bite as an expression of excitement. A strong negative emotional response by caregivers accompanied by putting down the infant generally leads to rapid extinction.

   c. The **second year of life** is normally a time when skills develop unevenly and there is a strong desire to act autonomously. Fledgling or delayed abilities in expressive language and fine motor skills serve to cause frustration and set the child up for aggressive outbursts. Under these circumstances, biting may be used to dominate, to acquire an object, or to express anger or frustration. Additionally, children undergoing stressful separation experiences (such as at daycare) may derive satisfaction from causing distress to others by biting. This phase of biting typically disappears quickly.

   d. Biting in children **over age 3 years** should occur only in extreme circumstances (e.g., if they are losing a fight or perceive their survival to be threatened).

II. Recognizing the issue.

A. History: Key clinical questions.

1. *"When did the biting start? What else was different around that time"?* Look for recent stress (such as new daycare or a new sibling).

2. *"In what situations does it occur?"* Look for situations in which frustration is common and the child has poor coping skills. This may be a clue to developmental weaknesses such as fine motor delay (e.g., if biting occurs when coloring is expected). Biting that only occurs before meals may suggest hunger as a cause.

3. *"How have you handled it so far?"* Determine the previous measures used to address the problem and whether there is any secondary gain for the child to continue to bite (such as increased attention).

4. *"What other concerns do you have about your child's behavior or development?"* Other signs of aggressive behavior or specific developmental delays may point to a more pathological process.

5. *"How is anger expressed in your home?"* Children may model other family members' behaviors around expression of anger and violence.

6. *"Have you had any concerns about how your child is cared for?"* Abuse, neglect, violence, or poor-quality care may contribute to the problem.

III. **Management.**

A. **Information for the family.** Adults view biting as a very primitive behavior that elicits strong emotional reactions, especially in daycare settings. Families need to understand that biting by toddlers is usually a normal developmental phase and does not predict later aggression.

B. **Treatment (see Table 29-1).**

1. **Determination of cause.** Before formulating a treatment plan, the clinician must determine the reason for the child's biting. Developmental assessment will dictate the need for management of specific delays. Children who are frustrated by their relative weaknesses in skills compared with peers, for example, often do better when placed with younger children or in a less demanding setting. Other children push themselves to perform beyond their abilities. Such children may need support by arranging same-age peer play, placement in smaller groups, and avoidance of difficult tasks.

2. **Aversive reinforcement and redirection.** The chronic biter will need to be observed closely so that appropriate social interactions can be praised and biting encounters interrupted quickly with a shout that declares the seriousness of the offense. The child should then be put in time-out, with a short explanation such as, "I know you are angry, but people are not for biting." Sympathizing with the victim is helpful and may also serve to avoid secondary gain for the biter. Later, the incident can be reviewed with the child and alternatives discussed for negotiating conflict and for expressing feelings. A teething ring to bite can be offered or attached to the clothing, allowing the child expression of the feelings through an acceptable alternative outlet.

3. **Parental attitudes toward aggression.** Parental attitudes toward aggression need to be discussed. Since corporal punishment is a contributor to persistent biting, it should be eliminated. Parents often need coaching to develop appropriate expression

Table 29-1 Techniques to diminish biting in toddlers

Directed to the child
- Provide close supervision
- Ensure attention to positive behaviors
- Redirect when anger or frustration appears
- Verbalize feelings for the child
- Assess all skill areas and habilitate deficiencies
- If a bite occurs, shout a loud "NO!" and place child in time-out
- Be sure the child receives no interaction in time-out
- Offer lots of positive attention to the bitee
- Offer teething ring or cloth to bite
- If most bites are toward a certain peer, separate the children
- If biting persists, remove to home or smaller daycare

Directed to the caregivers
- Set consistent limits, especially on aggressive acts
- Avoid physical punishment or exposure to violence
- Express negative emotions verbally and stay in control
- Do not bite back. This models the undesirable behavior, elicits fear and anger in the child, and makes the adult feel so guilty that his or her effectiveness in limit setting is diminished
- Ensure that the child is not the least competent in his or her group
- Ensure that all caregivers are properly responsive and not using physical punishment

Directed to the parents if the child is about to be removed from daycare
- Meet with daycare staff
- Determine exactly how incidents are being handled
- Establish a consistent plan for managing incidents (which does not include taking the child home, if possible)
- Consider a shorter day in the daycare if the child tires
- Negotiate a time-limited trial of intervention, documenting incidents to determine improvement
- If necessary, move the child to home or a smaller, closely supervised, structured setting or one with younger or less aggressive children, or staff who are more open to dealing with biting

of negative affect. Counseling regarding reasonable limits for the child's behavior and nonphysical ways to attain them are the centerpiece of treatment.

4. **Daycare setting.** When biting occurs in a daycare setting, a crisis often ensues. Having the parents of the victim meet the equally distraught parents of the biter (or even a meeting of the entire center) can help defuse these situations. The nature of the supervision and activities should be evaluated. Young children need an active curriculum focused on small-group play with responsive adults who are positive in their interactions and able to redirect untoward behaviors. There also should be enough toys to discourage disputes. Larger toys for shared play are associated with fewer struggles. A child in group care who persists in biting often will do better at home or in a family daycare setting.

BIBLIOGRAPHY

Block RW, Rash FC. *Handbook of Behavioral Pediatrics.* Chicago: Year Book, 1981.
Solomons HC, Elardo R. Biting in day care centers: Incidence, prevention and intervention. *J Ped Health Care* 5:191–196, 1991.

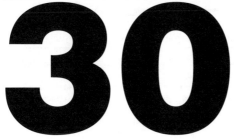

Breath Holding

Barry Zuckerman

I. **Description of the problem.** Breath-holding spells (BHS) involve the involuntary cessation of breathing in response to a painful, noxious, or frustrating stimulus. If prolonged, they can lead to loss of consciousness and/or seizures. There are no reported long-term adverse outcomes associated with breath holding.

A. **Epidemiology.**
- Simple breath holding without loss of consciousness may be seen in up to 25% of children.
- True BHS with loss of consciousness has been reported in approximately 4%.
- The peak frequency is between age 1–3 years, although they may begin in the newborn period.
- Breath-holding spells after age 6 years are unusual and warrant further investigation.
- They occur equally in males and females.
- There is a positive family history in approximately 25% of cases.
- 50% resolve by age 4; 90% by age 6.

B. **Etiology.** The etiology of BHS is speculative.
- Pallid spells may be facilitated by an overactive vagus nerve; cyanotic spells may be related to a more central CNS inhibition of breathing in response to stress.
- Hematologic differences (iron deficiency, transient erythroblastopenia) have been reported.

C. **Types.**
1. **Cyanotic spells.** The most common type of BHS is a cyanotic spell, which is precipitated by anger or frustration. A short burst of crying, usually less than 30 seconds, leads to an involuntary holding of the breath in expiration, resulting in cyanosis that can lead to a loss of consciousness and occasionally a seizure (Table 30-1).
2. **Pallid spells.** The second type is precipitated by fright or minor trauma (e.g., occipital trauma due to a fall). Following the precipitating event, there is an **absence of crying** or a single cry, followed by pallor and limpness. This sequence of events is thought to be due to a hyperresponsive vagal response that results in bradycardia (and even asystole), causing pallor and loss of consciousness. Some of these children (about 15%) go on to faint when they are injured or frightened as adults.

II. **Making the diagnosis.**
- The key to diagnosis is to differentiate breath-holding spells from seizures (Table 30-2).

Table 30-1 Progression of breath-holding spells

Cyanotic spell
Precipitating event (anger or frustration associated with temper tantrums)
Period of crying (frequently less than 20 secs)
Holding of breath in expiration
Cyanosis
Progressive loss of consciousness
Occasional twitching, opisthotonos, or clonic movements
Pallid form
Precipitating event (minor trauma, especially occipital trauma or fright)
Absence of crying or single cry
Bradycardia and often asystole
Simultaneous loss of consciousness and breath holding
Pallor
Occasionally generalized seizure or twitching

Table 30-2 Distinguishing breath-holding spells from seizures

	Severe breath-holding spells	Epilepsy
Precipitating factor	Always present	Usually not present
Crying	Present before convulsion	Not usually present
Cyanosis	Occurs before loss of consciousness	When it occurs, it is usually during prolonged seizure
Electroencephalogram	Almost always normal	Usually abnormal but may be normal
Incontinence	Uncommon	Common

The presence of a precipitating factor followed by crying and cyanosis before the loss of consciousness and/or seizure is specific to a breath-holding spell.
  • An electroencephalogram is rarely necessary unless a clear precipitating event is not apparent.
  • A blood count to rule out iron deficiency may be warranted in severe cases.

III. **Management**
   A. **Information for parents.** Breath-holding spells need to be explained and demystified for parents. The clinician should explain, in simple, concrete terms, the sequence of events leading to the loss of consciousness and seizure. The benign nature of these events should be emphasized because parental concerns about epilepsy, brain damage, or death are common.
   B. **Management strategies.**
      1. **Medications** are generally neither indicated nor helpful. Atropine has been tried in some cases of pallid spells. Iron supplementation may be tried in cases with hematologic abnormalities.
      2. For cyanotic spells, an **intense stimulus** (e.g., a cold cloth on the face) may terminate the breath holding if applied before or within the first 15 seconds of apnea. Although the window of opportunity for this intervention is brief, many parents find it comforting to have *something* to try, rather than just feeling helpless.
      3. If the event progresses for either type of breath-holding spells, the **child should be placed on the floor to prevent falling**.
      4. When the child awakes (usually immediately after the seizure or loss of consciousness) **parents should not fuss over the child** so that inadvertent secondary gain does not occur.

BIBLIOGRAPHY

DiMario FJ Jr. Breathholding spells in childhood. *Current Problems in Pediatrics.* 29(10):281–99, 1999.
Lombroso CT, Lerman P. Breathholding spells (cyanotic and pallid infantile syncope). *Pediatrics* 39:563–581, 1967.

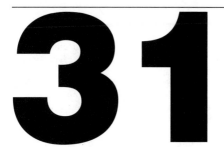

Bullying

Douglas Vanderbilt

I. **Description of the problem.** Bullying is the assertion of power through aggression. It involves one or more children repeatedly and intentionally targeting a weaker child through social, emotional, or physical means. The key features to this behavior are
- Power imbalance between the stronger bully and the weaker victim
- Intent to harm
- Repetition of the behavior toward a single victim

Bullying represents a continuum with teasing on one end and violent assault on the other. Teasing involves mild aggression and humor that creates social embarrassment, but does not have the intent to harm seen in bullying. Some behaviors such as physical assaults and "hate speech" are criminal and subject to the law. A bully-victim is often defined as one who has been bullied and then becomes a perpetrator of similar behavior.

A. **Bullying can come in two forms.**
1. **Direct bullying** is the overt type that occurs in the open. It can involve physical aggression such as hitting, stealing, and threatening with a weapon or verbal aggression, such as name calling, public humiliation, and intimidation.
2. **Indirect bullying** is the covert type that is relational in nature. It involves spreading rumors, social rejection, exclusion from peer groups, and ignoring. A subtype of this, emotional bullying, is an especially salient concern of youth today.

B. **Epidemiology.**
1. **Prevalence.**
a. 55% of 8–11-year-olds and 68% of 12–15-year-olds rated teasing and bullying as a big problems for kids their age.
b. 20%–30% of middle and upper school students are involved in bullying as perpetrators and/or victims.
c. Of 6th to 10th graders in one study in the US, 13% were identified as bullies, 11% as victims, and 6% report both being bullying and victims.
d. Among 6th graders of low socioeconomic status students in Los Angeles, 7% were bullies, 9% victims, 6% bully-victims, 22% borderline, and 56% uninvolved.
2. **Age.**
a. Bullying decreases with age in that it is highest in the 2nd grade and declines by the 9th grade.
b. Older children are less likely to talk about their victimization with only 50% of all children confiding in anyone.
3. **Gender.**
a. Boys are more likely to use and receive *direct* bullying.
b. Girls are more likely to use and receive *indirect* bullying.
c. Boys are twice as likely as girls to be bullies, greater than 3 times as likely to be bully-victims, and twice as likely to be victims.

C. **Etiology/contributing factors.**
1. **Settings.** Bullying occurs most frequently at school at any time or in any place where there is minimal supervision. Common times are during breaks, recess, and lunch. Common places are playgrounds, hallways, and en route to and from school. In addition to the real world settings of the school and neighborhood, the Internet is becoming another venue for this behavior to take place through mass emailing, chat rooms, and message boards.
2. **Risk factors.**
a. **Social.** Families may encourage bullying by showing a lack of consistent consequences, using discipline that is negative or physical, and modeling bullying behaviors in their children. Peer groups can also support bullying through acceptance and encouragement of the behavior. Schools have more episodes of bullying if they ignore or tolerate such behavior through weak supervision. Communities with more social chaos and community violence have worse problems. Media

images and societal values can promote aggression and violence as normative and appropriate methods of social behavior and conflict resolution.

b. Individual.

(1) Characteristics of victims. There are two types of victims: the **passive type** is physically weak and emotionally vulnerable. Although less prevalent, the **provocative** type is restless and fights back when attacked. They are more likely to have attention deficit hyperactivity disorder (ADHD) or oppositional defiant disorder (ODD). Overall both victim groups are anxious, insecure, lonely, and lack social skills but their external characteristics do not set them apart from others. Being bullied results in lower social status and higher social marginalization and isolation. They have more emotional disorders and suicides. Long-term consequences in adulthood of being bullied as a child include increases in depression, poor self-esteem, and abusive relationships.

(2) Characteristics of bullies. Bullies have higher rates of conduct disorders and social standing. They have the lowest rates of adjustment problems because of their higher social status/prestige but are avoided by peers. Bullies, who self-identify, have higher rates of depression and psychological distress as compared to those who deny their behavior. They have higher negative attitudes toward school and more use drugs. Childhood bullies have a four-fold increase in criminal behavior by their mid-20s. They are at higher risk of dropping out of school.

(3) Characteristics of bully-victims. This group has the highest risk group for psychiatric disorders with the most problems with peer relationships and have high rates of depression and loneliness. Equally troubling is the fact that amongst intended or conducted perpetrators of school shootings, two thirds were bullied and had violent ideation prior to their violent acts.

II. **Making the diagnosis.** The clinician has four roles when bullying is a concern.
1. Identify the problem
2. Screen for psychiatric comorbidities
3. Counsel the families and child
4. Advocate for violence prevention

A. Signs and symptoms.

1. **Identifying the victim.** Signs of a child being bullied include physical complaints such as insomnia, stomachaches, headaches, and new onset enuresis. Psychological symptoms may occur such as depression, loneliness, anxiety, and suicidal ideation and gestures. Behavioral changes are common such as irritability, poor concentration, school refusal, and substance abuse. School problems can also occur like academic failure, social problems, and lack of friends. Additional vigilance must be made for those children with chronic medical illnesses, physical deformities, and students in special education who may be potential targets.

2. **Identifying the bully.** Signs of a child being a bully are more difficult to discern due to the bully's desire to obscure the behavior. Children who are aggressive, overly confident, lack empathy, and are having conduct problems may need careful screening. These children are at high risk if they come from families who use physical punishment and model violent behavior in conflict resolution.

3. **Differential diagnosis.** Care must be made to not miss psychiatric disorder that pose safety issues such as suicidal ideation and plans, substance abuse, and risk-taking behaviors. The physical, behavioral, psychological, and school symptoms of bullying may overlap with other conditions such as medical illness, learning problems, and psychological disorders. Serious disorders may need psychiatric screening and management.

B. History: Key clinical questions (see Table 31-1).

III. **Management.** Management for bullying involves multifaceted interventions with parents, victims, bullies, and the school. Interventions should include giving information regarding the current research in bullying, supporting families, victims, and bullies, referring those children in need of further mental health services, and expecting behavioral change from the bully and social change from the school environment.

A. Individual.

1. **Victims.** The clinician should empathetically listen to the parent and child to help empower them. The child and family need reassurance; do not blame the victim or trivialize the child/parent's concern. For example
   - *"No one deserves to be treated this way."*
   - *"You are not alone."*
   - *"Your parents and I will work together to help things get better for you."*

Table 31-1 Sample questions to investigate whether a child is being bullied

Questions for Children
1. Have you ever been teased at school?
2. Do you know of other children who have been teased?
3. How long has this been going on?
4. Have you ever told the teacher about the teasing?
5. What kinds of things do children tease you about?
6. Have you ever been teased because of your illness/handicap/disability? For not being able to keep up with other children? About looking different from them?
7. At recess do you usually play with other children or by yourself?
8. Have you ever changed schools because you had problems with the other students?

Questions for Parents
1. Do you have any concern that your child is having problems with other children at school?
2. Does your child go to the school nurse frequently?
3. Has your child's teacher ever mentioned that your child is often by himself at school?
4. Do you suspect that your child is being harassed or bullied at school for any reason? If so, why?
5. Has your child ever said that other children were bothering him?

- "The bullying will stop very soon."

Suggestions should include having the child seek social support from teachers and friends and avoid situations where the bullying may occur. The phrase: *Walk, Talk, and Squawk* can help a child to deal with the bully. The child should "Walk" by ignoring the hurtful remarks; "Talk" by making confident yet nonprovocative statements to the bully; and "Squawk" by disclosing the episodes to adults. Role-playing can be helpful in problem solving these techniques with the child. Strategies can be used to help to bolster the child's insecurities and increase self-esteem, such as extracurricular activities like drama clubs and sports.

2. **Bullies.** Once a bully is identified and appropriate screening for risk factors is completed, the clinician should educate the parents and child about the seriousness of the behavior and its potential consequences. Care must be made to label the behavior and not the child as the problem. The first step in changing the bully's behavior is helping the family and child to acknowledge the behavior as hurtful. For example:
   - "Do you feel bad when other children hurt your feelings?"
   - "Bullying hurts other children's feelings."

   Interventions should include clear accountability of the child's behavior through observations at home and school.

B. **Systemic.** Bullying occurs in permissive and supportive environments. Adults in all aspects of children's lives have the responsibility to create safe and supportive environments that have explicit expectations of appropriate social behavior. The clinician must collaborate with the stakeholders in the community to inform practices and encourage interventions that change social norms and values.

BIBLIOGRAPHY

For Parents

Books

Olweus D. *Bullying at School: What We Know and What We Can Do.* Ames, IA: Blackwell Publishers, 1994.

Websites

Bullying Online www.bullying.co.uk/
Love Our Children USA http://www.loveourchildrenusa.org/bullying.php
National Education Association National Bullying Awareness Campaign http://www.nea.org/schoolsafety/bullying.html
National Mental Health and Education Center for Children and Families (NASP) http://www.naspcenter.org/factsheets/bullying_fs.html

U.S. Department of Health and Human Services/Health Resources and Services Administration *Take a Stand. Lend a Hand. Stop Bullying Now!* http://www.stopbullyingnow.hrsa.gov/index.asp

For Children

Books

Berenstein S, Berenstein J. *The Berenstein Bears and the Bully.* New York: Random House, 1993.
Romain, T. *Bullies are a Pain in the Brain.* Minneapolis, MN: Free Spirit Publishing, 1997.

Websites

http://www.bullying.org
http://bullystoppers.com

For Professionals

Websites

American Psychological Association http://www.helping.apa.org/warningsigns/recognizing.html
The Safetyzone www.safetyzone.org
Safe Schools/Healthy Students Action Center www.sshsac.org

32

Cerebral Palsy

Frederick B. Palmer
Alexander H. Hoon

I. **Description of the problem.** Cerebral palsy (CP) is a **disorder of movement and posture** caused by a static defect or lesion of the immature brain. Rather than a specific diagnosis, it encompasses a spectrum of neurodevelopmental syndromes characterized by **persistent motor delay, abnormal neuromotor examination, and often an extensive range of nonmotor-associated disabilities in cognitive, neurobehavioral, neurosensory, orthopedic, and other areas.** These associated disabilities reflect the fact that motor centers of the brain are rarely affected in isolation. Although the brain lesion is, by definition, **nonprogressive**, its motor and nonmotor manifestations can be expected to change with the child's development.

A. **Epidemiology.**
   - About 2/1,000 live births (1/2 born at term, 1/2 born preterm)
   - Increase in CP birth prevalence in very low birth weight babies (with a decrease in mortality in this group) in the 1980s and a possible decrease during the late 1990s

B. **Classification.** Clinical classification is based on the nature of the **movement disorder, muscle tone**, and **topography**. Classification by type is essential to management and anticipation of associated disabilities (Table 32-1) and future needs.

   1. **Spastic CP** (65% of children with CP). Most children with CP have spasticity, an upper motor neuron syndrome consisting of persistent velocity-dependent hypertonus (increased muscle tone of clasp-knife character), increased deep tendon reflexes, pathologic reflexes, spastic weakness, and loss of motor control and dexterity. Spastic CP is further classified based on topography as
      a. **Hemiplegia** (30% of children with CP). Primary unilateral involvement, often with the arm more involved than the leg.
      b. **Quadriplegia** (5% of children with CP). Four-limb involvement with legs often more involved than arms, but with functionally limiting arm involvement.
      c. **Diplegia** (30% of children with CP). Four-limb involvement with legs much more involved than the arms (which may show only minimal impairment and no functional limitation). Diplegia should be distinguished from paraplegia, which implies entirely normal arm function and suggests a spinal cord lesion, not CP.

   2. **Dyskinetic CP** (19% of children with CP). The other major physiologic category is designated dyskinetic due to the **prominent involuntary movements**, fluctuating muscle tone, or both. **Choreoathetosis** is the most common subtype. Most children with dyskinetic CP have relatively symmetric four-limb involvement and require no further topographic designation.

   3. **Ataxic CP** (up to 10% of children with CP). This type of CP has a relatively good motor prognosis.

C. **Etiology/contributing factors.** Despite 150 years of research, specific etiologic factors responsible for the motor impairment remain uncertain in most children with CP, especially in children born at term. Large studies have shown that brain injury occurring at birth is the cause in only 8%–12% of cases. **Developmental brain anomalies or prenatal insults are the most common etiologies.** In premature children, both prenatal and perinatal factors are felt to play a role in what is most commonly a spastic diplegia or quadriplegia. Postneonatal etiologies (e.g., traumatic brain injury, meningitis) account for about 10% of CP. Maternal and/or fetal infection has been recognized as an important antecedent of CP in term and possibly preterm infants. Thrombophilia, including the Factor V Leiden mutation, the most common cause of familial thrombosis in neonates, infants, and children, may be an important contributor to intrauterine stroke and hemiplegic CP. Advances in neuroimaging and molecular genetics offer continuing promise in improving our understanding of etiology and options for prevention.

II. **Making the diagnosis.** Attention should be given to both developmental diagnosis (type and severity of CP) and etiological possibilities.

Table 32-1 Selected nonorthopedic associated disabilities in cerebral palsy

Cognition
Mental retardation (present in 30%–77%)
The most important factor influencing habilitation
Hemiplegia and diplegia associated with higher cognition
Easy-to-underestimate cognition in choreoathetosis
Epilepsy associated with lower cognition
Language disorder, learning disability (present in about 40%)
    Heterogeneous group with deficits due to oromotor dysfunction, dysphasia, hearing loss
    Often "superimposed" on mental retardation
Very high risk for learning disability in child with CP and "normal" IQ
Neurobehavior (present in up to 50%)
Entire spectrum of neurobehavioral disorders (attention deficit hyperactivity disorder to
    autism) seen
No symptom typical
Behavior dysfunction may be primarily a neurologic symptom
Sensation
Visual disorders (present in 50%–90%)
    Most common ones amenable to treatment
    May have a bearing on education (acuity, field deficits)
    Hemianopsia in 25% of hemiplegia (easily missed as gaze may compensate to side of field cut)
    Refractive errors seen in 50% overall; 67% in diplegia; amblyopia develops in 14%
Hearing disorders (present in 10%)
    Easily missed
    Higher prevalence (45-60%) in postkernicteric choreoathetosis and TORCH etiologies
Somatosensation (present in up to 50% of hemiplegia)
    Deficits in otoreognosis most common
    May be the limiting factor in arm/hand functioning in hemiplegia
    Repeated clinical examination essential to recognition
    Associated with linear undergrowth but not muscular atrophy
Seizures (present in 30%–40%)
Often associated with spasticity and lower cognition
Growth failure
Undernutrition a frequent problem
Empiric nutritional goal of 10% weight for height
Multifactorial in origin: increased caloric needs, oromotor dysfunction, gastroesophageal reflux,
    chronic infection, "neurogenic," syndromic
Limb length asymmetry associated with hemisensory abnormalities
Other health problems
Genitourinary complaints common; pathogenesis unclear
Drooling a major cosmetic problem: may be exacerbated by antispasticity drugs; treatment with
    anticholinergics, surgery, and biofeedback disappointing

A. **Symptoms.** CP usually presents with significant motor delay, although the delay may
not be recognized in the first months of life. Other common presenting concerns include
poor head control, generalized hypotonia, hypertonia (especially during activities such
as bathing or diapering), early preferential hand use, absent weight bearing, and feeding
problems.
- The **nonprogressive** nature of "the lesion" is essential to the diagnosis. If etiology
is not clear or if the clinical picture is not static, then evaluation for a progressive
process (metabolic, structural, neurodegenerative, etc.) should be undertaken.
B. **Neurologic signs.**
1. Sole reliance on the neuromotor examination in diagnosing CP can lead to both
under- and over-diagnosis. Instead, the clinician should initially **focus on the presence or absence of motor delay. If there is no delay, CP is unlikely** even
if the neuromotor examination is abnormal (although children with such "minor
neuromotor dysfunction" may have other neurodevelopmental disabilities, such as
mental retardation or learning disability). An exception to this "no delay, no CP"
rule is seen in hemiplegia, in which the prominent upper extremity disability causes
substantial neuromotor asymmetry rather than gross motor delay.
2. On neuromotor examination, muscle tone may vary from excessive hypotonia to

hypertonia (spastic, dyskinetic, or mixed in character). Hypotonia may be manifest as head lag on pull to sit, slip through at the shoulders, or an exaggerated curve in ventral suspension. Early hypotonia may persist, normalize, or evolve into hypertonia. Persistent hypotonia with diminished deep tendon reflexes may suggest a different neurological etiology.

3. Recognition of abnormal spontaneous general movements during the first weeks of life may provide a sensitive tool for early detection of CP.
4. Spastic hypertonia may be brought out by rapid movement of the limb by the examiner.
5. The hypertonus seen in dyskinetic forms ("lead pipe rigidity") is variable in nature and can usually be "shaken out" by the examiner with rapid movements of the limb. Involuntary movements, such as choreoathetosis, dystonia, and tremor, are often associated. Facial and oromotor involvement are often prominent.
6. All children are born with a constellation of primitive (e.g., Moro) and "pathologic" (e.g., Babinski) reflexes, probably mediated at the brainstem level. In normal infants, brain maturation leads to the disappearance of these reflexes and the emergence of postural and equilibrium reactions that precede the attainment of motor skills. In infants with CP, **primitive reflexes are often increased in intensity and delayed in disappearance**. Recognition of these phenomena may aid in diagnosis, especially in the first 6–12 months of life when motor delay may be less apparent.
7. The examination should include a careful assessment, of **oromotor and ocular function** and a search for orthopedic abnormalities, including joint contractures. The general physical examination should focus on dysmorphic features, neurocutaneous signs, retinal abnormalities, organomegaly, and other findings that could suggest a specific etiology. Ophthalmologic and genetic consultations may be helpful.

C. **Tests.** Table 32-2 lists the indications for various tests in CP. Neuroimaging in the neonate and young infant known to be at risk for CP is an important step in the early detection of CP. An initial neuroimaging study in the older child may not directly affect management, but may provide a structural correlate of the motor impairment and insight into the timing of the brain insult. Often parents find this information quite useful as they try to come to terms with their child's impairment.
- In children with *atypical* clinical findings, especially choreoathetosis, metabolic disorders should be suspected. Plasma lactate, plasma amino acids, urinary organic acids, and selective use of other tests can be important. A karyotype may be revealing in children with apparent prenatal onset of CP and additional, even minor, malformations.

III. Management.
A. Primary Goals.
1. To allow the child with CP to **function as effectively and normally as possible** in **the home, school, and community**.
2. To provide a foundation for the child to **function independently as an adult**, within the constraints imposed by the neurodevelopmental and associated disabilities.
3. To **assist the parents** in accepting and assuming their roles as primary advocates for their child's needs.
4. To **coordinate the recommendations of the many medical providers** into an integrated healthcare plan. Table 32-3 outlines common clinical indications and goals for referral to nonmedical professionals. These guidelines and comments reflect personal experience rather than rigid rules and should be interpreted in the context of available resources.

B. General principles of treatment.
1. **The severity of disorder determines the aggressiveness of treatment.** For example, an infant with a motor quotient below 0.5 generally requires complete evaluation by a physical and/or occupational therapist and ongoing intervention. Children with milder delays (motor quotient 0.5–0.7) may only need a one-time consultation and suggestions for home management. The Gross Motor Function Measure (GMFM) and 5-level Gross Motor Functional Classification System (GMFCS) provide a standardized approach to determining motor prognosis.
2. Although most traditional interventions and motor therapies are not of clearly proved efficacy, they can be useful if used with clear indications and goals in mind.
3. Parents should be included in any therapy and should incorporate techniques into their everyday activities with the child.
4. Therapists and intervention programs should be kept informed about the child's health and, in turn, should keep the clinician informed of their activities.

Table 32-2 Suggested indications for diagnostic or screening tests in children with motor disorders

Magnetic resonance imaging of the brain
  Cerebral palsy or motor asymmetry
  Abnormal head size or shape
  Craniofacial malformation
  Loss or plateau of developmental skills
  Multiple somatic anomalies
  Neurocutaneous findings
  Seizures
  IQ<50
  Low birth weight infant at term age equivalent
Cytogenetic studies
  Microcephaly
  Multiple (even minor) somatic anomalies
  Family history of mental retardation
  Family history of repeated fetal loss
  IQ<50
  Skin pigmentary anomalies (mosaicism)
  Suspected contiguous gene syndromes (e.g., Prader-Willi, Smith-Magenis)
  Metabolic studies
  Dyskinetic CP (choreoathetosis, dystonia, ataxia)
  Episodic vomiting or lethargy
  Poor growth
  Seizures
  Unusual body odors
  Somatic evidence of storage
  Loss or plateau of developmental skills
  Sensory loss (e.g. retinal abnormality, hearing loss)
  Acquired cutaneous disorders

Adapted from Palmer FB, Capute AJ. Mental retardation. *Pediatr Rev* 15:473–479, 1994.

5. Clinicians must be familiar with available **local intervention programs, their services, and details** of eligibility, access, and **payment**.
6. Assistance in identifying needs and appropriate intervention options is often available through neurodevelopmental disability programs in tertiary centers.
7. Where tertiary services are not available or accessible, the physician should create and lead a virtual interdisciplinary team of available professionals to serve the child. Managed care gate-keeping roles require effective coordination by the primary care provider when tertiary services are not provided.

C. **Criteria far referral.**

1. An **orthopedic evaluation** is needed of any child with limitation in range of motion of any joint(s). Orthopedic surgery may be indicated when function is impaired, care is limited, or pain is caused by deformity, contracture, or muscle imbalance. Goals of surgery should be clearly understood by families. The common parental expectation for unreasonable functional gains should be anticipated. Orthopedic and neurodevelopmental pediatric consultants should work closely with physical and occupational therapists in nonsurgical interventions. They can assist in prescribing appropriate adaptive equipment and bracing. Such equipment includes seating and positioning devices and transportation implements.
2. **Neurosurgical interventions** in CP have a long history. Stereotactic ablation surgery and implanted stimulators have been unrewarding and are seldom indicated. Selective lumbar dorsal rhizotomy may offer help in lower extremity spasticity, especially spastic diplegia. However, long-term functional outcomes are unclear. Specific goals for functional improvement should be clear before deciding on surgery.
3. If **pharmacological adjuncts** are to be used, specific treatment goals are essential and should include functional improvement, not just reduction in tone. It is generally best to have the child's physical or occupational therapist assist in objective measurement of agreed on outcomes to avoid basing dosage decisions solely on "he's better [or worse] today" reports from family or treatment programs.
   - Medication is sometimes effective in reducing hypertonus in spastic and mixed forms of CP. However, striking functional improvement is rarely seen.

Table 32-3 Suggestions for use of nonmedical specialties

Service	Common useful indications	Comments
Special nutrition services	Weight for height less than 5% or declining Suspected insufficient caloric intake due to poor swallow, gastroesophageal reflux	Nutritional problems require extensive medical workups Significant gastroesophageal reflux common in severe CP Reactive airway disease in CP is chronic aspiration until disproved; pursue dysphagia and GE reflux Gavage or gastrostomy feeding may be needed to meet caloric requirements Ideal body weight is 10th percentile for height
Occupational therapy	Fine motor delay (DQ<0.50)^a Presence or risk of contractures in the upper extremities Overdependence on others for activities of daily living for child's cognitive level Oromotor dysfunction, excess drooling, poor oral intake, excessive feeding time Equipment needs	
Physical therapy helpful	Gross motor delay (MoQ<0.50)^b Difficult or inefficient ambulation in the absence of prominent delay Abnormalities of tone or reflexes interfering with function or management Presence or risk of contractures in the lower extremities Adaptive equipment needs	Videotaping motor function, or formal gait analysis, may be helpful in assessment Helpful to have physical therapist present for orthopedic evaluations Short term therapy for children with MoQ 0.50–0.70 may be useful
Audiology	All patients with CP due to high prevalence of hearing loss Recommend and apply amplification, if indicated	Office-based hearing screening is unreliable and insensitive BrainStem auditory evoked responses (BAERs) provide nonspecific measures of hearing loss in high-risk premature infants in the newborn period; more specific results using BAERs, behavioral audiometry, and acoustic impedance audiometry are obtained after 6 months of age Early treatment of hearing loss can significantly improve outcome
Speech and language	Global language delay Isolated expressive language delay Dysarthria May assist occupational therapy with feeding concerns	Receptive language may be surprisingly better than expressive language Language may be underestimated in patient with oromotor involvement Repeat evaluations necessary Isolated articulation lessons usually not rewarding

(continued)

- Benzodiazepines, especially diazepam, are most commonly used. Baclofen, a GABA agonist, is also used (usually in older children). Baclofen has been given by intrathecal pump with functional benefit. Botulinum toxin (Botox), a long-acting blocker of transmission at the myoneural junction, can be injected directly into the muscle and has resulted in reduction of tone. Again, functional goals should be identified and monitored in this intervention.
- Medications to control involuntary movements are sometimes useful as an effective

Table 32-3 Suggestions for use of nonmedical specialties *(continued)*

Service	Common useful indications	Comments
Psychometric testing	All children with CP due to high prevalence of cognitive disorder Reevaluate in patients with suspected plateau, degeneration, or difficulty in school	Academic achievement testing may be handled by school Parent and teacher input needed in assessing discrepancies between IQ and achievement Special testing methods for children with severe motor or sensory impairment
Special education (private or school based)	Upon entering first grade or when change in placement is suggested To develop an individualized educational plan (TEP)	Classroom teacher input is invaluable Evaluation in conjunction with psychometric testing advised May not be necessary to have a special education evaluation if IQ<55
Behavioral psychology	Parent or teacher difficulty in managing behavioral problems When caretakers use excessive physical punishment	Behavior techniques may be enhanced by medication (e.g., stimulants) Teachers and other caretakers should be involved in program Planned management should be adaptable to home, school, and community
Social work	Often useful at initial diagnosis When difficulties in parent adaptation are noted Suspected child abuse When services are not easily accessed	To aid the clinician in attending to the many details involved in supervising care by the intricate network of agencies Respite care services may enhance the long-term outlook for family-provided care Evaluation in suspected child abuse is essential

[a]Developmental quotient (DQ) = Fine motor age (mileston-based) divided by chronologic age.
[b]Motor quotient (MoQ) = gross motor age (milestone-based) divided by chronologic age.
Adapted from Rosenblatt M, Palmer EB. Cerebral palsy. In RT Johnson (ed), *Current Therapy in Neurological Diseases* (3rd ed). Philadelphia: Decker, 1991.

adjunct in severe dyskinetic CP. Dopamine agonists and anticholinergics have been employed in treating dystonia and rigidity.

BIBLIOGRAPHY

For Parents

Books

Batshaw ML. *Children with Disabilities (5th ed)*. Baltimore: Paul H Brookes, 2002.
Miller F, Bachrach SJ. *Cerebral Palsy: A Complete Guide for Caregiving*. Baltimore: The Johns Hopkins University Press, 1995.
Pueschel SM, Bernier JC, Weidenman LE (eds). *The Special Child: A Source Book for Parents of Children with Developmental Disabilities*. Baltimore: Paul H Brookes, 1988.

Organizations

American Academy for Cerebral Palsy and Developmental Medicine 6300 North River Road, Suite 727 Rosemont, IL 60018 847-698-1635 www.aacpdm.org
Association of University Centers on Disabilities 1010 Wayne Avenue, Suite 920 Silver Spring, MD 20910 301-588-8252 www.aucd.org
The Council for Disability Rights 205 West Randolph, Suite 1650 Chicago, IL 60606 312-444-9484 www.disabilityrights.org
Disabled Sports USA 451 Hungerford Drive, Suite 100 Rockville, MD 20850 301-217-0960 www.dsusa.org
Exceptional Parent Magazine 555 Kinderkamack Road Oradell, NJ 07649-1517 Also see www.eparent.com for an extensive online resource for parents of children with disabilities compiled by Exceptional Parent Magazine.

United Cerebral Palsy Associations 1660 L Street, NW, Suite 700 Washington, DC 20036 1-800-872-5827 www.ucp.org

For Professionals

Capute AJ, Accardo PJ. *Developmental Disabilities in Infancy and Childhood* (3rd ed). Baltimore: Paul H Brookes, 2005 (in press).

Cheney PD, Palmer FB. Cerebral Palsy. *Ment Retard Dev Disabil Res Rev* 3:109–219, 1997. [This volume contains 12 articles reviewing various aspects of CP including epidemiology, treatment, and neuroimaging.]

Hoon AH, Johnston MV. Cerebral Palsy. In: AK Asbury, GM McKhann, WI McDonald, et al. *Disease of the Nervous System: Clinical Neuroscience and Therapeutic Principles* (3rd ed). Cambridge, UK: Cambridge University Press, 2002.

Kuban KC, Leviton A. Cerebral palsy. *N Engl J Med* 330:188–195, 1994.

Ment LR, Bada HS, Barnes P, et al. Practice parameter: neuroimaging of the neonate: report of the Quality Standards Subcommittee of the American Academy of Neurology and the Practice Committee of the Child Neurology Society. *Neurology* 58:1726–1738, 2002.

Nelson KB. The epidemiology of cerebral palsy in term infants. *Ment Retard Dev Disabil Res Rev* 8:146–150, 2002

Nelson KB. Can we prevent cerebral palsy? *N Engl J Med* 349:1765–1769, 2003.

33

Chronic Conditions

Ellen C. Perrin

I. **Description of the problem.** A chronic health condition is defined as one that
- Lasts, or is expected to last, for 3 months or longer, *and*
- Affects the child's usual age-appropriate activities, *or*
- Results in extensive hospitalization, home health services, or utilization of medical care in excess of that generally considered appropriate for a child of the same age

A. **Epidemiology.** Children with chronic health conditions are of increasing interest and importance to primary care clinicians because of (1) their increasing prevalence; (2) the growing recognition that these children and their families are at higher than usual risk for family stress, social isolation, and difficulties with social and psychological adjustment; and (3) the additional challenges they present for comprehensive pediatric care and coordination.

B. **Prevalence.** The true prevalence of chronic health conditions in childhood is unknown because the inclusiveness of definitions of "chronic health conditions" has been extremely varied.
- Estimates from the National Health Interview Survey on Disability indicate that chronic conditions of *any type* affect 15%–18% of US children and adolescents, although these estimates may undercount some child and adolescent conditions, especially obesity and mental health conditions.
- Overall, the prevalence of chronic health conditions in children has increased considerably over the past 25 years.
- A few specific conditions have decreased in prevalence because of greater availability of prevention; others have increased because of improvements in survival; a few new conditions have emerged (e.g., HIV infection); but the largest proportion of recent growth has been driven by a few high-prevalence conditions.
- Asthma now affects almost 9% of children and adolescents; obesity well over 12%; and mental health conditions are now estimated at more than 15%.

II. **Salient issues.** There are considerable commonalities in the experiences of children who have a chronic health condition and the experiences of their families (Table 33-1). In addition to those issues they share, important characteristics of children themselves, of parents and families, and of the specific conditions have considerable effects on the experience of having a chronic condition (Table 33-2).

A. **Characteristics of children.**
1. The age at which a child develops a chronic health condition, and the child's age at any particular time, independently contribute to the child's experience of the condition and the particular issues associated with its management (Table 33-3). For example, congenital conditions generally are associated with greater resiliency than conditions whose onset is during early adolescence.
2. Children's ability to manage their condition is related not only to their age but also to their understanding of the illness. Children with chronic health conditions are no more sophisticated than their healthy peers in their conceptual sophistication about the processes of illness causation and treatment. Healthy children and their peers with a chronic condition gain conceptual understanding of the processes of bodily functioning and of the prevention, causation, and treatment of illness along a predictable sequence of developmental stages parallel to those described in other domains by Piaget and others (Table 33-4).
3. It is important to assess the level of the child's cognitive sophistication about illness prior to instituting specific health education efforts, providing information about the condition, or determining appropriate expectations for the child's participation in the care and management of the condition. The child's intelligence, temperamental style, locus-of-control beliefs, self-concept, gender, and ethnic background all contribute to his/her resiliency in adapting to the extra stresses of a chronic health condition.

Table 33-1 Issues common in the presence of chronic health conditions

For children

Limitations in usual childhood activities because of the condition itself and medical care
 requirements
Need for medications, other treatments
Experience with doctors, nurses, other providers
Pain and discomfort
Experience with hospitalization
Feeling different from peers
Loneliness
Worry about the future
Dependency, loss of control
Stigma

For families

Extra burden of care
Financial drain
Interactions with complex medical system
Multiple doctors, nurses, other professionals
Restricted social networks
Difficulties with child care, short and long term
Special requirements of school
Necessity to inflict pain and discomfort
Interference with needs of other family members and of family system
Worries about long-term care, insurance
Uncertainty in daily life planning
Loneliness
Guilt
Anger
Stigma

Table 33-2 Factors affecting children's experience of a chronic health condition

Characteristics of the child	**Characteristics of the family**
Age of onset	Marital status
Personality/temperament	Number and ages of children
Intelligence	Parents' education
Self-concept	Parents' occupations
Gender	Financial situation
Ethnic background	Strength of parents' relationship
Developmental level	Parents' self-esteem
Understanding of illness	Extended family support
Locus-of-control beliefs	Social support network
	Ethnic background
Characteristics of the illness	
Age of onset	
Stable or unpredictable	
Prognosis	
Interference with mobility	
Interference with normal activities	
Visibility	
Academic effects	
Medications and other treatments	
Intensity of care requirements	
Discomfort	
Nervous system involvement	

Table 33-3 Challenging tasks for children with chronic health problems

	Primary task	Challenges
Infants and toddlers	Development of trust and security	Parental grief Altered eating/feeding experiences Restriction of movement Hospitalizations Painful procedures Chronic discomfort
Preschoolers	Development of autonomy	Medication requirements Dietary restrictions Mobility restrictions Need for adult supervision Repeated separations Impaired limit setting Limitations on peer interactions Differences from peers
School-aged children	Development of sense of mastery	Dependence on medical care Restrictions on independence Requirements for adult monitoring Medication and dietary requirements Activity restrictions School absence Altered body image Decreased growth
Adolescents	Development of personal identity separate from family	Visible deformity Requirements of medical supervision Medication and dietary requirements Vocational limitations Challenges to sexuality Enforced dependency

B. Characteristics of conditions.
   1. Certain kinds of health conditions present children with greater risks for difficult adjustment than do others. Unpredictable conditions and those that involve the CNS or cognitive dysfunction appear to present special challenges to children and families.
   2. The adjustment of children, of their siblings, and of their parents cannot be predicted simply from the severity of the condition. Some children with only moderate disease experience a greater impact on their lives and challenges to their psychological and social adjustment than do children who are more severely affected. The confusing experience of marginality, in which a child is neither clearly sick (and in need of special services and attention), nor clearly well, may result when a health condition is not obvious to peers and important adults and does not interfere noticeably with normal activity but still requires a special diet, medication, or medical care.
C. Characteristics of families. Parents, siblings, and extended family interactions play a very major part in children's successful adjustment.
   1. Parental reactions to a diagnosis of a chronic health condition and their adaptation to its long-term implications affect the coping resources of the child and his siblings. The risk of parental discord and divorce is somewhat greater for families that include a child with a chronic health condition, reflecting the additional stresses presented by the parenting and care of these children.
   2. Siblings also are at risk to feel less important than the child towards whom so much worry and attention is directed.
   3. The development of children's positive views of themselves is supported by their family's perception of their health condition as an incidental difficulty requiring shared problem solving, rather than as an intrusion on the family's functioning. The

Table 33-4 Typical progression in children's understanding of illness concepts

Cognitive level	Approximate age, years	Understanding of illness	Typical responses to *How do children get sick?*	Typical responses to *How do children keep from getting sick?*	Typical responses to *How can children get better?*
1		No response; does not know; inappropriate or off-task response			
2	4–6	Phenomenism: circular or phenomenistic response	"By catching something", "sometimes you just do"; "from throwing up"	"Stay healthy"; "go to doctor for checkups"	"Go to the doctor", "take medicines"
3	7–9	External agents: concrete, external causes cited; no explanation of how the agents interact with the body to result in, prevent, or cure illness	"If you go out in the rain without your boots"; "eating bad foods"; "from other people"	"Get shots", "stay away from sick people", "eat good foods"; "rest enough"	"Eat foods that are good for you"; "rest a lot", "do what the doctor says"
4	10–13	Internalization: internalization and/or relativity in understanding of illness; once agent is internalized, illness follows invariably	"Germs get in and spread all over your body"; "when you breathe in sick people's germs"	"Take special vitamins that will keep your body strong"; "rest/food/exercise . . . give your body what it needs"	"Do different things for different illnesses"; "get more sleep than usual"; "take the right kind of medicine to give your body what it needs"
5	10–13	Interaction: interaction of host and agent described; some effect of agent on body	"Germs get in your system and start to eat/kill your cells"; "interference with normal body parts"	"If your body is strong from eating what you should, it will be able to resist the germs"; "exercising keeps the bones in place so they can work right"	"Resting allows your body not to waste its energy so it can fight the germs better"; "vitamins help the body to repair what's not working right"
6	>14	Mechanisms: processes of illness causation, prevention, or treatment described; includes notion of bodily response	"Germs take away food from the body and then the body has nothing to use for power"; "eat something that messes up your muscles so your heart doesn't work right"	"The right foods nourish the fighting cells so they are powerful enough to kill germs that get inside you"	"Good food/vitamins help your body to make more blood so the cells can fight off the germs"; "make your heart stronger so your body has better defenses"

family's ability to attend to each member's needs for nurturance and attention, to express and deal with conflict, to support the independence of all members, and to provide both structure and flexibility are critical to children's successful adaptation.

III. **Management.** Maintaining optimal growth and development in the presence of a chronic health condition is a challenge to families, to primary care clinicians, and to the children themselves. While there is a somewhat greater risk of psychological, social, and educational difficulties for children with chronic health conditions, most of them and most of their families adapt successfully to the extra challenges they confront.

   A. Primary care clinicians have the opportunity—and therefore also the responsibility—to be available to families over a long period of time. They are often the first professional person consulted about issues of concern to children and their parents. Thus, they are in a unique position to **support families and to help them to coordinate their child's care.** In addition to ensuring that these children receive all usual preventive and acute illness care and health supervision, the primary care clinician should serve as an effective interface among subspecialty and surgical teams, early intervention and family support programs, schools, third-party payers, nursing services, and a large variety of other care providers.

   B. Primary care clinicians also should provide regular **monitoring** of the child's development, the emotional and social adaptation of children, parents, and siblings, and **referral** for appropriate mental health services when indicated. Such comprehensive attention to overall health care supervision for children with ongoing health conditions has been made easier in some states with new coding guidelines that allow supplemental third-party reimbursement for extended office visits, case conferences, and sometimes lengthy telephone-assisted care.

   C. Primary care clinicians need to know the **resources available** in their own community. They should have, or be able to develop, effective contacts with local school systems, the resources of the department of public health, home nursing and respite care services, and sources of specialty medical and surgical care. In addition, they can provide community-specific information regarding supportive networks of children with health conditions and of their parents and their siblings.

   D. The clinician also has a responsibility to **assure appropriate education** of children and their families about the health condition and its management. In addition, they should help parents to plan for an appropriate school program, with attention to the integration of the child's medical and educational needs. Excessive school absences that result from the course of a condition itself and from requirements for its care can be made less disruptive by home tutoring services for long-term and for predictable short-term absences. Effective communication among the school system, the pediatric clinician, and the family can make overall healthcare management and transitions between school and home care efficient and effective.

BIBLIOGRAPHY

For Parents

National Information Center for Children and Youth with Disabilities (NICHCY). National information and referral center on disabilities and disability-related issues; offers state resource information.NICHCY P.O. Box 1492 Washington, DC 20013 1-800-695-0285 nichcy@aed.org www.nichcy.org

DisabilityInfo.gov. Information and resources for children and adults with special needs, and their families. Information on education, health, housing, technology, and much more. www.disabilityinfo.gov

Exceptional Parent. Monthly publication for families, addressing a wide range of topics related to children and youth with disabilities. 65 East Route 4 River Edge, NJ 07661 201-489-4111 1-800-535-1910 (library and information line) www.eparent.com

Family Village. Wide variety of specific resources for families who care for children and adults with disabilities. Spanish resources available throughout site. Waisman Center University of Wisconsin-Madison 1500 Highland Avenue Madison, WI 53705-2280 www.familyvillage.wisc.edu

Family Voices. National grassroots organization of families and friends of children with special health needs. State chapters and coordinators. Many publications on health care issues and resources. Spanish resources available throughout site. 3411 Candelaria NE, Suite M Albuquerque, NM 87107 1-888-835-5669 kidshealth@familyvoices.org www.familyvoices.org

Federation for Children with Special Needs. Provides advocacy and support for families in the areas of health, education, early childhood, and transition for children and young adults with special needs. 135 Tremont Street, Suite 420 Boston, MA 02120 617-236-7210 1-800-331-0688 (in MA) fcsninfo@fcsn.org www.fcsn.org

Beach Center on Families and Disability. Listserves and links to local and regional parent to parent organizations. 3136 Haworth Hall The University of Kansas Lawrence, Kansas 66045 785-864-7600 shttp://www.beachcenter.org/groups

For Professionals

Lavigne JV, Faier-Routman J. Psychological adjustment to pediatric physical disorders: a meta-analytic review. *J Ped Psych*, 17:133–157, 1992.

McMenamy JM, Perrin EC. Filling the GAPS: care of children with chronic health conditions in Pediatric Practice. *Ambul Pediatr* 4:(3)249–256, 2004.

Newacheck PW, Strickland B, Shonkoff JP, et al. An epidemiologic profile of children with special health care needs. *Pediatrics* 102:117–123, 1998.

Perrin EC, Gerrity PS. Development of children with chronic illness. *Pediatr Clin North Am* 31: 19, 1984.

Perrin EC, Schott J. Somehow We'll Make it Work: Interviews with Children with a Chronic Condition and Their Families. Available from the author (eperrin@tufts-nemc.org) as VHS tape (55 minutes) or in PowerPoint on CD.

Perrin EC, Lewkowicz C, Young MH. Shared Vision: concordance among fathers, mothers, and pediatricians about unmet needs of children with chronic health conditions. *Pediatrics* 105: 277–285, 2000.

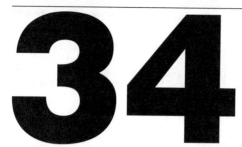

Colic

Steven Parker

I. **Description of the problem.** There is no reliably objective definition of colic. The most commonly accepted definition, Wessel's criteria, defines colic as crying for *more than 3 hours per day, for 3 or more days per week* for more than 3 weeks. By these standards, however, half of all infants would be classified as colicky. Additionally, parental tolerance for infant crying is quite variable: some are stoic in the face of constant crying, while others come to the primary care clinician for the occasional whimper. The best definition of colic may be a purely clinical one: colic is *any recurrent inconsolable* crying in a *healthy and well-fed infant* that is experienced by the parents or caregivers as a problem.

A. **Epidemiology.**
   - Estimates range from 7%–25%, depending on the criteria for diagnosis
   - No differences by gender, breast- vs bottle-fed, full-term vs preterm, or birth order
   - 2x increased risk if maternal smoking during pregnancy
   - Whites > nonwhites
   - Industrialized countries > nonindustrialized
   - More frequent the farther away from the equator
   - Increased incidence of physical abuse in colicky infants

B. **Clinical features.**
   1. Colic typically begins at **41–42 weeks gestational age** (including preterm infants).
   2. **Two patterns** of colic have been noted.
      a. **Paroxysmal fussing** typically occurs between 5–8 PM. The infant is contented and easily soothed at other times of the day. These infants do not cry more frequently over 24 hours; rather, they sporadically cry for a longer period of time.
      b. **The hyperirritable infant** is one whose crying occurs at all hours of the day, often in response to ambiguous external or internal stimuli. They may also exhibit increased tone and other signs of hyperarousal.
   3. Colic **stops as mysteriously as it starts,** by 3 months in 60% and by 4 months in 80-90% of infants.
   4. There are **no predictable long-term outcomes** (behavioral, temperamental, or psychological) that emerge from a colicky infancy.

C. **Etiology.** Theories of causation abound (Table 34-1), but evidence for any one is scant. It appears likely that there is no single cause of colic and that it represents the final common pathway for a number of etiologic factors.

II. **Making the diagnosis.**
A. **History: Key clinical questions.**
   1. *"When does the crying occur? How long does it last?"* The timing of the cry provides useful information. For example, if it occurs directly after a feeding, aerophagia or gastroesophageal reflux may be considered. If it occurs reliably 1 hour after feedings, a formula intolerance is possible. If the crying occurs only from 5–7 PM every day, it is difficult to posit an organic problem that would cause pain at only one time of the day.
   2. *"What do you do when your baby cries?"* It is important to determine how the parents have tried (successfully and unsuccessfully) to console the infant. In some cases, their techniques may have inadvertently worsened the situation (e.g., anxiously overstimulating a hypersensitive infant); in other cases, the technique may be inappropriate (e.g., giving half-strength formula).
   3. *"What does the cry sound like?"* Most parents can distinguish a cry of pain from that of hunger. Additionally, the description of the cry provides insight into parental distress, empathy, or anger with the cry.
   4. *"Tell me how and what you feed your baby."* Underfeeding, overfeeding, air swallowing, and inadequate burping have all been implicated in colic.
   5. *"How does it make you feel when your baby cries?"* History taking is an opportune time to begin the process of parental support. Opening up the subjects of parental

Table 34-1 Theories of the etiology of colic

Gastrointestinal

Cow's milk protein intolerance (an equal number of studies have found an association of cow's milk with colic as have not)

Gastroesophageal reflux

Lactose intolerance (higher breath H_2 level in some colicky infants)

Immature gastrointestinal system (ineffective peristalsis; incomplete digestion; gas)

Faulty feeding techniques (e.g., under- or overfeeding, infrequent burping)

Hormones causing enterospasm

Increased motilin levels (one study showed higher levels of motilin, but not vasoactive intestinal peptide or gastrin, in colicky infants)

Decreased cholecystokinin levels ($\rightarrow$ gallbladder contractions)

Hormonal

Increased circulating serotonin (hypothetical only but an attractive hypothesis because serotonin has a circadian rhythm in infancy, which could explain the curious timing of paroxysmal fussing)

Progesterone deficiency (one study in 1963, never repeated)

Neurological

Imbalance of autonomic nervous system (parasympathetric >> sympathetic)

Immature neurotransmittors

Nonestablished circadian rhythm

Temperamental

Difficult temperament (but there is poor correlation of colic and later temperament)

Hypersensitivity (crying at end of day represents discharge after a long day of shutting out intrusive environmental stimuli)

Parental handling

Most studies do not show a relationship between parental anxiety, psychopathology, and/or emotional difficulties and colic; at most, nonoptimal handling may exacerbate but not cause the symptoms

guilt, helplessness, and anxiety sends the message that these topics merit discussion. Some parents are especially worried about their anger toward the screaming child, believing that such anger is the mark of a bad parent. Others seek pediatric attention because they are afraid of actually harming the infant during a crying spell.

6. *"How has the colic affected your family?"* Colic is a *family* issue. In some cases it may disturb the parents' relationship with each other, cause distress in a sibling, or serve as a forum for blaming the parents (e.g., by grandparents).

7. *"What is your theory of why the baby cries?"* In order to support the family, their hypotheses for the crying must be understood. Some may view it as a curse, others as a rebuke to their parenting skills, and others as a sign that something is terribly wrong with the baby.

B. **Physical examination.** A thorough physical examination serves to rule out medical problems that cause pain or discomfort, as well as to reassure the parents that the infant is physically well. However, in only about 5% will a definable medical cause be found. Any problem that causes pain can lead to hyperirritability (but rarely to paroxysmal fussing).

- Infections (otitis media, urinary tract, oral herpes)
- Gastrointestinal (diarrhea, constipation, gastroesophageal reflux)
- Genitourinary (posterior urethral valves)
- CNS (intra- or extracranial hemorrhage, hydrocephalus)
- Ophthalmologic (corneal abrasion, glaucoma)
- Cardiac (supraventricular tachycardia)
- Narcotic withdrawal syndrome (especially methadone)
- Fracture, hernia, anal fissures
- Tourniquet (on toe or finger)

The diagnosis of colic is predicated on the infant being healthy and well fed. Only after a thorough history and physical examination do not reveal an obvious source of pain should the diagnosis of colic be considered.

III. **Management.**

A. **Shotgun approach.** Because the cause of colic is rarely clear, a shotgun approach is often helpful. Table 34-2 lists suggestions for parents to help them deal with colic. The

Table 34-2 Suggestions for parents to help colic

	Strategy	Comments
Feeding/ nutritional	Change formula from cow's milk to soy based	Emphasize to parent that it is a clinical trial, that it might not work, and that changing formulas does not mean that there is anything physically wrong with the baby
	Change formula from soy based to predigested	Expensive but sometimes effective
	If breast-feeding, have mother stop cow's milk, caffeine, etc.	One study showed increased bovine IgG in the breast milk of mothers of colicky babies
		Ask the breast-feeding mother which foods seem to be associated with increased irritability
	Change nipple or bottle; feed in upright position with frequent burping	Try to decrease air swallowing (e.g., by using bottle with a plastic liner)
Alternate sensory stimulation	Supplemental daytime carrying	One study found little benefit of supplemental carrying for truly colicky infants
	Front carrier (e.g., Snugli)	Allows hand to be free while carrying
	Car seat on dishwasher or drier	Must be observed, because the seat can shift
	Ride in the car	Not advisable in the middle of the night if driver is sleepy
	Change of scenery	New sights can distract from the distress
	Pacifier	In Herman Meyer's words, "If for no other reason than to obstruct the opening from which the cacophonous sound emanates"
	Swing	Rarely allows more than 30 min. of relief
	Belly massage	Use a lubricating lotion
	Swaddling	Especially good for babies who are hypersensitive to body movements or touch
	Heartbeat tape or white noise generator	Especially good for babies who are hypersensitive to noise
	Hot-water bottle on belly	Should not be too hot
	SleepTight (device that generates white noise and vibrates the bed)	Some pediatric practices have the device available to loan to patients. (Two controlled studies, however, have shown disappointing benefits)
	Warm bath	
Medications	Herbal tea (e.g., chamomile, spearmint, fennel)	A study of chamomile/verbena/licorice/fennel/mint tea found improvement in 57% of colicky infants
	Simethicone	Probably harmless, dubiously helpful
	Antispasmodics	**Should not be used.** Despite some evidence of efficacy, there have been case reports of respiratory arrests associated with their use in infants

history and physical examination may point to one line of treatment as potentially more useful than another. As a general rule, **most treatments for colic work in 30% of infants, but none works for all infants.** It is best to try only one or two interventions at a time. This allows for the effective measure to be more easily identified. Additionally, since *nothing* may work very well, it is helpful to keep a few suggestions in reserve, at least until the process runs its course at 3–4 months.

B. **Parental support.** Colic is a benign, self-limited problem with no untoward sequelae. Its impact on the early parent–child relationship should be of primary concern. Long after the crying abates, the consequences of an impaired parent–infant relationship can do damage. Therefore, the primary role for the clinician in the management of colic is to support the family through a difficult period and ensure that no untoward interactions are set up.

1. **Inform the family.** The mysterious but benign nature of colic should be reiterated. The family will need constant reassurance that nothing is physically wrong with the infant. This is best accomplished by frequent physical examinations to assure the family that nothing has been missed and an emphasis on the otherwise normal growth and development of the infant. The usual time course should be explained but not to downplay the family's current distress (e.g., *"I know how distressing it is to care for an inconsolable infant. I've seen a lot of colicky babies, and fortunately it almost always disappears by 3–4 months. In the meantime, let's see what we can do to help things here and now"*).

2. **Lessen parental feelings of guilt.** Most parents (especially inexperienced ones) feel that the crying occurs because of something that they are doing wrong. They require reassurance that this is not the case and that colic occurs with even the most attentive, loving, and experienced of caregivers. *"You aren't doing anything wrong. This is coming from your baby."*

3. **Empathize and depathologize parental feelings of resentment and anger.** Many parents are mortified by the ambivalent and frankly negative feelings engendered by their crying infant. They should be reassured that *all* parents feel some resentment and anger toward their colicky infant, that it does not make them bad parents, and that these feelings are short-lived. In some cases, parental fear of harming the baby during an episode should be taken seriously and a brief hospitalization may be indicated to provide respite. *"All parents have these feelings. Just let me know if you are ever so worried you could be at the breaking point and could get so mad you could hurt the baby."*

4. **Provide close and consistent follow-up.** Parents should call the clinician within 48 hours of the first visit to report on progress. If no progress is evident, a second visit can be scheduled within a week for further discussion and to reassure them that there is no organic problem. The parents need to be able to count on the clinician's availability during this difficult time. *"Let me see you back in a week to see how things are going. And call any time. Let me know how it is going. I have many tricks for colic up my sleeve. If one doesn't work, we'll try another. Don't worry, we'll get through this."*

5. **Remind the beleaguered parents that it is permissible to take breaks from the baby.** If the baby cries inconsolably despite all reasonable interventions, it is permissible to put the baby down and let him or her cry for increasingly longer periods of time before attempting another consoling maneuver. *"You've tried everything and she's still crying. Why not put her down for a while and let her cry without your holding her and see if she can calm down on her own."*

   • Parents can be reassured that crying is healthy for the lungs, that (especially since the infant is crying anyway) it is not emotionally damaging for the infant to cry alone for a while at this age, and that such isolation teaches some infants how to self-console. Some parents find letting their infant cry unattended to be intolerable. They should be supported in handling the problem in the way that is most comfortable to them.

   • Parents should also be encouraged to take breaks from the baby by letting a friend, family member, or babysitter attend to him or her for a few hours while the parents go out of the house for some unrestricted free time. They should be reminded that the crying is not as emotionally wrenching for a nonparent to hear and that they can best serve their baby when they themselves are refreshed. *"You know it's okay to leave her with someone else for a while. You both could use a break from each other every now and then."*

BIBLIOGRAPHY

For Parents

Websites

www.colichelp.com

For Professionals

Brazelton TB. Crying in infancy. *Pediatrics* 29:579–588, 1962.

Clifford TJ, Campbell MK, Speechley KN, et al. Sequelae of infant colic: evidence of transient infant distress and absence of lasting effects on maternal mental health. *Arch Ped Adolesc Med* 156:1183–1188, 2002.

Kilgour T, Wade S. Infantile colic. *Clinical Evidence* 7:321–330, 2002.

Wade S, Kilgour T. Infantile colic. *MJ.* 323:437–440, 2001.

Wessel MA, et al. Paroxysmal fussing in infancy, sometimes called "colic." *Pediatrics* 14:421–434, 1954.

35

Depression

Michael Jellinek

I. **Description of the problem.** Childhood major depressive disorder (MDD) is characterized by a significant, often recurrent emotional and behavioral change from baseline to a dysphoric or irritable mood, loss of pleasure or fun, and with decreased functioning in the home, in school and with peers.

A. **Epidemiology/incidence.** Incidence figures depend on criteria for diagnosis which are hard to measure precisely given age and subjective nature of this disorder. Estimates below are moderate to severe depression with dysfunction.

   1. **MDD in the pediatric population.**
      a. **Infants and preschoolers** : 1%. Seen as failure to thrive, as well as attachment, separation, and behavioral problems.
      b. **School age children** : 2%. Closer fit to adolescent/adult criteria. Typically heralds a more protracted, recurrent, or severe course. Suicide attempts and completions uncommon to rare.
      c. **Adolescents:** 5% +. Presents more like the adult syndrome and typically requires evaluation of suicidality and substance use.

   2. **MDD in specialized populations.**
      a. As many as 7% of general pediatric inpatients (especially with chronic disease) and 28% of child psychiatry clinic patients.

   3. **Comorbid diagnoses in children with MDD.** 60%–80% of children meeting criteria for MDD have additional or comorbid disorders, such as anxiety, attention deficit, substance abuse, and conduct problems, including lying, stealing, vandalism, and truancy. Comprehensive treatment planning must include and integrate comorbid disorders.

B. **Etiology/contributing factors.**

   1. **Genetic.** The biologic offspring of depressed adults are up to 3 times more likely to have MDD, which may present earlier and recur more frequently. Research suggests a polygenetic inheritance.

   2. **Environmental.** Distinguishing etiologic environmental factors that cause MDD from those that are coincidental to or a consequence of MDD is difficult. Children identify with, learn from, and share the mood of their parents and siblings. They are greatly affected by losses, especially parental death and divorce, and other stresses including trauma and abuse. The boundary between extended bereavement and MDD requires careful monitoring.

   3. **Organic.** It is hypothesized that a biochemical imbalance in norepinephrine may contribute to the fatigue of MDD; an imbalance in serotonin may cause the problems of irritability and anxiety. Many acute medical conditions (including toxic ingestions, metabolic disturbances, and CNS infections) and several chronic medical illnesses can lead to changes in appetite, weight loss, decreased energy, or irritable mood.

   4. **Developmental.** Adolescence is a time of change, of puberty, of separation, of transition from the familiar childhood family unit in the context of evolving autonomy. Intrapsychic depressive experiences become more differentiated and specific as emotional, language, cognitive, and social development proceed. Young children with MDD may simply experience a vague and overwhelming discomfort, while older children may come to use *stomachache, headache* or feeling fearful as words for internal mood states. Such abstract terms as depression and age-appropriate symptoms like *blue, bored, empty, down and bothered, angry or irritable* are more likely to be used in early adolescence.

   5. **Transactional.** The interaction of environmental contributions from school, home and peers differs at different developmental stages and is influenced by genetic and organic factors. Some factors such as a special skill, relationship or intellectual strength may foster resiliency; other factors such as family tension may act as a stressor. Some school-aged children with MDD lose their ability to concentrate in

school, causing performance and peer relationships to suffer. Other children are able to control their mood swings while at school, only to collapse into a depressed or irritable mood on safe arrival home.

II. **Making the diagnosis (see Table 35-1).**

   A. **Signs, symptoms and behavioral observations.** The new Diagnostic Statistical Manual for Primary Care (DSM-PC) gives an excellent range of presentations typical in primary care settings and is organized by symptoms rather than only by diagnosis.

      1. **Infant/toddler.** Both the persistently passive, unresponsive infant and the irritable, unsoothable, crying infant may suffer from the mood dysregulation associated with depression. Their clinical presentations may evolve into a quiet, inhibited toddler with arrested social development or an overactive, impulsive, and irritable pre-schooler.

      2. **School age.** In school-aged children with MDD, the expected pride associated with industry and enthusiasm may be overwhelmed by humiliation, defeat, irritability, and self-doubt. The child may become sad, isolated, rejected, and accident prone. Temper tantrums or morbid preoccupations with bodily injury, illness, abandonment, or death might emerge. There may be pediatric office visits for multiple somatic complaints. Bereavement may not gradually ease to normal functioning, but instead persist to a full depressive state.

Table 35-1 Criteria for child and adolescent major depressive episode

Depressed mood or loss of interests or pleasure in activities at home, at school, or with peers for at least 2 weeks or more than 50% of the time. Coincident with depressed mood, changes in *at least 4* of the following	Including sad, blue, bored, empty, oppositional, irritable, angry, and rageful feelings
Appetite or weight	In relation to expected weight gain; may present in infants and preschoolers as a feeding difficulty and in adolescents as anorexia or obesity
Sleep patterns	Including insomnia, hypersomnia, and frequent wakenings
Agitation	Including restlessness and aggressiveness; infants may be fussy and school-aged children hyperactive
Social withdrawal	In infants and preschoolers, problems of attachment and separation or loss of spontaneous play; in school-aged children, school reluctance, school phobia or a sudden drop in school performance or after-school activities
Energy loss	Including listlessness, fatigue, and lethargy
Self-esteem	In school-aged children, feelings of stupidity, clowning around, or engaging in self-reproachful boasting; in adolescents, expressions of guilt, self-deprecation, helplessness, or hopelessness
Concentration	In infants and preschoolers, speech and motor delays or regression; with children or adolescents in school, sustained change in ability to attend in class, complete assignments out of class, concentrate, or make decisions
Dangerousness	In infants, possibly head banging; in school-aged children, accident proneness; in adolescents, stealing, lying, and truancy
Somatic symptoms	In infants and preschoolers, failure to thrive and rumination; in school-aged children, enuresis, encopresis, and vague complaints; in adolescents, complaints of abdominal or head pain
Suicidal ideation	Recurrent thoughts or death or morbid preoccupation with illness, accidents and/or death
Substance use	

3. **Adolescents.** May have difficulty containing intense negative feelings. Experiencing a crushing defeat or rejection, they both have the passion and the means to act on self-destructive urges. They may have direct negative actions inward against themselves by disregarding food, sleep, and hygiene. Some turn to alcohol and drugs for numbing symptomatic relief or engage in destructive behaviors. Instead of appearing sad and eliciting sympathy (as adults with MDD might), adolescents with MDD often seem irritable, angry and resentful. Given the danger of depression and substance use, especially the high mortality of teenage accidents, this age group merits special attention, especially direct questions, in private, concerning their mood and behavior.

B. **History: Key clinical questions.**

1. *"How is your child's mood? How does the child feel about himself or herself? For how many days, weeks, months, has this been the case?"* Diagnosis of MDD requires at least a 2-week period of prominent mood related symptoms, but pediatric clinicians may see shorter periods of sadness or milder persistent symptoms. Parental depression can have an environmental as well as genetic impact on children; most parental depression goes unrecognized and untreated.

2. *"Has there been a recent change in your child's behavior, school performance, or peer relationships?"* A decrease in functioning or significant change in behaviors can be a key indicator of mood related stress and disability (and should be evident in all areas of daily functioning).

3. *"Does your child have a past history of feeling down, or has he ever seen a mental health professional in the past?"* Studies indicate a high risk for recurrence for MDD.

4. *"Does anyone in the extended family have a history of depression, mania, anxiety, attention deficits, or alcohol or substance use?"* Family psychiatric history is an important predictor of childhood risk. The incidence of depression in mothers, in general, is approximately 5%; mothers of young children or those facing marital discord are at higher risk.

5. *"Is your child often intensely worried? Profoundly anxious? Impulsive or inattentive? Prone to lie or steal?"* Identifying and clarifying comorbid diagnoses makes for more effective treatment.

6. *"If depressed, has your child ever brought harm to himself, even accidentally? Has the child ever talked or threatened to hurt himself or others?"* (And to the child: *"Have you ever felt so bad that you wanted to hurt yourself?"*). Self-destructive acts or threats must be taken seriously and should automatically lead to a careful suicide assessment and referral for psychiatric evaluation and follow-up. (See chapter on suicide.)

III. **Management.**

A. **Primary goals.** Most children with MDD can be safely cared for as outpatients. For mild to moderate depression, pediatric clinicians wishing to include this work in their practice, can consider assessing family history of MUD, noting short-term stressors and encouraging more support for the child. For moderate to severe MDD or where watchful waiting has seen the child's mood state persist or worsen, the comprehensive treatment of childhood MDD is beyond the expertise of most primary care clinicians and should be referred to a mental health professional. The primary care clinician should monitor the treatment through the ongoing relationship with the family. Urgent psychiatric consultation is indicated whenever the child or adolescent might be psychotic, acutely suicidal, abusing substances, or otherwise difficult to manage safely.

B. **Treatment strategies.** The strategies listed below are often integrated by experienced clinicians as clinically indicated. The pediatric clinician faces the difficult challenge of defining the symptoms, issues and convincing parents to accept and complete a mental health referral.

1. **Psychodynamic therapy** attempts to provide a safe and supportive environment for the child to explore, understand, and learn to express inner feelings and conflicts. It is often most effective for children and adolescents with low self-esteem. Play therapy is used in younger children who do not yet effectively use words to convey inner experiences.

2. **Cognitive-behavior therapy** reviews and challenges negative thoughts, actions, and feelings in a systematic and logical way.

3. **Family therapy** views the family as a system unto itself and attempts to identify behavioral patterns and alliances that keep the family from developing or changing. It is often best for multiply stressed families and can be an important avenue for early detection of depression in other family members.

4. **Group therapy** views the child in a social and interactive context. It is often useful for developing social skills and social support.
5. **Parent guidance** helps parents to learn to deal with depression in their children or in themselves. Parents who feel personally overwhelmed or confused by the parental role may find this approach helpful. Depressed parents should be referred for psychiatric evaluation.
6. **Environmental interventions** aim to support academic performance and raise a child's self-esteem through the use of role models and positive experiences that foster industry, responsibility and pride. A carefully chosen summer or after-school activity, hobby, or encouragement of a friendship can be invaluable.
7. **Medications** focus on correcting biochemical imbalances. Studies regarding the efficacy of desipramine and imipramine are inconclusive. Selective serotonin reuptake inhibitors (SSRIs) are increasingly being presented to children based on their efficacy with adults and seemingly low risk of side effects.However the high rate of placebo response in children makes distinguishing the efficacy of SSRIs difficult and only recently have studies demonstrated efficacy in adolescents (not yet in children). Parental responsiveness to a particular medication may be a guide for children with moderate to severe, recurrent depression. Currently there is concern for both underuse and overuse of SSRIs as well as little understanding of any long term side effects.

C. **Primary care follow-up.** The clinician should follow specific psychological symptoms over time, watch for side effects of medications, monitor patient compliance, and encourage appropriate child psychiatric follow-up.

BIBLIOGRAPHY

For Parents

CABF (Child and Adolesent Bipolar Foundation) www.bpkids.org
Greene R. *The Explosive Child: A new approach for understanding and parenting easily frustrated, "chronically inflexible" children.* New York, NY: Harper Collins, 1998.
Let's Talk Facts About Childhood Disorders, Manic-Depressive Disorder. Washington, DC: American Psychiatric Press, 1992.
National Institute of Mental Health
  http://www.nimh.nih.gov/HealthInformationdep/childmenu.cfm
Papolos D, Papolos J. *The Bipolar Child and reassuring guide to childhood's most misunderstood disorder.* New York, NY: Broadway books, 2002.

For Professionals

Coyle JT, Pine DS, Charney DS, et al. and The Depression and Bipolar Support Alliance Consensus Development Panel. Depression and bipolar support alliance consensus statement on the unmet needs in diagnosis and treatment of mood disorders in children and adolescents. *JAACAP* 42: 1494–1503, 2003.
McClellan JM, Werry JS. Evidence-based treatments in child and adolescent psychiatry: An inventory. *JAACAP* 42:1388–1400, 2003.
Rutter M, Taylor E (eds). *Child and Adolescent Psychiatry: Modern Approaches* (4th ed). London: Blackwell Scientific Publishers, 2002.

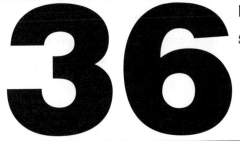

Down Syndrome

Siegfried M. Pueschel

I. **Description of the problem. Definition:** The child with Down syndrome has recognizable physical characteristics and limited intellectual functioning due to the presence of an extra chromosome 21 or part of a specific section of the long arm of chromosome 21.

A. **Epidemiology.**
- Estimated incidence of Down syndrome is between 1 in 800–1,200 live births.
- 3,000–5,000 children with Down syndrome are born each year in the United States.
- There has been a slight decrease in the birth prevalence due to the increased utilization of prenatal screening (alpha fetoprotein, unconjugated estriol, free beta human chorionic gonadotropin, PAPP-A, inhibin-A, and ultrasonography) and diagnostic techniques (chorionic villus sampling, amniocentesis, and other procedures), leading to subsequent termination of the pregnancy.
- There is a higher prevalence in the population because of an increased life expectancy.

B. **Genetics.** There are four main types of chromosome abnormalities in Down syndrome.
1. **Trisomy 21** is observed in the vast majority (93%–95%) of children with Down syndrome.
2. **Translocation** occurs in 4%–6% of children with Down syndrome. Most translocations involve the attachment of the long arms of the supernumerary chromosome 21 to chromosome 14, 21, or 22 . If a translocation is identified in a child with Down syndrome, the parents' chromosomes need to be examined, since in about one third of the cases a parent may be a carrier of the translocation. Genetic counseling is recommended.
3. **Mosaicism** occurs in approximately 1%–2% of children with Down syndrome.
4. A rare chromosome aberration, **partial trisomy 21**, is noted in some persons with Down syndrome.
5. Much progress has been made in molecular genetics. Recent genome studies revealed that there are more than 360 genes encoded on chromosome 21.

C. **Etiology.** Many etiologies of Down syndrome have been posited including radiation, viral infections, genetic predisposition, autoimmunue processes, and others. It is well known that advanced maternal age is a definite risk factor that may be associated with problems in production line, persistent nucleoli, hormonal imbalance, delayed fertilization, and relaxed selection. Most of these theories are tentative. Recent investigations suggest that the absence or reduced proximal recombination appears to predispose to nondisjunction in meiosis I and the presence or increase of proximal exchanges predisposes to nondisjunction in meiosis II. In addition, some studies indicate an increased incidence of Down syndrome in diabetic mothers and in females with only one ovary.

II. **Making the diagnosis.**

A. **Signs and symptoms.** There is a wide variability in the characteristics of children with Down syndrome. Some individuals have only a few signs, whereas others show most of the features as listed in Table 36-1.

B. **Differential diagnosis.** The main features of Down syndrome are often recognized by the clinician in the neonatal period. However, on rare occasions children with other chromosomal aberrations may display a similar phenotype (e.g., newborns with 49, XXXXX syndrome may have similar facial features). Conformation by chromosome analysis is mandatory.

C. **Medical concerns.** Some of the medical concerns of newborn children with Down syndrome may be life-threatening and require immediate correction, whereas others may only become apparent during subsequent days and weeks or in later life.
1. **Neonatal medical problems.**
   a. **Congenital heart disease** is diagnosed in 40%–50% of children with Down syndrome (most often atrioventricular canal, followed by ventricular septal defect, Tetralogy of Fallot, patent ductus arteriosus and atrial septal defect). All new-

Table 36-1 Percentage of phenotypic findings in a group of 114 infants with Down syndrome (abbreviated list)

Sagittal suture separated	98
Oblique palpebral fissures	98
Wide space between first and second toes	96
False fontanel (widening of sagittal suture at the parietal area)	95
Plantar crease between first and second toes	94
Increased neck tissue	87
Abnormally shaped palate	85
Hypoplastic nose	83
Brushfield spots	75
Mouth kept open	65
Protruding tongue	58
Epicanthal folds	57
Single palmar crease	53
Brachyclinodactyly	51
Short stubby hands	38
Flattened occiput	35
Abnormal structure of ears	28

borns with Down syndrome should be examined by a pediatric cardiologist and undergo echocardiography.

   b. Anomalies of the gastrointestinal tract including tracheo-esophageal fistula, esophageal atresia, pyloric stenosis, duodenal atresia, duodenal stenosis or webs, annular pancreas, aganglionic megacolon, imperforate anus and others occur in about 5%–12% of infants with Down syndrome. Many of these congenital anomalies require immediate surgical attention.

   c. Congenital cataracts are identified in approximately 3% of newborns with Down syndrome. These cataracts are usually very dense and need to be extracted soon after birth.

 2. Medical problems during childhood.

   a. Nutritional aspects. During infancy, feeding problems and poor weight gain may be observed, especially in infants with significant congenital heart disease. On the other hand, excessive weight gain often becomes a problem in later childhood and during adolescence. Parents need to be informed with regard to appropriate dietary practices, proper eating habits, avoidance of high caloric foods, and regular physical exercise starting in early childhood.

   b. Infections. Children with Down syndrome have a high prevalence of respiratory infections, especially those with congenital heart disease. Otitis media also has been noted to occur more frequently. Skin infections are often seen in adolescents with Down syndrome, mainly at the thighs, buttocks, and perigenital area.

   c. Dental concerns. Problems with tooth eruption, tooth shape, and sometimes absence or fusion of teeth are observed. The most devastating dental problems relate to gingivitis and periodontal disease. It is important that persons with Down syndrome practice appropriate dental hygiene, follow good dietary habits, and are examined regularly by a dentist.

   d. Visual impairment. Many children with Down syndrome have ocular disorders including blepharitis, strabismus, nystagmus, hypoplasia of the iris, and refractive errors. It has been reported that up to 40% of children are myopic and another 20% are hyperopic. Children with Down syndrome should be examined by a pediatric ophthalmologist annually.

   e. Audiologic dysfunction. Numerous reports from the literature indicate that about 60% of children with Down syndrome have some form of middle ear pathology, often resulting in a hearing deficit. Most of these deficits are due to a conductive hearing loss, and some children have neurosensory hearing impairment or a mixed hearing loss.

   f. Seizure disorders. There is an increased frequency (6%–10%) of seizure disorders in individuals with Down syndrome. Infantile spasms may be observed at a higher frequency in young children with Down syndrome during their first year of life, grand mal seizures as well as complex partial seizures are more often noted during adolescence and late adulthood.

    g. Sleep apnea. There have been several reports of sleep apnea due to upper airway obstruction in children with Down syndrome. These children usually present with noisy breathing, snoring, frequent apnea during sleep, sleepiness during daytime, and behavior disorders.

    h. Thyroid dysfunction. Up to 20% of children with Down syndrome have some form of thyroid dysfunction, usually compensated or uncompensated hypothyroidism. Also, hyperthyroidism has been observed in some children with Down syndrome. Because of the high prevalence of thyroid dysfunction, thyroid function tests should be carried out annually.

    i. Atlantoaxial instability. Atlantoaxial instability is due to increased ligamentous laxity at the upper cervical spine. Approximately 15% of children with Down syndrome have this disorder, although only 1%–2% have symptomatic atlantoaxial instability and usually require surgical intervention. Children with Down syndrome should have radiologic assessment of the cervical spine starting at the age of 2.5–3 years; before entering Special Olympics sport activities; and if indicated during adolescence. If asymptomatic atlantoaxial instability is present, it is recommended that the individual refrain from participating in sport activities that potentially could lead to injury of the neck and spinal cord compression. It is of utmost importance to prevent symptomatic atlantoaxial instability because of its devastating neurologic consequences.

    j. Orthopedic problems. There is an increased prevalence of hip dislocation, patellar subluxation, and metatarsus valgus in children with Down syndrome.

    k. Dermatological concerns. There are dermatological concerns such as alopecia, folliculitis, xerosis, cheilitis, onychomycosis, and others.

    l. Hematological diseases. Immunologic and hematologic issues (e.g. increased prevalence of leukemia) have been observed in children with Down syndrome.

    m. Gastrointestinal disorders. Gastroesophageal reflux and celiac disease occur at a higher frequency in children with Down syndrome.

III. Management.

    A. Primary goals. The main objective of appropriate management is to provide optimal medical and surgical care to all persons with Down syndrome. No form of treatment should be withheld from any child with Down syndrome that would be given unhesitatingly to a child without this chromosome disorder.

    B. Information for families

        1. Initial counseling. Although there is no completely satisfactory way of giving "bad news" to parents the clinician's positive approach, tact, compassion, and truthfulness will have a vital influence on the parent's subsequent adjustment. The clinician's style and manner of counseling parents during the initial traumatic period is of utmost importance and sets the tone for the atmosphere that will prevail in future years.

        a. Use proper terminology and inform both parents together in a sensitive and honest way as soon as the clinical diagnosis has been made.

        b. Time your remarks to coincide with increasing parental adaptation.

        c. Schedule follow-up sessions for review of basic considerations and communication of more details (chromosome analysis, developmental expectations, etc.).

        d. Spend extra time in talking about various health concerns and developmental issues that will make the parents aware of your sincere interest in helping them and their child.

        e. Stress that most observable characteristics do not cause significant disability in the child. For example, the slanting of the palpebral fissures and the presence of Brushfield spots do not interfere with the child's vision. However, other abnormalities such as congenital heart disease or duodenal atresia are serious and require prompt medical attention.

        2. Treatment. It is important to let parents know that there is no cure and no effective medical treatment available for children with Down syndrome at the present time. Numerous "medications" have been recommended to improve the mental capacity of children with Down syndrome, but none have been found to be of benefit.

        3. Education. Parents should be informed about early intervention programs and inclusive educational strategies in integrated school programs that are available to children with Down syndrome. With appropriate education and positive learning experiences, many children with Down syndrome will be able to function well in society. Most individuals will be able to hold a job and many will be gainfully employed later.

BIBLIOGRAPHY

For Parents

Organizations

National Down Syndrome Congress www.ndsccenter.org
National Down Syndrome Society www.ndss.org

Books

Pueschel SM. *A Parent's Guide to Down Syndrome: Toward a Brighter Future.* Baltimore: Brookes
Publishing, 2001.
Pueschel SM, Sustrova M. *Adolescents with Down Syndrome,* Baltimore: Brookes Publishing, 1997.

For Professionals

Cooley WC, Graham JM. Common syndromes and management issues for primary care physicians:
Down syndrome - An update and review for the primary pediatrician. *Clin Pediatr* 30:233–253,
1991.
Pueschel SM, Pueschel JK. *Biomedical Concerns in Persons with Down Syndrome.* Baltimore:
Brookes Publishing, 1992.

The Dysmorphic Child

John C. Carey

I. Description of the problem.

A. Epidemiology.

- Approximately 3%–4% of all infants have a medically significant congenital malformation (see Table 37-1 for definition of terms).
- About 28% of all children have a single minor anomaly.
- An additional 11% show two or more of these physical findings.

II. Making the diagnosis.

A. The diagnosis of a dysmorphic syndrome is significant for the child, the family, and the health care professionals, for a number of reasons.

1. **Recurrence risk in genetic counseling.** The recognition of an established disorder of known etiology provides information on cause and heritable aspects of the condition, as well as potential prenatal options for future pregnancies.

2. **Relative prediction of prognosis.** Each disorder has its own particular natural history, risks for problems, and outcomes.

3. **Appropriate laboratory testing and screening.** Precise diagnosis eliminates the need for unnecessary tests; appropriate screening can be planned according to natural history.

4. **Treatment and management issues.** Knowledge of the natural history of a condition allows for the establishment of guidelines for routine care, including suggestions for educational interventions.

5. **Coping with the disorder.** In some families, the knowledge of a condition helps in dealing with the uncertainty of the situation.

B. Data collection.
The importance of a thorough history in the evaluation of a child with a potential syndrome cannot be overemphasized. Information on the gestational and birth history should include history of fetal movement, drugs and medications taken during pregnancy, alcohol consumption, intrauterine positioning, status of amniotic fluid, and maternal medical history. Documentation of a complete family history with a three-generation pedigree (including inquiry regarding consanguinity) is suggested. Key clinical questions include:

1. Does the child in question have an **organized pattern of malformation** (i.e., a syndrome or sequence), or does the child exhibit a constellation of features that are consistent with the family and/or ethnic background (variant familial developmental pattern)?

    a. If the child has a pattern, do the findings consist of multiple **primary** malformations of dysplasias (a syndrome), or do the findings represent **secondary** manifestations (deformations or disruptions) comprising a sequence?

    b. If the child has a pattern, does the pattern represent a **known syndrome** (or sequence), or is it a **previously unidentified, provisionally unique pattern?**

2. What is the **date of the onset** of the physical abnormalities? Are they prenatal or postnatal? Some physical signs that are clues for syndromes are of postnatal onset and often provide signs for a metabolic disorder (e.g., the facial changes and joint contractures of the mucopolysaccharidoses).

C. Physical examination of the craniofacies.
The ability to **recognize and interpret minor anomalies and mild malformations** is the most important skill required in approaching the child with a potential syndrome. The practitioner needs to be observant and skilled in documenting physical variations and deciding what, in fact, is "normal" and what is not (Fig. 37-1). The **evaluation of the face and hands** is particularly important since most malformation syndromes have phenotypic variations in these areas. The common frustration of clinicians in approaching the potentially dysmorphic child probably helped lead to that pejorative, stigmatizing term, the "FLK" (funny-looking kid), which should be eliminated from clinical practice.

Table 37-1 Definitions of commonly used terms

Term	Definition
Malformation	A primary morphologic defect of an organ or body part resulting from an intrinsically abnormal developmental process (e.g., cleft lip)
Deformation	An alteration of the form, shape, or position of a previously normally formed body part caused by mechanized forces (e.g., club foot due to oligohydramnios)
Sequence	Pattern of multiple anomalies derived from a single known anomaly; a primary defect with its secondary changes (e.g., Pierre Robin syndrome)
Syndrome	A recurring pattern of multiple defects due to a single etiology (e.g., Williams syndrome)
Dysmorphic	Structurally abnormal or malformed; more conventionally, used to refer to the presence of multiple minor anomalies or mild malformations, as in *dysmorphic* facial features

Source: Adapted from the recommendations of the International Working Group. Spranger J, et al. Errors of morphogenesis: concepts and terms. *J Pediatr* 1982;100:160.

1. **The examination.** The clinician should examine the face as he or she would examine the heart or abdomen, looking at it in general and then examining each feature systematically (hair, forehead, eye slant, eyebrows, etc.) to determine what about this face makes it look different. Does one feature make the face look distinctive or unique, several features, or one area of the face? The gestalt should be noted (the whole is more than the sum of the parts). If the ears appear low set, the clinician should consider why they look that way. Are they small, posteriorly rotated, or overfolded, or does the low placement, in fact, represent an illusion?

2. **Classification.** Table 37-2 presents a classification of types of variations of the face. It is of note that most of the features of a child with Down syndrome fall into the minor anomaly category. This is the class of features that usually requires comparison to family members, especially parents and siblings, and also consideration of ethnic background. Photographing the patient is important for documentation. The pictures can be placed in the chart for future review.

3. **The approach.** Table 37-3 summarizes the practical steps that can be used in approaching the dysmorphic child.

   The most useful and easily available reference source for looking up features and attempting to make a diagnosis is *Smith's Recognizable Patterns of Human Malformation* by Jones. In addition, a number of computer programs have been designed to help in the diagnostic process.

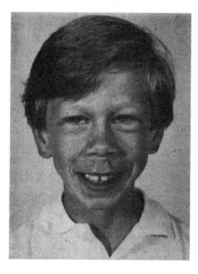

Figure 37-1. Child with Williams syndrome. Note the general facial gestalt, which is characteristic. Also, note that all of the features fall into the category of continuous features; none is a true malformation, minor or major. The mouth size measures above the 90%, but otherwise the features are not abnormal in the statistical or embryologic sense of the word.

Table 37-2 Types of variations and malformations of the craniofacies

	Definition
Major malformations	Medically significant defects (e.g., cleft lip, microtia)
Mild malformations	Structural alterations that have no intrinsic medical significance (occur in <4% of population, e.g., helical ear pit, cutis aplasia of the scalp)
Minor anomalies	
Continuous features with measurable alterations	Features that lend themselves to measurement and can be defined on standard curves (e.g., small ears) using the graphs in *Smith's Recognizable Patterns of Human Malformation*
Continuous features, not defined by measurements	Features that shade into normal variation and do not have a defined threshold (e.g., micrognathia, low nasal root, prominent nasal tip)

    D. Laboratory evaluation.

        1. After initial evaluation of the child, if no secure diagnosis has been reached and it appears that the child has multiple anomalies, a **chromosome study** should be performed. There is a 5% yield of positive chromosome studies among children with dysmorphic features and developmental delay. In most circumstances a routine G-banded karyotype is performed.

        2. If there is suspicion that the child's features are suggestive of the fragile X syndrome (Chapter 43), then a **fragile X study** is warranted.

        3. If one of the microdeletion syndromes is in question (e.g., Prader-Willi syndrome), then a **high-resolution study** or **FISH** (fluorescence in situ hybridization) is indicated.

        4. TORCH (toxoplasmosis, other, rubella, cytomegalovirus, herpes simplex) titers are usually not indicated in an infant who has multiple primary defects that are alterations in embryogenesis (e.g., cleft lip, polydactyly, or even minor anomalies).

        5. Amino acid studies are not indicated in an infant with multiple primary malformations since none of the known aminoacidopathies is consistently associated with structural anomalies of prenatal onset. However, there are some inborn errors of metabolism that will have associated congenital or early onset physical abnormalities that might raise the question of the child having a dysmorphic syndrome. Examples include the abnormal hair of an infant with Menkes syndrome and the dysmorphic features of the peroxisomal disorders. Imaging studies and referrals to subspecialists are indicated according to the presence of accompanying problems.

  III. Management.

    A. Specialty referral. Consultation with a dysmorphologist or clinical geneticist skilled in syndrome recognition is indicated for any child who appears to be dysmorphic. Referral for consultation is also appropriate for any family with questions about the diagnosis, the natural history of the disorder, the recurrence risk, prenatal options, issues of reproductive decision making, and psychological support.

    B. Health maintenance and anticipatory guidance. Once the diagnosis of a particular

Table 37-3 Practical steps in the approach to the dysmorphic child

1. *Examine the child's family members.* Compare features to parents' or siblings'. When possible compare to photographs of family members at the same age as the index case.
2. *Consider ethnic background.* Certain features have different frequencies in different ethnic groups (e.g., eye measurements are different in African Americans vs persons of Hispanic descent vs European Caucasians).
3. *Measure areas where standards exist* (e.g., ear size, palpebral fissure length). Do not trust the gestalt in deciding whether a feature is large or small; have plastic rulers available in the clinic setting.
4. *Look up the most distinctive and/or rarest defect for quick identification* (e.g., the white forelock suggesting Waardenburg syndrome).
5. *Become acquainted with the terminology and ways to describe the face and hands.*

syndrome is made, the clinician can review the natural history of the disorder and help establish a plan for follow-up and screening.

C. Psychological support. The process of ruling out a syndrome can, in and of itself, be overwhelming and even stigmatizing for the family. Families often perceive the meticulous detail of the examination as a "picking apart" process. Discussion of the reasons for making a diagnosis is helpful, and acknowledging these potential feelings are important in the initiation of the referral process.

IV. **Clinical pearls and pitfalls.**

- **The null hypothesis strategy.** The diagnosis of a syndrome should be approached in a hypothesis-generating manner. The clinician should state the null hypothesis—"This child does not have a dysmorphic syndrome"—and then review the evidence. This approach attempts to avoid overdiagnosis and puts the burden of proof on the person who makes the diagnosis. It also demands a certain amount of critical thinking about the use of the minor anomalies in the diagnostic thought process.
- **The eye doesn't see what the mind doesn't know.** This often-cited axiom underscores the importance of the knowledge of the disorder, as well as the need for astute observation. Recognition of the subtleties of physical variation, as well as clinical variability of a disorder, is crucial in the evaluation.
- Children with dysmorphic syndromes are not necessarily unusual or different in appearance. What is usually present is a **difference from their unaffected family members,** rather than a clear-cut abnormality. In many syndromes, the features are consistent and show difference from the family background but are not very distinctive or striking.
- "You know my method. It is founded upon the observance of trifles." Sherlock Holmes, *The Boscombe Valley Mystery.*

BIBLIOGRAPHY

For Parents

Alliance of Genetic Support Groups. Offers an updated catalog of support groups for various disorders. 35 Wisconsin Circle, Suite 440, Chevy Chase, MD 20815. 1-800-336-GENE

For Professionals

Aase JM. Dysmorphologic diagnosis for the pediatric practitioner. *Pediatr Clin North Am* 39 (1): 135, 1992.
Cohen MM. *The Child with Multiple Birth Defects.* New York: Raven Press, 1982.
Jones KL. *Smith's Recognizable Patterns of Human Malformations (4th ed.)* Philadelphia: Saunders, 1988.
POSSUM (Pictures of Standard Syndromes and Undiagnosed Malformations): An electronic reference. The program is found in many medical libraries and is often located in the office of a dysmorphologist or clinical geneticist. This is a very user-friendly system. Available through CP Export Pty. Ltd. 493 St. Kilda Road Melbourne, Victoria, 3004, Australia

38

Encopresis

Alison Schonwald
Leonard Rappaport

I. **Description of the problem.** Encopresis is defined as repeated passage of stool into inappropriate places in a child over 4 years old, chronologically and developmentally. The behavior is not due exclusively to the direct physiological effects of a substance (e.g., laxatives) or a general medical condition, except through a mechanism involving constipation.

A. **Epidemiology.**
  - Encopresis reportedly affects 2.8% of 4-year-olds, 1.9% of 6-year-olds, and 1.6% of 10–11-year-olds.
  - Usually presents in children under 7 years old.

B. **Etiology/contributing factors.**
  - More than 90% of encopresis is due to functional constipation where retained stool distends the rectum, resulting in stool leaking around a stool mass. Stretch receptors in a distended rectum do not seem to signal the child to defecate until soiling is nearly complete.
  - Encopresis is not generally caused by underlying psychopathology, but can be associated with emotional distress.
  - Rare cases of encopresis are due to damaged corticospinal pathways or anorectal dysfunction after pull through surgery.
  - A small subset of children with encopresis may impulsively pass stool due to anxiety or other emotional stressors, without underlying constipation.

II. **Making the diagnosis.**
A. **History: Key clinical questions.**
  1. *"Was there a time when the child's bowel movements seemed typical?"* History starts at birth with specifics surrounding bowel function and any treatments used. Past medical and surgical history may identify systemic diseases or medical causes of constipation that indicate treatments other than laxatives and maintenance of stool regularity.
  2. *"Did your child have a period of stooling into the toilet? How old was he or she? Did he or she feel the stool coming and get to the bathroom by her- or himself regularly?"* Distinguishing delayed toilet training, where the child never consolidated the ability to stool independently into the toilet, from encopresis is essential. Treatment will vary, depending on whether or not constipation underlies the stooling accidents, rather than toilet refusal (although toilet refusal is often associated with constipation as well).
  3. *"How often does your child stool and urinate into the toilet now? How often into underwear? Are the stools large? Hard? Liquid? Do they hurt?"* Review details of present urinary and bowel patterns, such as frequency of stool evacuation into the toilet, stool accidents, stool consistency, and the urge to defecate. More severe, prolonged constipation generally will require more aggressive treatment. Any history of abuse or other trauma should be sought as well. Children who have been abused may become incontinent in times of stress or as part of regressive behavior, and are less suitable candidates for rectal suppositories or enemas. They may also soil their underwear to keep someone away from them.
  4. *"Often stool problems are joined by urine problems. Has he or she had any urine infections? Does she or he have urine accidents in the day or at night?"* Urinary patterns, diurnal and nocturnal enuresis, and symptoms of urinary infection must be elicited, and may indicate neurological abnormalities or urine contamination. Constipation and encopresis may be associated with urine infections, especially in females, due to poor hygiene. Even without infection, enuresis can be caused by a dilated rectum pushing on and irritating the bladder, thus causing spasm.
  5. *"I see lots of kids who have poop accidents and don't like having them. If you and your parents help me figure out what is going on, I think I can help so the accidents get better."* History taking provides an essential opportunity to communicate with

the child. The child must be an active participant for treatment to be effective, and often children with encopresis are often overwhelmed and embarrassed when encopresis is discussed. Developing a sense of the child's perspective can create a connection between caregiver and patient, and should include questions about present school and family functioning.

B. Signs and symptoms. A child with functional constipation and consequent encopresis will report uncomfortable and infrequent stooling into the toilet with uncontrolled stool accidents into underwear or pull-ups. Physical exam of the child with encopresis includes:

- Growth parameters
- Attention to signs of systemic disease
- Neurological assessment
- Examination of the anal opening. Anal fissures will cause ongoing pain with defecation; tags may reflect inflammatory bowel disease, and an absent anal wink may indicate neurological abnormality
- Rectal examination can be useful in assessing for Hirschsprung disease, and may provide an indication of the degree of rectal impaction in order to guide treatment

C. Differential diagnosis. Any disorder that can cause constipation can cause encopresis. A detailed history and physical examination is required to rule out systemic or organic causes of constipation or incontinence, such as spinal cord dysplasia or tethering, hypothyroidism, and meconium ileus of cystic fibrosis.

D. Diagnostic assessment. For most children, no further diagnostic assessment is necessary beyond thorough, directed fact finding. Laboratory investigation is indicated only as history or physical examination suggests: rarely labs may include thyroid function tests, electrolytes, calcium, and magnesium. An abdominal radiograph may be useful when the history is vague or the child is uncooperative with examination. Lumbosacral spine films or MRI are indicated when lower extremity neurological exam is abnormal or sacral abnormalities are visualized.

III. Management.

A. Psychoeducation. Demystify the shame and blame around stool accidents. Use the child's abdominal radiograph or an illustrated explanation (or both) to review the process of retained stool that leads to a distended colon, allowing stool to sneak out without warning. Discuss that retained stool has to be cleaned out with medication and that there will likely be a lot of stool to clean out. Empathize with the stress and frustration, and emphasize the need to break the cycle of impatience that may have developed. Clarify that now the child truly cannot control the stool leaking out and should not be blamed.

B. The initial cleanout of retained stool. Children 7 and older without trauma history may opt for a fast and direct choice: a 14-day cycle of alternating bisacodyl pills, bisacodyl suppository, then Fleets® enema. Younger children (under 7) or those who cannot tolerate suppositories or enemas, may require polyethylene glycol without electrolytes, starting at one cap in 6 ounces of fluid per day. Impaction present for many months may require higher dosing or the addition of a stimulant such as senna or bisacodyl. During the initial cleanout, the child and family should expect a large amount of stool output and are reminded of the radiograph full of stool.

C. Regular bowel patterns must be established. This requires medication and a behavior plan. It makes sense to meet with the child and family after the clean out is complete to plan the next stage of treatment. One option is mineral oil titrated to efficacy, from 2 tablespoons per day to 6 tbsp twice per day. Polyethylene glycol without electrolytes is also used frequently, particularly for children who do not tolerate mineral oil's taste or have oil leakage. Maintenance dose of polyethylene glycol without electrolytes generally ranges from 1/2 cap every other day to 1 cap twice per day. Dosing is adjusted to maintain soft regular stools. As the child may not develop the urge to defecate for 6–9 months after constipation is treated, a regular sitting time is necessary.

The goal is to stool before the sensation of stool leakage develops. Sitting after breakfast and dinner for 5–10 minutes takes advantage of the body's gastrocolic reflex and can often be incorporated easily into the daily routine. The family must work to eliminate any negative associations around toileting that may have developed. Limiting conversation about toileting can be helpful, as can rewarding the child for sitting or taking care of his or her own bodily needs. Older children may benefit from having games or activities in the bathroom.

IV. Clinical pearls and pitfalls.

- Most families of a child with encopresis have never met anyone with the same problem. Reassuring them that encopresis is not so unusual and can be treated is a vital step.

- Constipation and encopresis are often long-term issues, recurring intermittently after great initial improvement. Children may require mineral oil, polyethylene glycol without electrolytes, and/or high fiber supplements for extended periods (months to years).
- Reviewing signs of backup (e.g., hard stools, skipping days, stomach aches, and/or smears) and developing a rescue plan (e.g., increased mineral oil, senna, increased sitting, and/or increased fiber) empowers the child and family to anticipate, tolerate and treat recurrences.

BIBLIOGRAPHY

For Parents

Websites

Children's Medical Center, University of Virginia http://www.people.virginia.edu/~smb4v/tutorials/constipation/encotreat.htm

For Professionals

Loening-Baucke V. Encopresis. *Curr Opin Pediatr* 2002;14(5):570–575.
Brazzelli M, Griffiths P. Behavioural and cognitive interventions with or without other treatments for defaecation disorders in children. *Cochrane Database Syst Rev* (4):CD002240, 2001.

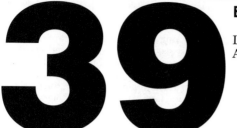

Enuresis

Leonard Rappaport
Alison Schonwald

I. **Description of the problem.** Enuresis is defined as a lack of urinary continence
  - Beyond age 4 years for diurnal (daytime) enuresis.
  - Beyond age 6 years for nocturnal (nighttime) enuresis, or
  - The loss of continence after at least 3 months of dryness
  A. **Epidemiology.** A universal definition remains elusive because the development of urinary continence varies by gender, cultural group, race, and country. Table 39-1 provides general guidelines for the attainment of urinary continence in the United States.
    1. **Subtypes.** Enuresis is divided into (1) **primary enuresis** (incontinence in a child who has never attained continence) and (2) **secondary enuresis** (when a child has attained continence for at least 3 months and begins to have episodes of incontinence). Enuresis is then further subdivided into **diurnal** (daytime) versus **nocturnal** (nighttime) enuresis. More than half of the children with diurnal enuresis also have nocturnal enuresis.
      a. Another classification distinguishes between nocturnal enuresis with and without bladder symptoms. **Monosymptomatic nocturnal enuresis** is bedwetting with normal daytime urination, while **polysymptomatic nocturnal enuresis** is bedwetting with severe frequency, urgency, or other signs of an unstable bladder.
      b. Secondary, diurnal, and polysymptomatic nocturnal enuresis are associated with a greater degree of organic pathology.
  B. **Familial transmission/genetics.** There is a genetic predisposition to enuresis. If one parent had enuresis, 40% of his or her children will have enuresis. If both parents had enuresis, 70% of their children will have enuresis. Identical twins have the highest concordance rate. Several genetic loci have been located by intensive family studies.
  C. **Etiology.** In the vast majority of cases, the etiology of enuresis is unknown. There are, however, causes that should be considered.
    1. **Nocturnal Enuresis.**
      a. **Known causes.**
        (1) **Increased bladder irritability.** The most common cause of secondary enuresis is increased bladder irritability, usually due to a urinary tract infection. Additionally, any mass impinging on the bladder (e.g., severe constipation) can increase bladder irritability. Recently, posterior urethral valves have been thought to be associated with diurnal enuresis in boys. The partial obstruction from the valves makes the bladder muscles hypertrophy and be less compliant and more irritable. It is unclear how commonly this occurs.
        (2) **Increased urinary output.** Any process that increases urinary output can cause enuresis (e.g., diabetes mellitus, diabetes insipidus, sickle cell disease).
        (3) **Bladder capacity.** Bladder capacity is decreased in children with enuresis compared to their non-enuretic siblings. This reflects differences in functional, rather than absolute, bladder capacity, with contractions occurring earlier in filling.
      b. **Contributing factors.**
        (1) **Maturational delay.** A commonly accepted but unproven cause of nocturnal enuresis, this refers to the enuretic child's inability to send, perceive, or respond to information about a filled bladder during the night. Support for this theory comes from the spontaneous cure rate.
        (2) **Sleep and arousal factors.** Originally it was thought that enuresis was a nonrapid eye movement dyssomnia (like sleepwalking and night terrors). Data suggest that enuresis occurs in *all* stages of sleep and that there is no difference in sleep patterns between children with enuresis and their non-enuretic peers. Additionally, many parents believe that their enuretic child sleeps more soundly than their other children. Of course, these parents only

Table 39-1 Prevalence of continence

Day	Night
50% by age 2½ yr	66% by age 3 yr
90% by age 4 yr	75% by age 4 yr
	90% by age 8 yr
	98% by ages 12–14 yr

attempt to awaken their children with enuresis so this is possibly a selection bias rather than a real finding. Recent studies suggest that some enuretic children may be more difficult to awaken than are age matched controls, particularly in the first half of the night, thus supporting caregiver reports. This may relate to an immature arousal mechanism, which prevents response to a distended bladder. Obstructive sleep apnea can be associated with nocturnal enuresis.

- (3) **CNS factors.** Continuing research has focused on the possible role of antidiuretic hormone (ADH) secretion in children with nocturnal enuresis, leading to an increase in urinary output. Much of the earlier research in this area pointing to a diminished surge of ADH during sleep in children with nocturnal enuresis has been called into question. This remains unproved.
- (4) **Psychopathology/stress.** There are no data to support enuresis as a neurotic disorder. Similarly, although stress may exacerbate or contribute to enuresis, it is not a primary etiologic factor.

2. **Diurnal enuresis.**
   a. **Known causes.**
   (1) **Increased bladder irritability**
   (2) **Micturation deferral.** The most common cause of daytime wetting in preschool children is due to holding of the urine and ignoring the urge to void, usually during play. Incontinence results when detrussor contraction cannot be suppressed. Children with short attention spans often fail to respond to body signals until it is too late.
   (3) **Abnormal sphincter control.** Although abnormal urinary sphincter control is rare, insidious pathology (e.g., spinal cord abnormalities) can cause abnormal sphincter control. Some hypothesize that there is a group of children with decreased sphincter strength without obvious cause who may have a higher incidence of diurnal enuresis.
   (4) **Structural abnormalities.** Girls with ectopic ureters which empty into the vagina, have constant wetting with no recognized episodes of incontinence. Partial labial fusion may develop after inflammation, allowing urine to collect in a pocket behind the fused labia minora and subsequently leak.
   (5) **Vaginal reflux.** Overweight girls who sit with their legs together when urinating can reflux urine into the vagina. The urine will then leak out over the next several hours without the urge to void. This causes almost constant daytime wetting without nighttime episodes.
   b. **Contributing factors.**
   (1) **Urge syndrome.** Children with daytime and nighttime wetting, as well as urgency and frequency, often have unstable detrusor contractions early in bladder filling. They often squat, sitting assymetrically on one heel in an effort to prevent a detrussor contraction. Symptoms resolve with time, usually by 10–12 years.
   (2) **Giggle incontinence.** Emptying the bladder entirely while laughing may be familial. It is common in school-age girls and generally resolves with maturity.
   (3) **Stress incontinence.** With increased abdominal pressure, such as during coughing, some children's bladders empty.
   (4) **Postvoid dribble syndome.** Children may sense wetness after a void but without actual incontinence.

II. **Making the diagnosis.**
   A. **History: Key clinical questions.** A complete history should be obtained with a particular focus on a family history of enuresis, the child's pattern of wetting, and the previous interventions.

1. *"Has the child ever been dry at night?"* It is important to differentiate primary from secondary enuresis.
2. *"Does the child have accidents during the day, as well as at night?"* Treat the daytime enuresis first if it coexists with nocturnal incontinence.
3. *"Has the child been constipated? How many days does he typically go between bowel movements? Are bowel movements hard, particularly large, or painful to produce?"* Treat constipation prior to more invasive investigation, unless history or physical exam suggests otherwise.
4. *"Was anyone else in the family late in achieving dryness at night or day?"* A positive family history may make the family more sympathetic to the child's feelings. It may be helpful to elicit the parents' own experience with enuresis and how it affects their response to their child.
5. *"What methods have you tried to fix the problem?"* Evaluate the positive and negative interventions. Determine if they were appropriately implemented and their secondary effects (e.g., on the child's self-esteem).
6. [To the child] *"How much of a problem is this to you?"* The child must be motivated to be cured if treatment is to be successful.

   B. **Physical examination.** A full physical examination should be performed, with emphasis placed on the spinal, neurologic, and genital examinations.
   C. **Tests.** The laboratory evaluation should be very limited. A urinalysis and urine culture should be obtained in all children. Further workup should be directed by findings in the history and physical examination. There is no indication for the use of imaging techniques or urodynamic studies unless suggested by the history or physical examination.

III. **Management.**
   A. **Primary goals.** The primary goals in the treatment of enuresis are to alleviate the problem and to limit its impact on the child's self-esteem and interpersonal relationships. Although a cure is possible for most children, a small percentage may have to learn to live with this problem. Initial interventions should be directed both at helping the child cope with the problem and working on a solution.
   B. **Information for the family.** The family should be told how common enuresis is and made to understand that it is usually a developmental problem over which the child has little to no control. Punishments only lower the child's self-esteem without improving the symptoms. Finally, parents should understand that effective treatments are available and that most treatments require cooperation between them, the child, and the primary care clinician.
   C. **Treatment strategies.**
      1. **Nocturnal enuresis.** The spontaneous remission rate for nocturnal enuresis is 15% per year. Table 39-2 lists the cure and relapse rates for the common treatments.
         a. **Alarms** have become the preferred treatment for nocturnal enuresis because of their high efficacy, low cost, ease of use, and low regression rate. However, their use requires a considerable commitment from the parents (at least for the first week or two) when the child may not awaken to the alarm. Children must be motivated, and are generally older than 7 years with the exception of younger, mature, highly motivated patients. The parents and child should be instructed in its use.
            • Use the alarm every night.
            • The child should be instructed to visualize the steps necessary before going to sleep at night, such as waking when the alarm sounds, going to the bathroom, changing into dry clothes, replacing the alarm, and pulling off wet sheets. The child should then act out these steps before going to sleep.
            • Parents should wake the child when the alarm rings and take the child to the bathroom (even if an accident has already occurred). After a week or two, the child usually will awaken independently when the alarm sounds.
            • Restart the alarm after the underwear is changed.
            • Use star or sticker chart for dry nights.
            • Most children who respond to alarms do so within 4 months. (See the list of alarm products at the end of the chapter.)
         b. **Medications.**
            (1) **Desmopressin acetate (DDAVP)** is a synthetic analog of 8-arginine vasopressin and has shown to be effective in the treatment of nighttime enuresis. Studies find longterm intranasal use (6 months) safe, but cost usually limits its use to short-term situations, such as overnight camp. Oral DDAVP at approximately 100 times the intranasal dose is an alternative effective

Table 39-2 Interventions for enuresis

Method	Initial success rate	Relapse rate
Nocturnal enuresis		
Alarms	70%	10%
Imipramine	50%	90%
Desmopressin acetate (DDAVP)	50%	90%
Bladder stretching	30%	?
Motivational	20%	?
Diurnal enuresis		
Urgency containment	75%	?
Alarms	?	?
Oxybutynin	?	?

treatment, though occasional nonresponders to the oral form respond to the spray. In both cases, relapse rate is very high. Patients should be instructed to avoid excessive fluid intake after the medication is taken to avoid water intoxication.

(2) **Imipramine,** a tricyclic antidepressant, has been shown to be successful in the treatment of nocturnal enuresis, although the mechanism for this improvement remains uncertain. There are two problems with imipramine in the treatment of enuresis: the high relapse rate when stopped and the very high toxic index if taken in overdosage.

c. **Bladder stretching exercises** are a moderately successful form of treatment. In these exercises, children are asked to hold their urine for as long as they can, as frequently as they can. In several studies, the children who increased their functional bladder capacity the greatest amount with these exercises had the greatest improvement in their enuresis.

d. **Motivational incentives** (e.g., star charts and other reward systems) generally provide a positive focus on a child's remaining dry at night. Their relatively low efficacy makes them a useful adjunct but not a primary treatment of nocturnal enuresis.

2. **Diurnal enuresis.** When a child has both nocturnal and diurnal enuresis, the daytime component should be addressed first.

a. **Urgency containment exercises.** Treatment for diurnal enuresis involves the use of bladder urgency containment exercises:
- The child goes into the bathroom when he has to urinate.
- Once there, he holds the urine for as long as possible.
- When the child does urinate, he is asked to stop and start the urine flow frequently.
- The objective is to increase the muscle strength of the sphincter, as well as to give the child confidence that he can control the urinary stream. In most children, the diurnal enuresis will resolve over several months.

b. **Contingent and noncontingent alarms** are helpful for some children. Contingent alarms go off when the child starts to wet, but these can be socially embarrassing. Noncontingent alarms involve wearing a watch that beeps about every 2 hours to remind the child to urinate.

c. **Medications** for diurnal enuresis are rarely indicated. Some believe that anticholinergic agents (e.g., oxybutynin chloride) have shown some efficacy, but there are limited trials supporting their use.

D. **Improving self-esteem/family function.** Self-esteem is best preserved by a nonpunitive response to the enuresis. The child should understand that enuresis is common and that it is usually not a sign of emotional, psychological, or medical dysfunction. The child can be empowered to take responsibility for dryness at night following an accident via the "double bubble" technique.
- Place a plastic sheet over the mattress, followed by the usual sheets and blankets.
- Place another plastic sheet over those sheets, again followed by another set of sheets and blankets.
- Keep a dry set of pajamas by the bedside.
- During the day, rehearse with the child how to take the wet set of sheets off the bed, uncovering the dry second set, and how to change pajamas.
- This technique can defuse family tensions by allowing the child to handle his own

needs at night and not awaken the parents. It is not for punishment, but to help the child take responsibility for his own bodily functions.
   E. **Criteria for referral.** The child should be referred to a urologist when genitourinary pathology is suspected. Psychological counseling should be sought when the child's social function appears to have been impaired by the enuresis or when the family's response appears to be unduly punitive.
IV. **Clinical pearls and pitfalls.**
   - *Always* complete a full history and physical when beginning the treatment of a child with enuresis, even if they are your primary care patient and you think you know them well.
   - Parents may have not shared with the clinician all the information pertaining to enuresis unless they are asked directly. Parents need to be asked about previous interventions and, in particular, how these interventions were instituted. Frequently parents will have tried an intervention inappropriately.
   - Success is contagious. A child who has had multiple failures in the treatment of enuresis might be helped by trying a medical therapy (e.g., DDAVP) to achieve some success immediately. A more definitive but difficult therapy (e.g., an alarm) can follow after the child and family have the sense that success is possible.
   - Involvement of the child is essential. No intervention will be successful without the motivation and commitment of the child.
   - Always pay attention to the evolution of the child's self-esteem. Punitive techniques should be avoided at all costs.
   - Don't forget to ask. Many families are ashamed to tell their pediatricians that their child has enuresis. Sadly, sometimes the more a family likes a pediatric clinician, the less likely they are to share a shameful subject.

BIBLIOGRAPHY

For Parents

Mack A. *Dry All Night.* Boston: Little, Brown, 1989.

For Children

Boelts M. *Dry Days, Wet Nights.* Morton Grove, IL: Albert Whitmen and Company, 1994.

For Professionals

Rappaport L. The treatment of enuresis: Where are we now? *Pediatrics* 1993;92:464.
von Gontard A, Schaumburg H, Hollmann E, et al. The genetics of enuresis: a review. *J Urology* 2001;166(6):2438–2443.
Wille S. Comparison of desmopressin and enuresis alarms for nocturnal enuresis. *Arch Dis Child* 1986;61:30.
Cayan S, Doruk E, Bozlu M, Akbay E, Apaydin D, Ulusoy E, et al. Is routine urinary tract investigation necessary for children with monosymptomatic primary nocturnal enuresis? *Urology* 2001; 58(4):598–602.
Robson WL, Leung AK. Daytime wetting. *J Pediatr* 2001;139(4):609–610.

Websites

American Academy of Family Physicians http://familydoctor.org/366.xml
American Academy of Family Physicians http://www.aafp.org/afp/20030401/1499.html

Selected Enuresis Alarms

Nite Train'r Alarm Koregon Enterprises 9735 Southwest Sunshine Court Beaverton OR 97005 1-800-544-4240
Nytone Medical Products 2424 South 900 West Salt Lake City UT 84119 801-973-4090
Wet Stop Alarm Palco Laboratories 8030 Soquel Avenue Santa Cruz CA 95062 1-800-346-4488

40

Failure to Thrive

Deborah A. Frank

I. **Description of the problem.** Failure to thrive (FTT) refers to children, usually under age 5 years, whose growth persistently and significantly deviates from the norms for their age and sex on the National Center for Health Statistics (NCHS) growth charts.

A. **Epidemiology.**
- Nutritional growth failure is seen in 8%–12% of low-income children. However, the prevalence of FTT in the general population is unknown.

B. **Family transmission/genetics.** Familial short stature may be considered when the child's weight is appropriate to height and when linear growth velocity parallels the normal curve on the growth chart. It is, however, perilous to assume that poor growth, particularly low weight for height, in children is secondary to familial predisposition for several reasons:
- Parental height may be a poor guide of the child's growth potential if parents themselves were nutritionally deprived as children and therefore did not attain their optimal growth (as is often the case with immigrant and impoverished families).
- The parents may have an eating disorder and be excessively concerned with obesity.
- The child may share an organic problem with the parents (e.g., lactose intolerance).

C. **Etiology.**

1. **"Organic" versus "nonorganic."** Traditionally, the etiology of FTT was considered either organic or nonorganic. However, this dichotomy is of limited use since children with so-called nonorganic FTT are suffering from malnutrition, a serious organic insult, while children with major organic diagnoses may, in part, have growth failure attributable to social and nutritional factors. Diagnostically and therapeutically, it is useful to assess each child and family along four parameters: (1) medical, (2) nutritional, (3) developmental, and (4) social. Problems in any or all of these areas may interact to produce growth failure. For example, a temperamentally passive child with lead poisoning may fail to receive frequent enough feedings from an exhausted mother who has other more demanding children.

2. **Psychosocial causes.**

   a. Child may fail to thrive in families of any social class **when parents' emotional and material resources are diverted or not available from for the care of the child**. This can occur because of poverty, parental depression, maladaptive parenting practices, family discord, another chronically ill family member, substance abuse, or losses (such as death of grandparent or unemployment).

   b. **FTT does not necessarily imply parental neglect or pathology**. Feeding disorders can develop when not eating serves other purposes (e.g., to express anger, to exert autonomy from overly intrusive caretakers, to gain the attention of otherwise abstracted caretakers, or to divert adults from conflict with each other).

   c. Children with **preexisting minor developmental deficits** (e.g., subtle oral motor difficulties, hypersensitivity to stimulation) may develop feeding problems that lead to nutritional FTT. Apathy and irritability associated with malnutrition may exacerbate parent–child interactional dysfunction and lead to further feeding difficulties.

   d. Children **living in poverty** are often at nutritional risk because of inadequate food supplies in the home, homelessness, overcrowding, and the inability of federal feeding programs (e.g., food stamps, supplemental food program for women, infants, and children [WIC], school meals) to reach many of the eligible families. In other cases, the benefit levels of such programs are insufficient to meet the nutritional needs of at-risk children.

3. **Medical causes.**

   a. The **organic causes** of FTT encompass a whole textbook of pediatrics. Usually most are suggested by a careful history and physical examination, but some are occult (Table 40-1).

Table 40-1 Often inapparent medical causes of FTT

Infectious
Giardiasis (other parasites, e.g., nematodes)
Chronic urinary tract infection
Chronic sinusitis
HIV
Mechanical
Adenoid hypertrophy
Dental lesions
Vascular slings
Gastroesophageal reflux with esophagitis
Neurologic
Oral motor dysfunction (gagging, tactile hypersensitivity)
Toxic/metabolic
Lead toxicity
Iron deficiency
Zinc deficiency
Gastrointestinal
Celiac disease
Malabsorption (various causes including cystic fibrosis)
Chronic constipation
Allergic
Food allergies (often presents as FTT with atopic dermatitis)

        b. Perinatal risk factors include prematurity and intrauterine growth retardation (IUGR). IUGR with dysmorphic features suggests a growth-retarding syndrome (genetic, congenital, or related to teratogen exposure).
    D. Long-term outcomes. FTT is a major risk factor for later developmental and behavioral difficulties, usually reflecting both the nutritional deprivation of the developing nervous system and the environmental experiences of the child.
  II. Making the diagnosis.
    A. Signs and symptoms. While there are no universally accepted anthropometric criteria, the following are frequently used:
      1. Weight less than 5th or 3rd percentile.
      2. Failure to maintain previously established growth trajectory, particularly after 18 months of age, with parameters crossing two major percentiles (e.g., 75th to below 25th).
      3. Decreased rate of daily weight gain for age (Table 40-2).
      4. Depressed weight for height, which always reflects inadequate nutritional intake for the child's metabolic requirements. (Short stature with a weight that is proportionate to height may reflect chronic malnutrition or may be genetic or endocrinologic in origin.)
    B. History: Key clinical questions. It is important first to scrutinize the growth chart to ascertain the timing of onset of growth failure.
      1. *"What were the changes in your family's or child's life around the time the child's growth slowed?"* Perhaps a parent returned to work and the child was placed in daycare at the time; perhaps there was a family loss.
      2. *"What, when (how often), where, why, and by whom is your child fed?"* It is useful

Table 40-2 Average daily weight gain for age

Age	Median daily weight gain (g)
0–3 mo	26–31
3–6 mo	17–18
6–9 mo	12–13
9–12 mo	9
1–3 yr	7–9
4–6 yr	6

to ascertain a 24-hour dietary recall. Additionally, the child's behaviors and affect at mealtime should be elicited.

3. *"How much low-calorie liquid (e.g., juice, soda, iced tea, Kool-aid, water) does your child drink each day?"*

4. *"Does your child choke on food, have trouble chewing or swallowing, vomit, or spit up?"* Oral motor problems and gastroesophageal reflux usually present with these symptoms.

5. *"What are your child's bowel movements like?"* Frequency and nature of stools may be a clue for occult gastrointestinal disease. Both constipation and diarrhea should prompt further evaluation and intervention.

6. *"Do you ever run out of food?"* If the clinician does not ask, the parents may never tell.

7. *"Does your child snore, even when there is no cold?"* Adenoidal hypertrophy is a frequently missed cause of poor oral intake.

8. *"Are there any foods to which your child is allergic or which he is not allowed to eat for religious or other reasons (e.g., vegetarian)?"*

9. *"Do you and the child's other caretakers see eye to eye about the growing and eating problem?"*

10. *"Are there any significant stresses in the house?"*

C. **Behavioral observations.**
1. The clinician can **observe the child while eating or being fed** in his or her office (or ideally during a home visit by trained observer):
   - Is the child adaptively positioned to eat?
   - Are the child's cues clear, and does the caretaker respond appropriately?
   - Are there oral motor difficulties?
   - Does the caretaker permit age-appropriate autonomy and messiness?
   - What is the affective tone at the feeding interaction for both the feeder and the child?
   - Is the child easily distracted during the feeding?
   - Is the child fed in front of television?
2. The clinician should also observe the **quality of the *nonfeeding* interactions**:
   - Is the caretaker irritable, punitive, depressed, disengaged, or intrusive?
   - Is the child apathetic, irritable, noncompliant, or provocative?

D. **Physical examination.** A careful physical examination should be performed to rule out medical causes of the FTT. Additionally, all children with FTT should have formal developmental testing.

E. **Tests.**
1. Testing should be performed on the basis of the history and physical examination. **Basic screening laboratory tests** should include CBC with differential, lead, FEP, urinalysis, urine culture, electrolytes, and a purified protein derivative (PPD). Clinicians should have a low threshold for obtaining urine cultures, HIV screening, sweat tests, and measurements of immunoglobulin A (IgA) and anti-transglutaminase antibody to rule out occult celiac disease.
2. If the child is a new immigrant or recent traveler, lives in a homeless shelter, has been camping, or is in daycare and has a history of diarrhea or abdominal pain, **evaluation for enteric pathogens** (e.g., *Giardia Lamblia, Heliobactor pylori*) should be considered and screening for hepatitis should be considered.
3. If the child is short but is an appropriate weight for height, a **bone age** may be useful to distinguish the constitutionally short child (with a bone age equivalent to chronological age) from a child with endocrine or nutritional derangement (with a delayed bone age).

III. **Management.**
A. **Primary goals.** The primary goal is for the child to attain catch-up growth at a rate faster than average for age in order to repair the growth deficit. This typically requires a calorically dense diet that provides 1.5–2 times the recommended daily allowance of calories. In addition, other identified socioemotional difficulties must be specifically addressed.

B. **Treatment strategies.**
1. **Instruct the parents in high-calorie/high-protein diet** (Figs. 40-1 and 40-2). This diet may violate current norms since increased fat may be necessary to provide adequate calories in small volume.
2. **Feed the child three meals and three snacks** on a consistent schedule.
3. Give a **multivitamin** with iron and zinc (and therapeutic dosages of iron if indicated).

Try to keep mealtimes and snack times about the same each day. Children work well with schedules.

Children need to eat often, not constantly. Offer something every 2–3 hours, to allow three meals and two to three snacks per day.

Make sure your child can reach the food. Use a high chair, telephone book, or a small table.

Allow your child to feed himself or herself. Try very small amounts at first. Offer seconds later. *Expect messiness.*

No force feeding, bribing, or cajoling! This will backfire.

Variety is not important. Total *calories* and *protein* are.

Offer solids before liquids.

Limit juice, water, and carbonated drinks. Offer milk or formula instead.

Offer foods that are easy for your child to handle: "finger foods" such as Cheerios, french fries, slices of banana, cut-up burger, hot dogs, or peas.

Add margarine, mayonnaise, gravies, and grated cheese. For snacks, use peanut butter, cheese, pudding, bananas, or dried fruit.

Junk foods (soda, doughnuts, candy, etc.) have little protein and fewer calories than some other food choices. Junk foods will not help growth; they only take up valuable space in the stomach.

Eat with your child when possible, or allow your child to eat with others, so meals and snacks can be fun.

Figure 40-1. Effective feeding checklist for parents.

4. **Meet with** *all* **caretakers** involved in feeding the child to reduce conflict, to prevent the child from playing one caretaker against another, and to ensure consistency in the feeding regimen.
5. **Discuss optimal feeding interactions** (e.g., allowing the child to self-feed even if messy, decreasing power struggles at meals, fewer distractions in the environment). Encourage turning off the television at mealtimes, eating with other family members, and pleasant conversation not related to food. Discourage grazing and constant sipping on low-calorie liquids.
6. **Ensure access to resources** (e.g., WIC, food stamps, food pantries).
7. **Give all immunizations** (including influenza vaccine); aggressively **treat intercurrent infections**; use **anti-microbial prophylaxis for recurrent otitis**.
8. **Follow growth weekly to monthly**, depending on age and severity of malnutrition. Success is manifested as faster than normal rate of weight gain for age.
9. Depending on the needs of the family, **mobilize community services,** including mental health, substance abuse treatment, housing advocacy, and job training.
10. **Ensure that the child receives developmental intervention** through Head Start, early intervention, or public school programs.

C. **Criteria for referral.**
1. Children whose **growth rate fails to respond in 2–3 months** should be referred to a multidisciplinary team in an appropriate center.
2. Children with **severe malnutrition, risk of abuse, serious intercurrent illness,** or **extreme parental impairment or anxiety** should be hospitalized.

IV. **Clinical pearls and pitfalls.**
- Failure to correct for prematurity in plotting growth may lead to a factitious diagnosis of FTT. The chronologic age should be corrected for prematurity until 18 months for head circumference, until 24 months for weight, and until 40 months for height. Even after correcting for prematurity, very low birth weight children may remain short for corrected age, but weight for height should be proportionate.
- Children with symmetrical intrauterine growth retardation whether from unknown causes or prenatal exposure to psychoactive substances may remain short but should not be underweight for height.

24-calorie per ounce formula
    1 can (13 oz) formula concentrate.
    8 oz. water.

Note: Don't make the formula more concentrated than this: overconcentrating can be harmful to a child's kidneys.

Super fruit
    1 jar (4 oz) strained fruit
    1 scoop formula powder

Super milk (use instead of whole milk; 28 calories per ounce)
    1 cup dry milk powder
    4 cups whole milk

Super pudding
    2 cups whole milk
    ½ cup dry milk powder
    1 pkg. instant pudding mix
Mix whole and dry milk together. Then follow package directions for making pudding. Yield: 4 servings. (116 calories per serving)

Super shake
    1 cup whole milk
    1 pkg. Carnation Instant Breakfast
    1 cup ice cream
Mix together in blender. (430 calories)

Note: If making any of these changes causes your child to have diarrhea, stop and call your pediatrician.

Figure 40-2. Recipes for children.

- Depressed height for age may be genetic, endocrine, or nutritional, but depressed weight for height always reflects primary or secondary malnutrition.

BIBLIOGRAPHY

For Parents

Texas Children's Hospital, article on high calorie diet.http://216.239.53.104/search?q = cache: fOjriwdNl_cJ:www2.texaschildrenshospital.org/internetarticles/uploadedfiles/ 145.pdf + CHILDREN + HIGH + CALORIE + FOODS&hl = en&ie = UTF-8

For Professionals

Bithoney WG, Dubowitz H, Egan H. Failure to thrive/growth deficiency. *Pediatr Rev* 1992;13: 453–460.
Chatoor I, et al. Nonorganic failure to thrive: A developmental perspective. *Pediatr Ann* 1984;13: 829–843.
Frank DA, Silva M, Needlman R. Failure to thrive: Mystery, myth, and method. *Contemp Pediatr* 1993;10:114–133.
Frank DA, Drotar D, Cook JT, et al. Failure To Thrive. In: Reece RM, Ludwig S (eds). *Child Abuse: Medical Diagnosis and Management.* Philadelphia: Lippincott Williams & Wilkins., 2001: 30–338.

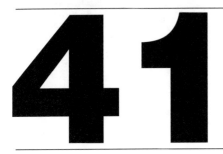

Fears

Marilyn Augustyn

I. **Description of the problem. Fear** is an unpleasant emotion with cognitive, behavioral, and physiological components. It occurs in response to a consciously recognized source of danger, either real or imaginary. From an evolutionary perspective, fear is a key to survival.

A phobia is a persistent and compulsive dread of and preoccupation with the feared object or event. Phobias may interfere with the child's functioning in a way that fears do not.

A. **Epidemiology.**
- Fears are present at various times in the lives of *all* children.
- Between 2–6 years, most children have experienced more than 4 fears.
- Between 6–12 years they experience an average of 7 different fears.
- Fears often peak at 11 years and then decrease with age.
- Studies of identical twins suggest a genetic predisposition to fearfulness in some children.
- Females report fears more often than do males.
- Mothers often underreport (by up to 40%) the fears of their children.
- Unconfronted fears are more likely to persist.
- Phobias are seen in 7% of adults (disabling phobias in 2%); the prevalence in children is unknown.

B. **Familial trends.**
1. **Fearful, anxious parents tend to have fearful, anxious children,** probably through a combination of genetic predisposition and social learning.
2. **Simple phobias appear to run in families,** although individuals rarely share the same specific phobic stimulus.

C. **Etiology/contributing factors.**
1. **Environmental.**
   a. Although fears in childhood reflect a universal developmental tendency, the **onset often relates to a triggering event.** For example, a child may become fearful of dogs following a startling experience with an unleashed large dog. The (perhaps) innate human fear of large animals is intensified by a developmental level that does not allow a nonthreatening explanation of the event.
   b. New **stimuli from the popular culture** join the roster of later childhood fears (e.g., parental divorce, physical assaults, sexual abuse, environmental toxins, terrorist attacks) even as old ones have dissipated (e.g., the Communists).
   c. Significant fears may reflect an **accurate assessment of a truly harmful situation** or represent a **displacement of feeling** from another environmental stressor (e.g., physical or sexual abuse).
2. **Developmental.** Fears change and evolve as cognitive development becomes more sophisticated. Fear of falling and loud noises are the only fears children have at birth. The emergence of other common fears reflect a child's increasing awareness of the world around him. Early childhood fears center on the environment. Exposure to real world dangers intensifies and expands fear. Table 41-1 provides the timing of selected fears throughout early development.

II. **Making the diagnosis.** The most useful way to differentiate a fear from a phobia is **the degree to which the fear interferes with the child's daily activities** (Table 41-2). If the child is developing normally in all other aspects, most often the behavior is a simple fear. If the fear impinges on important activities, it may have progressed to a phobia and requires specialized attention.

A. **History: Key clinical questions.** The primary care clinician must determine if the symptoms represent a simple fear, a response to significant environmental pathology, or a displacement of other stresses in the child's life.
1. *"Does your child's fear interrupt his or her daily schedule more than three times per day?"*

Table 41-1 Common fears in childhood and adolescence

Fear	Age (Years)							
	1	2	3	5	7	9	12	14
Separation	X	X			X			
Noises		X			X			
Falling	X				X		X	
Animals/insects	X		X	X				
Toilet training	X	X						
Bath	X	X						
Bedtime		X	X		X			
Monsters/ghosts		X		X				
Divorce				X				
Getting lost			X	X				
Loss of parent				X				
Social rejection						X		
War						X		
New situations						X		
Adoption						X		X
Burglars							X	X
Injections								X
Sexual relations								X

2. *"Can anyone recall a specific trigger to the fear?"*
    3. *"How do you [the parents] usually respond to the child's fear?"*
III. Management. Management will depend on whether the problem is a simple fear, a mild phobia, a debilitating phobia, or a response to environmental pathology. In most cases, simple parental support and empathy will suffice. Fears are ubiquitous throughout childhood. The goal is not to *banish* all of them but to help the child learn positive ways of coping with and transcending them. In the words of Selma Fraiberg, "The future mental health of the child does not depend upon the presence or absence of ogres in his fantasy life···. It depends upon the child's solution to the ogre problem."
   A. Information for parents. Parents should understand that simple fears are normal and do not necessarily represent a problem in the child or in the environment. The complexity and overwhelming nature of the world, coupled with a child's limited cognitive resources, conspire to create fears in *all* children, even those in the most secure and loving of homes.
   B. Supportive strategies. Parents can exacerbate children's fears by using them as a threat (e.g., *The doctor is going to give you a shot if you're not good*), by humiliating the child (e.g., *Only babies are afraid of bugs*), by indifference to the child's distress, by unrealistic expectations to master the fear, and by over-protectiveness (thereby confirming the child's hypothesis that the stimulus is to be feared). They should follow these guidelines:
   1. Parents should **respect the child's inclination to withdraw from that which is feared**.
   2. The parents and the clinician should not exaggerate the fear or belittle it. They should also not overreact.
   3. Support should be provided to the child as he develops an increased mastery of the fearful object. Don't cater to a fear. This may involve initial avoidance of the fearful stimulus, planned discussions about the fear with attempts to correct cognitive misconceptions, and a gradual introduction to the feared stimulus with much family support, "bibliotherapy", i.e., reading a book together about the feared stimu-

Table 41-2 Differentiation of fears and phobias

	Fears	Phobias
Response to reassurance	Yes	No
Plausible event as cause	Yes	No
Distractable	Yes	No
Impinges on play/development	No	Yes

lus can be useful. Watching reassuring videos together (such as *Monsters, Inc.*) can also lessen anxiety.

4. In young children, some fears cannot be reasoned away. **Parents may have to resort to comprehensible and concrete actions**, such as "monster proofing" the bedroom.

5. **Unconfronted fears can last.** Although many fears will disappear as quickly as they came, some persist and may become ingrained.

6. **Coping with a fear often involves breaking fear into its parts:** physical aspects, cognitive aspects, behavioral aspects. Different techniques may help in fear mastery for each but useful techniques for overcoming fear include: imagination, information, observation, and exposure.

C. **Criteria for referral.** The child/family should be referred to a mental health professional for a phobic condition when fears begin to generalize from the situation of origin or the fears significantly hamper the child's activities of daily living or if the fears are felt to represent a realistic response to a truly threatening environment. Mental health professionals may use such techniques as behavioral modification with systematic desensitization or psychopharmacology to treat severe phobias.

BIBLIOGRAPHY

For Parents

Books

Garber S, Daniels Garber, Spizman Freedman R. *Monsters Under the Bed and Other Childhood Fears: Helping Your Child Overcome Anxieties, Fears and Phobias.* New York: Villard Books, 1993.

Schachter R, McCauley CS. *When Your Child Is Afraid.* New York: Simon and Schuster, 1988.

Websites

American Academy of Pediatrics/Keep Kids Healthy
http://www.keepkidshealthy.com/cgi-bin/extlink.pl?l = http://www.aap.org/pubserv/fears.htm
http://www.keepkidshealthy.com/parenting_tips/fears.html

For Young Children

Dutro J. *Night Light.* New York: Magination Press, 1991.
Lankton S, Wiley N. *The Blammo-Surprise Book!* New York: Magination Press, 1988.
Wineman M, Marcus I, Marcus P. *Scary Night Visitors.* New York: Magination Press, 1990.

For Professionals

Egger H, Costello E, et al. School refusal and psychiatric disorders: A community study. *J Am Acad Child Adolesc Psychiatry* 2003;42(7):797–807.

Ollendick T, Neville J, Muris P. Fears and phobias in children: Phenomenology, epidemiology, and aetiology. *Child & Adolescent Mental Health.* 2002;7(3):98–106.

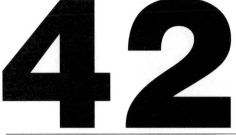

Fetal Alcohol Syndrome

Barbara A. Morse
Lyn Weiner

I. **Description of the problem.** Fetal alcohol syndrome (FAS) is a specific cluster of physical and neurobehavioral birth defects associated with maternal alcohol abuse during pregnancy. FAS represents the most severe end of possible damage. Fetal alcohol effects (FAE) or alcohol-related neurodevelopmental disorder (ARND) represent less severe forms of damage.

   A. **Epidemiology.**
   - FAS is variously estimated as occurring in 0.33–4.0/1,000 live births.
   - Among alcohol-abusing mothers, 10% will deliver a child with FAS and as many as 30%–40% will deliver a child with FAE.
   - FAS/FAE occur in all races and at all socioeconomic levels.
   - The risk for FAS/FAE may increase with greater parity or poor nutrition. Higher rates (1/250) are seen among certain ethnic groups (e.g., some Native Americans).

   B. **Etiology/contributing factors.**
   1. **Dose.** The more alcohol that is consumed, the greater the risk for FAS. Conversely, when consumption is reduced, so is risk.
   2. **Pattern.** Drinking patterns that produce very high blood alcohol levels, whether daily or weekly, pose the greatest risk.
   3. **Timing.** Effects vary by gestational stage of exposure. First trimester exposure poses risks to structural development; third trimester exposure has the greatest impact on CNS development.
   4. **Genetic sensitivity.** Dizygotic twins have demonstrated differential effects. There may also be racial or ethnic differences in the metabolism of and sensitivity to alcohol exposure.
   5. **Maternal metabolism.** Chronic heavy alcohol use impairs maternal hepatic function and reduces the mother's capacity to metabolize alcohol. Elimination of alcohol is slowed, acetaldehyde levels rise, and the potential for damage is increased.
   6. **Maternal nutrition.** Poor diet influences outcome. Chronic maternal alcohol use can deplete minerals and vitamins available to the fetus (notably magnesium, zinc, and folic acid).
   7. **Parity.** FAS is uncommon in a first pregnancy. The effects of alcohol become more severe with each child born.

II. **Making the diagnosis.**
   A. **Signs and symptoms.** Signs should be evident in each of these areas:
   1. **Pre- and/or postnatal growth retardation.** Weight, length, and/or head circumference are below the 10th percentile. Growth retardation persists throughout childhood, but improves substantially in adolescence. Initially, weight is more affected than height.
   2. **CNS involvement.** CNS problems may range from subtle to severe. Microcephaly, diminished cognition, developmental delays, neurobehavioral disorders, nonverbal learning disabilities, perceptual dysfunction, impaired memory and hyperactivity are common. Development may proceed erratically, appearing normal at times and delayed at others.

      About 30% of affected children have IQs below 70. The 40%–50% with IQs greater than 85 have fewer morphologic anomalies but have persistent neurobehavioral problems, including sleep disorders, sensory integration difficulties, language dysfunction and information processing difficulties. Logical and abstract thinking is often poor, and they may appear aggressive, oppositional, willful or lazy. Because their IQs are adequate and they appear "normal", making the case for services for this group is especially difficult.
   3. **Characteristic facial dysmorphology.** This may include
      - Microophthalmia and/or short palpebral fissures
      - A poorly developed philtrum

- A thin upper lip
- Flattening of the maxillary area
- A "scooped" nose, wide nasal bridge
- Low-set ears

These characteristics are most easily seen in severe cases and may be subtle in newborns, making diagnosis difficult. Sometimes these features become apparent only at age 2 or 3 years and often diminish in adolescence.

B. Signs of FAE. FAE is diagnosed when there are one or two of the signs noted for FAS in the presence of maternal alcohol abuse. Neurodevelopmental problems such as hyperactivity and learning disabilities and behavioral problems are most typically seen in FAE.

C. Differential diagnosis. A careful history that includes maternal alcohol use is needed to differentiate the effects of alcohol from those of other teratogens. The combination of growth retardation, facial dysmorphology, and CNS disturbance is not unique to FAS and may also be seen in other disorders (e.g., fetal hydantoin syndrome, Comelia de Lange syndrome, maternal phenylketonuria, Noonan syndrome).

D. History: Key clinical questions.
1. *"During this pregnancy, how many times a week did you drink beer, wine, or liquor? How many cans, glasses, or drinks each time?"* (Or in the case of a foster or adopted child, *"Do you know how much alcohol was consumed during this pregnancy?"*). FAS/FAE is associated with high blood alcohol concentrations and can be ruled out in children born to women known to have consumed small amounts.
2. *"Does your child show unusual sensitivity to touch (overreaction to injury, tags in the back of clothes, hugs), light, or sound (says things are too bright or too loud)? Does the child have difficulty behaving at large, noisy gatherings or at recess or lunch?"* Sensory hypersensitivity is a frequent but poorly recognized feature of FAS causing children to become easily overstimulated.
3. *"How does your child relate to peers?"* Many children with FAS read social cues very poorly and have few friends their own age. They may appear excessively friendly or fearless and exhibit poor judgment and impulse control.
4. *"Does your child understand cause and effect, abstract thinking? Can he generalize information learned in one context to another?"* Although their verbal skills make them appear superficially competent, people with FAS often fail to understand cause and effect, are unable to link consequences with their actions, to understand abstract ideas or generalize information.
5. *"How does your child react to a change in routine, such as a substitute teacher?"* Children with FAS rely on consistency. When a change occurs without sufficient preparation, they may react with frustration, aggression, or perseveration.
6. *Does your child seem to "learn" and "forget" the same piece of information over and over?"* A child's ability to retrieve cognitive information is often impaired in FAS/FAE.

E. Physical examination.
1. **Assessment** (both present and historical) of growth, CNS functioning, and facial dysmorphology is critical.
2. **Associated pathology** may be found in the following areas: cardiac (e.g., septal defects), renal (e.g., hypoplasia, hypospadias), ocular (e.g., intraocular abnormalities, strabismus, ptosis), ear (e.g., recurrent otitis media, deafness), skeletal (e.g., radioulnar synostosis, retarded bone growth), oral (e.g., poor suck, cleft palate) or immune system (increased infections, especially URI, nonspecific neoplasms).

F. Tests. There are no specific diagnostic tests for FAS. Neuropsychological and sensory integration assessment may assist in planning appropriate services.

III. Management.
A. Information for the family.
1. Symptoms are not the result of "poor parenting" or "a bad personality." The child is "unable," not "unwilling."
2. Children with FAS depicted in the media are often uniquely severe cases and do not represent the majority of children with FAS.
3. FAS/FAE is permanent but not degenerative. Some problems persist, while others improve. Diagnosis, intervention and treatment improve outcomes.
4. FAS results from chronic maternal alcoholism, not "a single drink before knowledge of conception."

B. Treatment.
1. **Medication.** Stimulants (methylphenidate, dextroamphetamine); serotonin reuptake inhibitors (SSRIs) (fluoxetine, fluvoxamine, sertraline); anti-convulsants (carbamaz-

epine, valproic acid); and anti-psychotics (thioridazine, risperidone) have all been used and reported anecdotally to have some success in improving focus, reducing activity levels, addressing depression or mood disorders, and controlling aggression or panic disorders. Working with a psychopharmacologist may be helpful.

2. **Sensory integration.** Sensory integration therapy (by specialized occupational therapists) can help a child's brain better handle tactile, auditory, and proprioceptive stimulation. Adaptations in the environment (e.g., nonrestrictive clothing, placement at end of line, sunglasses to reduce glare) help to avoid overstimulation and improve the child's ability to pay attention. Preparing the child for physical contact, loud noises, or bright lights can reduce overreactions. This therapy can also assist with sleeping and eating problems if they are sensory related.

3. **Social skills training.** The ability to read social cues is improved by teaching the child (using photographs and television) how to interpret facial expressions. Another strategy is to have the child practice specific expressions and communicative gestures in front of a minor or on videotape.

4. **Teaching cause and effect.** Repetition is the most effective way to teach cause and effect. Role playing the appropriate interpretation of ambiguous situations and appropriate reactions will also increase understanding. Children learn more quickly when external cues, such as pictures, are used.

5. **Adapting to transitions.** Adaptation to transitions is best achieved with explanations and ample warnings of an impending change in the routine or environment.

6. **Improving memory.** Learning can be improved by going beyond auditory and visual teaching methods and using tactile and kinesthetic strategies. Typewriters, computers, and tape recorders can compensate for poor memory or retrieval.

IV. **Clinical pearls and pitfalls.**
- Diagnosis (the earlier the better) is the single greatest factor to predict good outcome.
- For many affected children, facial features are subtle and may only be observed after the diagnosis has been suggested from other signs.
- Normal or average IQ is not a disqualifier for FAS/FAE, since the range of IQ is broad and at least 40% of those with FAS/FAE have IQs greater than 85. Severe mental retardation is rare.
- Sensory hypersensitivity is often misread as aggression or emotional liability; learning disabilities are misconstrued as behavioral problems.
- Many children with FAS suffer from low self-esteem due to their disabilities. Referral to a supportive therapist may be useful in such cases.
- Addressing primary disabilities (learning problems, etc.) is the best way to prevent secondary disabilities (substance abuse, school failure, mental illness).
- Behavioral problems (inappropriate sexual behavior, aggression, lying, involvement with the law) may escalate during adolescence.
- The clinician who suspects continuing addiction must be prepared to refer a parent for substance abuse evaluation and treatment. He or she can join with the parent's desire to help the child.
- The clinician can help the biologic mother to understand that she did not drink during pregnancy out of malice or with intent to damage and that both she and her child are victims of the disease of alcoholism.

BIBLIOGRAPHY

For Parents

Kleinfield J, Wescott S (eds). *Fantastic Antone Succeeds: Experiences in Educating Children with Fetal Alcohol Syndrome.* University of Alaska Press, 1993.

Kleinfeld JS, Morse BA, Wescott S (eds). *Fantastic Antone Grows Up: Assisting Alcohol Affected Adolescents and Adults.* University of Alaska Press, 1998.

Morse BA, Weiner L. *FAS: Parent and Child-A Handbook for Parent Raising Children with FAS. Available from the Fetal Alcohol Education Program, Boston University School of Medicine,* 1975 Main Street, Concord, MA 07142.

Streissguth, AP. *Fetal Alcohol Syndrome: A Guide for Families and Communities.* Baltimore: Paul R Brookes Publishing, 1997.

For Professionals

PM Medical Health News. 21st Century Complete Medical Guide to Fetal Alcohol Syndrome (FAS), Authoritative Government Documents, Clinical References, and Practical Information for Parents. CDROM:PRogressive Management, 2004.

Stratton K, Howe C, Battaglia F (eds). *Fetal Alcohol Syndrome: Diagnosis, Epidemiology, Prevention and Treatment.* Washington, DC: National Academy Press, 1996.

Websites for Parents and Professionals

The National Center on Birth Defects and Developmental Disabilities http://www.cdc.gov/ncbddd/fas/

I.   Description of the problem. Fragile X syndrome (FXS) is the most common inherited form of mental retardation. It causes a spectrum of developmental problems, ranging from learning disabilities and emotional problems (in those with a normal IQ) through all levels of mental retardation.

A. Epidemiology.

- Causes mental retardation in approximately 1 in 3,200 males in the general population and 1 in 6,000 females.
- Responsible for 30% of all cases of X-linked mental retardation.
- Approximately 1 in 259 females and 1 in 810 males in the general population carry the premutation.
- No known racial or ethnic differences; identified in all racial groups tested.
- Both males and females can be unaffected carriers although late onset tremor and ataxia can occur in male carriers >50 years.

B. Genetics. FXS is caused by a mutation in the fragile X mental retardation-1 gene (FMR-1), which is located on the bottom end of the X chromosome. The mutation causes a fragile site or break in the chromosome at that location. The FMR-1 gene was identified and sequenced in 1991. An unusual expansion of a cytosine, guanine, guanine (CGG) nucleotide repetitive sequence was found to be the mutation. Within the FMR-1 gene, normal individuals have a nucleotide CGG sequence that repeats up to 45 times, **carriers with a permutation have an expansion of the CGG sequence between 55–200 repeats**, and **individuals affected with FXS have a CGG repeat number greater than 200 (termed a full mutation)**. When this occurs, the gene usually becomes methylated or turned off so that little or no FMR-1 protein is made, and the full fragile X syndrome occurs.

A carrier male will pass his only X chromosome to all of his daughters, who will be obligate carriers and pass the mutation to 50% of their offspring. A significant expansion of the mutation will often occur in their children so that retarded male and significantly learning disabled female offspring are common. A detailed family tree must be drawn to sort out possible carriers and other extended family members who may be affected by FXS.

II.   Making the diagnosis. Both behavioral and physical features are included in the fragile X checklist (Fig. 43-1), which serves as a reminder for clinicians of the signs and symptoms of fragile X.

A. Signs and symptoms in males.

1. Early signs and symptoms.

- Infants with FXS may appear to be normal, although temperamental and feeding difficulties have been described.
- **Recurrent otitis media** begins in the first year of life for the majority of males affected by this syndrome.
- **Hypotonia** is also notable in young boys, with subsequent mild delays in motor milestones.
- Most boys with fragile X and significantly affected girls with fragile X **are delayed in the onset of language**. Phrases or short sentences are usually delayed until age 3 years or older. The language delays in addition to hyperactivity or tantrums are the typical initial concerns leading to medical consultation.
- **Prominent ears** with occasional ear cupping, **hyperextensible finger joints, double-jointed thumbs, flat feet**, and soft skin are seen in the majority of fragile X boys in early childhood. These physical findings are considered to be part of a connective tissue dysplasia that is related to the absence of the FMR-1 protein.
- Young boys with FXS may also have a broad or prominent forehead and a large head circumference.

2. Later signs and symptoms.

- **Macroorchidism** becomes prominent in males with fragile X during the early

	SCORE:	0	1	2
			Borderline or present	
		Not present	In the past	Definitely present
Mental retardation				
Hyperactivity				
Short attention span				
Tactilely defensive				
Hand flapping				
Hand biting				
Poor eye contact				
Perseverative speech				
Hyperextensible finger joints				
Large or prominent ears				
Large testicles				
Simian crease or Sydney line				
Family history of mental retardation or autism				

TOTAL SCORE _____

A score > 15 has a 45% chance of FXS

Figure 43-1. Fragile X checklist. Modified from Hagerman RJ, Amiri K, Cronister A. Fragile X checklist. *Am J Med Genet* 38:283–287, 1991.

stages of puberty. Usually the testicular volume is at least twice normal size, with an adult range in FXS of 40–100 cc. Although the spermatic tubules are tortuous by histological studies, fertility has been reported in several males with FXS.
- Additionally, a long **face and prominent jaw** are often noted after puberty.
- Other diagnoses such as Soto syndrome, Tourette syndrome, Pierre Robin sequence and other congenital defects such as cleft palate or hip dislocation may be associated with FXS because of the connective tissue problems and behavioral difficulties that occur in this disorder.
B. **Behavioral problems in males.** Behavioral problems are a common presenting complaint in young boys with FXS. These include hyperactivity; impulsivity; an extremely short attention span; perseveration in speech and actions; hand flapping with excitement; hand biting with anger or frustration; oversensitivity to touch, noises, and textures of food or clothing; shyness; poor eye contact; and tantrums. These behaviors are often described as "autistic-like," and 30% of boys with FXS have autism.
C. **Signs and symptoms in girls. Approximately 70% of females who carry the full mutation will have a borderline or retarded IQ.** The other 30% will have a normal IQ but may have significant learning disabilities, including attentional problems (with or without hyperactivity), math deficits, and language delays. **Significant shyness is** very common, often accompanied by poor eye contact. Females with FXS may be given a psychiatric diagnosis of avoidant disorder or autism because of their social deficits. Schizotypal features (i.e., oddness in social interactional skills and appearance), depres-

sion, mood lability, anxiety, impulsive behavior, attention deficit hyperactivity disorder (ADHD), or emotional problems have also been reported in women affected by FXS.

   D. Tests. All children with mental retardation or autism of unknown etiology should have **fragile X DNA testing.** If a learning disabled or carrier individual is suspected, fragile X (FMR-1) DNA testing should also be carried out. Once a proband is diagnosed with FXS, other family members should be assessed with FMR-1 DNA testing, including all siblings of the proband and of the carrier parent and grandparent. Premutation carriers, (older than 50 years, especially males, are at risk for the fragile X-associated tremor/ataxia syndrome (FXTAS) and should be referred to a neurologist if symptoms of tremor or gait instability occur.

III. Management.

   A. Goals and initial treatment strategies. The goals of the primary care clinician are to provide appropriate medical therapy and to coordinate a team of professionals who will provide optimal treatment for the child with fragile X. Speech and language therapy and occupational therapy are essential for all young children affected by FXS. A developmental preschool setting can usually provide these therapies, in addition to special education. Whenever possible, mainstreaming or full inclusion with normal peers is preferable since children with FXS usually model their behavior after their peers.

   B. Follow-up. Medical follow-up includes recognition and treatment of connective tissue problems and associated complications of fragile X syndrome (Table 43-1). **Since ophthalmological problems** are common, referral to an ophthalmologist prior to age 5 years will facilitate early treatment. Orthopedic referral is appropriate if scoliosis or joint dislocations occur. Mitral valve prolapse is usually noted in the older child or adult, so referral to a cardiologist for evaluation and echocardiogram is necessary if a murmur or click is heard in auscultation. Vigorous treatment of recurrent otitis media in early childhood is indicated and usually includes the use of pressure equalizing (PE) tubes, so that a fluctuating hearing loss does not interfere with optimal language development.

   C. Psychopharmacology. The most common behavioral problem is hyperactivity, which is seen in approximately 80% of affected boys and 30% of affected girls. Therefore treatment of ADHD symptoms in these children is a main focus of intervention (see Chapter 25). Folic acid in a dosage of 10 mg/day may be somewhat helpful for approximately 50% of young children. However, it is not as effective as stimulant medication, which is helpful for over 60% of children with FXS who are age 5 years or older.

   A common concern of families of adolescent children with fragile X syndrome is treatment of outbursts or aggression, a significant problem in approximately 30% of male adults and adolescents with FXS. Episodic dyscontrol usually occurs during or after significant environmental overstimulation (such as shopping in a busy store), or it may be precipitated by anger or frustration. A variety of medications have been used with some success (including clonidine, SSRIs, risperidone and anticonvulsants), but controlled studies have not yet been performed. Serotonin reuptake inhibitors (SSRIs) such as fluoxetine, sertraline, and cetalopram show the most promise; they have fewer side effects than antipsychotic medication and help to improve mood, obsessive-compulsive behavior, and anxiety. SSRIs have also been helpful to the majority of carrier females who have had significant problems with depression and anxiety.

   D. Other therapies. Sensory integration therapy by an occupational therapist with a specific focus on calming techniques may be helpful. Significant behavioral problems may also respond to a behavioral modification program organized by a psychologist who can also provide support and guidance for the parents. If autism is diagnosed, behavior intervention treatment for autism should be carried out.

Table 43-1 Associated medical problems in fragile X syndrome in males

Medical problem	Frequency in males
Flat feet	80%
Scoliosis	<20%
Mitral valve prolapse	50%–80% in adulthood
Recurrent otitis	60%
Strabismus	8%–30%
Nystagmus	Occasional
Refractive errors	20%
Seizures	20%
Macroorchidism	80% at puberty

E. **Criteria for referral.** All families with fragile X syndrome should be referred to a geneticist or genetics counselor for a detailed discussion regarding the inheritance of this mutation and an assessment of other family members, who require DNA testing to clarify their carrier status.

BIBLIOGRAPHY

For Parents

National Fragile X Foundation. Has produced many educational pamphlets, books, and videotapes regarding FXS; has resource centers associated with parent support groups in the United States and internationally; supports research and organizes conferences for parents and professionals. 1615 Bonanza Street, Suite 320 Walnut Creek, CA 94596 1-800-688-8765 www.FragileX.org

FRAXA Research Foundation. Has a network of support groups and funds research. P.O. Box 935 West Newbury, MA 01985-0935 978-462-1866 www.fraxa.org

Conquer Fragile X. This foundation funds international research on fragile X. 189 Bradley Place, Ste. 1 Palm Beach FL 33480 561-842-9219 www.CFXF.org

For Professionals

National Fragile X Foundation. Identifies laboratories that carry out DNA testing.1-800-688-8765 or 925-938-9300

Braden ML. *Fragile, Handle with Care: More About Fragile X Syndrome, Adolescents and Adults.* Dillon, CO: Spectra Publishing Co., 2000.

Glaser B, Hessl D, Dyer-Friedman J, et al. Biological and environmental contributions to adaptive behavior in fragile x syndrome. *Am J Med Genetics* 2003;117A:21—29.

Hagerman RJ. Medical follow-up and pharmacotherapy. In RJ Hagerman, PJ Hagerman (eds), *Fragile X Syndrome: Diagnosis, Treatment and Research (3rd ed).* Baltimore: Johns Hopkins University Press, 2002: 287–338.

Hagerman RJ, Leehey M, Heinrichs W, et al. Intention tremor, parkinsonism, and generalized brain atrophy in male carriers of fragile X. *Neurology* 2001;57:127–130.

Websites

National Fragile X Foundation http://www.fragileX.org
FRAXA Research Foundation http://www.fraxa.org
Conquer Fragile X http://www.CFXF.org
http://dante.med.utoronto.ca/Fragile-X/linksto.htm

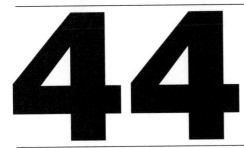

Gay, Lesbian, & Bisexual Youth

C. Wayne Sells
Gary Remafedi

I. **Description of the issue.** *Homosexuality* is defined as "a persistent pattern of homosexual arousal accompanied by a persistent pattern of absent or weak heterosexual arousal." *Sexual orientation* encompasses sexual fantasies, emotional and romantic attractions, sexual behavior, and self-identification. The heterosexual or homosexual direction of any of these dimensions may not be consistent, defying the simple categorization of individuals as heterosexual, homosexual, or bisexual. Sexual orientation, rather, should be viewed as a continuum between absolute heterosexuality and homosexuality.

A. **Epidemiology.**
- In a survey of almost than 35,000 junior and senior high school students, 1.1% described themselves as gay, lesbian, or bisexual. The percentage reporting predominantly homosexual attractions steadily increased with age, with a peak of 6.4% among 18-year-old students.
- In various studies, 1%–37% of youths have reported same-sex experiences.

B. **Familial transmission/genetics.** To date there have been three small studies examining the genetics of homosexuality. One had positive findings, one mildly positive, and one negative. No conclusive study has yet been done.

C. **Etiology/contributing factors.**
1. **Environmental/social process theory.** There is no scientific evidence that environmental stressors lead to a homosexual orientation. Additionally, it is now generally accepted that homosexual orientation is not due to parental influences, as had been suggested by the early "dominant mother–passive uninvolved father" theories.
2. **Organic/hormonal theory.** A biologic model involving hormonal influences and homosexuality has been postulated. However, assays of androgens, estrogens, and other hormones have not shown consistent differences between adult homosexual and heterosexual persons. Interestingly, an increased incidence of homosexuality in women with congenital adrenal hyperplasia (despite early detection and correction of androgen excess) has been observed. Neuroanatomic differences between homosexual men and heterosexual men and women have been noted in sexually dimorphic regions of the brain. Various studies also have found neurophysiological and neurobehavioral correlates of homosexuality. These observations support the hypothesis that factors operating early in development may have differentiated structures and functions of the brain that influence sexual orientation.

D. **Stages of acquisition of homosexual identity (Troiden). Stage I: Sensitization.** During childhood there is often a sense of being different from same-sex peers.

   Stage II: Identity confusion. Homosexual feelings create confusion and uncertainty about sexual identity. The adolescent may respond by trying to ignore homosexual impulses and activities or to view these behaviors as temporary.

   Stage III: Identity assumption. When the adolescent or young adult's confusion about sexual orientation is resolved, he or she is often able to share his or her identity with others ("coming out"). Close friends are usually informed before parents or professionals.

   Stage IV: Commitment. Stage IV is generally reached during adulthood when the individual experiences self-acceptance, emotional intimacy, and an unwillingness to alter sexual orientation.

II. **Making the diagnosis.**
A. **Recognizing gay, lesbian, and bisexual youth.** Homosexual youth have many of the same medical concerns and needs as heterosexual teenagers. However, they are at greater risk for both psychosocial and medical problems because of the experience of growing up gay, lesbian, or bisexual.
1. **Psychosocial issues.**
   a. **Homophobia** is an irrational, distorted fear of homosexuality or homosexual individuals. This fear may be manifested as discomfort, prejudice, verbal abuse, or

psychological or physical hostility. In the face of disapproval from friends or family, the teenager may internalize feelings of guilt and shame, contributing to poor self-image.

b. Depression and suicidality are potential consequences of the teenager's sense of isolation in an openly hostile environment. In various studies, 20%–40% of gay, lesbian, and bisexual youths have reported suicide attempts. They may be at greatest risk when first acknowledging their bisexuality or homosexuality, often before having told others or internalized homophobia (self-loathing). In a large population-based study, gay and bisexual males were 7 times more likely than heterosexual males to attempt suicide; but there was no significant association between sexual orientation and attempted suicide in young women. The findings suggest that suicidality is not caused by homosexuality, but might be mediated by other factors that particularly disadvantage males.

c. Homelessness and prostitution. Many gay, lesbian, or bisexual youths leave their homes because of parental disapproval or rejection. The teenager's desperation, poor self-esteem, lack of education or job skills, and social isolation without adult or peer role models may leave few options but to engage in sex for survival (i.e., prostitution).

d. Substance abuse may represent an attempt to ease the pain of isolation, condemnation, and rejection. An increased frequency of alcoholism among lesbians when compared to heterosexual women has been reported. Similar trends exist with males but the association is not as strong.

2. Medical issues.

a. Tobacco. Gay, lesbian, or bisexual youth are more likely to initiate tobacco use at a younger age and to report ongoing tobacco use than their heterosexual peers.

b. Eating disorders. It has been theorized that both gay men and heterosexual women are predisposed to weight dissatisfaction and eating disorders by a desire to appear physically attractive to men. In a population-based study of adolescents, one quarter of gay youth reported a poor body image, and about 1 in 10 dieted frequently or purged. As compared to heterosexual males, all indicators of disordered eating were more prevalent among gay youth. By contrast, lesbian adolescents reported a better body image than heterosexual females, without significant differences in eating disorder behaviors.

c. HIV and sexually transmitted infections (STIs). Gay youth who have multiple partners and engage in high-risk behaviors are at greatest risk for sexually transmitted infections (STIs) and human immunodeficiency virus (HIV). In a recent (2000) study of HIV seroprevalence, 7% of 3,492 15–22-year-old men who have sex with men (MSM) living in seven US cities were HIV seropositive. The initial optimism of the 1980s that the epidemic in gay communities could be contained by massive behavioral change is fading with new reports that youths have not been reached by preventive messages. Among subpopulations of teenage MSM, HIV seroprevalence is highest among youth of color. Lesbian teenagers with only same-sex partners are at lower risk for STIs than either gay or heterosexual youth.

d. Traumatic Injuries related to sexual intercourse. Primarily consists of anorectal trauma secondary to anal intercourse or use of foreign objects for anal intercourse.

B. Differential diagnosis.

1. Transient sexual orientation ambiguity. Given appropriate information and support, individuals generally will resolve uncertainty about sexual orientation by late adolescence through self-exploration of feelings, fantasies, and experiences. Paroski (1987) describes an 18-month process consisting of: realization of same sex desire; guilt and shame for those feelings; attempts to change to heterosexuality through altering behavior or fantasy; failure to alter sexual orientation with the subsequent development of poor self-esteem; investigation into homosexual lifestyle through various methods, including sexual activity, acceptance, and development of positive homosexual identity.

2. A transvestite is a person who derives pleasure by dressing in clothing of the opposite sex. Typically, this person's sexual orientation is heterosexual.

3. Transsexual individuals feel that their anatomic gender does not correspond to psychological gender identity.

C. History: Key clinical questions. Establish confidentiality. Establish a "need to know": tell the patient that there will be personal questions asked and although the patient dose *not have* to answer all questions, honest answers will result in the best medical care. Ask all questions nonjudgmentally.

1. *"Have you ever dated?"* Asking "Do you have a girlfriend?" of a gay male teenager may suggest that the health provider is not open to a discussion of the youth's boyfriend.
2. *"There are many different ways of being sexual with another person: hugging, kissing, touching genitals, intercourse. Have you begun having sexual relations?"* It is important to understand the extent of the teenager's sexual activity.
3. *"Are these relations with men, women, or both"?* Although the teenager may not readily discuss homosexual behaviors or feelings, he or she now knows that there are others with similar feelings and that the health provider is approachable.
4. *"Have you ever had oral sex? Vaginal intercourse? Rectal intercourse."* Once an individual has acknowledged homosexual sexual behaviors, it is important to inquire about specific sexual experiences. Detailed information (e.g., receptive vs. insertive intercourse) will help assess risk factors for HIV/STIs.
5. *"How do you protect yourself against pregnancy and sexually transmitted infections, including HIV?"* It is important to determine the teenager's knowledge of pregnancy, STIs, and AIDS in order to help the youth with risk reduction.
6. *"Do you consider yourself heterosexual (straight), bisexual, gay, or lesbian"?* Sexual activity alone may be a poor indicator of sexual orientation.
7. *"Do you have any concerns about your sexual feelings, attractions, or the things you are doing?"* The youth should know that it is permissible to discuss his or her concerns.
8. *"Have you discussed your sexual attractions with your friends? Parents? Other adults?"* It is important to know if the teenager has a support system with which he or she can discuss openly these very personal feelings.

   D. **Behavioral observations.** Observation of gender-atypical behaviors is not a reliable indicator of sexual orientation. The healthcare provider should avoid stereotyping the effeminate male and tomboy female.
III. **Management.**
   A. **Primary goals** include the promotion of healthy physical, sexual, social, and emotional development. The teenager must develop a positive gay, lesbian, or bisexual self-image in which he or she is seen as a respectable, lovable, and competent person with the ability to enjoy emotional and safe physical intimacy with persons of the same gender. Many youths will experience significant confusion, guilt, fear, and anxiety as they raise questions about their sexual orientation. These feelings are common and need to be discussed and understood. There is no need for the youth to make an immediate decision concerning sexual orientation; over time, sexual orientation will become clear.
   B. **Information for the family.** Parents of gay, lesbian, or bisexual teenagers may experience a multitude of emotions, including anger, guilt, grief, and fear. It is important to explore these feelings. In many cases, the primary care provider can help the family view homosexuality as an acceptable variation of sexual orientation. The teenager's potential for a happy, healthy, and productive life need not be limited by his or her sexual orientation.
   C. **Specific care.**
   1. **Initial strategies** emphasize patient and parent education concerning development and sexuality, including HIV prevention information. Healthy adult and peer role models, in addition to social support groups, are extremely important to youth. Support groups for parents are also very useful.
   2. **Anticipatory guidance** is extremely important for gay and lesbian youth. Many youth will have difficult and extremely complicated questions (e.g., with whom, how, and when to discuss their sexual orientation).
   3. **Psychosocial development** should be carefully monitored. Both the teenager's and the family's adjustment should be followed. Additional services and support may be needed, including alternative schools; gay or lesbian sensitive mental health and social services; foster home placement; prostitution diversion programs; special programs for adolescents with human immunodeficiency virus (HIV); and gay and lesbian community clinics.
   4. **High-risk behaviors.** The clinician should assess the patient's symptoms and high-risk behaviors, inquiring about depression; suicidality; conflict with family and peer; faltering academic and job performance; substance abuse; and unsafe sexual behaviors.
   5. **Contraception and sexually transmitted infection (STI) prevention.** Not all gay, lesbian, and bisexual youth need a full STI evaluation. The level of evaluation depends on the teenager's sexual behaviors. It is important that the provider creates a safe environment in which the youth feels comfortable discussing personal information. It is always important that the provider remember that the youth's sexual orientation does not necessarily correlate with sexual behaviors. Thus, gay and lesbian youth may also need access to effective contraceptives.
   D. **Criteria for referral** include severe psychiatric symptoms (e.g., suicidal ideation, depres-

sion; serious social problems (e.g., prostitution, homelessness, school dropout, chemical dependency); or problems of personal or family adjustment that do not respond to education and social support.

IV. Clinical pearls and pitfalls.

- When coming out, isolated adolescents may exhibit severe psychiatric symptoms (e.g., extreme anxiety, depression, cognitive impairment, emotional liability) which may resolve quickly when appropriate information and social support are provided.
- Most teenagers are aware of their attractions before having sex. Discourage sexual experimentation as a litmus test for sexual orientation.
- In order to avoid embarrassment and judgment, gay and lesbian adolescents often tell healthcare providers that they are unsure of their sexual feelings or that they are "experimenting" with bisexuality.
- When a professional says that an adolescent is confused about sexual orientation, more often than not it is the professional who is confused because of lack of information or misinformation.
- Regardless of sexual orientation labels, young men who have unsafe sex with men require intensive HIV prevention services, which should not await the determination of sexual identity.
- Because of the risks of rejection and discrimination, the clinician should encourage careful forethought and planning prior to disclosure of homosexuality to family and friends.
- Even if initially vitriolic, parents' first reactions to a child's homosexuality often temper with time.
- Young lesbians and gay men often experiment with partners of the opposite sex. The clinician should inquire about heterosexual experience and the need to protect against pregnancy and HIV/STIs.
- Efforts to change sexual orientation over time are unsuccessful.

BIBLIOGRAPHY

Organizations

Bisexual Resource Center (BRC) P.O. Box 1026 Boston, MA 02117-1026 617-424-9595 www.biresource.org

Gay, Lesbian, Straight Educational Network (GLSEN) 121 West 27th Street, Suite 804, New York, NY, 10001, 212-727-0135 http://www.glsen.org/templates/index.html

National AIDS Hotline 1-800-342-2437 http://www.ashastd.org/nah/

National Federation of Parents and Friends of Lesbians & Gays, Inc. lpar;P-FLAG) 1726 M Street, NW Suite 400 Washington DC 20036 202-467-8180 www.pflag.org

National Gay and Lesbian Task Force 1325 Massachusetts Ave NW, Suite 600 Washington DC 20005 202-393-5177 www.ngltf.org

National Youth Advocacy Coalition (NYAC) 1638 R Street NW, Suite 300 Washington, DC 20009 1-800-541-6922 http://nyacyouth.org

For Teenagers and Young Adults

Books

Bass E, Kaufmann K. *Free Your Mind.* New York: Harper Collins, 1996.

Bauer MD (ed). *Am I Blue? Coming Out From the Silence.* Minneapolis: Harper Collins Children's Books, 1994.

Heron A (ed). *Two Teenagers in Twenty – Writings by Gay and Lesbian Youth.* Boston: Alyson Publications, 1994.

Pollack R, Schwartz CH. *The Journey Out – A Guide for and About Lesbian, Gay, and Bisexual teens.* New York: Puffin Books, 1995.

Rench JE. *Understanding Sexual Identity: A Book for Gay Teens and Their Friends.* Minneapolis: Lerner, 1990.

For Parents

Books

Bernstein R. *Straight Parents, Gay Children: Keeping Families Together.* New York: Thunder's Month Press, 1995.

Chandler K. *Passages of Pride.* New York: Times Books, Random House, Inc., 1995.

For Professionals

Frankowski BL, and the Committee on Adolescence. American Academy of Pediatrics, Clinical Report. Sexual Orientation and Adolescents *Pediatric* 2004 June;113(6):1827–1832.

Stonski Huwiler S, Remafedi G. Adolescent Homosexuality. *Advances in Pediatrics* 1998;45: 107–144.

Meininger E, Cohen E, Neinstein L, et al. Gay, Lesbian and Bisexual Adolescents. In LS Neinstein, (ed), *Adolescent Health Care: A Practical Guide (4th ed)*. Philadelphia: Lippincott Williams & Wilkins, 2002.

Mondimore F. *A Natural History of Homosexuality*. Baltimore: The Johns Hopkins University Press, 1996.

Paroski PA Jr. Health Care Delivery and the Concerns of Gay and Lesbian Adolescents. *Journal of Adolescent Health Care* 1987 Mar;8(2):188–192.

Perrin E. *Sexual Orientation in Children and Adolescents: Implications for Health Care*. New York: Kluwer Academic/Plenum, 2002.

Ryan C, Futterman D. Lesbian and Gay Youth: Care and Counseling. *Adolescent Medicine: State of the Art Reviews*. Philadelphia: Hanley Belfus, Inc., 1997.

45

Gender Identity Issues

Ellen C. Perrin

I. **Description of the issue.**
A. **Gender variance** is a behavioral pattern of *intense, pervasive, and persistent interests and behaviors characterized as typical of the other gender.* These gender-variant behaviors include play activities, toys and hobbies, clothing and external appearance, identification with role models, preference for other-gender playmates, and statements that indicate a wish to be of the other sex. This pattern is described in the Diagnostic and Statistical Manual (DSM-IV) as "Gender Identity Disorder" (GID), although some question whether this diagnostic label is appropriate based on current knowledge.

Boys with gender variance may, for example, be consumed by an interest in Snow White, or want nothing for their birthday except a new Barbie doll. Their interests tend to be restricted to typically feminine ones. They may show observable discomfort with typically masculine pursuits and avoid rough-and-tumble play. Similarly, girls with marked gender variance typically show distinct discomfort with activities that are typically associated with girls, they may refuse to wear skirts and dresses, and insist that they "want to be a boy."

B. **Natural history of gender variance.** This pattern of gender variance typically begins before or during the preschool period. Longitudinal data suggest that the majority of boys with marked gender variance early in childhood later identified themselves as gay. A smaller percentage (about 6%) identified themselves as "transgender" and about 25% eventually identified themselves as "heterosexual." It is not, however, possible at this time to predict which boys will take which course. Very little research has been done on girls.

Health professionals see fewer girls than boys with this type of gender variance. This pattern may reflect a true difference in prevalence, but it is also impacted by the fact that the range of acceptable behaviors in most modern societies is broader for girls than for boys.

II. **Significance of the issue.** Children referred for so-called "gender identity disorder" are reported by their parents to have both **internalizing** and **externalizing** symptoms in greater number than their peers, especially after 6 years of age. Why? There is no intrinsic disadvantage caused to a boy by wearing dresses and makeup, nor to a girl with short hair competing in contact sports. Girls and boys with atypical play and playmate preferences confront **stigma** from peers and adults. They may be isolated and teased. Their parents may face stigmatization also and may feel embarrassed, conflicted, and insecure, which in turn may lead to critical and punitive responses. Emotional and behavioral symptoms are likely to be a reflection of this distress.

III. **Management.** While the adult sexual orientation of individual children with gender variance cannot be safely predicted, many of these children will identify themselves as gay, lesbian, or transgender as adults. The serious risks gay, lesbian, and transgender adolescents typically face may be at least partly averted if children have the clear knowledge early in childhood that they are loved and accepted for who they are and as they are. Therefore, an important role of the pediatric clinician can be to provide their parents with information and support for diversity in sexual orientation from early childhood onward. Although heterosexual parents may initially know little about and/or harbor negative views about homosexuality, many, if not most, will be able to modify their attitudes to become affirming, which in the long run will boost the child's self esteem and his/her ability to cope with social stigma. Parents who maintain persistently negative and harsh judgmental beliefs should be counseled about the potential effects of their attitudes on their children's long-term well-being.

When parents initially express concerns about their child's gender-variant behaviors, pediatric clinicians generally have offered reassurance ("Don't worry, he'll outgrow it"), hoping that these behaviors are evidence of the child's greater-than-average behavioral flexibility. But this approach may not be in the best interest of the child and the family.

Denial of the child's differentness deprives families of an opportunity to develop a more authentic view of the child and to be actively affirming in case he is gay or she is lesbian.

It is also important to not to minimize the considerable challenge of parenting a gender-variant child in most families and communities. Siblings, grandparents, aunts, and uncles also may need information, support, and guidance to come to a new understanding and acceptance of the gender-variant child.

Parents of a child with GID, and the professionals to whom they look for advice, face considerable uncertainty with regard to helpful action. Some principles seem clear.

1. It is likely beneficial.
   a. To help children feel more secure about their gender identity as a boy or a girl
   b. To work to diminish, as much as possible, peer ostracism and social isolation
   c. To identify and treat evidence of associated behavioral/emotional distress
2. Attempts to alter the early developmental pathway towards a homosexual or a heterosexual orientation are unlikely to be effective and very likely to send of message of disapproval and nonacceptance to a child who has little or no real control over his/her gender-variant behaviors.
3. The best advice for parents is what it always is—to support their children, to foster their strengths, and to model desired behavior. The positive and nurturing qualities of both parents, and their contentment with their own gender roles, should be made evident to their children.
4. Families can help children learn techniques of recognizing and combating the damaging effects of stigma. For example, they can explain that particular behaviors are not typical of boys/girls of his/her age, that he/she may be unfairly criticized, and provide strategies and language to help children resist teasing and criticism.
5. Discussion with a pediatric clinician about their young child with atypical gender role behavior can provide a helpful opportunity for parents to consider how they might feel if their child were to be gay or lesbian as an adult. Most families can come to accept a homosexual son or daughter, especially if given adequate time and support to come to such acceptance. Clinicians can be influential as a source of support, information, and guidance for all members of the family.
6. Parent-to-parent support may be invaluable, either locally or using electronic technology. Table 45-1 provides further suggestions for parents who are faced with the challenge of supporting a gender-variant child.

Table 45-1 Suggestions for parents

1. Create an atmosphere of acceptance so your child feels safe within your family to express his or her interests.
2. Identify and praise your child's talents.
3. Encourage your child to develop activities that help him/her to "fit-in" socially but still respect his or her interests and talents.
4. Strengthen your child's relationship with an adult role model of the same sex (e.g. a parent, aunt/uncle, close friend).
5. Help your child learn specific language and strategies to counteract criticism and stigma.
6. Use gender-neutral language in discussing romantic attachments.
7. Watch TV programs and movies together that include gay and lesbian adults and families.
8. Read books about gay and lesbian heroes in history and in fiction.
9. Discuss news stories about gay and lesbian issues with compassion and explicit acceptance.
10. Highlight personal experiences and news stories of discrimination and negative stereotyping as inappropriate.
11. Describe particular activities and interests concretely rather than labeling them as "girlish" or "boyish".
12. Educate others in your child's life. Be sure to let your child's siblings, your parents and siblings, neighbors and friends know that you love and support your child unconditionally.
13. Encourage classroom discussions about diversity and tolerance.
14. Ensure that school and community libraries have reading materials (both fiction and nonfiction) that include evidence of the diversity of sexual orientations.
15. Ask your primary care clinician to provide reading materials and contact information for organizations of other parents and children with similar questions.
16. If indicated, arrange a referral to a psychotherapist with expertise in issues related to sexual orientation.

Most children will respond to their parents' acceptance and encouragement, referral to a mental health specialist is appropriate if the child is anxious, depressed, angry, exhibits self-destructive behavior, or if the child experiences significant social isolation, and these problems do not improve with short-term counseling. Therapists who are competent in dealing with other childhood issues do not necessarily have the competence to deal with gender variance. Parents may need clarification that psychotherapy does not change sexual orientation or gender identity.

BIBLIOGRAPHY

For Parents

Fanta-Shyer M, Shyer C. *Not Like Other Boys*. Boston: Houghton-Mifflin, 1996.

Cantwell MA. *Homosexuality: The Secret a Child Dare Not Tell*. Chicago: Rafael Press, 1998.

Rottnek M (ed). *Sissies and Tomboys: Gender Non-conformity and Homosexual Childhood*. New York: New York University Press, 1999.

Richardson J, Schuster MA. *Everything You Never Wanted Your Kids to Know About Sex (But Were Afraid They'd Ask)*. New York: Random House, 2003.

"If You Are Concerned About Your Child's Gender Behaviors."A parent guide, available at www.Dcchildrens.com/gendervariance. Printed copies can be ordered at pgroup@cnmc.org. This Website also provides information on how to access a discussion group for families of gender-variant children.

For Children

de Paola, Tomie. *Oliver Button Is a Sissy*. 1979. New York: Voyager Books, Harcourt Brace. (Reading levels 4–8.)

Fierstein, Harvey and Henry Cole (illustrator). *The Sissy Duckling*. New York: Simon & Schuster, 2002. (Reading levels 4–8.)

Harris, Robie. *It's Perfectly Normal*. Candlewick Press, 1994. (Ages 10 and up.)

Bell, Ruth, et al. *Changing Bodies, Changing Lives*. New York: Random House, 1998. (Teenage level.)

Movies/Videos

Ma Vie en Rose (My Life in Pink) [video]. A film by Alain Berliner; Sony Picture Classics. (For older children and adults.)

The Dress Code [video/DVD]. A film by Shirley MacLaine; MGM/UA Studios. (PG-13).

Oliver Button Is a Star [video]. Directed by John Scagliotti and Dan Hunt, with Tomie de Paola and others. www.oliverbuttonisastar.com

For Professionals

Menvielle EJ, Tuerck C, Perrin EC. The Beat of a different drummer: Children who do not follow gender-typical expectations. *Contemporary Pediatrics* 2004 (in press).

Perrin EC. Sexual Orientation in Child and Adolescent Health Care. New York:Kluwer/Plenum, 2002:43–69.

Zucker KJ, Bradley SJ. *Gender Identity Disorder and Psychosexual Problems in Children and Adolescents*. New York: The Guilford Press, 1995.

46 The Gifted Child

Eve Colson
Neil Schechter

I. **Description of the issue.** The definition of "giftedness" is controversial. Initially giftedness was thought to be synonymous with an IQ in the top 1%. However, a linear relationship between high IQ and eventual societal contribution and productivity has not been found; creativity and task persistence, among other factors, appear to play a critical role. The newer definitions of giftedness include the notion that a gifted person shows (or could have the potential to show) exceptional performance in one or more domains, such as the traditional "school-house" learning, but also other areas such as outstanding leadership skills or creative thinking.

Since socioeconomically advantaged children tend to score higher on IQ tests than poorer children and because some schools rely exclusively on IQ tests to define giftedness, children from higher socioeconomic backgrounds are more likely to be classified as gifted. Current recommendations avoid this bias by suggesting that giftedness is a relative construct and that each community should create its own standards to determine who qualifies for programs aimed at such children. In most school systems and communities, about 5%–10% of children are considered to be gifted. Unlike special education for children with handicapping conditions, there is no federal mandate to provide unique educational programming for gifted children.

II. **Making the diagnosis.**
   A. **Signs.**
      1. **Early childhood.** Parents may raise the issue of giftedness in infancy and early childhood if their child appears precocious at mastering developmental milestones. Retrospective studies of gifted children suggest that early language development and early reading were frequently present. In one study, nearly half of the group later identified as gifted had learned to read before entering first grade; 20% could read before age 5 years.
         • Prospective studies, however, suggest that there is little relationship between milestone acquisition or developmental testing before age 4 years and the IQ score achieved at age 7 years. Precocious infants do not necessarily become precocious children.
      2. **School age.** Giftedness among school-aged children is less likely to be recognized by the primary care clinician and more likely to be recognized by the school system. Occasionally, parents may wonder if their child's behavioral or academic problems in school stem from his or her boredom with the curriculum.
   B. **Characteristics.** Children with extraordinarily high IQs (those over 180 or developmental functioning at twice their chronological age) may have social difficulties, in part due to the disparity between their intellectual acumen, their social development, and their chronological age. For example, these children may have a difficult time identifying an appropriate peer group or engaging in age-appropriate activities. Other gifted children do not seem to routinely have the same social difficulties. In fact, some studies suggest that these children may be quite popular among their peers. Additional characteristics often seen among gifted children can be found in Table 46-1.

III. **Management.**
   A. **Identification.** If questions are raised about whether or not an infant or young child might be gifted, it is important to explore what such a diagnosis would mean to the parents. It should be explained to the parents that testing in infancy or early childhood will not accurately predict subsequent academic high achievement and in fact may result in the inappropriate labeling of the child.

   In older children, intellectual testing may be more helpful. Schools are not obligated to test or provide services for gifted children, but some school systems are willing to evaluate such children and offer specialized services for those identified as gifted and talented. Given the inherent ambiguity in the definition of giftedness, some parents may place undue pressure on schools to label their children as gifted. Clinicians should

Table 46-1 Characteristics of gifted children

Asynchrony across developmental domains
Advanced language and reasoning skills
Conversation and interests like older children
Insatiable curiosity; perceptive questions
Rapid and intuitive understanding of concepts
Impressive long-term memory
Ability to hold problems in mind that are not yet figured out
Ability to make connections between one concept and another
Interest in patterns and relationships
Advanced sense of humor (for age)
Courage in trying new pathways of thinking
Pleasure in solving and posing new problems
Capacity for independent, self-directed activities
Talent in a specific area: drawing, music, games, math, reading
Sensitivity and perfectionism
Intensity of feeling and emotion

Adapted with permission from Robinson NM, Olszewski-Kubilius PM. Gifted and talented children: Issues for pediatricians. *Pediatrics in Review* 17:427, 1996.

attempt to help parents separate their own desires, goals, and aspirations for their children from their children's actual abilities and potential.

  B. Home.
    1. Parents may be prone to overstimulate their children either to foster giftedness or to meet its challenges. Parents need not feel pressured to provide an elaborate intellectual enrichment program for their child in fear that their "gifts" will wither if not appropriately stimulated. In fact, undue pressure may prove injurious to their children's long-term development. Stimulation for children identified as academically talented and gifted should be individualized and focus on activities of the children's interests.

    2. Siblings of children who are academically precocious often feel inferior, especially if they are chronologically older but academically less capable. The label "gifted" should not be flaunted in front of siblings, nor should siblings continuously be compared to the gifted children. All children should be treated equally (e.g., with age-appropriate expectations for chores) and encouraged to cultivate their own areas of uniqueness.

    3. Friendships may be problematic for some gifted children, especially for children who are extremely intellectually advanced. Attempts should be made to encourage gifted children to play with same-age peers so that social skills will develop appropriately. However, there may be specific friendships that emerge with older children who have interests or expertise in similar areas to the gifted children. Parents of gifted and talented children may benefit from support groups for gifted children and their parents.

  C. School. There remains significant controversy about how to educate gifted and talented children. Some school systems urge acceleration and place children in advanced grades that parallel the child's ability rather than chronological age. Other systems cluster academically advanced children in substantially separate classrooms in which they receive an advanced program. More typically, gifted and talented programs exist within school systems and not as a separate curriculum. Such programs provide a designated period for children to focus on a specific area in greater depth and in a more creative way than typically allowed by the curriculum.

BIBLIOGRAPHY

For Parents

Organizations

The Council for Exceptional Children www.cec.sped.org
National Association for Gifted Children www.nagc.org

Website

Gifted Child Today www.prufrock.com (epub)

For Professionals

Gifted Child Quarterly National Association for Gifted Education 1707 L Street, NW Suite 559 Washington, DC 20036 www.nagc.org/Publications/GiftedChild

National Research Center on the Gifted and Talented http://www.ucc.uconn.edu/~wwwgt/nrcgt.html

ERIC Clearinghouse on Disabilities and Gifted Education www.eric.ed.gov

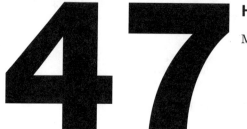

Headaches

Martin Stein

I. **Description of the problem.**
  A. **Epidemiology.**
  - Headaches represent the most common recurrent pain pattern in childhood and adolescence.
  - 40% of children and 70% of adolescents have experienced a headache at some time.
  - Chronic recurrent headaches occur in 15% (2.5% classified as "severe") and migraine headaches in approximately 3% of all children by age 15 years.
  B. **Etiology.** Children experience headaches from many causes, but only a few pathologic mechanisms induce head pain.
  - Inflammation, traction, and direct pressure on intracranial structures.
  - Vasodilation of cerebral vessels.
  - Sustained contractions, trauma, or inflammation of scalp and neck muscles.
  - Sinus, dental, and orbital pathologic processes.
  - The brain parenchyma, most of the dura and meningeal surfaces, and the ependymal lining of the ventricles are insensitive to pain. Central nervous system (CNS) causes of headache result from stretching or inflammation of a limited number of pain-sensitive intracranial structures.

II. **Making the diagnosis.** Most headaches are brief and do not significantly alter a child's life. Recurrent headaches may be accompanied by fears and anxieties about brain tumors and other life-threatening diseases. The diagnostic challenge for the primary care clinician is multifaceted.
  - To differentiate benign, self-limited headaches from those that suggest a serious organic disease.
  - To explore the potential relationship between headaches and a child's home, school, and social environment.
  - To recognize patients with headaches secondary to internal stressors (depression, anxiety, phobias) and those with environmental causes.
  - To develop a therapeutic plan consistent with the cause, severity, and significance of the headaches for the child and family.
  A. **Differential diagnosis.** A useful clinical model to differentiate the large variety of headaches in children and adolescents focuses on four categories: (1) tension headaches, (2) migraine headaches, (3) extracranial headaches, and (4) intracranial headaches (Table 47-1). **Tension-related and migraine headaches occur most frequently.** An alternative model of headaches in children deemphasizes the migraine-tension dichotomy and places greater emphasis on a headache continuum with migraine with associated anatomic nervous system symptoms at one end of the continuum and muscular tension headache at the other. Symptoms and signs of both tension and migraine headaches in children are often nonspecific compared to the less common causes. Headaches in younger children, especially infants and toddlers, are more likely to have a specific organic cause. A focused clinical interview, coupled with age-appropriate behavioral observations and a comprehensive physical examination, will result in the probable diagnosis at the initial office visit for most patients.
  B. **History: Key clinical questions.** Whenever possible, questions should be directed to the patient. Parents can then be queried only after the child or adolescent has had an opportunity to describe the headache to the clinician. With the knowledge that most recurrent forms of pediatric headaches are associated with a behavioral diagnosis (in the presence or absence of migraine), the astute provider should guide the clinical interview in a manner that raises questions simultaneously about both organic and nonorganic causes.

    The clinical interview begins the therapeutic process. Detailed, focused, and empathic questions give the child and family a sense of security that the symptoms are being evaluated by a concerned, knowledgeable clinician. It also gives the child and parents the opportunity to explore the interpersonal, educational, and family aspects of their lives that may provide insight into the headache formation.

1. *"Tell me about your headaches. What do they feel like?"* The child who has difficulty describing the headache can be asked to "draw a picture of what the headache feels like." The child's description of the drawing, as well as the parents' and clinician's emotional responses, may provide useful information about the nature of the pain. Features in the drawings consistent with migraine included pounding pain, nausea/

Table 47-1 Classification of headaches

	Mechanism	Features/etiology
Tension headaches (muscle contraction headaches)	Contraction of scalp and neck muscles	Sensation of tightness or pressure over frontal, temporal, occipital regions, or generalized Life-event change/stress: home, school, social relations, activity overload, depression Normal physical examination (occasional tightness or tenderness of posterior cervical muscles)

Migraine headaches	Vasoconstriction and/or vasodilation of cerebral vessels	Family history (70%–80%)
		
		Paroxysmal attacks
		Gender: in childhood, boys and girls equally; in adolescence, girls more than boys
		Common migraine
		  Unilateral or generalized
		  Throbbing or aching
		  Nausea/vomiting
		  No aura
		Classic migraine
		  Aura (visual)
		  Nausea/vomiting
		  Unilateral
		  Throbbing
		Complex migraine
		  Ophthalmoplegia
		  Hemiparesis
		  Acute confusional state
		  Cyclic vomiting
		  Paroxysmal vertigo

Extracranial sources	Inflammation or trauma of structures or sustained contracture of scalp and neck muscles	Typically regional pain in area of pathology but often generalized in young children Otitis media and mastoiditis Sinusitis (chronic purulent rhinorrhea and/or nocturnal cough) Dental infection Tonsillopharyngitis (streptococcal) Refractive errors and strabismus Cervical spine osteomyelitis or discitis Systemic infection with fever Temporal-mandibular joint syndrome Severe malocclusion

(continued)

Table 47-1 *(continued)*

	Mechanism	Features/etiology
Intracranial sources	Inflammation	Meningitis, encephalitis, cerebral vasculitis, subarachnoid hemorrhage
	Traction	CNS tumor
		Cerebral edema
		Abscess
		Hematoma
		Postlumbar puncture
		Pseudotumor cerebri
	Toxic substances	Lead alcohol
		Carbon monoxide
		Hypoxia
		Foods and food additives (nitrates, nitrites, monosodium glutamate, phenylethylamine)
		Paint, glue (including model glue)
		Oral contraceptives
		Renal disease
	Direct pressure	Hydrocephalus
		Trauma
	Vascular (nonmigraine)	Hypertension
		Arteriovenous malformation
		Fever
	Miscellaneous	Noise
		Sensory overload

    vomiting, desire to lie down, periorbital pain, photophobia and visual scotoma. Images of sadness or crying are found in both migraine and nonmigraine headaches.

2. *"When do the headaches tend to occur? Is there a recognizable pattern?"* In infants and toddlers, nonspecific symptoms may reflect a headache (e.g., irritability, inconsolability, sleep disturbances, poor appetite, head banging, or repetitive placing of a hand to the head or face). In older children and adolescents, an open-ended question may yield important information about the location, quality, onset, duration and frequency of the headache.

3. *"What seems to bring on a headache?*[or] *What are you doing when the headache starts?"* The emotional or physical environment in which the headache occurs may provide a clue to etiology.

4. *"What do you do to stop the headache?"* Common migraine typically resolves with sleep. Tension headaches resolve gradually during an awake state.

5. *"Do others in your family experience headaches?"* A history of episodic throbbing headaches in adults will suggest familial migraine headaches. Positive or negative reinforcement of headaches within the family may give an important clue to the etiology of recurrent headaches.

6. *"What is a headache?"* [To the preschool child:] *"Where do headaches come from?"* [School-aged child:] *"What causes your headache?"* [Adolescent:] *"Why do you think you get headaches?"* These developmentally appropriate questions give a clue to the child's explanatory model of headache formation. Responses provide clinical insight into a patient's development, a clue to cognitive adaptation to the headache, and a source for improved communication between clinician and child through empathic connections.

7. *"Why do you think that your headaches are more frequent or more severe?"* For most children who experience headaches, it is helpful to explore the child's developmental understanding of headaches. A perceived cause of a headache will be linked to the child's cognitive and developmental stage (Table 47-2). The child is given an opportunity to reflect on the symptoms. The response may provide a clue to self-esteem, ego integration, superego formation, and interpersonal relationships.

8. *"How are things going at school ⋯ at home ⋯ with your friends?"* The structure of the family (and a family medical history), friendships, and the school environment

Table 47-2 Developmental conceptions of headache

Cognitive stage	Answer to "How do people get headaches?"
Prelogical (3-6 yr)	
Phenomenism	*From God* or *From the weather*
Contagion	*From foods, like chocolate*
Concrete-logical (7–12 yr)	
Contamination	*From running and getting hot*
Internalization	*Eating or doing certain things that make inside your head hurt* or *From thinking too hard in math class*
Formal-logical (>13 yr)	
Physiological	*From things happening to you that cause too much blood flowing to your head; that's why it feels like a hammer pounding in your head*
Psychophysiological	*When people get nervous or do too much, this causes their body to react with a headache*

Modified with permission from Marcon RA, Labb EE. Assessment and treatment of children's headaches from a developmental perspective. *Headache* 9:586–592, 1990.

are critical to understanding the etiology of and response to the headache, and potential therapeutic interventions.

 a. **Family stress.** Is the child living with someone who experiences headaches? The family constellation should be explored for recent changes in parental relationships, a new sibling, emotional illness in family members, economic stress (lost job, homelessness, and child support), and family violence.

 b. **Social stress.** When factors such as inherent shyness, bullies, class and racial differences, and physical or mental dysfunction affect social relationships, psychophysiologic reactions are common. Recurrent frontal, generalized, or temporal headaches (both with and without associated symptoms of pallor, malaise, nausea, and vomiting) are seen in these situations. Importantly, common migraine headaches as well as tension headaches may be associated with social or familial stress.

 c. **School stress.** Stress that originates in the classroom may be associated with headache formation. The school may act as an environmental stressor by placing demands on both cognitive achievement and social behavior. Children's adaptive potential to a variety of school pressures varies significantly. The clinical interview should explore the nature of the classroom (number of students, where the child sits), the relationship between the child and the teacher, the quality and quantity of academic work, the child's response to homework, and the parents' attitudes about learning. Parents can be asked when they last spoke to the child's teacher, the content of the conference, whether the child is learning, and if the child is happy at school.

 9. *"What do you think we can do together to help the headaches go away?"* This question engages the child in a therapeutic alliance and opens the possibility of managing the problem together.

 C. **Physical examination and further testing.** Narrating normal physical findings to the child during a comprehensive physical examination is reassuring and helps to demystify the medical evaluation. Organic causes for a child's headaches are usually apparent after a complete history and physical examination. Routine diagnostic studies are not indicated when the clinical history has no associated suggestive risk factors (e.g., recent onset of severe headaches, absence of a family history of migraine) and the physical/neurologic examination is normal. When the signs and symptoms of organic causes of headache are vague or subtle and a specific diagnosis remains elusive, a specialty consultation may be useful.

III. Management.

 A. **Primary goals.** The clinician's goals for management should be to provide a developmentally appropriate understanding of the cause of headaches for both parent and child. The working assumption is that through a greater understanding of the physical and behavioral causes and triggers for headaches, both the child and the parent will be able to cope with and adapt to the pain as well as collaborate in recommended therapies.

 B. **Treatment strategies.**

 1. **Information.** When migraine or tension headaches are present, the anatomic mechanisms of pain should be illustrated by means of a descriptive narrative and schematic

drawings. Visual images of the abnormal anatomic structures may help some children to gain control over the symptoms. Simple drawings of a blood vessel contracting and dilating with an explanation of pain-sensitive nerve endings within the blood vessel illustrates the physical nature of migraine headache and the associated symptoms.

2. **Relaxation exercises.** For tension headaches, children may respond to a progressive relaxation exercise that teaches them to relax specified areas of the body. The exercise may be followed by teaching the child to focus on a pleasant image of his or her choosing. Other children respond to an explanation directed at "tight muscles around the head" that cause pain at times of stress and tension ("worry," "nerves," and "daily hassles"). The clinician can demonstrate this phenomenon by tensing her biceps and asking the child to mimic that maneuver. This should be followed by an explanation that the biceps muscle is similar to the thin muscles around the head, which tighten at the point where the headache occurs. The child can learn to image—through visual imagination—the tense, painful cranial muscles' relaxing gradually and voluntarily as the pain diminishes.These forms of voluntary relaxation follow the principles of self-regulation that have been successful in the elimination of migraine and tension headaches in school-aged children and adolescents.Controlled studies of children with headaches have shown that relaxation therapy and imaging (with or without biofeedback) decrease headache frequency up to 88% with lasting effects. It is a safe and simple intervention that can be practiced by the primary care clinician.

3. **Headache diary.** A headache diary may be a useful adjunct intervention. The older child or parent is asked to chart the headaches (time of day, intensity on a 1–10 scale, associated symptoms, intervention, and duration) and record any stressful events that occur in the life of the child or family around the time of the headache. This exercise may encourage parents and children to talk about environmental triggers for headaches specifically and improve parent–child communication in general. Following an initial treatment period, it may be useful to shift the emphasis of the diary to headache-free days, which can shift family focus to successes rather than failures.

4. **Medication.** A pharmacologic approach to acute, chronic, and recurrent headaches may be beneficial for pain relief and prevention. Most children and adolescents with occasional migraine and tension-related headaches respond to acetaminophen or ibuprofen when the pain is of mild to moderate severity. Parenteral medication is available for the very severe migraine. Severe recurrent migraine headaches respond to prophylactic suppression therapy, although there are few controlled drug studies in children. This headache pattern is uncommon in children and adolescents seen in primary care practice.

C. **Follow-up.** In general, a child with recurrent headaches should always be followed up within 2–4 weeks after the initial office evaluation. Support for behavioral interventions, monitoring of headache frequency and functional severity, and reviewing the parent–child understanding of the symptoms are the goals for the follow-up visit. New information or clinical observations may either alter the initial diagnosis or provide a new direction for management.

BIBLIOGRAPHY

For Parents

Websites

The National Headache Foundation http://www.headaches.org/consumer/educationalmodules/childrensheadache/chhome.html

For Professionals

American Academy of Neurology and the Practice Committee of the Child Neurology Society. Practice parameter: Evaluation of children and adolescents with recurrent headaches. *Neurology* 58, 1589–1596, 2002.

Holden EW, Levy D, Deichmann MM, et al. Recurrent pediatric headaches: Assessment and intervention. *Dev Behav Pediatr* 1998;19,109–116.

McGrath PS, Reid GJ. Behavioral treatment of pediatric headache. *Pediatr Ann* 1995;24:486–491.

Solomon GD. The pharmacology of medications used in treating migraine *Semin Pediatr Neural* 1995;2:165–177.

48

Hearing Impairment

Laurel M. Wills
Karen E. Wills

I. **Description of the condition.** Deafness or hearing loss is more than an audiologic condition. It must be understood in terms of its developmental, linguistic, and sociocultural implications. Children who are deaf or hard of hearing require individualized management decisions that take into consideration the following characteristics.

A. **Degree or severity of hearing loss.**
- "Normal" hearing is considered to be the ability to detect a full range of speech sounds at a whispering volume of 10–20 decibels (dB).
- Typical conversational speech registers at roughly 50 dB.
- **Mild** (25–40 dB range), **moderate** (41–55 dB), **moderately severe** (56–70 dB), **severe** (71–90 dB), and **profound** (>90 dB) degrees of deafness are associated with diminishing capability to detect and discriminate speech and environmental sounds (Figure 48-1).
- The exact "configuration" or profile of hearing loss varies for each child, with better hearing in certain frequencies and less in others.
- Hearing acuity may also differ between the right and left ears.
- Deafness is not simply "turning down the volume" on normal hearing; generally, it also involves *distortion* of speech sounds that are heard.
- The audiogram does not always directly match the functional listening level, because there are individual differences in "listening skills," e.g., one child with moderate hearing loss might be able to decode and comprehend what she hears better than a second child with only mild hearing loss.

B. **Type of hearing loss.** This refers to the affected anatomic location along the auditory pathway causing the child's hearing loss.
- **Conductive** losses commonly result from middle ear effusions, cholesteatoma, or other problems with the functioning of the eardrum or ossicles that leave the hearing nerve intact.
- **Sensorineural** losses represent a dysfunction of the cochlear hair cells or auditory nerve (8th cranial nerve).
- **Mixed hearing losses** involve both.
- **Central hearing losses** involve the auditory cortex or brainstem nuclei.
- **Auditory neuropathy** refers to involvement of the 8th nerve, with an otherwise normally functioning cochlea.

C. **Age of onset of hearing loss.** A congenitally deaf child or one who loses his hearing prior to acquiring spoken language ("pre-lingual deafness") will usually be at a communicative disadvantage relative to a child who loses hearing after being exposed to or becoming fluent in a spoken language ("post-lingual deafness"). The child with pre-lingual deafness lacks stimulation to the auditory pathways during sensitive language learning years, until hearing aids or cochlear implants are supplied. These children also may lack stimulation to the brain's language-learning systems, which process both spoken and signed languages, if early parent–child communication is lacking. Good, reciprocal, early, parent–child communication, via signed or spoken language or both, is strongly associated with better outcomes for children with pre-lingual deafness.

D. **Age of identification and intervention.** Children whose hearing loss is identified as a newborn or young infant and for whom amplification and developmental services are initiated immediately, usually fare better than late-identified youngsters. The 10% of deaf babies who are born to deaf parents and who have accessible, fluent Sign Language models from birth, tend to fare well developmentally. The more severely deaf child is likely to prompt referral earlier by showing symptoms such as not responding to sound, not talking, or "not listening." Children with unilateral (one-sided) hearing loss, on the other hand, may be overlooked until well into their elementary school years. Universal newborn hearing screening programs, strongly advocated for by the American Academy

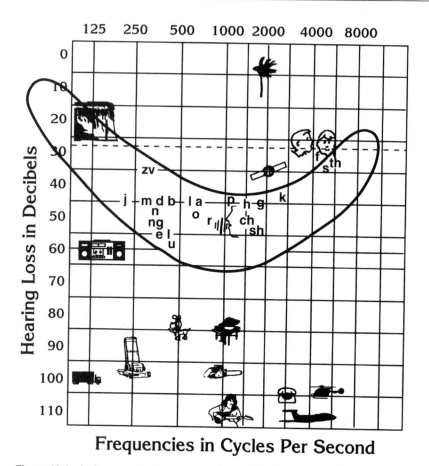

Figure 48-1. Audiogram showing a comparison of the frequency and intensity of various environmental and speech sounds.

of Pediatrics and other professional groups, have made a significant difference in the rates of early detection and intervention.

E. **Presence of additional disabilities.** Approximately one third of children with hearing loss will have additional medical or neurological diagnoses. These tend to be the children for whom deafness is caused by prenatal infections, meningitis, or other etiologies that also confer neurodevelopmental risk. Problems with learning, language, attention, or behavior, as well as physical problems, are more prevalent in this group. The other two thirds of children tend to be healthy, neurologically intact youngsters with "isolated" or uncomplicated hearing loss, usually genetic in origin.

F. **Psychosocial experience and home environment.** Positive adjustment and social-emotional well-being among deaf children is closely linked to the quality of parent–child communication, as well as to warmth and developmentally appropriate expectations within the parent–child relationship. Hostility, chronic frustration, and chaos in the home are linked to aggression and noncompliance in deaf children. Since 90% of deaf children are born to hearing parents who know little about deafness, the diagnosis of deafness is a crisis that tries the family's coping resources, demanding support systems within their extended family and community, as well as support from healthcare and education professionals.

II. **Epidemiology.**
- 20 million Americans of all ages have a hearing loss.
- Roughly 1 million children and adolescents have a "communicatively significant" hearing loss.

- 1–2/1,000 live births will have severe or profound deafness.
- 6–10/1,000 will have milder degrees of hearing loss.
- Males and females are equally affected.
- Preventative medical advances such as vaccines against rubella, *Hemophilus influenza* B, and pneumoccal disease and treatment of otitis media and hyperbilirubinemia have markedly reduced the incidence of childhood hearing loss in developed countries. However, still roughly one third of school-aged deaf and hard of hearing children have other medical, neurological, psychiatric, and/or vision problems.
- Academic underachievement, functional illiteracy, and underemployment remain significant concerns for this population.

III. **Etiology.**
   A. **Genetic** deafness, most often of an **autosomal recessive** type, accounts for roughly 50%–60% of children and youth with isolated hearing loss. Laboratory testing by DNA molecular analysis is now available for some of the more common gene mutations, such as Connexin 26. A variety of congenital syndromes associated with hearing loss, and often other physical findings, account for another 10%. Malformations of the cochlea or other inner ear structures can result in hearing loss and, in some children, problems with balance or equilibrium. Other examples include Usher syndrome (sensorineural deafness associated with progressive vision loss from retinitis pigmentosa), Treacher-Collins syndrome (conductive or mixed hearing loss, associated with dysmorphic facies), and Waardenburg syndrome (sensorineural deafness and pigmentary changes of the hair and irises).
   B. **Nongenetic or "acquired" hearing loss** can be separated into prenatal, perinatal, and postnatal etiologies.
      - **Prenatal:** Maternal infections, most commonly including cytomegalovirus (CMV), toxoplasmosis, and rubella should be considered in the setting of a newborn with microcephaly, intrauterine growth retardation, seizures, or unusual eye findings. Newborns with CMV or toxoplasmosis may also be asymptomatic. Deafness from congenital CMV infection may be present at birth or can emerge and progress during early childhood.
      - **Perinatal:** Severe hyperbilirubinemia, also relatively rare in developed countries, can result in damage (kernicterus) to the auditory nuclei and other "retro-cochlear" neurologic regions. Neonatal sepsis or severe neonatal cardiorespiratory compromise often requires treatment with ototoxic antibiotic or diuretic medications, thus newborn intensive care unit (NICU) graduates and premature babies have a much higher incidence of hearing loss than full term healthy neonates.
      - **Postnatal:** Chronic suppurative otitis media or other types of middle ear pathology can result in a transient or permanent conductive or mixed hearing loss. Bacterial meningitis, though much less common in this vaccine era, remains a common cause of acquired hearing loss. Ototoxic medications also include certain chemotherapeutic agents used in pediatric cancer therapy. Noise trauma or physical trauma can result in conductive or mixed hearing loss. Rare in childhood, acoustic nerve tumors can also cause deafness, usually unilateral.
      - **Unknown etiology:** 20%–30% of children have a hearing loss of undetermined etiology, despite thorough evaluation.

IV. **Making the diagnosis.**
   A. **Developmental screening tools,** used during well child visits to pediatric and family medicine primary practices, query parents about speech and language milestones or concerns (see American Academy of Audiology Website chapter on language). Parental concerns should be taken seriously in order to make the diagnosis of hearing loss early.
   B. **History and physical examination.** A thorough prenatal and birth history, past medical, developmental, family (genetic), and noise exposure history will be necessary to attempt identification of the cause of deafness, and any additional health conditions. On the physical examination, particular attention should be given to facial features and other potentially syndromic markers (e.g., skin and hair pigment changes), appearance of the external and middle ear, eye exam and vision screen, and a complete neurologic exam, including muscle tone, coordination, gait, and balance.
   C. It is important to realize that no infant is too young to have his hearing acuity tested. The testing methods discussed are performed or supervised by qualified audiologists who have specific pediatric training:
      1. **Physiologic measures** (require no cooperation). Universal newborn hearing screening relies on noninvasive **physiologic** methods such as **otoacoustic emissions (OAE)** and/or **brainstem auditory evoked response (BAER or ABR)**. OAE testing is performed by presenting a click stimulus via a soft-tipped probe in the external

ear canal. The computer receiver then detects the "acoustic emissions" or echo-like sounds produced by the hair cells of the cochlea. False-positive OAE tests can result from middle ear fluid or vernix in the external canal at birth.

- If these emissions are not detected, the baby or child is referred on for BAER testing, the current "gold standard" physiologic measure of hearing acuity. BAER testing involves placement of scalp electrodes to measure electrical waveforms produced along the auditory pathway in response to a sound stimulus, presented by an earphone. These physiologic tests are often necessary for evaluating children with global developmental disability or autism spectrum disorders.

2. **Behavioral measures testing** (requires active participation). These include **visual reinforcement audiometry** (useful with older infants and toddlers), **conditioned play audiometry** (useful with older toddlers and preschoolers), and **routine behavioral audiometry** (useful with school aged children and adolescents). **Informal office methods can be deceptive and inaccurate**, such as watching for a baby's response to a hand clap or bell ringing, since the baby may react to a visual cue, vibration, or movement, and the decibel level of the noise presented is uncontrolled.

   a. **Visual reinforcement audiometry** is performed by having the toddler sit facing outward on a parent's lap in a sound-treated room. The audiologist presents a series of tones at specific frequencies and volumes from a speaker at one or the other side of the room, watching for the child's reaction. Visual reinforcement is offered (e.g., with a dancing toy in one or the other corner of the room) when the baby localizes and looks toward the sound source.

   b. **Conditioned play audiometry** is performed in a sound-treated room in which the preschooler is taught or "conditioned" to respond with a play activity (e.g., put a block in a box) in response to hearing a specific tone. When the child is too young or unable to tolerate headphones, hearing acuity can only be determined for "the better ear in a sound field", as opposed to more precise measures of hearing in each ear made possible by using headphones in older children and adolescents.

   c. **Routine behavioral audiometry** involves the older child simply raising a hand when a tone is heard through the right or left side of the headphones. School- and clinic-based hearing screens are useful tools, but can miss milder degrees of hearing loss. Referral to an audiology clinic is recommended whenever hearing status is questioned, even for a child who has passed routine screening.

   d. **Tympanometry and pneumatic otoscopy** are measures of eardrum mobility and middle ear disease performed by many primary care offices. It is not uncommon for parents to mistake an office-based tympanogram for a hearing test. For example, a child with profound sensorineural deafness may have normal tympanograms.

3. The audiologist will also perform **measures of speech detection and discrimination**, in addition to "pure tone" audiometry, at the initial assessment and later, when testing hearing aid function. It is important to make the distinction among speech detection (knowing when one is being spoken to), speech discrimination (being able to recognize certain speech sounds or words), and comprehension of "connected" speech (being able to listen and understand the meaning of spoken words and sentences in conversation).

4. In addition to audiological testing, children with hearing loss require **assessment of communicative competence,** i.e., thorough evaluation of spoken, signed, and gestural communication abilities, by an experienced Speech-Language Pathologist.

V. **Management.**

A. **Role of the primary care practitioner.** Pediatric management starts by creating a compassionate and conscientious "medical home" for the child with hearing loss and for his or her parents. A thorough history, physical exam, and laboratory workup may elucidate the underlying etiology of the child's hearing loss and any associated conditions. Fostering a realistic, but hopeful sense of the future is critical in energizing parents for the challenges ahead.

B. **Role of medical and audiological specialists.** Valuable medical input regarding diagnosis and treatment options can be obtained from pediatric otolaryngologists and clinical geneticists and/or genetic counselors. All deaf and hard of hearing children should have regular, thorough eye and vision examinations by a pediatric ophthalmologist, since visual acuity is so crucial to communication via speech-reading and visual-manual methods (e.g., ASL, Cued Speech). Additionally, the ophthalmologist may need to evaluate specifically for colobomata, chorioretinitis, or retinitis pigmentosa, depending on the individual patient's history. The vast majority of children will need regular follow-up with a "primary" audiologist in order to detect and document any change or progression in the hearing loss and to assess for proper functioning of hearing aids, cochlear implants, or other assistive listening devices, for example, used at school.

C. **Cochlear implants.** A cochlear implant is a surgically implanted electronic device that has two main parts: an internal portion comprised of an array of microelectrodes inserted into the turns of the cochlea, and an external portion that receives, processes, and transmits speech sounds to the internal portion via an ear level attachment. The FDA has approved the surgery in babies as young as 12 months of age since the cochlea is essentially full-sized at birth. Evaluation of potential candidates for this procedure involves a specialized team of medical and audiology professionals, along with deaf education teachers, speech-language clinicians, and clinical psychologists who can thoroughly evaluate the child's medical and developmental status and the family's expectations and ability to follow through with the intensive process of auditory (re)habilitation and speech therapy. Children with additional disabilities may be candidates, but the prognosis may be more guarded. Children who receive implants often continue to use and benefit from either American Sign Language or Cued Speech communication, but intensive therapy to develop listening skills and speech production is a critical part of the postsurgical plan. School speech therapists, as well as those in private agencies, should be supported by consultation and collaboration with hospital-to-school liaison staff on the cochlear implant team.

D. **Communication options.**
   1. **American Sign Language (ASL)** is often considered the "native or natural language" of the Deaf Community in the United States. ASL uses hands, arms, face, and body position and movement to convey meaning, with sign order and grammatical rules that are visually based and therefore quite different from English. Manually Coded English (including various systems such as Pidgin Signed English and Signing Exact English) are a variety of signing systems that "transliterate" speech, that is, English word order and grammar, generally using one sign per spoken word. These systems, though much less efficient or "natural", enable one to sign and speak simultaneously, which is referred to as Total Communication or Simultaneous Communication (Simu-Comm).
   2. **Cued Speech** is a system of hand positions ("cues"), used while speaking, which clarify the distinction between sounds (such as /p/ and /b/) that look alike to the lip-reader. Even deaf persons who are proficient lip-readers, or more accurately "speech-readers", comprehend only about 40%–50% of what is spoken, and "piece together" meaning from the context of the conversation. One common example is the similar appearance on the lips of the words "red" and "green". Cues can remove the ambiguity for the "listener". Cued speech is becoming more popular in schools because it seems to help children with hearing loss grasp important phonemic distinctions, an important foundation for literacy.
   3. **Oral** communication emphasizes intensive instruction and practice with speech, listening, and speech-reading skills. This modality clearly works better for children who have milder hearing losses or better aided hearing, or cochlear implants, than with children who have severe to profound deafness.

E. **Education and psycho-educational evaluation.** With such great individual differences among children who are deaf, there is no one-size-fits-all educational program. School programs differ in the **communication options** that they offer (see above). They also differ in the extent to which children are **mainstreamed or congregated**.
   1. Deaf and Hard-of-hearing (D/HH, in educational parlance) children may be included within a regular classroom, perhaps using an **Oral, Cued Speech, Signed English, or ASL interpreter** to better understand the teacher and classmates.
   2. Many students use assistive listening devices, such as an **FM system**, in which the teacher wears a microphone that transmits speech sounds directly to the child's hearing aid. **CART (computer assisted real time) captioning**, in which a typist transcribes a lecture using a computer, is becoming a popular option for D/HH high school and college students who can also study the printed English transcript of a lecture.
   3. **Psychological or psycho-educational evaluation** of deaf children should be done by a clinician who is knowledgeable about cultural, educational, linguistic, and developmental issues associated with deafness; and, ideally, who is conversant in the child's primary communication mode. Tests of reasoning and problem solving, using visual patterns and pictures are usually the most appropriate way to measure general intelligence in children who are deaf. Verbal question-and-answer tests may be useful to assess the child's proficiency with conceptualizing problems and articulat-

ing solutions in English—keeping in mind that their exposure to English language-based concepts and culture may be limited.

- Care must be taken *not* to attribute a child's struggles with English speech or literacy to low intelligence. On the other hand, children with deafness, especially those who have other neurologic compromise, can also have developmental and learning disabilities. Teachers and caregivers may mistakenly assume that a child's problems with learning, language, memory, attention, or emotional self-regulation occur "just because of his deafness." These children should be evaluated by a psychologist who is familiar with normally developing deaf children, who can assess whether the presenting concerns simply "come with the territory" or represent an additional, potentially treatable, condition.

F. **Community building and social support.** Parents need to understand that there are a variety of choices, but no "one right way" to raise a deaf child. However, parents should be forewarned that some professionals, other parents, books and media, will strongly advocate for one or another "right way." Parents are likely to need professional help and support to learn about, and select, communication options and educational programs for their child who is deaf. The National Dissemination Center for Children with Disabilities, State Resources pages (www.nichcy.org) list contact information for parent-to-parent support groups and agencies that help parents make these decisions. Additional resources are listed in the Bibliography.

G. **Mental Health.** In general, the parenting attitudes and skills that promote mental health, strong self-esteem, and prosocial behavior in all children, also are associated with positive adjustment among children who are deaf. Specifically, a supportive, warm, family environment is associated with better social skills and happier mood in the child. The presence of harsh, critical, aggressive, or lax and inconsistent parenting is associated with children's aggressive and rule-breaking behavior.

VI. **Clinical pearls and pitfalls.**

- A baby is never too young to test hearing acuity. If a parent or grandparent raises concern about hearing in a child, refer the family to a pediatric audiologist as soon as possible.
- Comprehensive evaluation of a deaf or hard of hearing child is a multidisciplinary pursuit, best performed by clinicians experienced in working with deaf children and ideally proficient in or knowledgeable about various communication modalities.
- Early identification of hearing loss can radically improve developmental outcome. Engage the family with local early intervention or D/HH educational services.
- Terminology in this field can be tricky. Many individuals take offense at the clinical term, "hearing *impaired*" (often because of the view that the signing Deaf Community represents a healthy, linguistic minority, rather than a disability group), while others do not like "hearing *loss*" when the condition has been present from birth. Thus, it is best to simply ask parents or older patients what words they use to describe themselves or their children.
- Think "eyes", not just "ears", when thinking about deaf children. They will learn about their world through their eyes, as much or more than hearing children, whether they communicate using speech-reading or manual-gestural methods. All deaf and hard of hearing children need to see the eye doctor for a thorough exam. Special services exist in many areas for children with deaf-blindness.
- Parent-to-parent support is vitally important as the parents of a child with hearing loss are coming to terms with the diagnosis and exploring treatment options, which can be confusing and controversial. Reliable, unbiased national parent resources, as well as local parent networks exist in many regions. Forewarn parents that some professionals, agencies, books, and other parents may be strongly biased towards the view that there is only "one right way" to raise, educate, and communicate with a child who is deaf. Try to provide parents with a more balanced view, such as is represented in the bibliography that follows.

BIBLIOGRAPHY

For Parents and Clinicians

Books

Candlish PM. *Not Deaf Enough: Raising a Child Who Is Hard of Hearing With Hugs and Humor.* Alexander Graham Bell Association, 1996.

Frazier-Maiwald V, Williams LM. *Keys to Raising a Deaf Child.* New York: Barron's, 1999.

Medwid DJ, Chapman Weston D. *Kid Friendly Parenting with Deaf and Hard of Hearing Children.* Gallaudet University Press, 1995.

Ogden PW. *The Silent Garden: Raising Your Deaf Child.* Washington, DC: Gallaudet University Press, 1996.

Schwartz S (ed). *Choices in Deafness: A Parents' Guide to Communication Options.* Bethesda, MD: Woodbine House, 1996

Websites

Alexander Graham Bell Association http://www.agbell.org/information/brochures.cfm

American Academy of Audiology http://www.audiology.org/professional/tech/eihbrochure.php

American Society for Deaf Children www.deafchildren.org

BEGINNINGS, For parents of children who are deaf and hard of hearing, Inc. www.beginningssvc-s.com

Boy's Town National Research Hospital www.babyhearing.org

Cochlear implant information: http://www.listen-up.org/implant.htm

Council on Education of the Deaf Kent State University "Facilitate informational sharing and collaborative activities within the field of Deaf Education" www.deafed.net

Deaf/Blind Education Resources http://www.ibwebs.com/region4.htm#MN

Early Hearing Detection and Intervention (from Centers for Disease Control) http://www.cdc.gov/ncbddd/ehdi/default.htm

Laurent Clerc National Deaf Education Center (Gallaudet University) http://clerccenter.gallaudet.edu/InfoToGo/117.html

National Association of the Deaf www.nad.org

National Dissemination Center for Children with Disabilities (formerly the National Information Clearinghouse for Handicapped Children and Youth) www.nichcy.org The "State Resources Sheets" are an invaluable list of agencies in every state that provide parent support and governmental oversight of services related to hearing loss.

The National Center for Hearing Assessment and Management http://www.infanthearing.org/familysupport/

National Institutes on Deafness and Other Communication Disorders, in collaboration with Children's Hospital of Philadelphia. www.raisingdeafkids.org.

Self Help for Hard of Hearing People, Bethesda, Maryland www.shhh.org

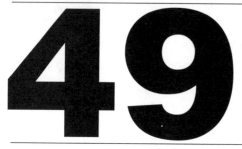

Language Delays

James Coplan

I. **Description of the problem.**
  • **Language** is a symbol system for the storage or exchange of information
  • **Expressive language** refers to the ability to generate symbolic output. This output may be either visual (writing, signing) or auditory (speech).
  • **Receptive language** refers to the ability to decode (i.e., extract meaning from) the language output of others. Receptive language encompasses visual (reading, sign language comprehension) and auditory (listening comprehension) skills.
  • **Speech** refers to the mechanical aspects of sound production.
  • **Language disorders** encompass any defect in the ability to encode or decode information through symbolic means.
  • **Speech disorders** encompass any deficit in the production of speech sounds. Children with disordered language may have normal speech. Similarly, children with disordered speech may have normal language (as in the case of dysarthria or deafness).
  A. **Epidemiology.** Delayed speech or language development are the most common developmental disorders of childhood, occurring in approximately 10% of preschool children (Table 49-1).
  B. **Development of language.**
    1. Language acquisition results from a complex interplay of innate biological capabilities and environmental stimulation. Infants acquire language through observation and through listening to speakers in their environment. Early efforts at imitation tend to be stimulus driven (i.e., automatic or unconscious), but by the latter half of the first year of life, infants appear capable of deliberate imitation of others' language. Parents and caretakers usually strongly reinforce and model linguistic behavior in order to create a linguistically enriched environment.
    2. By age 12 months, normal infants have grasped the notion that an arbitrary set of sounds (a word) symbolically represents a specific object or action. Likewise, a 12-month-old knows that he or she can signify a desired object by pointing to it rather than reaching for it. This ability to represent objects or actions in symbolic form constitutes the central feature of language.
    3. Language proficiency correlates closely with overall cognitive development in normal children and in children with global developmental delay (mental retardation). Some consider language development to be a special aspect of overall cognitive development. Alternatively, language acquisition may represent the emergence of a parallel but independent set of skills, which develop at the same time as general cognitive ability.
  C. **Etiology of language delays.**
    1. **Environmental.**
      • In an average home with average parents ("the ordinary expectable environment" with "good enough parents"), lack of stimulation is seldom, if ever, the cause of language delay. Suggestions that such parents become "more stimulating" may do more harm than good, either by inspiring misplaced parental guilt or by delaying a search for an underlying organic disorder as the basis for the child's delay.
      • Bilingual upbringing does not cause language delay. The bilingual child may intermix the vocabularies of both language, but total vocabulary size and length of utterance should be normal by age 2–3 years.
      • Birth order does not cause language delay.
      • Although language delay is frequently observed in association with social or environmental risk factors (e.g., poverty, lack of parental stimulation), these social and environmental risk factors are frequently intertwined with organic risk factors such as nutritional status, low-level lead exposure, low-grade iron deficiency, and parental genetic endowment. Thus, a child may receive a genetic "hit" leading to language impairment, compounded by the fact that the child's environment is language-poor because the parent also has a subtle developmental issue.

Table 49-1 Causes of delayed speech or language

Etiology	Prevalence (per 1,000 children)
Hearing loss	?
Permanent, mild to moderate	10
Intermittent, mild to moderate otitis media (OME)	*
Mental retardation (MR)	30
Developmental language disorders (DLD)[†]	50
Autistic spectrum disorders (ASD)	2–4
Dysarthria[‡]	1–3

*Up to 25% of children have chronic/recurrent otitis media with effusion during the first 3 years of life. The "attack rate" for speech and language delay due to OME remains unknown.
[†]Focal impairment of brain systems serving language, with sparing of the rest of the CNS.
[‡]Usually encountered within the context of cerebral palsy.

2. **Organic.** Speech or language delay may be primary (as in the case of developmental language disorders, or DLD), or secondary to some other developmental disability, such as hearing loss (HL), mental retardation (MR), autistic spectrum disorders (ASD), or dysarthria. DLDs are clinically heterogeneous, and may involve some combination of phonologic development (speech sound production), semantics (meaning), syntax (sentence structure) and pragmatics (use of language as a tool for social interchange).

3. **Developmental.** Laziness, twinning, and tongue-tie do not cause language delay. So-called twin speech is often indicative of the fact that both twins have an organically based language disorder, rather than a private language.

   • **"Constitutional delay"** implies a normal long-term developmental outcome. Although constitutional delay of speech acquisition exists, this is a diagnosis that can be established only in retrospect. If a preschool child's speech pattern is deficient based on comparison with age norms, then action is called for. Adopting a wait-and-see attitude in the hope that the child will "outgrow" the problem is inappropriate.

II. **Making the diagnosis.**

   A. **Signs and symptoms.** Parents may express concerns regarding "delayed speech." The practitioner must determine whether it is the child's speech and/or the child's language, that is delayed (Table 49-2). The pattern of speech and/or language delay, coupled with an appraisal of development in other domains (fine motor, adaptive, play, personal/social), will often suggest a specific developmental diagnosis. Note the value of visual language development as a distinguishing feature: visual language development is delayed in mental retardation and autism but normal in hearing loss, DLD, and dysarthria.

   B. **History.** A well-taken developmental history is the most important diagnostic measure. The language history should encompass auditory expressive, auditory receptive, and visual language milestones. The Early Language Milestone Scale (ELM Scale-2; see Appendix E) is one useful guide for normal language development in very young children. The developmental history should also cover general cognitive development (tool use, self-care skills), personal-social development (atypicality), and motor development.

   C. **Physical examination.** Elements of the history and physical examination pertinent to the assessment of the child with language delay are listed in Table 49-3.

Table 49-2 Signs of speech or language delay by type of disability

Language Feature→ Etiology ↓	Auditory Expressive Content	Auditory Expressive Intelligibility*	Auditory receptive	Visual
Hearing Loss	↓	↓	Variable	Normal
Mental retardation (MR)	↓	↓	↓	↓
Developmental language disorders (DLD)	↓	↓	Variable	Normal
Autistic spectrum disorders (ASD)	↓	Normal	↓	↓
Dysarthria	Variable	↓	Normal	Normal

*Clarity of speech. Unfamiliar adult can understand 25% of a 1-year-old, 50% of a 2-year-old, 75% of a 3-year-old, and 100% of a 4-year-old.

Table 49-3 Assessing the child with language delay

Medical history
- Teratogenic exposure (alcohol, prescription or recreational drugs)
- Fetal growth (weight, length, head circumference, and percentile values)
- Risk factors for HL (neonatal intensive care unit; recurrent otitis media)

Developmental history
- Oromotor: Problems with sucking, swallowing, chewing, excess drooling
- Fine motor/adaptive: Age at acquisition of tool use (spoon, crayon)
- Language: Auditory expressive, auditory receptive, visual
- Play: Banging and mouthing (9 mo); casting (12 mo); stacking and dumping (14 mo); scribbles with crayons (16–18 mo); imitative play ("helps" with housework, 24 mo); make-believe (36 mo); rule-based play (board games; 48 mo)
- Personal/social: Eye contact; rigid behavior, stereotypical movements, fascination with certain objects, sensory issues

Family history
- Educational attainment of parents and siblings
- Language delay, hearing loss, or other developmental disability

Physical examination
- Length, weight, head circumference, and percentile values
- Dysmorphic features
- Submucous cleft palate/bifid uvula
- Neurocutaneous lesions
- Neurologic exam: Hyper- or hypotonia, hyperreflexia, cognitive level

D. **Tests.**
   1. **Office screening of language development.** The ELM Scale-2 (Appendix C) covers language development from birth to age 36 months and intelligibility of speech from ages 24 to 48 months. It is designed for childcare professionals with varying degrees of expertise in early child development and demonstrates excellent test-retest and inter-observer reliability. Screening tests for ASD are now available as well.
   2. **Hearing.** Screening audiometry procedures used by physicians are prone to yield false-negative results or are inappropriate for the very young child. Therefore, **all** speech- or language-delayed children should have their hearing tested by a certified audiologist, regardless of the clinician's subjective impression of how well the child seems to hear.
   3. **Formal developmental testing.** Language, cognitive, and behavioral function should be assessed with an eye toward the following questions: (1) "What is the child's overall cognitive level, and is the child's language ability commensurate to his overall cognitive level?" (2) "Are there any atypical features (poor socialization, impaired pragmatics, repetitious behaviors or stereotyped movements, sensory aversions or attractions)?"
   4. **Referral.** The primary care clinician should not hesitate to refer children with suspected language delays for evaluation and treatment. If the results are negative, everyone will be appropriately reassured; if the results are positive, developmental intervention can be implemented in a timely fashion.
   5. **Medical assessment.** All children with speech or language delay need formal audiologic evaluation. Additional testing may include cytogenetic and metabolic studies (in the case of MR or ASD). CNS imaging and EEG are seldom informative, the principal exception being children with autistic regression or Landau-Kleffner syndrome (epileptic aphasia).

E. **Prognosis.**
   1. Children with primarily speech or language delay due to DLD typically present with impaired intelligibility of speech and delayed emergence of single words, phrases and sentences. Comprehension often appears normal, at least initially. Speech gradually improves, and most children become functional oral communicators by the time of school entry. As speech improves, evidence of underlying deficits in language production or comprehension often becomes evident (e.g., word-finding difficulties, problems with short-term auditory memory). Children with DLD are at increased risk for language-based learning disabilities. The prognosis for children with secondary speech or language delay is a function of the severity of the underlying disability (hearing loss, MR, ASD, cerebral palsy).

Table 49-4 Do's and don'ts for parents to promote language development

Don't

Try to make your child speak; it's unhelpful and demoralizing.

Use complicated language. Instead, expand a little bit on whatever your child says (e.g., Child: "Cookie!", Parent: "Oh, you want a cookie.")

Criticize pronunciation or grammatical errors.

Do

Talk to your child. Narrate daily events as you do them (e.g., "Okay, now I'm cleaning the floor. Oh, it's dirty. Can you see the dirt?").

Respond whenever your child speaks. It's important to reward every utterance.

Ask your child a lot of questions (e.g., "What's that? Where should we put that?").

Accompany your words with gestures to make them more comprehensible.

Read books aloud to your child.

Keep communication fun!

III. **Management.**
   A. **Primary goals.** The primary goal of management is to minimize frustration for the child and parents, while promoting optimal development of language. Table 49-4 lists suggestions for parents to provide a linguistically enriched environment.
   B. **Reading aloud.** Information on reading-aloud programs is usually available through the local public library. Not infrequently, a recommendation that parents read aloud with their child will lead the clinician to discover that the parent is semiliterate or illiterate. A remedial reading program for the parent can sometimes be instituted in conjunction with the reading-aloud program for the child.
   C. **Information for the family.** Do not rush to judgment, giving parents either false reassurance ("Don't worry, your child will grow out of it") or needless anxiety ("He or she will never be able to⋯"). On the other hand, do not procrastinate once the outcome seems clear. If there is a developmental disability, this should be explained to the parents in a straightforward yet compassionate manner. ("Why didn't our doctor tell us before now?" is a common complaint). Above all, listen to the family. ("We tried to tell our doctor there was a problem, but the doctor wouldn't listen to us" is another equally common complaint.) Following identification of a developmental disorder, the primary care clinician serves a key role by ensuring that the consultants who are involved have appropriately explained the issues and by regularly monitoring the child and the family's progress. With the explosion of information available on the World Wide Web, there are specific resources and support groups for virtually all developmental disorders. Connecting the family to other parents of similarly affected children is a source of great strength and comfort to most families.
   D. **Treatment.**
   - Treatment of speech or language delay is primarily educational. Infants and toddlers up to age 36 months are typically served in home-based programs.
   - Enrollment in a special education program administered by the child's school district is often the best option for children age 36 months or older, since a classroom setting will provide not just language instruction but practical experience in the use of language in a social setting.
   - For all children with speech or language disorders, the first priority is to enable the child to *communicate*—whether verbally or by some other means. Signing or picture card systems are commonly employed for children with severe speech delay due to DLD, as well as for children with autism, who are typically visually oriented. Parents can be assured with confidence that signing does not delay speech. On the contrary, sign language exposure may actually promote oral language development.
   - Language therapy for the child with MR will be integrated into an overall program stressing adaptive, play, and social development, in addition to language.
   - Augmentative communication devices are also widely available for children with persistent, severe deficits of speech and language due to cognitive or motor impairment.
   - Therapy for the child with hearing loss will vary, depending on the degree of hearing loss, but may include some combination of orally based speech therapy plus sign language, as well as amplification or cochlear implantation.
IV. **Clinical pearls and pitfalls.**
   - Parents will often say, "My child's speech is delayed, but he understands everything." On the contrary, the child with delayed language often does not understand everything

that is being said but relies instead on contextual cues and set routines, or depends on the parents to break everything down into a series of one-step commands. These strategies may be highly adaptive for a child with limited comprehension, but the ability to follow even a very large number of 1-step commands is no better than approximately 18–24 months, developmentally.

- Clinical detection of hearing loss, even severe to profound loss, is astonishingly difficult on physical examination, since children "cheat" by observing visual cues. If the child's speech or language is delayed or if the parents question hearing loss, the clinician should get an audiogram, no matter how well the child seems to hear in the office.

BIBLIOGRAPHY

For Parents

Beginning with Books. Information on reading aloud. Carnegie Library of Pittsburgh Homewood Branch 7101 Hamilton Avenue Pittsburgh PA 15208 412-731-1717

Websites

http://www.cherab.org/information/speechlanguage/delayresources.html

For Professionals

Light JC, Drager KD. Improving the design of augmentative and alternative technologies for young children. *Assist Technol* 14(1):17–32, 2002.

Rapin I. Practitioner review: developmental language disorders: a clinical update. *J Child Psychol Psychiatry* 37(6):643–655, 1996.

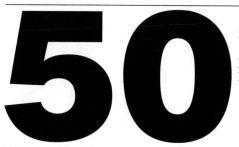

Lying, Cheating, & Stealing

Nerissa B. San Luis
Martin T. Stein

I. **Description of the problem.** The significance of three related behaviors in children—lying, stealing, and cheating—should be understood in the context of developmental tasks: imagination and symbolic thinking in the preschool child with the formation of a conscience, understanding cause and effect, and self-esteem in a school-age child. These developmental challenges determine and modulate the meaning of these behaviors. Every child lies and cheats at some time and many children steal something before adolescence. The challenge for the pediatric clinician is to unravel the significance of these events for an individual child and for her family—to clarify what might be a developmentally normal (albeit distressing) behavior from one that is disruptive and developmentally inappropriate.

A. **Epidemiology.**
   1. These behaviors are seen occasionally in all children. A precise prevalence is unknown for the normal population.
   2. 3–4 times more common in boys.
   3. When occurring frequently in association with aggressive behaviors and impacting adversely on development and function, may be a symptom of a more serious diagnosis.
      a. Oppositional defiant disorder (incidence 2%–16%)
      b. Conduct disorder: males (6%–16%); females (2%–9%).
      c. Significant stealing: (5%)
   4. Risk factors: inappropriate parental response to behavior, family disharmony, coercive discipline, difficult temperament, excessive exposure to violence (in home, community, television, movies), cognitive deficiency.

B. **Etiology/contributing factors.**
   1. **Environmental.** The child's immediate environment may be a contributing factor. When a preschool child expresses a developmentally appropriate "untruth," parental overreaction (e.g., expression of guilt or excessive discipline) may contribute to repetition of the behavior. Situational stress may come from school (recent change in grade, new school, bullying or victimization), home (parental unemployment, poor housing conditions, parental illness, exposure to violence), or community (child abduction, natural disaster, violence in media).
   2. **Developmental.**
      a. Temperamental factors may increase the likelihood of lying, stealing and cheating. Both behavioral inhibition and the "difficult child" may predispose to these behaviors, especially in the context of a parent or teacher whose own temperament is not adaptable to the child.
      b. Characteristics of a developmental stage clarify many behaviors
         • In the **3- and 4- year old**, an active imagination can generate "tall tales" or "white lies." They reflect developmentally appropriate processing of events. Young children cope with stressful situations by reflection—how a child wishes things were or how they should be. **Stealing** may begin with a preschool child whose actions are guided by egocentrism and who does not understand that taking something that does not belong to him is wrong.
         • In the **school-age child**, there is an awareness of societal expectations and the gradual emergence of a conscience with the cognitive and emotional maturity to differentiate a truth from an untruth. **Cheating** is seen occasionally in the school-age child and more often in middle school. Winning games and academic success in school may overcome the child's sense of what is right and desire to be part of a team. In school-age children, isolated stealing is usually an impulsive act. At this age and in middle school, stealing may develop from the child's desire for possessions or a result of attention seeking or revenge. It may reflect poor parent role modeling or ill-defined rules/boundaries.

3. **Parenting and other role models.** Considering the frequency of lying, stealing and cheating during early development, the parental response to such an event is perhaps the most critical factor. Each of these behaviors presents a potential opportunity to teach a child about their role in society—a preschool child who steals a candy bar, a school-age child who lies about a grade, or a middle school youth who cheats on an exam. The manner in which parents, teachers, and other adults respond to these events is important. In addition, the way parents live their own lives models significant behaviors for children each day.

4. **Organic.** Neurobehavioral disorders may be associated with poor self-regulation and lead to excessive lying, cheating and stealing. It may be seen in children and youth with oppositional behaviors as a component of depression, anxiety, or conduct disorder.

II. **Making the diagnosis.** The assessment should take place in a supportive environment that allows for a thorough history and physical examination, review of pertinent supporting documents (i.e., teacher narratives, past psycho-educational testing) and time to address specific parental concerns. The pediatric clinician can be instrumental in helping the parents perceive the disruptive behavior as part of a developmental process and advise them on the next step.

A. **Signs and symptoms.** Parents and clinicians usually (or eventually) know when a child has lied, cheated or stolen something. The recognition of these behaviors begins the process of a behavioral diagnosis. An isolated symptom in the absence of other behavior problems or developmental delay suggests that the behavior may be consistent with normal developmental expectations. Assessment should include

1. **Developmental milestones** with an emphasis on language, cognitive capacity and social interactions. Developmental mastery at specific stages is protective against persistent disruptive behaviors

2. **Family role modeling** and **parental response to behaviors**

3. **Experience with peers** in context of social role models; peer pressure

4. **Educational achievement**, including family and child's expectation for performance

5. **Low self-esteem**

B. **Differential diagnosis.** When the behaviors cannot be explained in the context of normal developmental stages, consider more pervasive type of disorders. Lying, cheating and stealing may be associated with a specific behavioral disorder, including oppositional defiant disorder, conduct disorder, attention deficit hyperactivity disorder, anxiety, depression, post-traumatic stress disorder, an adjustment disorder, or pervasive developmental delay. These behaviors may reflect aggression manifested by words or actions that seem intended to harm another person or oneself. Lying, for example, is seen in bullying behavior and stealing may be a part of retaliatory behavior.

C. **History.** Start with an inventory of possible risk and protective factors.

1. **Individual risk factors.** Prenatal history (exposure to drugs, alcohol, cigarettes, lead), birth history (resuscitative events or prolonged neonatal ICU experience), quality of early attachment experiences, temperament (poor adaptability, distractible, intense reaction to change), immature social skills, vulnerable peer groups, developmental regression.

2. **Familial and relational risk factors.** Poor temperament match between parent and child, ineffective parenting practices, marital conflicts, parental separation, divorce, domestic violence, family history of psychopathology (e.g., alcoholism, depression) especially in parents, child abuse/neglect.

3. **Community factors.** Neighborhood and media violence exposure, availability of firearms.

4. **Protective factors/patient strengths.** Strong and stable social support in home or community, child's special talents, academic success, temperament of child and parents.

5. **Key clinical questions. For the family:**
   - *"Has there been any major change or other stress in the life of the child or family?"* Lying, cheating or stealing may manifest as a new behavior after a significant shift in the child's life and may impact the ability to cope with a new situation or event. Assess the different environments—home: parental conflict, birth of a new sibling; school: change in school or poor adjustment to new academic level, problems with friends or bullying; community: exposure to negative role model, unstable parental employment.
   - *"How often does the behavior occur?"* If it happens infrequently, examine the cir-

cumstances immediately preceding, during, and following the event. Does it occur only in certain settings? Assess patterns in the behavior, including an increased intensity or severity. If the behavior is chronic, consider depression, anxiety, conduct disorder.

- *"How do the parents respond to the behavior?"*

For the child: (it may be helpful to separate the child from the parent)

- *"What happened immediately before the event?"*
- *"What were you feeling when you····.?"* Assess motivation and insight.
- *"How did you feel afterwards?"* Regret or remorse reflects moral development. (Lack of remorse may indicate a conduct disorder.)
- *"How do you feel about it now?"*
- *"What makes you angry? What helps you to calm down?"*
- *"How do you think you could have handled the situation differently?"*

D. Behavioral observation. Observational data in the office may be helpful in assessment. Observe the child's interactions with the parent, with you and during self-play. A clinical assessment of temperament should be recorded as well as activity level, impulsivity, affect, cognitive functioning and social responses. Observed behaviors should be interpreted in the context of the child's developmental stage.

E. Tests. To determine the contextual aspect of the behaviors, a daily behavioral diary may prove helpful. Ask the family to document the antecedents of the behavior (what was going on), the behavior (what the child did or said), and the consequences (what happened after the event). Clues to specific diagnoses associated with these behaviors will surface during a comprehensive behavioral-developmental and family history. In specific situations, behavioral questionnaires or psychoeducational testing may define the problem with greater precision.

III. Management.

A. Information for the family. Educating the family is the initial step toward effective collaboration with the pediatric clinician. When addressing negative behavioral issues, begin the discussion by pointing out the patient's and family's strengths. Guide parents to an understanding of how these qualities support a positive outcome. Framing the behavior in context of developmental principles should lead to an understanding of the behavior and insight into the child's temperament, motivation, and responses to the environment. Discuss the child and family vulnerabilities that may be associated with the behaviors.

B. Helpful behavioral management tips for the family.

1. **Lying.** Consider the context in which it occurs and do not accuse or label the child as a "liar." The 3- to 4-year-old child processes experience with magical, egocentric thinking; the preschool child is in the early stage of understanding right from wrong. By 8 or 9 years old, the conscience is more developed and becomes an internal moral guide. Help parents to use this knowledge to respond to their child. After an episode of lying, discuss the reasons for the behavior in an open manner. Reassure the child you will always love him or her. Reassurance can help ease a child's anxieties and help her share feelings and reasons for lying.

2. **Stealing.** A clear explanation about possessions and the concept of ownership should be given to the child. Firm limits should be in place. Modeling appropriate behavior, such as "let's return the toy back to your friend" or "let's go say sorry and pay for the candy" should be used. Do not overreact since this may frighten the child. Forcing the child to confess may only push the child to lie. Parents should begin to talk about ownership, sharing and asking for what he or she wants as early as toddler age. If stealing is repetitive, seek additional help.

3. **Cheating.** Parents can talk about how cheating hurts other people's feelings and ask the child if there is a better solution. Approach the child in a gentle manner and refrain from harsh punishment. Explain consequences in a calm, matter-of-fact way.

C. Criteria for referral.

1. When lying, cheating or stealing is frequent and not responsive to education and behavior management, consider referral to a mental health professional.

2. Domestic violence or child abuse should be reported to an appropriate agency as mandated by law.

3. Ongoing parental–child conflicts, a significant temperament mismatch, or underlying psychopathology should be managed concurrently with a mental health professional.

4. Social issues such as parental unemployment and lack of adequate childcare may be addressed by referral to a social worker or case manager involved with a community-based organization.

BIBLIOGRAPHY

For Parents

Brazelton, TB, Sparrow JD. *Touchpoints: Three to Six: Your Child's Emotional and Behavioral Development.* Cambridge, MA: Perseus Books, 2001.

Pruitt DB. *Your Child: What Every Parent Needs to Know About Childhood Development from Birth to Preadolescence.* New York: Harper Collins, 1998.

Spock B, Parker SJ, Needlman R. *Dr. Spock's Baby and Child Care (8th ed).* New York: Pocket Books, 2004.

For Professionals

Dixon SD, Stein MT. *Encounters with Children: Pediatric Behavior and Development (3rd ed).* St. Louis, MO: Mosby, 2000.

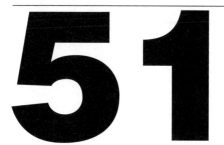

Masturbation

Ilgi Ozturk Ertem
John Leventhal

I. **Description of the problem.** Sexual health has been defined by the World Health Organization as the "integration of the somatic, emotional, intellectual, and social aspects of sexual being, in ways that are positively enriching and that enhance personality, communication and love." Childhood sexuality is as much a part of a child as are physical health, growth, and other aspects of development. It is within this framework that the clinician should address parental concern with masturbation, one of the early manifestations of the sexual development of the child.
   - The term *masturbation* is derived from the Latin words for "hand" (*manus*) and "defilement" (*stupratio*). It is defined as a deliberate self-stimulation that results in sexual arousal.
   - At least since the time of Hippocrates (400 BC), masturbation has evoked negative attitudes within societies. For example, during the 18th century, two thirds of all human illnesses were attributed to masturbation. Various treatment regimens, such as disciplining the patient, mechanical preventions, cautery of genitals, clitorectomy, and castration, were established and practiced until the mid-20th century. It is still true that parents' and teachers' responses to sexual behavior in children are largely influenced by cultural patterns. Some societies condone and encourage self-stimulation during childhood; others condemn it. In general, Western societies take a more restrictive view of masturbation.
   A. **Epidemiology.** Masturbation is universal and intentional in children of both sexes by age 5–6 years. Almost all boys and 25% of girls have masturbated to the point of orgasm by age 15 years.
   B. **Environmental, developmental, and transactional factors in etiology.** Masturbatory activity has been observed in the male fetus in utero. In the first months of life, infants of both sexes learn to experience the sensations associated with diapering and the cleansing of genitals. A developmental progression toward adult erotic responsiveness proceeds from these early pleasurable sensations. This includes the differentiation and appreciation of genitals, inclusion of sexual parts in the body concept, "exhibitionism" to test adult reactions, mastery of a variety of self-elicited sensations, and the integration of sexual function into the emerging self-concept.
   C. **Signs and symptoms.** Most commonly, masturbatory activity in infants and toddlers involves a particular posturing, tightening of the thighs, handling of the genitals, and symptoms of sexual arousal (e.g., flushing, rapid or irregular breathing). Masturbation may also involve less obvious acts such as leaning the suprapubic region on a firm edge, stiffening of the lower extremities, or rocking movements in various positions. These may be accompanied by brief bouts of crying or sweating and may last from minutes to hours at a time.
II. **Making the diagnosis.**
   A. **Differential diagnosis.**
      1. **Masturbatory actions may be misdiagnosed as seizures** because of the abrupt onset of the episodes, the tonic posturing, facial flushing, irregular breathing, and the child's preoccupation. During masturbation, there may also be blank stares or tremulous movements. The child may resume his or her previous play or activity after the event or may appear drowsy and fall asleep, mimicking children in the postictal phase. Tonic posturing with crossing of the thighs has been reported to occur as early as 3 months of age. Masturbatory activity in children has been associated with unnecessary investigations for organic disease such as seizures, epilepsy, paroxysmal dystonia, carcinoid syndrome, or urinary tract infections. The symptoms of masturbation also have been confused with abdominal pain or the "retentive" posturing that occurs in children who withhold stool. This is manifested as episodic tightening of the buttock and thighs, often accompanied by facial flushing and grunting.
      2. **The clinician should consider the diagnosis of sexual abuse** in children with com-

pulsive masturbation, especially if accompanied by other sexualized behaviors. In Western societies, searching for and responding to body contact has been shown to occur frequently in daycare centers for healthy preschoolers. However, obsessive masturbation without pleasure or causing pain, using objects against own or other child's genitals/anus, attempting to make an adult touch the child's genitals or touching an adult's genitals occurs very rarely. These sexualized behaviors should alert the clinician to the possibility of sexual abuse.

B. History: Key clinical questions. A thorough history is key to an appropriate diagnosis and effective management. Since masturbation is not harmful, it should be considered a problem only when it causes distress to the child, parental anxiety, or social condemnation.

1. *"Tell me what you've noticed about your child's touching his or her genitals. Where does this happen? In school? At home?"* This elicits the method the child uses and the frequency and the context in which the child engages in masturbation and other sexualized behaviors.

2. Parents have different thoughts and feelings when their children touch their own genitals. *"Can you tell me how it is for you? What do you do when this happens?"* The meaning of masturbatory behavior to the parents and their responses to the behavior should be understood.

3. *"When you respond like that, how do you think he or she feels?"* The parents' perceptions of the consequences of their responses and the outcome of the behavior are important.

4. *"Are there any significant stressors for family and/or child, and /or developmental delays?"*

C. Physical examination. Clinical circumstances may dictate exploration of a more pathologic interpretation of the masturbatory behaviors. Masturbation may begin with genital irritation or discomfort. If the behavior is especially compulsive and of acute onset, consider the possibility of sexual abuse. A child who has been sexually abused may have physical findings suggestive of or consistent with genital trauma. Also, children may insert objects in their genitalia during sex play. Therefore, the anus, genitalia, and perineum should be examined as part of a general physical examination.

D. Tests. Laboratory tests are almost never required during a work-up for masturbation. However, causes of irritation such as pinworm infestations or urinary tract infections will require appropriate diagnosis and treatment. Home-video recordings have been shown to be effective in the evaluation of paroxysmal events in children. The widespread availability of home-video recordings may provide the opportunity to examine in detail the child's activity and may prevent the use of unnecessary investigations and referrals.

III. Management.

A. Anticipatory guidance. A clinician who, from the beginning of a relationship with parents, is open to discussing issues of sexuality is more likely to receive questions about sexual development, behaviors, and problems as the child grows older. Parents are less likely to be anxious, confused, or scornful of masturbatory behavior in their child if they have been told in advance that this behavior is normal, universal, and healthy. Such anticipatory guidance should be offered early in life, when infants begin to explore their bodies. During a review of developmental milestones or during a genital examination, parents can be asked in a matter-of-fact manner whether their child has discovered his or her genitals and whether he or she plays with them. Parental feelings and attitudes can then be explored and information on how they would react to the situation can be obtained.

B. When masturbation is viewed as a problem behavior:

- The clinician should not simply dismiss parental concerns about the issue by flatly stating that "masturbation is normal." Rather he or she should attempt to understand the level of parental discomfort and the social and psychological consequences of the behavior for the child, with the goals of alleviating parental anxiety and diminishing feelings of fear, anxiety, guilt, and shame in the child.

- A detailed history will not only establish the diagnosis but also give the parents a chance to discuss their fears and worries. Examples of parental concerns include fear that their child has an organic disease, has been sexually abused, is experiencing conflict with a family member or teacher/caretaker, will develop promiscuity, or will be mentally handicapped. The masturbatory behavior may evoke a parent's own conflicts about sexuality, and the parent may withdraw attention and/or affection from the child. In the majority of cases, after such concerns and attitudes are explored, reassurance will be sufficient.

- Parents should be advised not to overreact to the child's behavior. It should be emphasized that punishing and scolding can be harmful to the child's self-esteem and long-term sexual development.

- Parents can tell their preschool child that masturbation is a private behavior that is best not done in public (e.g., "There are some things that we do around other people. This is one of the things that we do in private").
- Behavioral modification techniques, such as positive reinforcement, have been helpful in cases of compulsive masturbation (especially in children with mental retardation).

C. **Criteria for referral.**

1. When appropriate counseling by the clinician elicits complaints by the parents that the **child is in psychologic distress.**
2. When **unusual manifestations or excessive masturbation impede self-esteem** and adaptive functioning of the child and/or cause social problems.
3. When **other family or interpersonal pathology** is recognized by the clinician to contribute to the problem.
4. When there are accompanying **developmental/behavioral or affective disturbances** in the child.

BIBLIOGRAPHY

For Parents

Sex Education: A Bibliography of Educational Materials for Children, Adolescents, and Their Families. Available from American Academy of Pediatrics, Department of Publications, 141 Northwest Point Blvd., P.O. Box 927, Elk Grove Village, IL 60009.

What Kids Want to Know about Sex and Growing Up. From Children's Television Workshop, One Lincoln Plaza, New York, NY 10023.

For Professionals

Finkelstein E, Amichai B, Jaworowski S, Mukamel M. Masturbation in prepubescent children: a case report and review of the literature. *Child Care Health Dev* 1996;22(5):323–326.

Friedrich WN, et al. Normative sexual behavior in children. *Pediatrics* 88(3):456–464, 1991.

Leung AK, Robson WL. Childhood masturbation. *Clin Pediatr* 32(4):238–241, 1993.

Lindblad F, Gustafsson PA, Larsson I, Lundin B. Preschoolers' sexual behavior at daycare centers: an epidemiological study. *Child Abuse Negl* 1995;19(5):569–577.

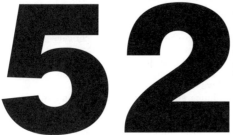

Mental Retardation: Behavioral Problems

Theodore Kastner
Kevin Walsh

I. **Description of the problem.**
   A. **Epidemiology** The incidence of behavioral disorders in children with mental retardation is greater than in children without mental retardation because any brain damage or dysfunction appears to increase the likelihood of behavioral or psychiatric disorders.
   - 40% of people with mental retardation experience a period of disturbed behavior and function at some time in their lives.
   - The epidemiology of behavioral problems among children with mental retardation is unknown because of their cognitive and communicative limitations and because appropriate diagnostic tools are not yet available.
   - It is estimated that diagnosable psychiatric disorders exist in 5%–10% of children with mental retardation.

   B. **Etiology.** There are four major causes of severe, challenging behaviors in children with mental retardation: adaptive dysfunction, psychiatric disorders, medication side effects, and organic causes. In many cases, the etiology is of multiple origins (e.g., a psychiatric disorder accompanied by family dysfunction).
      1. **Adaptive dysfunction** is a mismatch between the needs, abilities, and goals of the child and that of the environment (usually the school and/or family unit). In this model, the potential *communicative* nature of the behavior is often considered. For example, does a behavioral outburst always accompany a request to accomplish difficult tasks? In this case, the behavioral problem may be due to unrealistic environmental expectations. Adaptive dysfunction can often be distinguished from mental illness or an organic cause by a lack of vegetative signs (weight loss or sleep problem) and a consistent relationship between the behavior and antecedent events.
      2. **Psychiatric disorders** are more common in children with mental retardation than in the general population. The most common psychiatric disorders associated with mental retardation in children may be the mood disorders, such as depression and bipolar disease (often in atypical forms, e.g., rapid cycling and chronic mania). Mood disorders in children with mental retardation can often be recognized by the presence of a sleep disturbance, change in weight or eating habits, overactivity or motor restlessness, mood lability (crying or laughing), and a behavioral history of cycling. Less commonly, anxiety disorders, psychosis, Tourette syndrome, attention deficit hyperactivity disorder, and obsessive-compulsive disorder are seen.
      3. **Medication side effects** are a common cause of behavioral morbidity among children with mental retardation. For example, in a study of 209 people with mental retardation who presented with behavioral complaints, undiagnosed medication side effects were noted in 7%. These included akasthisia, tardive dyskinesia, and other side effects typically associated with the use of major tranquilizers.
      4. **Organic causes.** Occult medical illnesses have been found in about 20% of behaviorally disordered children with mental retardation. The high prevalence is due to their greater health care needs, communication barriers around symptomatology, and a lack of effective healthcare services. Perhaps the most common medical cause of disturbed behavior is unrecognized or poorly treated epilepsy, especially partial complex seizures. Interictal irritability, for example, can exacerbate aggressive or self-injurious behaviors. Other undiagnosed medical causes of behavioral problems include thyroid dysfunction, premenstrual syndrome, and cardiac disease.

II. **Making the diagnosis.**
   A. **Signs and symptoms.** Behavioral problems in children with mental retardation include aggression, self-injury, overactivity, and sleep disturbances. In addition, rumination, elopement, property destruction, and other behaviors are occasionally seen.
   B. **Behavioral questionnaires.** Inventories or behavioral scales can be used to facilitate the evaluation of behavioral problems in children with mental retardation. These include the Reiss Screen for Maladaptive Behavior, the Reiss Scales for Children's Dual

Table 52-1 Formulating a Diagnostic and Mental Retardation and Behavioral Problems

1. Rule out the presence of a medical disorder.
2. Evaluate the presence of environmental supports and stressors.
3. Look for a complex of behavioral symptoms.
4. Establish a psychiatric diagnosis using standard or modified criteria.
5. Develop treatment goals.
6. Monitor treatment with a predetermined methodology.
7. Establish a treatment end point.

Diagnosis, the Psychopathology Instrument for Mentally Retarded Adults (PIMRA), and the Aberrant Behavior Checklist. It is frequently of benefit to use two or more inventories and to have more than one caregiver complete the instrument.

C. Physical examination. The physical examination should be comprehensive and thorough. If an organic cause of behavioral problems (e.g., hypothyroidism in a child with Down syndrome) is missed by the clinician, it is unlikely that the disorder will be recognized by another childcare provider. Laboratory testing should be based on clinical suspicions aroused by the history and physical examination. Even when these produce no clues, however, the clinician should remain ever vigilant to the possibility of an occult medical problem.

D. Diagnostic hypotheses. The clinician should formulate a psychiatric diagnosis or etiologic hypothesis before prescribing a treatment. Steps needed to develop a diagnosis and treatment plan for children with mental retardation and behavioral problems are outlined in Table 52-1>.

Strict diagnostic criteria for psychiatric disorders may not be met due to a number of features related to mental retardation, especially cognitive and communicative deficits. Frequently, a clear diagnosis cannot be made, and the clinician may resort to empirical trial-and-error treatments. The general points in Table 52-2 should be noted when considering the use of psychotropic medication in children with mental retardation.

III. Treatment. The treatment of behavioral problems in children with mental retardation may require changes in the caretaking environment, psychoactive medications, medical interventions, or any combination of the three.

A. The environment. If the social milieu is nonoptimal, the behavior of the child with mental retardation may represent an attempt to control or alter that environment. Behavioral problems may then be reduced or eliminated as the child is taught appropriate replacement behaviors that can serve the same function. This intervention begins with *functional analysis* and is best conducted as part of a comprehensive diagnostic process that includes traditional medical and psychiatric evaluations.

B. Psychoactive medications. Given the vast number of psychoactive medications on the market, it is wise to be familiar with one or two drugs in each of the major classes of medications. This is generally sufficient to allow the clinician the flexibility to make appropriate choices between treatments. Specifically, the interested clinician should be comfortable using anticonvulsants (carbamazepine, valproic acid), antimanic drugs (lithium carbonate), tricyclic antidepressants (desipramine and imipramine), stimulants (methylphenidate and dextroamphetamine), antianxiety drugs (propranolol and buspirone), serotonin reuptake inhibiting antidepressants (sertraline and fluoxetine), and atypical neuroleptics (risperidone and quetiapine). The general indications for use of many of these medications are included in Table 52-3.

Table 52-2 Clinical Concerns When Using Psychopharmacology in Children with Mental Retardation and Behavioral Problems

The diagnosis should guide treatment.

The more severe the behavior or the degree of mental retardation, the more likely it is that the problem is biologically based and will respond to appropriate medication.

Anticonvulsants (such as carbamazepine and valproic acid), and antihypertensives (such as beta-blockers) are powerful psychotropic agents.

Treat multiple diagnoses with a single medication if possible (e.g., treat epilepsy and depression with carbamazepine; treat attention deficit hyperactivity disorder and anxiety with a tricyclic antidepressant).

The end point in a trial of medication is behavioral remission or intolerable side effects.

Table 52-3 Behavioral Symptoms Suggesting Psychiatric Diagnoses and Treatment

Behavioral symptoms	Possible diagnoses	Potential psychoactive therapy
Overactivity, decreased sleep, poor attention, self injury, aggression	Bipolar disorder	Mood stabilizers or atypical neuroleptics
Overactivity, poor attention, autism, self injury, aggression	Anxiety disorders	Propranolol, buspirone, atypical neuroleptics, or selective serotonin reuptake inhibitors
Poor attention, fragile X syndrome	Attention deficit hyperactivity disorder	Methylphenidate, tricyclic antidepressants, clonidine
Stereotypic behavior, self injury, aggression	Obsessive compulsive disorder, depression	Atypical neuroleptics, or selective serotonin reuptake inhibitors
Social withdrawal, abnormal sleep pattern, poor attention, self injury, aggression, rumination	Depression	Mood stabilizers, antidepressants

Many of the medications have multiple effects. Carbamazepine is an effective anticonvulsant with antidepressant, antimanic, and neuralgic effects. It can be an excellent first choice in the treatment of aggression and/or self-injury, particularly in the presence of overactivity or a sleep disorder. In addition to depression, selective serotonin reuptake inhibitors are valuable in the treatment of anxiety disorders and obsessive compulsive disorder. The atypical neuroleptics are often a good first choice of treatment during an acute problem, although every effort should be made to find alternative treatments because of long-term side effects.

C. **The family.** The level of family stress and the family's ability to use the resources of the extended family or obtain alternative community supports are important predictors of outcome. For example, a recent study of children with epilepsy noted that family function was one of the most important predictors of behavioral problems. The primary care provider should always remember that a strong family is a more effective treatment partner.

D. **Follow-up.** Interventions for children with mental retardation and behavioral problems should be accompanied by careful follow-up. The behavioral response to the treatment plan should receive careful scrutiny. Children taking psychoactive medication may require periodic screening for drug levels, side effects, and behavioral changes, depending on the medication used. In addition, the diagnosis may need to be reconsidered in the light of the response to treatment. For example, when a trial of stimulant medication causes a worsening of behavior or ever-increasing dosages are required to maintain therapeutic effect, the diagnosis of bipolar disorder should be considered.

BIBLIOGRAPHY

For Parents

Books

Batshaw M, Perret Y (eds). *Children with Disabilities (4th ed).*Baltimore: Brookes 1997.

Websites

The Arc (formerly called the Association for Retarded Citizens) http://www.thearc.org/info-mr.html Developmental Disabilities Health Alliance, Inc. www.ddha.com

For Professionals

Books

Matson J, Mulick J. *Handbook of Mental Retardation (2nd ed).* New York: Pergamon, 1991.
O'Neill R, et al. *Functional Analysis of Problem Behavior: A Practical Assessment Guide.* Sycamore, IL: Sycamore Publishing Co., 1990.

Rubin L, Crocker A, eds. *Developmental Disabilities: Delivery of Medical Care for Children and Adults.* Philadelphia: Lea & Febiger, 1989.

Newsletters/Reviews

Habilitative Mental Health Care Newsletter
P.O. Box 57
Bear Creek NC 27207

Behavioral Questionnaires

Aberrant Behavior Checklist
Slosson Educational Publications
P.O. Box 280
East Aurora NY 14052
1-800-828-4800
Reiss Screen for Maladaptive Behavior Reiss Scales for Children's Dual Diagnosis, and Psychopathology Instrument for Mentally Retarded Adults
International Diagnostic Systems
P.O. Box 389
Worthington OH 43085
1-800-876-6360

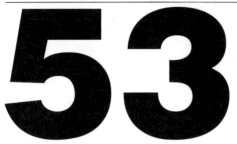

Mental Retardation: Diagnostic Evaluation

David L. Coulter

I. **Description of the problem.** According to the American Association on Mental Retardation (AAMR), mental retardation is defined as follows:

A. **Definition.** "Mental retardation is a disability characterized by significant limitations both in intellectual functioning and in adaptive behavior as expressed in conceptual, social, and practical adaptive skills. This disability originates before age 18." (Luckasson et al. 2002)

1. Significant limitation in intellectual functioning means an IQ score that is more than two standard deviations below the mean for the IQ test used.

2. Significant limitation in adaptive behavior means a score that is more than two standard deviations below the mean for the adaptive behavior test used.

3. Classification of individuals with mental retardation should not be based solely on the IQ score, and categories of mild, moderate, severe, and profound mental retardation (which were based solely on the IQ score) are no longer used. Instead, *classification is based on the types and intensities of supports and services needed by the individual.* These are categorized as: "Intermittent", "Limited.", "Extensive", or "Pervasive".

B. **Etiology.** Mental retardation may be the end result of *one or more* of the following categories of risk.

1. **Biomedical.** These are factors that have had a deleterious impact on the child's CNS (e.g., genetic disorders, environmental toxins, infections).

2. **Social.** Inadequacies in the social and/or family environment (e.g., inadequate stimulation, social unresponsiveness) can diminish cognitive and social growth and functioning.

3. **Behavioral.** The damaging behavior of others (e.g., trauma, maternal substance abuse) can lead to mental retardation.

4. **Educational.** The availability and quality of educational and training programs can affect intellectual development and influence whether or not a child functions in the range of mental retardation.

5. **Interactions between risk factors.** In any given case, multiple risk factors may be present and may interact at different ages or stages of development. This concept reflects the transactional approach to human development, in which reciprocal interactions between individuals and their environment influence the developmental outcome. Some risk factors may be more significant (principal or primary cause of mental retardation), and others may be less significant (contributing or secondary cause), but the interaction between them is almost always important. For example, a child with phenylketonuria (biomedical risk factor) may function at a lower level because of both environmental deprivation (social risk factor) and poor parental compliance with the prescribed diet (behavioral risk factor).

II. **Making the diagnosis.**

A. **Signs and symptoms.** Mental retardation should be suspected in any child who is significantly below the normative developmental milestones for his age. Additionally, children with *established* risk (e.g., Down syndrome) are very likely to have mental retardation.

B. **Evaluation of the etiology.**

1. An understanding of the etiology of mental retardation begins with a **complete medical and psychosocial history** and a **complete physical and neurologic examination.** This preliminary assessment results in a list of possible causes or differential diagnosis, which should include consideration of any and all potential risk factors.

2. The differential diagnosis should be thought of as a set of **hypotheses about the etiology**, so that the subsequent workup is designed to test the most reasonable hypotheses. Table 53-1 is designed to help the primary care clinician design an appropriate workup based on the most likely hypotheses in a particular case. This table lists a series of possible hypotheses based on whether the potential risk occurred

Table 53-1 Hypotheses and Strategies for Determining Etiology of Mental Retardation

Hypothesis	Possible strategies
Prenatal onset	
Chromosomal disorder	Extended physical examination
	Referral to geneticist
	Chromosomal analysis, including fragile X study and high-resolution banding
Syndrome disorder	Extended family history and examination of relatives
	Extended physical examination
	Referral to clinical geneticist or neurologist
Inborn error of metabolism	Screening for amino acids and organic acids
	Quantitation of amino acids in blood, urine, and/or CSF
	Analysis of organic acids by GC-MS or other methods
	Blood levels of lactate, pyruvate, carnitine, and long-chain fatty acids
	Arterial ammonia and gases
	Assays of specific enzymes
	Biopsies of specific tissue for light and electron microscopic study and biochemical analysis
Developmental disorder of brain formation	CT or MRI scan of brain
	Detailed morphologic study of brain tissue (e.g., biopsy)
Environmental influences	Growth charts
	Placental pathology
	Maternal history and physical examination of mother
	Toxicologic screening of mother at prenatal visits and of child at birth
	Referral to clinical geneticist
	Review maternal records (prenatal care, labor and delivery)
Perinatal onset	
	Review birth and neonatal records
Postnatal onset	
Head injuries	Detailed medical history
	Skull x-rays, CT or MRI scan (for evidence of sequelae)
Infections	Detailed medical history
Demyelinating disorders	CT or MRI scan
Degenerative disorders	CT or MRI scan
	Evoked potential studies
	Assays of specific enzymes
	Biopsy of specific tissue for light and electron microscopy and biochemical analysis
Seizure disorders	Electroencephalography
Toxic-metabolic disorders	See "Inborn error of metabolism"
	Toxicologic studies
	Heavy metal assays
Malnutrition	Body measurements
	Detailed nutritional history
	Family history of nutrition
Environmental	Detailed social history
	Psychological evaluation
	Observation in new environment

prenatally, perinatally, or postnatally. A set of possible strategies for testing each of these hypotheses is then suggested.

3. **There is no single diagnostic workup that is appropriate to all cases.** In some cases the workup will be very simple (as in chromosomal analysis when Down syndrome is suspected). In most cases, however, the etiology will not be obvious, and a careful workup will be needed. Such an evaluation, however, will result in identification of the principal or primary cause of mental retardation in only about one third of cases. Because new diagnostic measures for mental retardation are emerging rapidly, the

etiologic evaluation of idiopathic mental retardation should be considered an ongoing process that can take advantage of the newest research.

The Child Neurology Society recommends the following studies for evaluation of the child with global developmental delay:

a. **High-resolution chromosomal analysis and fragile X studies** are recommended because not all chromosomal abnormalities lead to obvious physical signs (diagnostic yield approximately 5%–6%).

b. **Radiologic imaging of the brain** is recommended, and MRI is preferred (diagnostic yield 55%) to CT (diagnostic yield 39%).

c. **Metabolic screening** for amino acid and organic acid disorders has a low diagnostic yield but may identify potentially treatable disorders, and so is recommended particularly when genetic studies and neuroimaging are unrevealing.

III. **Management.**
   A. **Conveying the diagnosis and prognosis.**
      1. **Diagnosis.** Primary care clinicians are often present when the diagnosis is first made. Unfortunately, parents often have unpleasant memories about how the diagnosis was first conveyed to them. To avoid this and to help ensure that the diagnosis is conveyed sensitively, clinicians can follow these guidelines:
         a. **Listen to what the parents say about the child.** This will give the clinician a sense of their level of sophistication, understanding, and emotional acceptance of the child's problems.
         b. **Ask the parents about which particular aspects of their child's problems bother them the most.** This will help to address the issues *most important to them.*
         c. **Review the results of the evaluation in a way that is easily understandable and unambiguous.** Avoid technical jargon and overly complex explanations. Assess parental understanding by asking them to rehearse how they will explain their child's problem to a family member.
         d. Parents will be all too eager to assume the responsibility and guilt for their child's problem. **Consistent and persistent reassurance that the condition was not their fault is always indicated.**
         e. **The clinician should respect the parents' preference for using an alternative term to "mental retardation"** (such as "special needs" child). However, it may be useful for them to understand that their child meets the diagnostic criteria for mental retardation when such a designation provides eligibility for important supports and services.
      2. **Prognosis.** The primary care clinician should help the family to prepare for the future. This requires an understanding of the child's prognosis for functioning as an adult. In general, pediatric clinicians tend to *underestimate* the level at which adults with mental retardation can function in the community. The clinician must achieve the delicate balance of not giving overly optimistic predictions of the child's potential capabilities (thereby engendering intense disappointment over time) and not underestimating his long-term potential (thereby creating a negative self-fulfilling prophecy). The clinician should ensure, over time, that the family accepts the prognosis, incorporates it into their family planning (e.g., for guardianship and financial trusts), and has realistic expectations for the child's future.
   B. **Clinical issues.**
      1. Primary care issues include **health supervision, immunizations, nutrition and growth, gynecologic care, and sex education**. Some children with mental retardation also have other problems that may require referral to a specialist (e.g., neurologist, psychiatrist, orthopedist, or physiatrist). The primary care clinician should work collaboratively with the family and with any specialists involved in the child's care.
      2. The primary care clinician should closely monitor the **academic progress of the child** with mental retardation. A young child (age<3 years) should be referred for early intervention services as soon as a developmental problem is identified (often before the diagnosis of mental retardation is actually made). An older child should be referred to the public school system to ensure that a comprehensive evaluation is done and an appropriate educational plan is developed.
      3. As the child gets older, the clinician will need to anticipate concerns about the **transition to adult living**: guardianship, living arrangements, work, sexuality, and family planning, among others.
      4. The primary care clinician understands better than most specialists that the child with mental retardation belongs to a family that may be extended and/or nontraditional. Improving the child's quality of life requires improving the family's quality

of life. Particular attention should be paid to helping siblings of the child with mental retardation understand and accept their role, which may become prominent during adulthood.

BIBLIOGRAPHY

For Parents

The Arc (formerly called the Association for Retarded Citizens). The largest organization for parents of children with mental retardation. Many local Arc's have parent support groups as well as case advocacy and specific supports and services.

Every state has a government agency responsible for providing services to people with mental retardation. 301-565-3842 www.thearc.org

For Professionals

Associations

American Association on Mental Retardation. Conducts workshops and publishes journals and books on mental retardation.
1-800-424-3688
www.aamr.org
Association of University Centers on Disability. Coordinates a network of regional training and service programs.
301-588-8252
www.aucd.org

Publications

Coulter DL. Prevention as a form of support. *Mental Retardation* 34:108–116, 1996.

Dykens EM, Hodapp RM, and Finucane BM. *Genetics and Mental Retardation Syndromes: A New Look at Behavior and Interventions.* Baltimore: Paul H Brookes, 2000.

Luckasson R, et al. *Mental Retardation Definition, Classification and Systems of Supports, 10th ed.* Washington, DC: American Association on Mental Retardation, 2002. [See especially Chapter 8 on Etiology and Prevention.]

Shevell M, Ashwal S, Donley D, Flint J, et al. Practice parameter: Evaluation of the child with global developmental delay. *Neurology* 60:367–380, 2003.

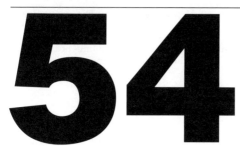

Motor Delays

Peter A. Blasco

I. **Description of the problem.** Delayed motor milestones are the highest-ranked concern of parents with children between ages 6–12 months. Related complaints include vague references to tone abnormalities ("too stiff" or "too weak"), perceived structural abnormalities (most commonly the legs or feet), or an awkward/clumsy gait in the ambulating child.

   A. **Epidemiology.**
   - The prevalence of significant motor delays in the general pediatric population is not established. By statistical definition, 2%–3% of infants will fall outside the range of normal motor milestone attainment. A minority of these milestone-delayed children (15%–20%) will prove to have a significant neuromotor diagnosis, most commonly cerebral palsy or a birth defect, rarely some progressive nervous system or muscle disease.
   - Early motor delays in the remainder of children often represent a marker for subtle neurologic dysfunction, which manifests itself more definitively in later childhood as troublesome awkwardness, attention deficit syndromes, and/or specific learning disabilities.

II. **Making the diagnosis.**
   A. **Evaluation.** The clinician should organize data gathered from the history, physical examination, and neurodevelopmental examination into three domains: motor developmental milestones, the classic neurologic examination, and markers of cerebral neuromotor maturation (primitive reflexes and postural reactions).

   1. **Motor milestones** are extracted from the developmental history, as well as from observations during the neurodevelopmental examination (Tables 54-1 and 54-2). Milestone assessment is best summarized as a single (or narrow) motor age for the child. The motor age can be converted to a motor quotient (MQ) giving a simple expression of deviation from the norm: MQ = motor age/chronologic age × 100.

Table 54-1 Gross Motor Development Timetable

Prone	
Head up	1 mo
Chest up	2 mo
Up on elbows	3 mo
Up on hands	4 mo
Rolling	
Front to back	3–5 mo
Back to front	4–5 mo
Sitting	
Sit with support ("tripod" sitting)	5 mo
Sit without support	7 mo
Get up to sit (unassisted)	8 mo
Walking	
Pull to stand	8–9 mo
Cruise	9–10 mo
Walk with 2 hands held	10 mo
Walk with 1 hand held	11 mo
Walk alone	12 mo
Run (stiff-legged)	15 mo
Walk up stairs (with rail)	21 mo
Jump in place	24 mo
Pedal tricycle	30 mo
Walk down stairs, alternating feet	3 yr

Table 54-2 Fine Motor Development Timetable

Retain ring (rattle)	1 mo
Hands unfisted	3 mo
Reach	3–4 mo
Hands to midline	3–4 mo
Transfer	5 mo
Take 1-in. cube	5–6 mo
Take pellet (crude grasp)	6–7 mo
Immature pincer	7–8 mo
Mature pincer	10 mo
Release	12 mo

A motor quotient above 70 is considered within normal limits. Those falling in the 50–70 range are suspicious and deserve further evaluation (although most of these children will turn out to be normal). An MQ below 50 is unequivocally abnormal and warrants subspecialty referral.

2. **Neurologic examination.** Motor milestones are purely measures of function and do not take into account the *quality* of a child's movement. The motor portion of the **neurologic examination** includes assessments of tone (passive resistance), strength (active resistance), deep tendon reflexes, and coordination plus observations of station and gait. The best clues often come from observation, not handling.

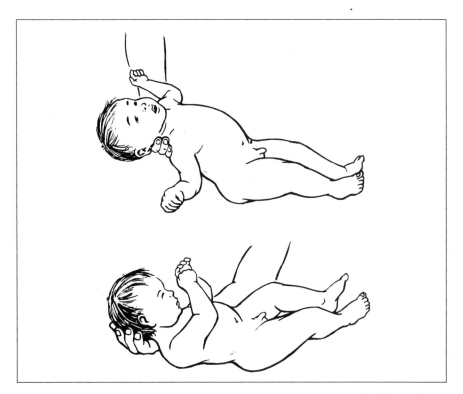

Figure 54-1. Tonic labyrinthine reflex. In the supine position, the baby's head is gently extended to about 45 degrees below horizontal. This produces relative shoulder retraction and leg extension, resulting in the "surrender posture." With head flexion to about +45 degrees, the arms come forward (shoulder protraction) and the legs flex. (From Blasco PA. Normal and abnormal motor development. *Pediatr Rounds* 1(2):1–6, 1992.)

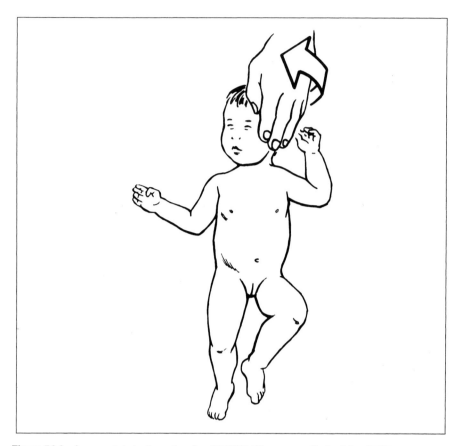

Figure 54-2. Asymmetric tonic neck reflex (ATNR). The sensory limb of the ATNR involves proprio-ceptors in the cervical vertebrae. With active or passive head rotation, the baby extends the arm and leg on the face side and flexes the extremities on the occiput side (the "fencer posture"). There is also some mild paraspinous muscle contraction on the occiput side producing subtle trunk curvature. (From Blasco PA. Normal and abnormal motor development. *Pediatr Rounds* 1(2):1–6, 1992.)

    a. Tone. Spontaneous postures (e.g., frog legs seen with hypotonia or scissoring with spasticity) provide visual clues to tone abnormalities.
    b. Strength. Spontaneous or prompted motor activities (e.g., weight bearing in sitting or standing) require adequate strength. A classic example is the Gower's sign (arising from floor sitting to standing using the hands to "walk up" one's legs), which indicates pelvic girdle and quadriceps muscular weakness.
    c. Station refers to the posture assumed in sitting or standing and should be viewed from anterior, lateral, and posterior perspectives, looking for body alignment.
    d. Gait refers to walking and is examined in progress. Initially, the toddler walks on a wide base, slightly crouched, with the arms abducted and elevated a bit. Forward progression is more staccato than smooth. Movements gradually become more fluid, the base narrows, and arm swing evolves, leading to an adult pattern of walking by age 3 years.
  3. Primitive reflexes are movement patterns that develop during the last trimester of gestation and generally disappear 3–6 months after birth. Each requires a specific sensory stimulus to generate the stereotyped motor response.
    The Moro, tonic labyrinthine, asymmetric tonic neck, and positive support reactions are the most clinically useful (Figs. 54-1, 54-2, and 54-3). Normal babies and infants demonstrate these postures inconsistently and transiently, whereas those with neurologic dysfunction show stronger and more sustained primitive reflex pos-

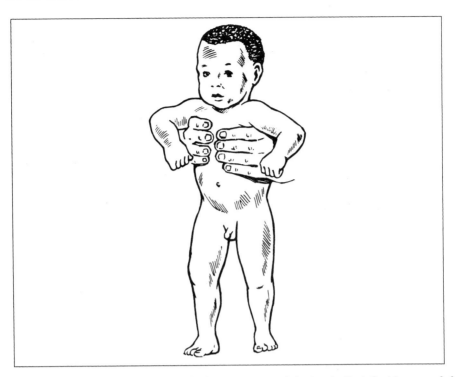

Figure 54-3. Positive support reflex. With support around the trunk, the infant is suspended and then lowered to pat the feet gently on a flat surface. This stimulus produces reflex extension at the hips, knees, and ankles so the subject stands up, completely or partially bearing weight. Children may go up on their toes initially but should come down onto flat feet within 20–30 seconds before sagging back down toward a sitting position. (From Blasco PA. Normal and abnormal motor development. *Pediatr Rounds* 1(2):1–6, 1992.)

turing. Although primitive reflexes are somewhat tricky to gauge, even in expert hands, the clinician should keep attuned to four factors:

    a. Some form of primitive reflex response should be clearly elicitable in the newborn through ages 2–3 months.

    b. Symmetry of response is important, especially with the Moro.

    c. An obligatory primitive reflex is abnormal at any time. This is the situation where the child remains "stuck" in the primitive reflex posture as long as the stimulus is imposed and breaks free only when the stimulus is removed.

    d. Visible primitive reflexes **should no longer be present after ages 6–8** months.

  4. Postural reactions consist of countermovements, which are much less stereotyped than the primitive reflexes and involve a complex interplay of cerebral and cerebellar cortical adjustments to a barrage of proprioceptive, visual, and vestibular sensory inputs. They are not present at birth but sequentially develop between ages 2–10 months. Postural reactions are sought in each of the three major categories: righting, protection, and equilibrium (Fig. 54-4). Although easy to elicit in the normal infant, they are markedly slower in their appearance in the baby with nervous system damage.

B. Classification of motor impairments.

  1. Static central nervous system disorders indicate some type of non-progressive brain damage. The insult may have arisen during early fetal development, resulting in a CNS anomaly. Alternatively, a brain developing in a normal fashion can be damaged before, during, or after birth by a wide variety of infectious, traumatic, and other insults. When a motor impairment is due to a brain anomaly or to a static lesion that occurs before cerebral maturation is complete (roughly age 16 years), the disorder is

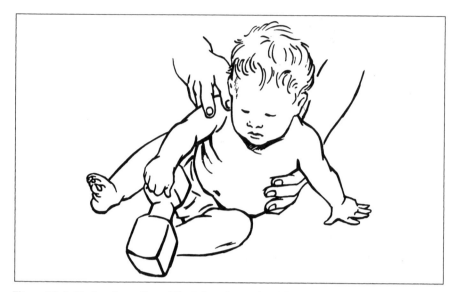

Figure 54-4. Postural reactions. The infant is comfortably seated, supported about the waist if necessary. The examiner gently tilts the child to one side noting righting of the head back toward the midline (coming in at 2–3 months), protective extension of the arm toward the side (coming in at 6–7 months), and equilibrium countermovements of the arm and leg on the opposite side (appearing at 5–6 months). (From Blasco PA. Normal and abnormal motor development. *Pediatr Rounds* 1(2):1–6, 1992.)

referred to as *cerebral palsy*. This group represents the largest number of children with disabling motor problems.

2. **Progressive diseases** of the brain, spinal cord, the peripheral nerves, or the muscles produce motor impairment that worsens with time (e.g., Duchenne muscular dystrophy, Werdnig-Hoffman spinal muscular atrophy, nervous system tumors). Children with progressive conditions initially experience a period of normal or near-normal development. Evidence of a progressive disease is determined by careful history and/ or by repeated examinations over time. The fraction of all motor-impaired children with progressive diseases is small. Uncovering the specific diagnosis helps one anticipate the rate of progression, provides other prognostic information, and forms the basis for accurate genetic counseling.

3. **Spinal cord and peripheral nerve disorders** are all static conditions except for the rare instances of an intrinsic spinal cord tumor or a progressive extrinsic compression syndrome. The largest single group in this category consists of children with myelodysplasia.

4. **Structural defects** refer to conditions in which an anatomical structure is missing or deformed (e.g., a limb deficiency) or in which the support tissues for nerves and muscles are inadequate (e.g., connective tissue defects, abnormal bones). On the mildest end of the spectrum, there exist a wide variety of fairly common orthopedic deformities, which may or may not affect early motor milestones (club feet, developmental hip dysplasia, etc.). More severe disorders in this category include osteogenesis imperfecta and some varieties of childhood arthritis.

III. **Management.** Direct treatment for the child with a motor disability falls into five categories: (1) counseling and support for the child and family, (2) hands-on therapy, (3) assistive devices, (4) medication, and (5) surgery. A subspecialty team should be consulted to provide state-of-the-art evaluation, treatment services, and counseling in all needed disciplines. Professionals skilled in different disciplines need to work together and *in concert with the parents*. The primary clinician's roles include seeing to the patient's general health, monitoring overall development, helping the child and family cope with many stresses (especially at anniversary and transition times), promoting the child's self-esteem and long-term adaptation to disability, and helping parents keep the multitude of subspecialty inputs in perspective.

BIBLIOGRAPHY

For Parents

Hanson MJ, Harris SR. *Teaching the Young Child with Motor Delays.* Austin TX: Pro-Ed, 1986.

For Professionals

Publications

Baird HW, Gordon EC. *Neurological Evaluation of Infants and Children.* London: Heinemann Medical Books, 1983.

Blasco PA. Normal and abnormal motor development. *Pediatr Rounds* 1(2):1–6, 1992.

Shapiro BK. The pediatric neurodevelopmental assessment of infants and young children. In AJ Capute, PJ Accardo (eds), *Neurodevelopmental Assessment of Infants and Young Children.* Baltimore: Brookes, 1:311–322, 1996.

Websites

Pathways Awareness Foundation www.pathwaysawareness.org

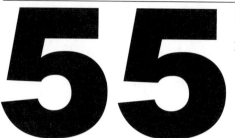

Neglect

Howard Dubowitz

I. **Description of the problem.** Child neglect is usually defined as **parental omissions in care, resulting in actual or potential harm to a child**. Child Protective Services (CPS) typically requires evidence of harm, unless the risks are serious (such as when very young children are left home alone). Some states exclude situations attributed to poverty.

An alternative and broader view of neglect is from a child's perspective, defining neglect as **occurring when a child's basic needs are not adequately met**. Basic needs include adequate health care, food, clothing, shelter, supervision/protection, emotional support, education, and nurturance. However, it is often difficult to establish at what point any of these needs are "adequately" met and thresholds may be rather arbitrary. Usually, the "neglect" label is applied to clearly worrisome circumstances. Less serious circumstances may still require intervention, perhaps without labeling them as "neglect".

There are several advantages to this child-focused definition. It fits with the broad goal of ensuring children's health and safety. It is less blaming and more constructive. It draws attention to other contributors to the problem (discussed later) aside from parents, and encourages a broader range of interventions. Clearly, many neglect situations may require intervention (e.g., a child with failure to thrive due to an inadequate diet), but may not warrant or meet criteria for CPS involvement. Practitioners, however, need to be aware of the laws and regulations in their area and factor these into their practice.

A. **Epidemiology.** Neglect is the most common form of child maltreatment, accounting for over half of all cases reported annually to CPS. It is a factor in approximately half the estimated 1,200 deaths each year due to child maltreatment. Due to ambiguity in diagnostic criteria and underreporting, accurate prevalence data are impossible to determine. One study in 1993 identified 30 cases of neglect per 1,000 children in the population, but it is likely that these are very conservative estimates, as neglect is a problem that frequently occurs "behind closed doors".

B. **Manifestations of possible neglect.** Aside from direct observation, the possibility of "neglect" should be considered in the following circumstances.
   - Noncompliance (nonadherence) with healthcare recommendations
   - Delay or failure in obtaining medical, mental health or dental care
   - Hunger, failure to thrive, and unmanaged morbid obesity
   - Drug exposed newborns and older children
   - Exposure to hazards in the home: ingestions, recurrent injuries, exposure of children with pulmonary disease to second hand smoke, access to guns, exposure to intimate partner violence
   - Exposure to hazards outside the home, failure to use car seat/belt, not wearing bike helmet
   - Emotional concerns (e.g., excessive quietness or apathy in a toddler), behavior issues (e.g., repetitive movements) and learning problems (especially if not being addressed), extreme risk-taking behavior (*may* reflect inadequate nurturance, affection, or supervision)
   - Inadequate hygiene, contributing to medical problems
   - Inadequate clothing, contributing to medical problems
   - Educational needs not being met
   - Abandoned children
   - Homelessness

C. **Etiology.** There are often multiple *and* interacting contributors to child neglect, including:
   - *Child*: disability, chronic illness, prematurity, difficult behaviors or temperament
   - *Parent:* depression, substance abuse, low IQ, limited nurturing as a child
   - *Family:* intimate partner violence, father uninvolved, many children in the family
   - *Community:* social isolation, violence, lack of treatment or support programs
   - *Society:* poverty, lack of health insurance

D. Assessment.
   1. The first questions to address are: *Is this neglect?* Does it seem likely that a child's basic needs have not been met? Also, has this resulted in harm, or, the risk of significant harm? If neglect is a concern, it is important to ascertain the duration of neglect, the frequency of incidents, the severity (based on actual and potential harm), and the possible co-occurrence of other forms of maltreatment, including abuse.

   Often one is confronted with the concern about *potential harm*. For example, epidemiological data may be factored into the equation (e.g., the risk of head injury if a bike helmet is not worn) or the child's specific risks (e.g., knowing that a child with severe asthma is likely to be readmitted if the treatment regimen is not followed). Consideration of potential harm needs to weigh both the likelihood of harm and the seriousness of the possible outcomes.

   2. The second key issue involves the assessment of **safety—Is it reasonably safe to send this child home?** Child health professionals often defer to CPS when this concern arises. However, primary care providers are best positioned to judge this when there are concerns about medical care. In general, out of home placement is considered when there appears to be a risk of "imminent harm" with states often requiring that it be "life-threatening." In addition to the nature of the neglect, two other issues are germane to assessing safety:
      a. **The vulnerability of the child,** based on age, developmental, socio-emotional, and health status.
      b. **The "controllability" of the situation.** This is assessed by consideration of the parent's willingness and ability to cooperate, their mental health, experience with prior interventions, and the availability of services. For example, it is difficult to control a situation where the mother has a substance abuse problem, prior drug treatment has not been successful, and there are no available treatment slots.

   3. The third assessment issue is to probe the **underlying situation**, the contributors, and the protective factors, such as a parent's wish for the child to be healthy, which may offer a "hook" for effective management. Understanding this context of neglect is key to tailoring the intervention to the specific needs of the child and family. For example, if the child is not receiving the medical treatment prescribed, one needs to know what is contributing to the problem. There may be health professional–patient factors (e.g., unclear communication), issues pertaining to the disease (e.g., complacency when the patient feels well), and reasons pertaining to the treatment plan (e.g., cost of medications).

II. Management. Addressing potential issues of neglect with families is often complex and difficult:
   - **Convey concerns** to the family, kindly but forthrightly. It is important to apprise them of the child's needs, your concern, without being confrontational or judgemental.
   - **Express your interest in helping,** or suggest another pediatric clinician. Establishing good rapport is a critical ingredient of effective interventions.
   - **Ensure continuity of care** as primary healthcare provider.
   - **Address contributory factors** based on a good understanding of what's underpinning the problem. Prioritize those most important and amenable to being remedied (e.g., recommending treatment for mother's depression). "Multiproblem" situations can be overwhelming, but tackling even one key element can tip the balance, helping ensure a child's needs are more adequately met.
   - **Begin with the least intrusive approach** (usually not CPS). This hinges on the severity of the specific situation, safety concerns, as well as state law and regulations.
   - **Establish specific objectives** (e.g., family will always use a car seat), with **measurable outcomes** (e.g., family reports routine use of car seat at next visit).
   - **Engage the family** in developing the plan, solicit their input and agreement. This process helps ensure the plan is reality-based, and accepted.
   - **Build on protective factors and family strengths;** there are always some (e.g, a parent's wish to see their child do well).
   - **Encourage informal supports** (i.e., family, friends). Most people receive most of their support from these sources, rather than from professionals.
   - **Consider support through a religious affiliation**. This can be particularly helpful for families who are socially isolated, a factor in neglect. In addition, parents who are averse to professional mental health care may accept pastoral counseling.
   - Consider the need for **concrete services** (e.g., Medical Assistance, Temporary Assistance to Needy Families [TANF], WIC). These are often major problems in families where neglect is a concern.

- Be knowledgeable about **community resources**, and facilitate referrals.
- **Consider the need to involve** *CPS*, particularly when there is serious harm or risk, or when less intrusive interventions have failed.
- **Recognize that neglect often requires long term intervention**, support, follow-up. Many of these families require more frequent visits than those in the AAP or Early Pediatric Screening, Diagnostic and Treatment (EPSDT) periodicity schedules.
- Provide **support, follow-up, review of progress, and adjust plan** if needed.

BIBLIOGRAPHY

DePanfilis D. How do I determine if a child is neglected? In: Dubowitz H, DePanfilis D, eds. *Handbook for Child Protection Practice.* Thousand Oaks, CA: Sage Publications, 2000; Ch. 25,

Dubowitz H, Giardino A, Gustavson E. Child neglect: A concern for pediatricians. *Pediatrics in Review* 21(4):111–116, 2000.

Dubowitz H, Black M. Medical neglect. In: Berliner L, Myers J, Reid T, Jenny C, eds. *The APSAC Handbook on Child Maltreatment.* Newbury Park, CA: Sage Publications, 2002.

56

Nightmares and Night Terrors

Barry Zuckerman

I. **Description of the problem.**

   A. **Night terrors.** Children with night terrors bolt upright from their sleep and cry inconsolably for 5–20 minutes (in rare cases, even longer). They usually occur 15–60 minutes after going asleep. Night terrors are associated with autonomic signs including a rapid pulse, increased respiratory rate, and sweating. The child has a glassy-eyed stare, which is due to the fact that the child is in rapid-eye-movement (REM) sleep and not actually awake. Following resolution, children easily return to sleep and have amnesia for the event in the morning.

   1. **Pathophysiology.** Night terrors are a *disorder of arousal,* occurring during an abrupt (rather than the usual slow) transition from stage 4 non-REM sleep to REM sleep.

   2. **Epidemiology.** Occurs in approximately 3% of children.

   B. **Nightmares.** Nightmares are upsetting dreams that occur during REM sleep. Nightmares and night terrors are compared in Table 56-1. Nightmares are a universal occurrence in childhood and usually not due to a significant problem.

II. **Management.**

   A. **Night terrors.** Because of the inconsolable crying and glassy-eyed stare, parents are usually terrified that something is wrong with their child. After the child returns to sleep, the parents may remain awake with their own terrors.

   1. The primary goal in management is to **reassure the parents** of the benign nature of these episodes. Management involves demystifying night terrors by explaining the physiologic basis of the behavior. Using an analogy like a myoclonic jerk during light sleep can help parents understand the physical nature of the night terrors. Most important, parents need to be assured that night terrors are not due to psychopathology or horrible life events. When parents know that there is nothing wrong with their child, they can usually tolerate periodic episodes.

   2. When the episodes are frequent and/or disrupt the sleep of others (especially siblings), **the child can be awakened prior to the time the episode usually occurs.** This is thought to alter the sleep cycling and prevent a night terror from occurring.

   3. **Diazepam,** which should be used only rarely, will stop the attacks by suppressing REM sleep and provide the beleaguered family with temporary relief.

   B. **Nightmares.** While night terrors are more frightening for parents to witness, nightmares are more distressing for the child. Although children may know that the nightmare is a dream, they remain frightened nevertheless.

   1. Parents need to **accept the child's fear** and not dismiss it as "just a bad dream."

   2. Parents should **comfort and stay with the child** until the child's distress has abated.

   3. Parents should **empathize with the child's fright** and tell him or her that while they cannot personally banish scary dreams, they will always come whenever the child is afraid.

   4. **While dreams have magical properties, so do parents.** They should assure the child that nothing will harm him or her. They can use magic of their own, like sprinkling anti-monster dust around the room.

   5. **Transitional objects** (e.g., teddy bear, favorite blanket) should be at the ready; a nightlight may be comforting. Ask the child what (besides a parent) is comforting after a nightmare.

   6. In selected instances **parents may have to remain with the child** or even take the child to their own bed.

   7. Parents should **discuss the nightmares and explain what nightmares are with the child** in the comforting light of day.

   8. Parents may consider reading a book in which the subject of the dream is resolved, with the child during the day to help increase their cognitive understanding of the fears.

251

Table 56-1 Comparisons of nightmares and night terrors

	Night terrors	Nightmares
Stage of sleep	Non-REM	REM
Consolability	Poor	Good
Amnesia for event	Yes	No
Interest in returning to sleep	High	Low

REM, rapid-eye-movement.

BIBLIOGRAPHY

For Parents

Books

AAP Editors. *Guide to Your Child's Sleep.* Chicago: AAP Press, 2000.
Leuck L, Buelner M. *My Monster Mama Loves Me So.* Harper Collins, 1999.

Websites

Yahoo!Health http://health.yahoo.com/health/centers/sleep_disorders/136

For Professionals

Schmitt BD. Dealing with night terrors and sleepwalking. *Contemp Pediatr* 6:119–120, 1989.

57

Obesity

Lawrence Hammer

I. **Description of the problem.** Commonly accepted definitions of obesity in childhood are based on the presence of excess body fat in relation to total body weight or lean body mass. Diagnostic criteria are described later in Making the Diagnosis. The clinical assessment of obesity must include consideration of the impact of the child's weight on his general well-being, relationships with peers, and family function.

   A. **Epidemiology.**
   - 15% of children and adolescents 6–17 years of age were considered overweight, based on 1999–2000 data from the National Center for Health Statistics.
   - In childhood, obesity is more common among upper socioeconomic groups. This trend remains true in adult life, except among upper income Caucasian women, who tend to be thinner than lower income women.

   B. **Familial transmission/genetics.** Obesity clearly "runs in" families, but familial transmission usually involves both genetic and environmental influences. Adoption and twin studies point to a strong genetic component. Roughly 80% of children in families with two obese parents will become obese, while only 40% of children in families with one obese parent are likely to become obese.

   C. **Etiology/contributing factors.**
   1. **Environmental.** Numerous studies have reported minimal differences in food intake and physical activity between obese and nonobese children. However, small differences in daily food intake or physical activity, when extended over long periods of time, may account for the excessive weight gain of some children. In clinical practice, the diet history of obese children almost always reveals either regular or periodic intake of excessive calories and high fat foods. The intake may be excessive in portion size or due to high calorie food selection.
   2. **Organic.** Obese children do not have lower basal metabolic rates than their nonobese peers. However, studies of metabolic rate and energy expenditure following exercise or meals do reveal a lower rate in obese versus nonobese adults. A number of medical conditions may contribute to obesity, especially those causing restrictions in physical activity. Finally, there are children with abnormalities of appetite or satiety, due to CNS lesions, who may be predisposed to the development of obesity.
   3. **Developmental.** There is a developmental pattern to the deposition of body fat through childhood and adolescence. Critical periods in the development of body fat occur prenatally, during the adiposity rebound, and during early puberty.
      - During the first year of life, children tend to accumulate "baby fat," followed by a relative reduction in body fatness over the next several years as the child gains proportionally greater height than weight.
      - Most children again begin to accumulate body fat at ages 5–6 years. This rebound in adiposity continues at a steady rate until puberty, after which there is a slower trend toward increasing fat deposition. Investigators have noted that children whose rebound in adiposity occurs earlier than age $5\frac{1}{2}$ years tend to have a higher likelihood of obesity during adolescence.

II. **Making the diagnosis.**
   A. **Signs and symptoms.** The easiest clinical approach to making the diagnosis of childhood obesity is direct observation and examination. The child who appears to be obese probably is obese. In order to confirm the diagnosis, an assessment of the child's fatness must be performed.
   - Weight alone is not a sufficient criterion for obesity in childhood, as weight varies with age and height.
   - The child's body mass index (BMI) should be calculated and a BMI growth curve used to find the child's percentile BMI for age and sex (BMI = Weight (kg) / height (m)^2).
   - BMI can be plotted on a percentile curve (Fig. 57-1). A BMI of 95th percentile or above

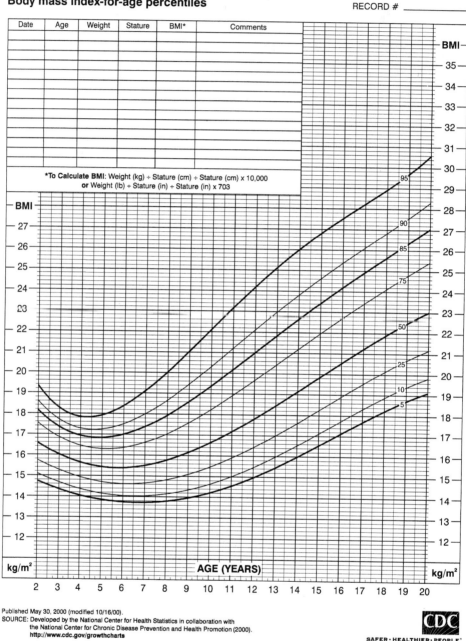

2 to 20 years: Boys
Body mass index-for-age percentiles

NAME _____

RECORD # _____

*To Calculate BMI: Weight (kg) ÷ Stature (cm) ÷ Stature (cm) x 10,000
or Weight (lb) ÷ Stature (in) ÷ Stature (in) x 703

Published May 30, 2000 (modified 10/16/00).
SOURCE: Developed by the National Center for Health Statistics in collaboration with
the National Center for Chronic Disease Prevention and Health Promotion (2000).
http://www.cdc.gov/growthcharts

Figure 57-1. CDC Growth Charts: United States. (A) Body Mass Index for age percentiles: Boys 2, 2 to 20 years. (B) Body Mass Index for age percentiles: Girls 2, 2 to 20 years. Developed by the National Center for Health Statistics in collaboration with the National Center for Chronic Disease Prevention and Health Promotion (2000). Available for download from the CDC at http://www.cdc.gov/growthcharts/.

2 to 20 years: Girls
Body mass index-for-age percentiles

NAME _____

RECORD # _____

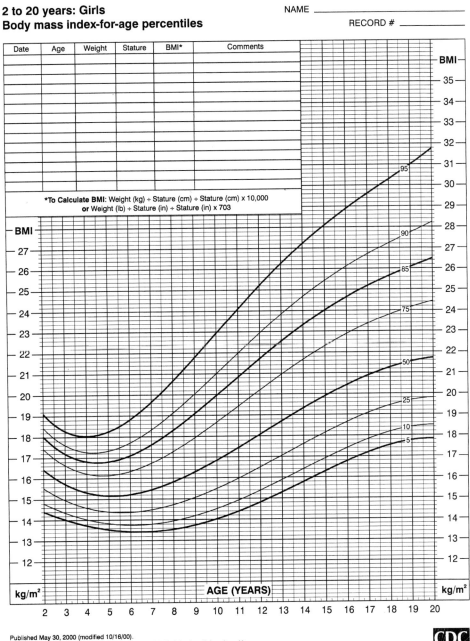

*To Calculate BMI: Weight (kg) ÷ Stature (cm) ÷ Stature (cm) x 10,000
or Weight (lb) ÷ Stature (in) ÷ Stature (in) x 703

Published May 30, 2000 (modified 10/16/00).
SOURCE: Developed by the National Center for Health Statistics in collaboration with
the National Center for Chronic Disease Prevention and Health Promotion (2000).
http://www.cdc.gov/growthcharts

Figure 57-1. Continued.

is considered to be indicative of **overweight** in the assessment of children, while BMI values between the 85th and 95th percentile indicative of "at risk of overweight."
- Serial measurements of BMI are useful in monitoring a child over time. Among adults, BMI values of 30 and above are indicative of **obesity** and values between 25 and 30 are considered **overweight**.
- One of the problems with using weight and height as diagnostic criteria for obesity is their inability to distinguish between two children who have the same weight and height but are different in fatness or muscle mass.
- A skinfold thickness measurement may add additional valuable information to the diagnostic assessment of the child, although measurement of subcutaneous fat is not directly proportional to total body fat.

B. Differential diagnosis. Only about 5% of obese children have an underlying endocrinopathy or genetic syndrome. The endocrinopathies that are associated with child obesity include hypothyroidism, Cushing syndrome, pseudohypoparathyroidism, and growth hormone deficiency. Syndromes associated with child obesity include Prader-Willi, Alström, Carpenter, Cohen, and Laurence-Moon-Bardet-Biedl.
- Children with endocrinologic disorders or clinical syndromes manifest clinical histories and physical findings that distinguish them from children with idiopathic obesity. One key difference in such children is the presence of shorter-than-expected stature for the child's age and weight. In fact, a careful history and physical examination can successfully rule out these underlying disorders in the vast majority of children. Laboratory examination is rarely necessary except to confirm a clinically suspected diagnosis or to pursue further evaluation of associated conditions, such as type 2 diabetes mellitus or polycystic ovary syndrome.

C. History: Key clinical questions.

1. *"What was the child's weight at birth and at subsequent points during childhood?"* The clinician should plot the child's weights on a growth chart from birth to the present time. It is important to identify the child who has had an unusual pattern of weight gain, a sudden increase in weight, or a pattern that suggests an increase in the risk of long-term obesity, such as an early adiposity rebound.

2. *"Are there any factors that may have influenced your child's weight gain at particular periods in his life?"* The parents should contribute their thoughts regarding the child's excessive weight gain.

3. *"Does your child's pattern of weight gain appear similar to that of others in the immediate or extended family?"* The parents should describe other members of the family with weight problems and describe their own patterns of weight gain.

4. *"What is it about your child's weight that concerns you?"* This question provides an opportunity for parents to describe their concerns and motivation for seeking evaluation or treatment.

5. *"How does your child's weight influence him directly or indirectly?"* Does the child's weight seem to get in the way of physical activity, participation in school activities, performance in sports, interaction with peers, and other elements of social development and maturation?

6. *"How does your child's weight influence the family?"* Parents and child should discuss ways in which concern for the child's weight may influence family activities, such as vacations, outings, or physical activity, and describe the impact of the child's weight on their relationships with each other. For example, many parents shield their children from the impact of obesity by avoiding situations in which the child's obesity is more public. Parents may describe their conflicts over the importance of the child's weight problem, its severity, and their differing approaches to it.

7. *"What might happen if your child's obesity becomes a life-long problem?"* This question encourages parents to express their deepest fears about the impact of the child's obesity on his life and to discuss ways in which their own experiences with weight may have influenced their decision to seek help with this problem. Many parents seek to protect their children from the misery they themselves have experienced in relation to their weight.

8. *"I would like to learn a little bit about your child's regular eating habits. Please try to recall each of the meals and snacks that your child has eaten over the last 24 hours and give me as much detail as possible about them. Please let me know if you would call this a typical eating day for your child or if there are any differences that I should be aware of. Are there any times when your child appears to 'lose control,' leading to a binge eating or overeating?"* These questions introduce the notion that dietary intake is relevant and fulfills the parents' expectation that modification of dietary intake may be part of the approach to the problem. It is helpful to point

out that although the child may not appear to have excessive dietary intake, there may still be an opportunity for dietary modification as part of the overall approach to the problem.

9. *"Do you consider your child to be physically active on a regular basis? Please describe some of the vigorous physical activities that your child participates in. How often and for what period of time does your child participate in these activities? Is your child part of an organized sports program? Do you and your child ever exercise together? Please describe your own physical activity."* This question opens up discussion of the child's physical activity and gives the clinician insight into the parents' perception of their own physical activity and level of exercise. Opportunities for ways to increase regular physical activity may be discovered during the discussion.

10. *"Does your child have any difficulties with sleep?"* Children with severe obesity may have secondary sleep problems, such as daytime somnolence and obstructive sleep apnea. These children should be evaluated by a sleep disorder specialist for central hypoventilation and obstructive sleep apnea.

D. **Behavioral observations.** During the process of evaluating the obese child and his family, it is useful to observe the interaction of family members and observe their expression of concern, criticism, or support of the child in dealing with this problem. It is also important to note parents' responses to the child's requests for food during the visit. Although overeating may not be the primary factor contributing to the child's obesity, interactions with food are often salient to the evaluation and treatment process.

E. **Physical examination.** A careful general physical examination is useful in the evaluation of the obese child. Such an examination yields identification of physical findings that may suggest an underlying endocrine syndrome or genetic disorder. The physical examination should include an overall assessment of the child's body habitus and notation of the pattern of fat distribution.
- Careful measurement of the height and weight of the child is important to rule out underlying short stature, which may indicate an associated endocrine or genetic abnormality.
- The presence of a buffalo hump, moon facies, short stature, and hypertension may suggest Cushing syndrome (although many normal obese children have extra fat deposition over the upper back).
- Hypogonadism is present in a number of syndromes (Prader-Willi, Laurence-Moon-Bardet-Biedl, and Carpenter).
- Short stature, short metacarpals and metatarsals, subcutaneous calcifications, and retardation are present in pseudohypoparathyroidism.
- Presence of acanthosis nigricans should be noted, particularly in relation to the presence of menstrual irregularity and hyperandrogenism in adolescent girls with the polycystic ovary syndrome and in boys or girls with features of type 2 diabetes mellitus.

F. **Tests.** Laboratory tests should be used to confirm suspected underlying diagnoses rather than as routine screening. Obese children who are tall, of normal intelligence, and without stigmata of underlying syndromes do not require routine thyroid screening, for example.

III. **Management.**

A. **Primary goals.** It is reasonable to establish a target weight for the child. This does not imply that the child must lose weight. Rather, taking into account appropriate rates of growth, the child's weight should fall into a healthy range for height and age, defined as below the 85th percentile for BMI. The process of establishing a goal weight or BMI goal for the child should be revised periodically, depending on the child's age and the family's ability to participate in the treatment program.
- For many children, particularly those who are prepubertal, weight loss may be a less desirable goal than maintenance of weight at a particular level or reduction in the rate of weight gain. For children who are beyond puberty, it may be more appropriate to establish goals for weight loss. A reasonable rate of weight loss for children under age 12 years is 0.5–1 lb/week. Adolescents may safely lose 1–2 lb/week while still maintaining adequate nutritional status.
- In addition to weight loss, it is important to emphasize associated goals of improved fitness, self-esteem, social interaction, and family harmony.

B. **Information for the family.** The family's involvement is critical to the evaluation and management of childhood obesity. A focus on the impact of the child's obesity on the family and on the child can lead to effective intervention. For example, rather than using the dietary history as a means of proving the presence of excessive dietary intake, the provider should use the dietary history as a means of identifying opportunities for dietary change. In discussing the child's regular physical activity, it should be possible to identify opportunities for increasing this activity.

- The clinician can approach intervention as a process of gradually modifying the child's eating behavior and physical activity over time, in the context of the whole family.
- It is critical that the family engages in this process in an active way and agrees to initiate and maintain change in the whole family's food and exercise habits. Attempts to modify the child's diet in isolation rarely succeed and lead to an environment of blame.

C. Treatment.

1. Initial strategies. Intervention for child obesity begins during the evaluation process. Involving the family in the evaluation gives the message that they are part of the solution. In the course of evaluation, if the family appears to be dysfunctional, it is appropriate to delay the implementation of behavioral strategies until the family has had more extensive evaluation and entered into family counseling. Referral to a family therapist, particularly one familiar with many of the issues associated with obesity, can be extremely helpful.

For families who are capable of supporting the child's efforts, the initial strategies are focused on gradual alterations of the child's eating and physical activity. There are a number of behavioral strategies that are useful in the office-based approach to child obesity (Table 57-1).

Intervention does not require calorie counting or specific calorie intake. An alterna-

Table 57-1 Behavioral Strategies for Weight Loss

Establish goals for behavior change	Establish goals for small changes in the diet and physical activity on a weekly basis to increase the likelihood of success.
Self-monitor diet and physical activity	Self-monitoring provides the child with a heightened awareness of his efforts and successes.
Record review and parental reinforcement	One-on-one review of the record with the child provides an opportunity for parents to provide positive feedback for demonstrable change.
Establish a behavioral contract and use a simple reward system	By setting realistic goals each week, the parent and child can contract for a limited reward system.
	Expensive rewards, or those that can be achieved only after a significant period of time, are less effective than rewards that can be delivered immediately or soon after the demonstrated behavior change.
	A dual-level reward system may be useful in providing initial reinforcement for short-term change and greater levels of reinforcement for long-term success. This reward system can later be extended to the maintenance period so that reinforcement is delivered periodically for maintenance of behavior change. Simply rewarding weight loss alone should be discouraged.
Praise	Parents can use praise very effectively to reinforce and maintain desired behavior change.
	Criticism and punishment are ineffective and counterproductive.
Environmental control	Identify and eliminate factors within the environment that tend to promote overeating. For example, remove high fat, high calorie foods from the household, increase the availability of cut-up vegetables rather than chips or pretzels for snack time, avoid television viewing during mealtimes, reduce the amount of time indoors during daylight hours, and increase the expectation for daily physical activity.
Cognitive restructuring	Identify and reject thoughts that may be demeaning, degrading, or pessimistic. Emphasis should be placed on successes, not failures.

tive approach is to categorize foods as more or less desirable and to set goals for the reduction of less desirable foods and encouragement of more desirable foods.

- One such system of categorization is described in *The Stoplight Diet for Children,* which categorizes food as "red light," "yellow light," and "green light." By identifying foods in this way, parents can support the child's efforts to reduce intake of "red light" foods and increase intake of foods from the other categories. Gradual reduction in intake of "red light" foods can be rewarded and sustained in association with goals of weight loss or maintenance.
- The use of pharmacotherapy as an adjunct to behavioral treatment is being investigated in the adolescent population. At least one clinical trial involving adolescents has demonstrated the benefit of adding sibutramine, a neurotransmitter reuptake inhibitor, to standard behavioral treatment. Orlistat, a lipase inhibitor, received FDA approval in 2003 for use in the treatment of overweight adolescents 12 years of age and older.
- Although still considered quite controversial in the management of severe obesity in teenagers, bariatric surgery using a roux-en-Y procedure is being investigated in clinical trials in some pediatric centers for patients whose BMI exceeds 40 in the presence of obesity-associated comorbidity and in patients with BMI greater than 50. With FDA approval, the laporascopic band procedure may also become available for this population.

  2. **Follow-up.** The primary care provider should provide regular follow-up for the child who is involved in either an office-based or a group treatment program. This follow-up can include periodic monitoring of the child's weight and height, review of the child's self-monitoring records for diet and physical activity, and encouragement to persevere.

D. **Criteria for referral.** Most obese children and their parents who are interested in participating in a treatment program can benefit from the peer support available through a group treatment program. The primary care clinician should investigate the options that are available in the community and provide that information to the family. The family that is too dysfunctional to participate in an office-based or group-based program should be referred for family evaluation and therapy. The family may benefit from such additional professional involvement as it struggles to help the child overcome the effects of obesity.

IV. **Clinical pearls and pitfalls.**
- Obesity is a problem that develops over time and is not easily treated. Unless the patient is experiencing life-threatening complications due to severe obesity, the problem should be approached in a non-emergent fashion.
- Obesity rarely occurs in isolation. There are commonly other family members who have struggled with weight and whose experience can be valuable in helping to develop a realistic set of goals for the child and family.
- The tendency for families to feel defeated by obesity comes from their unrealistic expectation of dramatic and continued change. In order to avoid the trap of setting unrealistic goals and expectations, the family should be encouraged to identify situations in which their attempts at change have been successful. Once these small victories are identified, they can be used to help identify other opportunities for change and to create an environment of positive expectation.
- Obesity is not the child's problem alone. The child lives within the family environment, and the family must be drawn into the process of evaluation and change.

BIBLIOGRAPHY

For Parents

Books

Epstein LH, Squires S. *The Stoplight Diet for Children: An Eight-Week Program for Parents and Children.* Boston: Little, Brown, 1988.
Satter, Ellyn. *Secrets of Feeding a Healthy Family.* Kelcy Press, 1999.

Websites

The National Institutes of Health, National Institute of Diabetes and Digestive and Kidney Disease; part of the Weight-Control Information Network, especially targeted for parents. http://www.niddk.nih.gov/health/nutrit/pubs/parentips/tipsforparents.htm

For Professionals

Barlow SE, Dietz WH. Obesity evaluation and treatment: expert committee recommendations. *J Pediatr* 102(3):e29, 1998.
Rosenbaum, M, Leibel RL. Pathophysiology of childhood obesity. *Adv Pediatr* 35:73–138, 1988.
Rosner B, Prineas R. Loggie J, Daniels SR. Percentiles for body mass index in U.S. children 5 to 17 years of age. *J Pediatr* 132:211–222, 1998.
Committee on Nutrition, American Academy of Pediatrics. Prevention of pediatric overweight and obesity. *Pediatrics* 112:424–430, 2003.

Websites

American Academy of Pediatrics http://www.aap.org/obesity/
The AAP's official policy statement on obesity. http://www.aap.org/policy/s100029.html
Resources from the Centers for Disease Control http://www.cdc.gov/nccdphp/dnpa/obesity/index.htm, including links to a Body Mass Index Calculator http://www.cdc.gov/nccdphp/dnpa/bmi/index.htm, and to the CDC's growth charts, which can be downloaded from http://www.cdc.gov/growthcharts/

58

Physical Abuse

Christine E. Barron
Carole Jenny

I. **Description of the problem.** Child physical abuse is defined as **acts of commission involving physical violence that result in injuries**. These injuries may include fractures, bruises, burns, head trauma, and internal injuries. When making the diagnosis of child physical abuse, one needs to consider the age of the child, the plausibility of the history, alterations in the history, delays in seeking medical care, possible mechanisms of injury, potential eyewitnesses, and other possible causes within the differential diagnosis.

  A. **Epidemiology.** Despite almost certain underreporting, physical abuse accounts for approximately 23% of substantiated cases of child maltreatment in the United States. Although certain social and demographic factors have been identified as risk factors, children can be victims of physical abuse regardless of their age, gender, ethnic and socioeconomic backgrounds. In fact, cases without these identified risk factors are more likely to be misdiagnosed.

  B. **Etiology/contributing factors.** There are many identified risk factors for child physical abuse, including:

   1. **Unrealistic expectations.** Often the lack of understanding a child's developmental abilities and needs results in caregivers establishing unrealistic developmental and social expectations. These unrealistic expectations can lead to frustration and anger, which may result in abuse.

   2. **Social Isolation.** Lack of parenting skills often combine with inadequate parenting models and additional life stressors, and limited resources from family, friends, and community to increase the risk of abuse.

   3. **Domestic Violence.** Children who live in homes where domestic violence is present are more likely to be victims of physical abuse (up to 15 times the national average).

   4. **Substance Abuse.** The most frequently reported cause for neglect and abuse of children is parental substance abuse.

II. **Making the diagnosis.**

  A. **Signs and symptoms.** Child physical abuse has variable presentations and should be considered when:

   1. A child presents with unexplained injury or pattern injuries.

   2. A nonmobile child present with injuries.

   3. Illogical or changing explanations are offered by a parent to account for an injury.

   4. A child presents with multiple injuries with different stages of healing.

   5. There is a delay in seeking medical care.

  B. **Differential diagnosis.** The history and physical examination are beneficial in excluding the many competing diagnostic possibilities that can mimic child physical abuse.

   Table 58-1 identifies possible differential diagnosis, but is not an exhaustive list.

  C. **History: Interviewing guidelines.** Interviews should be conducted in a nonjudgmental manner, acknowledging that everyone's goal is to simply ensure the safety of the child. Open-ended questions should be asked to determine how an injury occurred. Specific notations should be made for changing histories or for blaming injuries on child themselves or siblings.

   1. **Interviewing the parents.**

     a. All caregivers should be interviewed separately.

     b. The interview should obtain information regarding:
       • The sequence of events that resulted in the injury
       • Identification of all caregivers during the time of injury
       • Any other potential witnesses to the injury, including verbal children
       • Information regarding past medical history, developmental history and social history should be obtained
       • Social history including questions that identify any potential risk factors such as domestic violence, substance abuse, and limited support system

     c. Record parents information, using exact quotes when possible.

Table 58-1 Possible Differential Diagnosis

Findings	Differential Diagnosis
Bruising	Accidental bruising in mobile children
	Blood diathesis—hemophilia, idiopathic thrombocytopenic purpura, von Willebrand disease, vitamin K deficiency, leukemia
	Dye or ink
	Birth mark—Mongolian spots, café au lait spots
	Phytophotodermatitis
	Ehlers-Danlos syndrome
	Infectious—meningococcemia, Henoch-Schonlein purpura,
	Folk medicine—cao gao
	Contact dermatitis
Burns	Accidental
	Car seat or seat belt burns
	Infectious—impetigo, epidermolysis bullosa, staphylococcal scalded skin syndrome
	Folk medicine—cupping, moxibustion
	Fixed drug reactions
	Phytophotodermatitis
Fractures	Birth trauma
	Congenital syphilis
	Accidental trauma
	Osteogenesis imperfecta
	Leukemia
	Infectious—osteomyelitis, septic arthritis
	Scurvy
	Rickets
	Menkes syndrome
Intracranial bleeding	Motor vehicle crash
	Aneurysm
	Epidural hemorrhage
	Glutaric aciduria Type 1

  2. Interviewing the child.
   a. Verbal children should be interviewed separately. It is important to **ask open-ended questions** and to completely avoid asking direct or leading questions such as "Your father hits you doesn't he?" Children should be interviewed at eye level, using age-appropriate language. If a child makes a disclosure, ask further questions such as "Can you tell me more about that?"
   b. Record child's disclosures **using exact quotes**.
   c. Further detailed interviews should be completed by trained professionals in response to a report of suspicious injuries to the child welfare agency.
 D. Physical examination.
  1. The examination should be completed in a child-friendly examination room with adequate lighting and with the goal of putting the child at ease.
  2. An entire examination should be completed, *not* simply focusing on areas of obvious injury.
  3. All children should be examined in a gown, with inspection of entire skin surface.
  4. Clear documentation of any injuries should be completed using photographs and drawings to describe location, size and pattern of injuries. Table 58-2 covers specific areas of detail to be noted.
 E. Tests. Radiological tests may be necessary.
  1. Occult skeletal injuries.
   a. Children under 2 years of age with possible physical abuse require a complete skeletal survey to identify any occult osseous trauma.
   b. Children with acute injuries should also complete a second skeletal survey 2 weeks later.
  2. CNS imaging for suspected head trauma.
   a. CT scan completed to identify acute CNS injuries; MRI to identify deep structure injuries and aid in determination of aging of intracranial injuries.

Table 58-2 Physical Examination

Examination	Findings
Growth parameters	Obtain and plot growth parameters
General	Altered level of consciousness
	Distress or discomfort
	Behavior during examination
HEENT (head, ears, eyes, nose, throat)	Traction alopecia
	Subgaleal hemorrhages
	Facial bruising
	Subconjunctival hemorrhages
	Retinal hemorrhages (ophthalmology consult may be necessary)
	Pinnae injuries
	Hemotympanium
	Nasal-septal injuries
	Frenulum injuries
	Dental injuries
	Dental impressions on mucosal surface of upper lip
Chest/back	Crepitus from rib fractures
	Bruises
Abdomen	Bruises (lack of bruising on the abdominal wall does not rule out abdominal trauma)
	Distension, tenderness (pediatric surgery consult may be necessary)
Genital	Bruising
	Bite marks
Extremities	Soft tissue swelling
	Tenderness to palpation
	Bruising
	Deformities
Skin	Location of injuries
	Recognizable patterns
	Bilateral injuries
	Circumferential injuries
	Multiple injuries in different stages of healing

    3. Imaging of intraabdominal injuries for suspected abdominal trauma
        a. Abdominal CT scan, upper GI, ultrasound.
  III. Management.
    A. Primary goals. The goal for the clinician in addressing possible child abuse is to make the diagnosis, provide needed treatment, report suspicious injuries to child welfare agencies, and ensure the safety of the patient and other children within the same environment.
    B. Initial strategies. Primary care clinicians are responsible by law for reporting suspicion for abuse to child welfare agencies. These cases require a multidisciplinary approach from medical personnel, child welfare authorities, and law enforcement officials.
  IV. Clinical pearls and pitfalls.
- Obtain all information in a nonjudgmental manner.
- All states have laws that require mandatory reporting of suspicious injuries.
- Nonmobile children with unexplained bruising should have a workup completed for possible child physical abuse.
- Rely on history and physical examination findings to narrow the differential diagnosis.
- Skeletal survey for children under 2 years of age should be completed at time of presentation and repeated in 2 weeks.

BIBLIOGRAPHY

For Parents

Parents Anonymous (check local telephone directory). Childhelp USA 1-800-4-A-CHILD www.childhelpuse.org

For Professionals

Kleinman PK. *Diagnostic Imaging of Child Abuse (2nd ed)*. St. Louis, MO: Mosby, 1998.

Ludwig S, Kornberg AE (eds). *Child Abuse: A Medical Reference*. New York: Churchill Livingstone, 1992.

Reece RM (ed.) *Child Abuse Medical Diagnosis and Management*. Baltimore: Williams and Wilkins, 1996.

Sugar NF, Taylor JA, Feldman K. Bruises in Infants and Toddlers: Those Who Don't Cruise Rarely Bruise. *Arch Pediatr & Adolesc Med* 153(4):399–403, 1999.

Organizations

American Professional Society on the Abuse of Children (APSAC) 332 South Michigan Ave, Suite 1600 Chicago, IL 60604 312-554-0166 http://www.apsac.org

I. **Description of the Problem.** Picky eating occurs on a continuum. Aside from the rare instances in which nutrition is negatively impacted, there is no clear cut-off for when it becomes problematic. Therefore, the best definition of picky eating incorporates parental concern: *an unwillingness to eat familiar foods or try new foods, severe enough to interfere with daily routines to an extent that is problematic to the parent, child, or parent–child relationship.*

A. **Epidemiology.**
   - Approximately one third of toddlers are described by their parents as "picky eaters." Additionally, nearly two thirds of parents report one or more problems in eating with their toddler (e.g., 54% are not always hungry at mealtime, 33% do not seem to enjoy mealtimes, 34% have strong food preferences, 26% frequently refuse to eat, 21% request specific foods and then refuse them, and 42% try to end a meal after a few bites).
   - Children who are picky eaters more often have negative temperamental traits and are more often behaviorally inhibited (shy) and anxious. Their parents may report more difficulties in the parent–child relationship.
   - The most commonly rejected foods are vegetables. Picky eaters have lower dietary variety, but no significant difference in overall nutrient intake.
   - It is unclear if picky eating varies by gender, culture, socioeconomic status, ethnicity, or a history of breastfeeding.
   - Pickiness seems to decline with age. If children are still described as picky after about age 9 years, they are likely to be picky for the rest of their lives.

B. **Evolutionary framework.** Picky eating seems to increase as children gain mobility. Some theorize that children are "wired" for pickiness to protect them from eating potentially poisonous substances in the environment; children who are inherently reluctant to eat an unfamiliar food or to eat a variety of foods will not "wander into the bush and eat a poison berry".

C. **Etiology.**
   - People reject foods because they: (1) dislike the sensory characteristics (flavor and appearance); (2) have a fear of negative consequences (e.g., it causes stomach upset upon eating); or (3) are disgusted by the food (due to contamination or the thought of where it came from, which does not begin until 7 years of age).
   - Pickiness often runs in families, but it is unclear if this is primarily due to "nature" or "nurture".

II. **Making the diagnosis.**

A. **History: Key clinical questions.**
   1. *"Tell me which foods he won't eat."* A pattern of refusal, such as only refusing milk products or certain textures, raises the question of food allergies/intolerances or oral hypersensitivity.
   2. *"Tell me what he ate yesterday, starting with breakfast."* A diet history can give a flavor of how picky the child is and open a discussion about what and how foods are presented to the child, and what is done when the child rejects them.
   3. *"What do you do when he rejects a food at dinner? What sort of rules do you have in your house around eating?"* Obtaining a history that the child is required to remain at the table until his plate is clean, or that the child is coerced to eat a particular food, is important. Neither of these methods has been shown to result in a long-term improvement in picky eating, and both likely simply add stress and negativity to the family mealtime.
   4. *"What worries you the most about your child's eating?"* Frequently parents are concerned the child will develop a growth or vitamin deficiency. Reassurance that the child is growing adequately (try showing the parent a growth chart) is often helpful, as is demystifying the behavior by describing how common it is and the theories as

to why it is present (see Evolutionary Framework). Explaining that a multivitamin with iron can replace vegetables in the diet often assuages a great deal of parental concern.

5. *"Is there anyone else in your family who is a picky eater?"* This question (to which the answer is nearly universally "yes") often opens the door to talking about the natural course of picky eating and may provide some insight into why the parent views the behavior as so problematic.

B. **Physical exam and laboratory testing.** Careful measurement of weight and height, with plotting on the appropriate growth chart, is important. If growth deficiency is present, a different approach should be taken, which includes an exhaustive history with directed laboratory testing. If the child's diet is particularly restricted in iron-rich foods, testing for iron deficiency anemia is warranted. Children should also be screened by history and physical for constipation. The picky eater's diet is often low in fiber and constipation can result in abdominal discomfort that only worsens the eating behavior.

Table 59-1 Strategies to Suggest to Parents to Reduce Picky Eating

Strategy	Comments
Functional analysis What are the properties of preferred foods the child likes?	If child likes food a particular temperature or texture, try expanding the repertoire of foods with similar foods first.
Discount parental medical/nutritional concerns	Explain to the parents that this is a common problem and that unless growth is adversely affected, the child will suffer no consequences from the pickiness. Giving the child a daily vitamin as "insurance" reinforces this view.
Mealtime atmosphere Calm, pleasant meals can improve willingness to try new foods. Food tastes better when it is eaten in a positive social context. Avoid mealtime power struggles!	Children who are prone to anxiety or overstimulation may benefit from a calm eating atmosphere.
Social cues Modeling eating a food by a parent is helpful, but peers are more powerful.	If child has the opportunity to eat meals with other children (such as in preschool), this may be an opportunity to expand the child's repertoire of foods.
Positive reinforcement Providing verbal praise for trying a new food may be helpful in sustaining the behavior and result in increased liking for the target food. Parents should not provide material or food rewards for eating, and children should never be punished for refusal to try a new food.	When children are given a material or food reward (dessert) for eating a food (a vegetable), they eventually learn to like the food they were rewarded for eating (the vegetable) less over time (not the desired goal).
Repeated exposure Increased familiarity results in increased liking. Foods typically must be introduced 10 times before they are accepted.	If the family wishes for the child to accept a vegetable, choose a generally mild, palatable vegetable to be served at dinner repeatedly.
Forced exposure The "try one bite" rule has been shown to result in an increased willingness to try other new foods over time.	If the child has a difficult temperament, however, and requiring the child to take a bite is disruptive to mealtime, this method should be abandoned.
Providing information For older children, providing information about a food's flavor will increase willingness to try the food.	If younger children don't grasp the meaning of "flavor words" (i.e., sweet, salty, sour), or have not yet developed a vocabulary of "food words," this method may not be effective.
Combining foods Combining a nonpreferred food (a meat) with a preferred food (ketchup) may be helpful—even in seemingly illogical combinations.	If a child wants to dip carrot sticks in soup, and this increases his willingness to eat the carrots, this should be accepted (in lieu of disallowing it because it is "bad manners").

C. Differential diagnosis.

- Lactose intolerance or food allergies can present with refusal of specific types of foods.
- Gastroesophageal reflux disease, as evidenced by frequent vomiting or pain after eating, can result in problematic eating behavior.
- Children can present with oral hypersensitivity, the etiology of which is not always clear. These children respond negatively to oral stimuli, and have particular difficulty with textured foods.
- Escalating negative affect in the mother and child, or an unusually strong focus on the issue may signal an interactional problem. Picky eating may be the presenting complaint of a larger problem with power struggles.
- Unrealistic parental expectations about the quantity and range of food that a child will eat may be present. Expecting the child to eat every food presented at the dinner table every evening (including spicy or bitter flavors) may be a goal that cannot be met by all children.
- Limitation of resources—the family may not have adequate financial resources to supply a range of palatable foods at each meal. Parents may be concerned that the child's picky eating, in combination with limited choice, is affecting the child's health.

III. **Management.** The mainstay of management is to explain to parents that picky eating is, in most cases, a behavior that worsens during the toddler and preschool years and then begins to improve through the early elementary years. In other cases, it can be seen as a quirky personality trait. Either way, there is rarely a medical indication for intervention. Behavioral interventions should be recommended only when parents are eager to put effort into modifying the behavior. Interventions must be benign and simple, and should never be continued if they result in increased stress or discord at mealtimes. Some strategies that could be suggested to parents that request them are listed in Table 59-1.

IV. **Clinical pearls and pitfalls.**

- Parents who are concerned about a child's picky eating may be articulating the eating as the problem, when it is really a discrete symptom of an overarching concern: a difficult temperament.
- Although picky eating occurs on a continuum and is a "normal" behavior, parental concerns should not be minimized. Helping the parent to understand the child's temperamental qualities, and how the picky eating is a symptom of them, will likely be most helpful in the long term in the parent–child relationship.

BIBLIOGRAPHY

For Parents

Dietz WH, Stern L, ed. *The American Academy of Pediatrics Guide to Your Child's Nutrition: Making Peace at the Table and Building Healthy Eating Habits for Life.* Elk Grove Village, IL: American Academy of Pediatrics, 1999.

Your Child: Development and Behavior Resources, University of Michigan Health System http://www.med.umich.edu/1libr/yourchild/

Ellyn Satter has published several books for parents and professionals about childhood eating and feeding behavior, and maintains a Website http://www.ellynsatter.com/

Satter EM. *Child of Mine: Feeding with Love and Good Sense,* Boulder, CO: Bull Publishing Co., 2000.

For Professionals

Birch L, Fisher J. Appetite and eating behavior in children. *Pediatr Clin N Am* 42:931–954, 1995.

Jacobi C, Agras W, et al. Behavioral validation, precursors, and concomitants of picky eating in childhood. *J Amer Acad Child Adolesc Psychiatry* 42(1):76–84, 2003.

Reau N, Senturia Y, et al. Infant and toddler feeding patterns and problems: normative data and a new direction. *J Dev Behav Pediatr* 17:149–153, 1996.

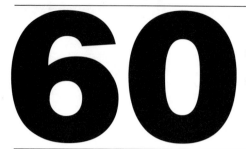

Posttraumatic Stress Disorder (PTSD) in Children

Glenn Saxe

I. **Description of the problem.** Trauma exposure is an international public health problem. Large-scale epidemiologic studies have reported extraordinarily high percentages of exposure to trauma. A national representative study found up to 40% of children have experienced a traumatic event. This rate is much higher among inner-city children. Studies of the prevalence of posttraumatic stress disorder (PTSD) have varied widely depending on the type of trauma and the child's proximity to it. Additionally, the likelihood of a child getting PTSD if traumatized depends on many factors independent of the trauma itself. Consequently, the research literature has increasingly focused on constitutional factors within the child that determine resiliency or vulnerability to trauma.

A. **Epidemiology.** Prevalence studies suggest between 5%–70% of traumatized children qualify for a diagnosis of PTSD. Depending on the study, exposure to sexual assault or abuse yields a prevalence of PTSD between 40%–60%, disasters between 5%–70%, injuries 10%–30%, and war 20%–70%.

B. **Etiology/contributing factors.**

1. **Genetic.** Studies using twin registries of Vietnam veterans have found higher concordance rates in monozygotic twins. There is no doubt, however, of a complex polygenetic vulnerability to the effects of environmental trauma. Recent research has focused on a series of candidate genes, particularly the genes that code for the serotonin transporter.

2. **Environmental.** Children with PTSD frequently grow up in environments saturated with ongoing stressors, including parental mental health and substance abuse problems, marital stress, exposure to ongoing community and family violence. Each of these appears to increase the risk for contracting PTSD.

3. **Organic.** A number of biochemical and neuroanatomical correlates to PTSD have been identified. For each, the research does not always distinguish which may be a *cause* of PTSD versus a *consequence* of PTSD. For example, a number of studies have found smaller hippocampal sizes in adults with PTSD. It remains undetermined whether this smaller hippocampal size is preexisting and predisposes an individual who is traumatized to get PTSD or whether this smaller hippocampal size is a consequence of PTSD (and some of the biochemical changes that occur with it). This *cause* or *consequence* problem is found in the other organic correlates of PTSD, such as lower levels of cortisol, hypersupression of cortisol with dexamethasone, and higher noradrenergic levels.

4. **Developmental.** PTSD has been diagnosed in children as young as 1 year. An alternative criteria set for PTSD has been developed for preschool children which relies far less on verbal report of the child and more on report from the parent and on behavioral observations of the child. Younger children's reactivity to traumatic reminders is much more likely to be observed in their behavior. School-aged children will begin to talk about their fears and anxiety. Adolescents will begin to focus on the meanings of the trauma for themselves, their world, and their future.

II. **Making the diagnosis.** Symptoms can look different depending on the developmental age of the child. See Table 60-1 for DSM-IV criteria.

A. **Signs, symptoms, and behavioral observations.**

1. **Infant/toddler.** Infants and preschool children are often unable to describe internal states or to know how or why they are responding to the environment. Accordingly, PTSD is assessed by observing behaviors in infants and toddlers. Very young children with PTSD will become **aggressive, withdrawn, or very distressed at reminders of the trauma**. Frequently, children will repeatedly play about the trauma (**posttraumatic play**). There may be **significant sleep disruption** including nightmares (which may or may not be about the trauma).

2. **School age.** School-aged children may more easily talk about the trauma and its impact on them. Children of this age group are particularly vulnerable to the **feel-**

Table 60-1 DSM-IV Criterion for PTSD

A. The person has been exposed to a traumatic event in which both of the following were present:
   (1) the person experienced, witnessed, or was confronted with an event or events that involved actual or threatened death or serious injury, or a threat to the physical integrity of self or others.
   (2) the person's response involved intense fear, helplessness, or horror.
B. The traumatic event is persistently reexperienced in one (or more) of the following ways:
   (1) recurrent and intrusive distressing recollections of the event, including images, thoughts, or perceptions.
   (2) recurrent distressing dreams of the event.
   (3) acting or feeling as if the traumatic event were recurring (includes a sense of reliving the experience, illusions, hallucinations, and dissociative flashback episodes, including those that occur on awakening or when intoxicated).
   (4) intense psychological distress at exposure to internal or external cues that symbolize or resemble an aspect of the traumatic event.
   (5) physiological reactivity on exposure to internal or external cues that symbolize or resemble an aspect of the traumatic event.
C. Persistent avoidance of stimuli associated with the trauma and numbing of general responsiveness (not present before the trauma), as indicated by three (or more) of the following:
   (1) efforts to avoid thoughts, feelings, or conversations associated with the trauma.
   (2) efforts to avoid activities, places, or people that arouse recollections of the trauma.
   (3) inability to recall an important aspect of the trauma.
   (4) markedly diminished interest or participation in significant activities.
   (5) feeling of detachment or estrangement from others.
   (6) restricted range of affect (e.g., unable to have loving feelings).
   (7) sense of a foreshortened future (e.g., does not expect to have a career, marriage, children, or a normal life span).
D. Persistent symptoms of increased arousal (not present before the trauma), as indicated by two (or more) of the following:
   (1) difficulty falling or staying asleep.
   (2) irritability or outbursts of anger.
   (3) difficulty concentrating.
   (4) hypervigilance.
   (5) exaggerated startle response.

From American Psychiatric Association. *Diagnostic and Statistical Manual of Mental Disorders.* 4th ed, text rev. Washington, DC: American Psychiatric Association, 2000.

ings of helplessness often elicited by experiencing a trauma and becoming overwhelmed with traumatic stress symptoms. Often school-aged children respond to memories of the trauma with behavioral reactions (e.g. **aggression, withdrawal, avoidance**).

3. **Adolescence.** Adolescents are better able to describe their internal states and properly attribute these states to the traumatic event, which helps facilitate treatment. Adolescents are often highly focused on the **social stigma of the trauma**, particularly sexual trauma. Adolescents can also be very focused on the **interpersonal, societal, or spiritual meanings** of the traumatic event and being a victim of it. Puberty is a particularly difficult time for a child who has experienced sexual trauma.

B. **Comorbid and differential diagnoses in children with PTSD.**
   1. It is clear that PTSD is not the only diagnosis related to trauma. Other psychiatric diagnoses that have been associated with trauma include mood disorders, conduct disorders, attention deficit disorders, dissociative disorders, somatoform disorders, eating disorders, and substance abuse. Additionally, exposure to trauma has been associated with chronic health problems, educational problems, and youth violence. Regarding psychiatric diagnoses, the issue of what is comorbidity and what is differential diagnosis is a complex clinical problem as there is diagnostic overlap between symptoms of PTSD and other disorders.

C. **History: Key clinical questions.** The affirmative answers to at least 2 of these questions suggest that the child is at high risk for PTSD. If these questions are asked in the days after the child is exposed to a trauma they predict the eventual development of PTSD.

1. *"Does your child have **physical** symptoms (headaches, stomach aches, sick feelings, etc.) when reminded of the trauma?"*
2. *"Does your child avoid **talking** about the trauma?"*
3. *"Does your child have a **startle** reaction when he hears a loud noise or see something suddenly?"*
4. *"Does your child get **distressed** when he is reminded of the trauma?"*

The mnemonic for remembering these screening questions is PTSD:

- **P–Physical** symptoms
- **T–Talking** avoidance
- **S– Startle** reactions
- **D–Distress** on reminders

D. **Physical examination.** Physical examination is useful to rule out medical illness as a cause of the symptoms.

E. **Tests.** Screening laboratory tests should be performed only when suggested by the history and physical examination.

III. **Management** Children with PTSD require treatment that **focuses on safety**. Children will need to develop skills that will help them to manage emotional states, to talk about the trauma in a safe way, and to be less consumed by the past and more focused on the future. There are a number of different models of intervention. Most help by addressing the aforementioned goals. This treatment usually requires a trained mental health professional and can be conducted in an outpatient setting. **Family involvement** is usually required to help the family support the child's emotional regulation capacities and work towards limiting stresses and reminders in the environment. When families are unable to do this, home-based intervention is often helpful. Treatment frequently will involve some case management and integration of mental health care with other service systems such as school, social services, and medical system.

The primary care clinician can be extremely helpful to monitor treatment progress and to facilitate the families' engagement in care across the service system. Urgent psychiatric consultation is indicated whenever the child or adolescent is thought to be psychotic, or engaging in violent or self-destructive behaviors. Psychopharmacology will occasionally be required to help the child manage emotional states. Currently, selective serotonin reuptake inhibitors (SSRIs) are considered first line. Psychopharmacology should always be conducted in coordination with psychosocial interventions.

BIBLIOGRAPHY

For Parents

National Child Traumatic Stress Network has handouts and other literature for families that can be downloaded at www.nctsnet.org.

For Professionals

American Academy of Child and Adolescent Psychiatry. Practice parameters for the assessment and treatment of children and adolescents with posttraumatic stress disorder. *J Am Acad Child Adolesc Psychiatry* 37(10 Suppl):4S–26S, 1998.

Cicchetti D, Lynch M. Toward an ecological/transactional model of community violence and child maltreatment: Consequences for children's development. *Psychiatry* 56:96–118, 1993.

Scheeringa MS, Zeanah CH, Myers L, Putnam FW. New findings on alternative criteria for PTSD in preschool children. *J Am Acad Child Adolesc Psychiatry* 43:561–570, 2003.

Saxe GN, Chawla N, Stoddard F, et al. The Child Stress Reaction Checklist: A measure of ASD and PTSD in children. *J Am Acad Child Adolesc Psychiatry* 42:972–979, 2003.

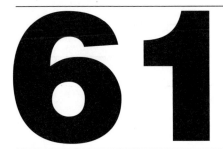

Prematurity: Primary Care Follow-up

James A. Blackman
Robert J. Boyle

I. **Description of the problem.** Infants born before the 37th week of gestation are at risk for chronic medical, neurodevelopmental, and behavioral problems. The shorter the gestation and greater the number of associated medical and psychosocial complications, the higher the risk and need for close primary care surveillance.

A. **Epidemiology.**
- Approximately 9% of all births are premature.
- 2% have a gestational age less than 32 weeks.
- While the incidence of prematurity has not declined over the past decade, mortality and morbidity risk for this group has declined dramatically (Table 61-1).
- The births, often premature, of multiples due to popularity of in-vitro fertilization has increased dramatically.

B. **Risk factors for developmental and behavioral problems.** Risk factors mandating especially close developmental surveillance include
- Very low birth weight (<1500 g)
- Gestational age <28 weeks
- Intrauterine growth retardation
- Neonatal seizures
- Persistent head ultrasound/CT/MR abnormalities, including ventricular dilatation or asymmetry, periventricular leukomalacia, or porencephalic cysts
- Chronic lung disease
- Persistent feeding problems (e.g., need to gavage feed beyond 34 weeks postconceptual age)

Biological risk alone does not determine outcome. Rather, it is the interaction of those risks with social and environmental factors that best predicts long-term functioning (Figure 61-1). In the first 2 years, biological factors are strong predictors of developmental function, especially in the motor domain. However, after age 2 years, socioenvironmental factors assume a prominent role in determining cognitive outcome and school success. The primary care clinician is not able to change the preexisting organic insults, but can alter and improve a child's developmental and behavioral functioning by supporting the social environment.

II. **Evaluation.**

A. **Common health problems of the premature infant.** Since chronic medical problems and developmental and behavioral difficulties are inextricably linked, meticulous management of these problems will enhance the likelihood of good outcomes.

1. **Neurologic.** Maintain good seizure control through judicious use of anticonvulsant medications. Anticonvulsants for neonatal seizures often are weaned during the first year of life.

2. **Ophthalmologic.** Many premature infants leave the neonatal ICU with retinopathy of prematurity that is not fully resolved. Strabismus and myopia are more common among premature infants. Ensure follow-up by a pediatric ophthalmologist.

3. **Audiologic.** Newborn hearing screening is mandatory in many states. Be certain that hearing has been tested or that screening failures are followed-up. Infants with a history of persistent pulmonary hypertension, ECMO therapy, hyperbilirubinemia requiring exchange transfusion, or congenital infection are at risk for progressive or later-onset hearing deficits. They should be retested at 6 months of age.

4. **Respiratory.** Pulmonary symptoms can impede developmental progress. In concert with specialists in chronic lung disease, optimize pulmonary function.

B. **Growth and feeding.** High-risk infants often come home from the hospital with continuing feeding problems: tube dependency, inadequate caloric intake, or volume intolerance due to cardiopulmonary disease. Good nutrition provides the necessary substrate for optimal brain growth and developmental gain. Premature infants should remain on special care formulas for 9–12 months. Key questions to ask include the following.

Table 61-1 Risk by birth weight

Birth weight	Mortality	Major morbidity of survivors[a]	Minor morbidity of survivors[b]
< 800 g	50–60%	20–30%	20–30%
800–1000 g	30–40%	15–20%	15–20%
1000–1500 g	5–10%	10–15%	10–15%

[a]Includes developmental quotient below 70, cerebral palsy, epilepsy, and blindness.
[b]Includes learning disabilities, borderline cognitive function, attention deficits, and poor school achievement (5–10% in the general population) among children without major morbidity.

- Is weight gain appropriate?
- What is the caloric density of the formula?
- What is the daily caloric intake?
- How long does it take to feed the child?
- Does the child have difficulty sucking or swallowing?
- Are the feeding techniques appropriate, given the child's development and capabilities?

Growth patterns should be interpreted from a longitudinal perspective using standard growth charts. For premature infants, measurements can be plotted on special growth charts for premature infants or, after age adjustment (chronological age in weeks minus number of weeks premature), they can be plotted on a regular growth chart. Beyond ages 18–24 months, continued age adjustment is unnecessary.

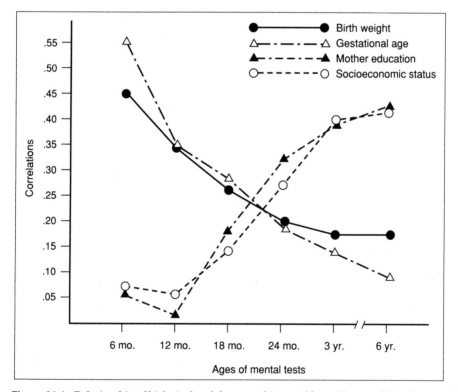

Figure 61-1. Relationship of biological and demographic variables with mental development. Prematurity exerts a potent but short-lived influence on mental development; heritage and home environment have a more lasting effect beyond age 2 years. (Reprinted with permission from Wilson RS. Risk and resilience in early mental development. *Dev Psychol* 21:797, 1985. Copyright 1985 by the American Psychological Association.)

1. **Growth trends.**
   a. **Dropping growth percentiles** or moving further below the 5th percentile. This may be secondary to medical, nutritional, environmental, or neurologic factors. Further investigation is warranted.
   b. **Catch-up growth** or forward movement across percentiles. Catch-up growth may begin slowly and continue over the first 2 years of life.
   c. **Growth parallel to 5th percentile.** The child may continue to be small or catch up in future years. This pattern is often seen following extreme low birth weight and/or intrauterine growth retardation.
   d. **Rapid head growth.** Catch-up head growth is a good sign. However, when head circumference crosses percentiles more rapidly than length or weight, head ultrasound evaluation for hydrocephalus should be considered. Extra axial fluid collection (external hydrocephalus) is usually a benign and transient condition. Babies with grade III–IV intra-ventricular hemorrhages occasionally have late-onset hydrocephalus requiring a shunt.
   e. **Head growth lagging behind other parameters.** This is an ominous sign, often associated with mental retardation.
C. **Behavior and development.**
   1. **History: Key clinical questions.**
      a. *"Are you concerned that your baby is too passive or overly irritable?"* Premature babies may be especially passive or irritable due to CNS injury or the prolonged hospital experience. Infants with CNS injury manifest the same problems as all other infants (e.g., colic, night wakening, temper tantrums), but they tend to be more intense or prolonged.
      b. *"Do you see your child as especially fragile or vulnerable?"* It is sometimes difficult for parents to modify their perception of the child from "fragile" to "healthy." Although it may take months (or years) for the child to achieve medical stability, it may take parents even longer to accept this reality. Common pediatric illnesses may be over interpreted as evidence of continuing vulnerability. (See Chapter 99)
      c. *"Does your child seem either stiff or floppy?"* Hypotonia is fairly common among premature infants and usually resolves. While persistent hypertonia may be a sign of cerebral palsy (CP), CP in preterm infants typically begins with a period of persistent hypotonia, which then evolves over several months into hypertonia.
      d. *"Does your child have any unusual movement patterns?"* Dragging the legs along in crawling, body rolling (instead of crawling), or seat scooting may be manifestations of neuromotor abnormalities. Early hand preference is abnormal and may indicate injury to subcortical white matter or the corticospinal tract contralateral to the less used upper extremity. In such a case, a head imaging (MR) study is indicated.
   2. **Assessment.** Although developmental surveillance is recommended for all children, careful and regular assessment is even more important for premature children. Healthy premature infants tend to catch-up to their like-aged peers in developmental functioning over the first years of life. Furthermore, the older the child gets, the less relevance 2–3 months correction has.
      • To correct for prematurity when assessing developmental milestones, a practical compromise is to use a one half correction approach: subtract one half the weeks premature from the child's chronological age and use this result as the expected level of developmental attainment.
      • Some developmental screening tests recommend full correction until age 2–3 years.
      • If the child is not achieving age-appropriate skills, an in-depth assessment by a developmental specialist or early intervention program is warranted.
D. **Psychosocial issues.**
   1. **Family dynamics and stress.** Shortened gestation interrupts the normal psychological preparation for life with a newborn. The long, uncertain intensive care experience can drain the family's physical and emotional stamina. Parents take home a normal but fragile, slow-starting, or clearly abnormal infant. The clinician should schedule an early "decompression visit" for the parents to discuss the neonatal intensive care unit experience and to give vent to their frustrations and fears. Counseling or family support groups may be helpful.
   2. **Day care issues.** Due to the increased morbidity from respiratory infection in premature infants with a history of chronic lung disease, day care settings with extensive

exposure to other children with respiratory illnesses should be avoided if possible. Families may need assistance and guidance with appropriate daycare arrangements.

III. **Management.** Each infant should have an identified "medical home" where primary care and regular developmental screening occur. The clinician must be aware of the infant's and family's needs and assist the family in obtaining and coordinating other necessary services. Follow-up should be seen as a multidisciplinary team function, with the primary care clinician, other medical specialists, early intervention services, and other therapies (occupational or physical) participating as needed.

IV. **Clinical pearls and pitfalls.**
- Beware of overwhelming the family with services or appointments. Simplification and coordination of services as well as family involvement in the process will decrease family stress and ensure better overall compliance and satisfaction.
- Do not assume that an infant will "outgrow" any identified problems. Appropriate evaluation and correction for the degree of prematurity should allow the clinician to make an informed judgment about the infant's status.

BIBLIOGRAPHY

For Parents

Organizations

American Association for Premature Infants www.aapi-online.org
Parents of Preemies www2.medsch.wisc.edu/childrenshosp/parents_of_preemies/index.html
Premature Baby/Premature Child www.prematurity.org
Parents of Premature Babies, Inc www.preemie-l.org

Publications

Garcia-Prats JA, Hornfischer SS. *What to Do when your Baby is Premature: A Parent's Handbook for Coping with High-Risk Pregnancy and Caring for the Preterm Infant.* Three Rivers, MI: Three Rivers Press, 2000.
Linden DW, Paroli ET, Doron MW. *Preemies: The Essential Guide for Parents of Premature Babies.* New York: Pocket Books, 2000.
Madden SL, Sears W. *The Preemie Parents' Companion: The Essential Guide for your Premature Baby in the Hospital, at Home, and through the First Years.* Boston: The Harvard Common Press, 2000.

For Professionals

Bernbaum J. *Preterm Infants in Primary Care: A Guide to Office Management.* Columbus, OH: Abbott Laboratories, 2000. Available from Ross Products, Abbott Laboratories.

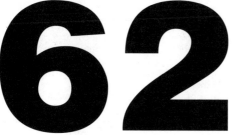

62 School Avoidance

Barton D. Schmitt

I. **Description of the problem.** Children with school avoidance repeatedly stay home from school or are sent home from school for physical symptoms of emotional origin. In the classic case, the child awakens with a stomachache on Monday morning, is allowed to stay home, and feels fine by midmorning. The terms *school refusal, school avoidance,* and *school phobia* are often used interchangeably.

   A. **Epidemiology.**
   - School avoidance is the most common cause of vague physical symptoms in school-aged children.
   - Approximately 5% of elementary school children and 2% of middle school children have this disorder.
   - The incidence of school refusal may be decreasing because of the increasing numbers of working mothers, which requires most children to master their separation fears long before entering kindergarten.
   - The home-schooling movement shelters many of these children.

   B. **Etiology.** There are two basic types of school avoidance syndrome:
   1. **Anxiety-related school avoidance.** These children are excessively worried (e.g., about grades, being rejected by peers, marital discord). Most of these children also have persistent separation anxiety, which most children have mastered by ages 3–4 years. Many have a shy and sensitive temperament. Frequently there is an overprotective parent who worries too much about the child's experiencing stress in the neighborhood and school. These children are good to excellent students and cause no behavioral problems in the classroom. Girls outnumber boys, and the onset usually occurs in kindergarten. Approximately 20% of this group also have an acute precipitating event (e.g., being teased by someone at school).
   2. **Secondary-gain school avoidance.** These children do not manifest any symptoms of anxiety. Their poor school attendance often follows an acute illness that seems to stretch on and on as they get further behind in their schoolwork. The desire to stay at home is also perpetuated by the sympathy they receive and the amount of television they are allowed to watch. They often have a lenient parent who does not place much value on education. Boys outnumber girls in this group, and often they are poor students.

II. **Making the diagnosis.**

   A. **Signs and symptoms.** Table 62-1 reviews common presenting symptoms. Most children with school avoidance complain of physical symptoms at the time of departure for school. The children with the anxiety-related type usually have physiologic manifestations of

Table 62-1 Presenting symptoms for school phobia

1. General—**insomnia**, excessive sleeping, fatigue, "always tired," "fever," "always sick.
2. Skin—**pallor**
3. Eye—blurred vision
4. ENT—recurrent sore throats, recurrent sinus problems, constant colds, dysphagia
5. Respiratory—**hyperventilation**, coughing tics, **vocal cord dysfunction**
6. Cardiovascular—**palpitations**, chest pains
7. Gastrointestinal—**recurrent abdominal pains, anorexia, nausea, recurrent vomiting, diarrhea**
8. Renal/genital—**frequency-urgency syndrome**
9. Skeletal—bone pain, joint pain, back pain, "fibromyalgia"
10. Neuromuscular—**headaches, dizziness, syncope**, "weakness," "always tired"
11. Pervasive symptoms—acute anxiety attack or **panic reaction**

The **symptoms** are physiological manifestations of anxiety. The other symptoms may be fabricated or exaggerated.

anxiety (e.g., headache, recurrent abdominal pain). The children with the secondary-gain type of school refusal usually fabricate or exaggerate symptoms (e.g., sore throat, leg pain).

B. **Confirming the diagnosis.** School avoidance is a diagnosis of inclusion that can be confirmed by documenting four diagnostic criteria:

1. **The child complains of recurrent vague, mysterious physical symptoms.**

2. **No physical cause** is found on careful evaluation, including a physical examination and appropriate laboratory tests. *The discrepancy between how sick the child sounds and how well the child looks is a hallmark of this disorder.*

3. **Physical symptoms predominate in the morning** and are accentuated when the family tries to send the child to school. Often the symptoms clear by 10:00 AM.

4. **The child has missed 5 or more days of school because of these physical symptoms.** By comparison, children with chronic physical diseases often have excellent school attendance records.

C. **Differential diagnosis.** Each physical symptom listed in Table 62-1 has a specific and lengthy differential diagnosis.

- The primary care clinician is obligated to rule out any physical disease as a cause of the school refuser's symptoms. Excessive or chronic school absence also can have other causes (Table 62-2).
- Some parents keep a child at home for a prolonged period of time because of mistaken beliefs regarding the need for bed rest or isolation (e.g., keeping a child home 10 days for streptococcal pharyngitis).
- Children with chronic physical disease or learning disabilities may become reluctant to attend school because they are unable to adapt well to the academic environment or to the other children.
- A *truant* is a youngster who is neither at home nor at school during school hours. These children are at risk for becoming school dropouts. The acute onset of school avoidance may relate to a precipitating event, such as a change of schools or the loss of a school chum. Other precipitants include:
- **Family stresses** (e.g., acute marital strife, the father's loss of a job, a sick mother, the birth of a sibling)
- Stresses that occur **en route to school** (e.g., a bully at the bus stop)
- **Academic stresses** (e.g., an impending test, a requirement to recite in class, a poor report card)
- **School-based stresses** (e.g., bathroom restrictions for children with small bladders, physical fitness requirements for overweight or clumsy children, teasing on the school grounds)

D. **History: Key clinical questions.**

1. *"How much school has your child missed because of these symptoms?"* It is a mistake to assume that the parents will bring up poor school attendance to the clinician. They often believe that everyone keeps "sick" children at home and in bed.

2. *"How many days of school did your child miss last year?"* This information is needed when parents blame the problem on some illness or stress that began during the current school year.

3. *"When are the symptoms worse?"* In school avoidance, the symptoms are usually worse on Sunday nights, early mornings, Mondays, during September, and following holidays. Often the onset of symptoms dates to entering kindergarten or first grade.

Table 62-2 Chronic school absence: a differential diagnosis

School refusal
  Anxiety-related type (school phobia)
  Secondary-gain type (school avoidance)
Overresponse to minor illnesses
Chronic physical disease with poor adaptation
Learning disability with poor adaptation
Truancy
Substance abuse
Depression
Psychosis
Teenage pregnancy
Family dysfunction

4. *"What do you think is causing the symptoms?"* or *"What is the worst diagnosis your child could have?"* The parents may fear a specific disease that the child does not harbor.

5. *"Have any major changes occurred in your family?"* This question may help the family acknowledge stressors they had initially overlooked or denied.

6. *"Does your child ever stay overnight with friends at their homes?"* An inability to be away from parents at night supports separation issues.

7. *"What is the worst possible thing that could happen if you sent your child to school with these symptoms?"* The parents may fear that the child will emotionally decompensate at school, have embarrassing symptoms, or be teased.

E. **Physical examination.** The physical examination of these children should be completely normal. The performance of a meticulous examination is reassuring to the parents, as parents place an inordinate amount of faith in the ability of the examination to uncover hidden disease. During the examination, the clinician should discuss normal findings rather than proceed in silence. He or she can provide double reassurance for more skeptical parents by asking a partner to confirm the findings and comment briefly.

F. **Tests.** Each specific physical symptom will determine which laboratory studies (if any) are appropriate.

III. **Management.**

A. **Primary goals.**

1. Convince the parents that their child is in excellent physical health.
2. Convince the parents that their child has school avoidance
3. Return the child to full-time school attendance.

B. **Information for the family.** The main barrier to successful treatment is changing the family's focus from an organic to a nonorganic etiology:

1. **Explain what school avoidance is and that stress can cause real physical symptoms.** Explain the difference between physical symptoms and physical disease. Explain that pain is real, even when it has an emotional origin. Point out that everyone's body has a certain physical way of responding to emotional stress.

2. **Clarify for parents that school avoidance occurs in normal children and normal homes.** Mention that it is a "stress-related," not a "psychiatric" problem. Support the parents as being good caregivers.

3. **Clarify that the child is in excellent physical health.** Pronounce the child *unequivocally* physically well. Do not leave the parents hanging with statements such as, "He probably has school avoidance, but we can't be certain." If a clinician is unwilling to call the cause stress-related, he or she can at least attribute the symptoms to some benign physiologic process, such as gas pains, a sensitive stomach, growing pains, or tension headaches.

4. **Tell parents why the symptom is not the result of physical disease.** Justify the nonorganic diagnosis by pointing to the timing of the symptoms, the age of onset that coincides with school entry, the presence of the symptoms during previous school years, the normal physical examination, and normal laboratory tests.

5. **Reassure parents that you can effectively treat this condition.** The primary care clinician can promise to provide a treatment plan that will reduce the symptoms in the majority of cases. The minimal goal of this discussion should be to get the parents to agree to regular school attendance pending additional observations, even if they cling to the idea that their child may have some rare disease.

C. **Initial treatment strategies.**

1. **The mainstay of treatment is returning the child to regular school attendance.**

2. **Talk with the parents.** Once the primary care clinician has convinced the family that the youngster is physically well, he or she must insist on an immediate return to school. Being in school is intrinsically therapeutic and breaks the vicious cycle that occurs when a child gets out of step with schoolwork and friendships. Parents will need to be firm in the morning for several weeks. On any morning that the "child has to stay home for illness," the clinician is needed to reassess the child and send him or her to school if the condition is minor or a psychosomatic symptom.

3. **Talk with the child.** The clinician should reassure the youngster that she or he is in good physical health and in no physical danger. The symptoms can be blamed on worrying too much about competition, grades, bad things happening, or catching up with schoolwork. The clinician can offer a face-saving way to accept the diagnosis (e.g., headache from worrying too much) and emphasize that daily school attendance, a non-negotiable requirement, will help the child feel better.

a. **Secondary-gain school refusal.** Simply state, "You can't miss any further school

because it is illegal to do so." This type of refusal responds quickly to this warning and limit-setting.
  b. **Anxiety-related school refusal.** More sympathy is in order. If the child has severe symptoms at school, promise the availability of lying down in the nurse's office for 5–10 minutes. Clarify, however, that he cannot go home because of these symptoms.
  4. **Contact the school staff.** Communication between the primary care clinician and the school nurse is essential. The clinician should be called if the child's attendance remains poor or if the child is in the nursing station and wants to go home. The clinician and school nurse can then work together to decide whether the child should stay in school. School staff can also help to make the return to school as nontraumatic as possible, (e.g., cancelling some of the make-up work).
  5. **Treat contributory stress factors.** Most school stresses can be dealt with by the parent, school principal, special education teacher, or the primary care clinician. Correction of most of these factors alone may produce little improvement in school attendance, because they only partially account for the child's preference for staying home. Changing to a different class or a different school generally is of no benefit except in those rare situations in which an unstable teacher is mistreating one or more children.
  6. **Providing follow-up visits.** Follow-up visits are essential for monitoring attendance. Children with school avoidance should have return visits in approximately 1 week, 1 month, and again approximately 2 weeks into the following school year. These parents also need to call their clinician on the first day of acute illnesses to help decide whether the child needs to stay home.
  D. **Criteria for referral.** The primary care clinician needs to refer the child with more severe, intractable emotional problems to a child psychiatrist, psychologist, or social worker. Most children who have been on prolonged bed rest should also be referred. Most of all, patients who are unresponsive to pediatric counseling need referral

IV. **Clinical pearls and pitfalls.**
  - Ask about school attendance whenever you evaluate a child for recurrent or persistent symptoms.
  - Suspect school avoidance by the symptom's pattern because no organic disease has this profile or keeps this timetable.
  - Don't be misled because the child "likes school," is a good student, or "wants to go back."
  - If in doubt about the diagnosis, request a 7-day symptom diary. It will be more helpful than any imaging study.
  - Protect these children from unwarranted laboratory tests, procedures, prescriptions, hospitalization, and surgery.
  - Request that children return to school, even while the evaluation is in process. The response will be either diagnostic or therapeutic.

BIBLIOGRAPHY

For Parents

Schmitt BD. When your child has school phobia (a parent information sheet). *Contemp Pediatr* 7(8):41–42, 1990.

Websites

American Family Physician http://www.aafp.org/afp/20031015/1563ph.html
American Academy of Child and Adolescent Psychiatry http://www.aacap.org/publications/factsfam/noschool.htm

For Professionals

American Academy of Pediatrics: Committee on School Health. Home, hospital, and other non-school-based instruction for children and adolescents who are medically unable to attend school. *Pediatrics* 106:1154–1155, 2000.
Egger HL, Costello EJ, Angold A. School refusal and psychiatric disorders: a community study. *J Am Acad Child Adolesc Psychiatry* 42:797, 2003.

King NJ. School refusal in children and adolescents: a review of the past 10 years. *J Am Acad Child Adolesc Psychiatry* 40:107–205, 2001.
Schmitt BD. School refusal. *Pediatr Rev* 8:99–105, 1986.

Websites

American Academy of Family Physicians http://www.aafp.org/afp/20031015/1555.html

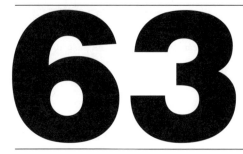

School Failure

Paul H. Dworkin

I. **Description of the problem.** Over 10% of schoolchildren in the United States are receiving special education and other services because of difficulties with school performance. School failure is a complex issue that defies traditional methods of pediatric evaluation and management. While learning problems are of obvious multidisciplinary concern, the primary care clinician plays a vital role in clarifying the reasons for school failure and facilitating appropriate evaluation and intervention.

   A. **Reasons for school failure.** A wide variety of causes may contribute to a child's failure in school. A simple classification scheme identifies **intrinsic** or child-related causes (e.g., specific learning disabilities, attention deficits) and **extrinsic** or environmental-related causes relating to either the home (e.g., parental separation or divorce) or the school setting (e.g., poor instruction). In most cases, school failure is not due to a single factor but rather the result of a **complex interaction of child-, family-, and school-related variables**.

   D. **Spcoific causes**.
      1. **Learning disabilities (LD).** As defined by federal legislation: *Specific learning disability means a disorder in one or more of the basic psychological processes involved in understanding or in using language, spoken or written, which may manifest itself in an imperfect ability to listen, think, speak, read, write, spell, or to do mathematical calculations.*

         The term includes such conditions as perceptual handicaps, brain injury, minimal brain dysfunction, dyslexia, and developmental aphasia. The term does not include children who have problems that are primarily the result of visual, hearing, or motor disabilities, or mental retardation, emotional disturbance, or of environmental, cultural, or economic disadvantage.

         Learning disabilities are characterized by a **discrepancy between ability (as measured by intelligence tests) and actual academic achievement**. Their prevalence is estimated **at 3%–15% of schoolchildren**. While most learning disabled children have underlying weaknesses in language function, weaknesses in other higher-order cognitive functions (so-called metacognitive skills) have been increasingly recognized. Such children may have difficulties with reasoning, memory, or focusing their attention and have been described as "passive learners" because of their difficulties with selecting strategies for problem solving.
      2. **Attention deficits** (see Chapter 25). There exists significant overlap between children with LD and attention deficit hyperactivity disorder (ADHD). From a clinical standpoint, distinguishing between children with an intrinsic deficit of attention and those with attention deficits secondary to other developmental and behavioral dysfunctions (e.g., language impairment, depression) is often difficult.
      3. **Mental retardation (MR)** (see Chapters 52 and 53). Mild MR is often not identified until children are confronted with the cognitive demands of school. At that time, a slow learning rate and ultimate acquisition of academic skills up to the fifth- or sixth-grade level is typically seen.
      4. **Sensory impairment.** Hearing loss results in a significant educational handicap because language acquisition and communication skills are impaired. Such students typically experience difficulties in reading, arithmetic reasoning, and problem solving. They may exhibit classroom maladjustment, behavioral problems, and social immaturity. The prognosis directly relates to the age at which identification occurs. In comparison, blind children usually fare better within the classroom. Visually impaired children who experience school failure tend to have additional handicaps.
      5. **Emotional illness.** From 30%–80% of emotionally disturbed students have problems with academic achievement and classroom behavior. Emotional problems such as

low self-esteem and poor self-image often exacerbate school failure brought on by other causes, such as LD or ADHD.

6. **Chronic illness.** 50%–65% of chronically ill students have problems with academic achievement (see Chapter 33). Possible adverse influences on school performance include limited alertness or stamina, chronic pain, medication side effects, absenteeism, emotional maladjustment, low intelligence (primarily children with certain neurologic disorders), the inferior quality of alternative classroom placement, and inappropriate or unrealistic expectations by teachers and parents. Additionally, certain chronic diseases (e.g., epilepsy, cerebral palsy, myelomeningocele) are associated with an increased incidence of LD.

7. **Temperamental dysfunction** (see Chapter 77). The temperamentally "difficult" student may become easily frustrated and angry when confronted with material not easily mastered. The initial reluctance to participate and tendency to withdraw of the "slow-to-warm-up" child may be misinterpreted as anxiety or as a limited capacity for learning. Although the temperamentally "easy" student usually fares well, problems may arise when expectations for behavior markedly differ between home and school. For example, a student's mild intensity of reaction to situations or stimuli may be misinterpreted within the classroom as a lack of interest or motivation.

8. **Family dysfunction and social problems.** Family issues that contribute to school failure include parental separation and divorce, child abuse and neglect, the illness or death of an immediate family member, parental psychopathology, early parenthood, substance abuse, and poverty.

9. **Ineffective schooling.** School *processes* are more important determinants of students' performance than such features as whether schools are public or private, class size, the age and spaciousness of school buildings, and student teacher ratio. Rather, the school's academic emphasis, expectations for attainment, amount of homework, teachers' actions during lessons, use of group instruction, and the use of rewards and praise are major influences on students' performance. Aspects of the school's social environment (such as the amount of praise offered to children) may be particularly important for children from disadvantaged homes in which less emphasis is placed on academic attainment and standards for classroom behavior.

II. **Making the diagnosis.** If psychoeducational evaluation has already identified the reasons for a student's school failure (e.g., LD or mild MR), the goal of pediatric evaluation is to exclude medical problems as contributors to poor classroom performance. Additionally, the primary care clinician's familiarity with the child and family may be helpful in identifying social or emotional factors that further impair school performance. For the child with newly recognized school failure, the pediatric clinician must identify such conditions as sensory impairment or chronic illness, while searching for medical, neurophysiologic, and psychological correlates of such other conditions as LD, MR, and emotional illness.

Possible components of the evaluation of children with school failure include:

A. **History.** Important historic information should be sought from parents, teachers, and the child. Review of the student's perinatal and past medical history, developmental milestones, past and present behavior, and family and social history may yield findings with possible implications for school failure (Table 63-1).

B. **Key clinical questions.**
   1. *"Which subjects are particularly difficult for the child?"* The pattern of delays may suggest a specific etiology; for example, children with an LD typically have discrete difficulties in select subjects, while students with mild MR have more pervasive academic delays.
   2. *"How does the child behave in the classroom?"* Classroom behavior may suggest ADHD, poor self-image, or conduct disorder.
   3. *"How many days has the child missed school?"* Poor school attendance may be due to chronic illness, school phobia, or poor motivation due to LD.
   4. *"Has past testing been performed?"* Past educational or psychological testing may have identified causes of a child's school failure.
   5. *"What special services has the child received?"* Responses to different instructional techniques ("diagnostic teaching") may suggest reasons for school failure.

C. **Physical examination.** The physical examination has a limited, but important, role in the evaluation of children with school failure. Certain specific aspects deserve special emphasis (Table 63-2).

D. **Mental status examination.** Simple projective techniques may suggest emotional issues such as depression, anxiety, or poor self-image as the cause or, even more likely, the consequence of school failure. Examples include
   1. *"If you had three wishes, what would they be?"*

Table 63-1 The role of history in the evaluation of school learning problems

Aspect	Findings suggestive of learning disorders
School functioning	
Academic achievement	Discrete delays in select subject (e.g., language)
	Adequate early performance, with difficulties emerging later (e.g., mathematics, writing)
Classroom behavior	Long-standing, pervasive problems with inattention, impulsivity, overactivity
	Disorganization and poor strategy formation
	Depression, moodiness
Attendance	Excessive absenteeism
	School avoidance
Past psychoeducational testing	Discrepancy between cognitive abilities and academic achievement
Special required school services	Response to "diagnostic teaching"
Perinatal history	Clusters of adverse events
	Maternal alcohol or drug intake
Medical history	Recurrent and/or persistent otitis media
	Iron deficiency anemia
	Lead poisoning
	Seizures
	Frequent injuries
	Chronic medication use
Development	Delayed or disordered language acquisition and communication skills
	Subtle delays in select milestones
	Uneven pattern of skills and interests
Behavioral history	Long-standing, pervasive problems with attention span, impulsivity, acting out, overactivity
	Sadness
	Poor self-esteem
Family history	Learning problems
	School failure among first-degree relatives
Social history	Child abuse or neglect
	Other stressors

Reproduced with permission from Dworkin PH. School learning problems and developmental differences. In: Hoekelman RA, et al., eds. *Pediatric Primary Care,* 4th ed. St. Louis, MO: Mosby, 2001:778.

Table 63-2 The physical examination and evaluation of school learning problems

Aspect	Findings suggestive of learning disorders
General observations	Sadness, anxiety
	Short attention span, impulsivity, overactivity
	Tics
Phenotypic features	Stigmata of genetic syndromes (e.g., sex chromosome abnormalities, fetal alcohol syndrome)
	Minor congenital anomalies
Skin	Multiple café au lait spots
	"Ash-leaf" spots, adenoma sebaceum
Tympanic membranes	Signs of recurrent or chronic otitis media
Genitalia	Delayed sexual maturation in boys
Growth measurements	Short stature
	Microcephaly and macrocephaly
Sensory screening	Poor hearing or vision

Reproduced with permission from Dworkin PH. School learning problems and developmental differences. In: Hoekelman RA, et al., eds. *Pediatric Primary,* 4th ed. St. Louis, MO: Mosby, 2001:779.

2. *"If you could make three changes in your life, what would they be?"* The sad or anxious child may be unwilling to offer wishes or hope for changes in family or school circumstances.

3. *"Draw a picture of your family"* may suggest concerns with family composition or reveal anxiety or uncertainty regarding the child's status within the family.

E. **Neurodevelopmental assessment.** Surveying the child's abilities in different areas of development may help to identify weaknesses contributing to school failure. For example, the developmental profile of a child with a LD is typically characterized by an uneven pattern, with discrete areas of relative strength and weakness. The significance of minor neurologic indicators ("soft neurologic signs") is controversial; such findings should not serve as a basis for diagnosing a LD.

F. **Laboratory studies.** No laboratory studies are routinely indicated in the assessment of school failure (except perhaps screening for lead poisoning). Rather, tests should be performed based on specific indications.

G. **Further investigations and referrals.** Psychoeducational evaluation is critically important in the evaluation of children with school failure.

1. **Goals.** The goals of such evaluations include
   a. **To examine the student's academic strengths and weaknesses.**
   b. **To determine the child's cognitive ability,** including such higher-order functions as abstract reasoning, problem solving, and learning style.
   c. **To assess perceptual strengths and weaknesses.**
   d. **To examine communicative ability.**
   e. **To assess social and emotional adaptation.**

2. **Performance.** Ideally, such evaluations are performed by the child's school system, in accordance with state and federal mandates. There is no one standardized evaluation appropriate for all children, and the specific tests used depend on the preference and expertise of the examiner and the child's needs. Examples include intelligence tests; tests of general learning abilities; academic achievement tests; diagnostic reading, math, and writing tests; tests of perceptual and motor function; and such informal techniques as diagnostic teaching. School personnel performing such evaluations may include psychologists, special educators, learning disability specialists, speech-language pathologists, and social workers.

III. **Management.** For learning disabilities, mild mental retardation, and other common causes of school failure, educational intervention is the most crucial. Nonetheless, a variety of important primary care roles are both feasible and important in the management of school failure:

A. **Specific medical intervention** is the most traditional of pediatric roles. Examples include
   1. **The treatment of underlying medical conditions,** such as asthma or a seizure disorder, that influence school performance.
   2. **Pharmacologic management** of ADHD.

B. **Counseling** is a traditional mode of pediatric intervention. Aspects may include:
   1. **Clarification of a student's strengths and weaknesses and demystification of any diagnosis such as learning disability, mental retardation.**
   2. **Anticipatory guidance regarding commonly encountered school difficulties** and the consequences of school failure (e.g., low self-esteem).
   3. **Alleviation of guilt and anxiety.**
   4. **Explaining the legal rights of students and families.**
   5. **Guidance regarding the lack of effectiveness of nontraditional treatment strategies** (e.g., dietary manipulation, optometric training).
   6. **Offering advice regarding specific behavior management strategies,** such as time-out and positive reinforcement.

C. The primary care clinician can assume an active role in monitoring the progress of children with learning problems. Office visits provide important opportunities to monitor self-esteem, search for signs of depression, and offer encouragement and praise for progress.

BIBLIOGRAPHY

For Parents

Organizations

Council for Exceptional Children (CEC) Division for Learning Disabilities (DLD) 1920 Association Drive Reston, VA 22091-1589 703-620-3660 www.dldcec.org

Council for Learning Disabilities (CLD) P.O. Box 40303 Overland Park, KS 66204 www.cldinternational.org

Learning Disabilities Association of America 4156 Library Road Pittsburgh, PA 5234-1349 412-341-1515 www.ldanatl.org

Schwab Foundation for Learning 1650 South Amphett Boulevard, Suite 300 San Mateo, CA 94402 650-655-2410 www.schwablearning.org

Books

Levine M. *A Mind at a Time.* New York: Simon and Schuster, 2002.

For Professionals

American Academy of Child and Adolescent Psychiatry. Practice parameters for the assessment and treatment of children and adolescents with language and learning disorders. *J Amer Acad Child Adolesc Psychiatry* 37(10 Suppl):46S–62S, 1998.

Capin DM. Developmental Learning Disorders: clues to their diagnosis and management. *Pediatr Rev* 17:284, 1996.

Dworkin PH. *Learning and Behavior Problems of Schoolchildren.* Philadelphia: Saunders, 1985.

Dworkin PH. School failure. *Pediatr Rev* 10:301–312, 1989.

64

School Readiness

Margot Kaplan-Sanoff

I. **Description of the problem.** *School readiness* is the term used to describe those characteristics which are considered prerequisites for a child to be ready to succeed in a school setting. Table 64-1 lists the criteria most often identified as necessary for academic success in kindergarten or first grade. The question of school readiness also raises emotional concerns for both parents ("unfamiliar people will be judging my child and, by extension, my parenting") and children ("can I meet the challenges of the BIG school?"). There are a number of social, emotional, motoric, and cognitive factors to consider when assessing school readiness:

A. **Ability to master new experiences.** The ability to grapple with and master new experiences defines the initial task of school success. Children are asked to listen and relate to unfamiliar adults, to follow specific rules, to interact with a large group of children, and to manage daily tasks by themselves. Children who can build on familiar experiences and who can pick out the novel features of a new experience and compare the "new" with the known will quickly gain mastery of the new situations required by school. On the other hand, children who are easily overwhelmed, who panic at new experiences, and who are unable to bring knowledge of the familiar to bear on new demands may have a difficult time assimilating new knowledge into a coherent context. Each new piece of learning disorients them and they are unable to understand how to manage successfully in school.

B. **Lack of experience.** Some children simply lack the experience of being in a group of children of their own age. Others may lack access to books and learning materials in their homes. Due to the enormous burdens of poverty, family trauma and stress, domestic violence, inappropriately low expectations for preacademic development, or diverse cultural backgrounds, these children are unfamiliar with the tasks required for success in school (such as waiting in line, sharing materials, taking turns, or following verbal directions).

C. **Ability to tolerate separations from primary caregivers.** The relationships which children develop with teachers are different from their relationships with parents and extended family. Children are expected to establish and maintain the teacher's attention in a large group through such socially acceptable ways (e.g., waiting to be called on, or holding up their hands to answer a question or make a request).

D. **Independence in most activities of daily living.** Separated from primary caregivers, children are required to be independent in such caregiving functions as eating, toileting, napping, dressing and taking care of their possessions.

E. **Ability to control impulses.** To succeed in school, young children need to be able to sit in a circle without bothering other children, to attend to adults for a limited amount of time (5–10 minutes), and to listen to and follow adult directions, some of which might be delivered from the other side of a busy room. Children are required to delay their own needs, urges, and feelings: to defer snack when they are hungry, to modify their wishes or accept alternatives to the plans they want to pursue, and to tolerate the feelings of others without resorting to inappropriate outbursts.

F. **Appropriate play skills.** Early school success is dependent, in part, on the child's ability to get along with peers, to manage in a group, and to engage in developmentally appropriate play. Children should be able to play with other children without resorting to hitting, biting, or yelling to resolve conflicts. They should be able to manage the give and take of peer relationships, both within a structured play activity like a board game and in fantasy play. Children should also be able to differentiate fantasy play and stories from reality.

G. **Developmental delays.** Specific cognitive or learning problems, receptive or expressive language delays, and visual motor or sensory integration problems may make it difficult for a child to succeed in a regular school classroom. Yet these are the very children who benefit most from a more formal learning environment. They should be evaluated

Table 64-1 School readiness skills

Kindergarten
Knows color names
Counts to 10
Retells a story
Cooperative play with peers
Identifies some printed letters
Draws a person
Prints name
First Grade
Identifies upper and lower case letters
Identifies numerals to 10
Copies letters and numerals
Demonstrates conservation of mass, length, and volume
Knows address and birth date
Reads simple sight words
Works cooperatively with groups of children

by the school department and placed in the least restricted learning environment within the school, perhaps in a transitional classroom or a resource room program with placement in a regular classroom. Children who do not possess sufficient school readiness skills due to developmental delays will not benefit from "another year" at home or in childcare waiting to be ready for school. They are legally eligible for school services after three years of age and should be provided with specific educational placements which maximize their strengths and address their problems.

II. **Making the diagnosis.** The skills listed in Table 64–1 constitute the "how" of school readiness. Such specific cognitive and motor tasks (e.g., knowing the ABCs, printing one's name, skipping, or tying one's shoes) are highly idiosyncratic milestones and do not automatically correlate to the actual tasks of school learning. For example, knowing the alphabet by singing the ABC song is a far less powerful predictor of reading success than is the child's understanding of the power and function of the written word.

A. **History taking.** Involving both parents and child in a developmental history taking can provide the clinician with a great deal of information pertinent to the issue of school readiness. Input from the child's childcare provider can add an additional perspective to the diagnosis. The following clinical inquiries can be used to guide the discussion and trigger the need for additional information:

1. *"Has the child followed an age appropriate developmental trajectory in language, cognitive, social and motor development?"*
2. *"How does the child respond to unusual events at home or in child care such as a substitute provider or a change in the daily routine?"*
3. *"Has the child had any preschool or group care experience? How has he done in these settings?"*
4. *"Were there any developmental or behavioral concerns during those experiences in group care?"*
5. *"Does the child play well with peers? Or does the child consistently choose to play with younger children?"*
6. *"Does the child cling to behaviors more appropriate for a younger child (e.g., continual thumb sucking, frequent toileting accidents, tantrums)?"*
7. *"Can the child identify colors, shapes, letters, and numbers?"*
8. *"Is the child's speech understandable and can he converse with the clinician about everyday topics of interest?"*
9. *"Does the child sit and listen to stories and look at picture books by him/her self?"*
10. *"Has the child developed a dominant hand?"*

B. **Issues within the family.** In some situations, children's behavior and development might be hampered by patterns within the family such as domestic conflict, alcohol or substance abuse, parental depression, crisis within the extended families, loss and grief. In other families, developmental expectations might be based on gender, birth order, or learning problems within the family. Inappropriate family expectations for school success or differences between family members about school readiness should be discussed. Questions assessing the level of family functioning and the support systems which are available to the family can be helpful to a diagnosis of school readiness:

1. *"Have there been any changes within the family such as a move, change in employment, unemployment, illness or death within extended family or friends? Have you noticed any changes in your child's behavior as a result?"*
2. *"All couples have their ups and downs. Would you say that currently your relationship is up, down or in the middle? How do you and your partner resolve conflicts?"*
3. *"How is your health and the health of family members? Has that changed recently?"*
4. *"What was your experience in school? Were you happy and successful in school or was it a difficult experience for you? For your partner?"*
5. *"Are you getting any pressure from family members to send or not to send your child to school?"*
6. *"What are your expectations for this child in school?"*
7. *"What schools have you considered?"*
8. *"With whom have you discussed these decisions?"*

C. **Physical examination.** During the routine physical examination, place emphasis on handedness, coordination of gross, visual motor and fine motor activities, and the presence or absence of excessive overflow movements. Examine the child's vision, hearing, neurologic status, sensory integration, and neurodevelopmental maturation.

D. **Developmental assessment.** Unfortunately, there are currently few good developmental screening tests that are predictive of school success. Most instruments available to the pediatric clinician are not equipped to detect subtle learning disabilities or a more complicated diagnosis. If assessment is warranted because of parental, school or pediatric concern, a referral should be made, either to the school district for an evaluation, or to an independent specialist such as a neuropsychologist, learning disabilities specialist, or developmental and behavioral pediatrician.

III. **Management.**

A. **Children with specific learning or developmental problems.** Children with identified learning problems should be referred for a complete evaluation by the school department or by an independent evaluator. Under federal law, children with special learning needs are required to receive appropriate services within "the least restrictive environment". Parents may opt to provide additional independent services such as speech or sensory integration therapy if these are not provided in the child's individual education plan (IEP). Clinicians should monitor the child's progress carefully to determine the accessibility and effectiveness of the particular therapy or educational plan. For children with identified problems or global delays (such as mental retardation or attention deficit disorder), school entry can be a particularly challenging time for parents who may have been able to deny the extent of their child's learning problems during the preschool period. Parents often look to clinicians for projections about their child's future, thus it is important to provide realistic, but hopeful, parameters for families.

B. **Behavioral issues.** School placement for children who present with either acting out, impulsive behaviors or extremely shy, inhibited behaviors should be carefully considered. Some school settings are a bad fit for these children. Due to overcrowding, inadequate teaching, or the overwhelming needs of the larger school population, withdrawn or inhibited children who cause no trouble can be ignored as attention goes to more aggressive or demanding children. Similarly, disruptive children or those with impulse control problems can be quickly identified as difficult students even if they are quite bright. Parents and clinicians must be vigilant in addressing the issues behind the labeling so that the label does not become a self-fulfilling prophecy for the child.

C. **Is the school ready for the child?** Perhaps the most challenging task for clinicians is to help families negotiate school entrance when the school does not have appropriate options for children with particular special needs. Although schools are required to educate all children within the least restrictive environment, they are often unable to provide carefully planned learning experiences for children with significant emotional or technological needs. Some schools cannot provide the developmentally appropriate experiences needed by children who have experienced such trauma as extreme poverty, child abuse, domestic violence or substance abuse. Finally, many schools do not have the resources to cope with the increasing linguistic demands of children who have recently immigrated to this country. Clinicians have tremendous untapped power to advocate on behalf of these children. They need to join voices with the families to persuade schools to provide appropriate educational experiences for the children.

D. **Waiting another year.** School entrance deadlines are arbitrarily set, based as much on demographics and finances (how many young children are in the upcoming kindergarten cohort and does the school have the space and teaching resources to provide for them if the cutoff date is June or November?) as they are on best practice. There is no magic age when all children are optimally ready for school. It is important to support parents of "late summer and fall" babies as they think through the options available to them and their child, by exploring:

1. "Will there be appropriate social and learning peers for the child?"
2. "Will there be adequate new challenges for the child?"
3. "Are the child's physical appearance and social skills in line with the proposed preschool placement? This may differ for boys and girls."
4. "Do both parents agree with the decision to retain the child in preschool?"
5. "Does the program agree with the parents' decision to retain the child for another year?"
6. "What is the community norm? Do many parents hold back their 'fall' children?"
7. "What does the child expect to happen? Will the child perceive staying in preschool as a failure if everyone else goes on the kindergarten?"
8. "If needed, will supplemental interventions and extra support such as speech therapy by provided?"

If the parents decide to send the child on to elementary school:

1. "What options might be available now for preparing the child for school entry?"
2. Parents can ask for the upcoming class list and arrange for their child to spend time with a few children who will be in the same class. Seeing familiar faces when entering a new school can be extremely reassuring, especially to shy or slow-to-warm-up children.
3. "Does the school have options for additional support for the child such as a transitional classroom, a second year of kindergarten if warranted, resource room support or afterschool programming?"

If the child begins to have serious problems in school, it is important to acknowledge the placement mistake early on, rather than continuing to push the child ahead in the hope that he or she will catch up. It is much easier to retain a child for a second year in kindergarten or first grade than it is to repeat the fourth grade where serious learning problems may prevent the child from keeping up. Many parents report that their young or immature children do all right in the first half of the school year when much of the work is review, but that they encounter significant and disheartening failure during the second half of the school year as teachers push children to master the required curriculum. Because school learning and success are so closely related to lifelong self-esteem, initial placement decisions should be taken seriously and careful thought given to possible retention if the child is struggling in kindergarten or first grade.

BIBLIOGRAPHY

For Parents

Ryan B. *Helping Your Child Start School: A Practical Guide for Parents.* Citadel Trade, 1996.

Walmsley BB, Walmsley SA. *Kindergarten: Ready or Not?: A Parent's Guide.* Heinemann Publishing, 1996.

For Children

Cohen M, Hoban L. *Will I Have a Friend?* Aladin Paperbacks, 1986.

Wing N, Durrell J. *The Night Before Kindergarten.* Grosset & Dunlap, 2001.

For Professionals

American Academy of Pediatrics Policy, "The Inappropriate Use of School Readiness Tests". http://www.aap.org/policy/00694.html

Palfrey JS, Rappaport LR.School Placement. *Pediatr Rev* 8:261–270, 1987.

ReadyWeb http://readyweb.crc.uiuc.edu/library.html

65

Selective Mutism

Naomi Steiner

I. **Description of the problem.** Selective mutism is a **childhood anxiety disorder** and can be seen as the symptomatic expression of social anxiety in an **extremely shy child**. It is characterized by:
- A child's **inability to speak in certain social settings** (such as daycare, school) where speaking is expected, **despite speaking in other, usually more familiar, settings** (such as at home).
- Onset **usually before age 5 years**, although it may not come to clinical attention until school entry
- **Lasting for at least 1 month** (not including the first month of school or child care, during which many children may be shy or reluctant to speak).

A. **Epidemiology.**
- Limited research reports a **prevalence of 0.1%–0.7 %** in the general population and 1% of children in mental health centers.
- At least **90% of these children also have social phobia** (social anxiety disorder).
- Girls outnumber boys 2 to 1.
- Although selective mutism usually lasts for only a few months, it may persist longer and may even continue for several years.

B. **Etiology/contributing factors.**
1. **Genetic predisposition.** There is often a first degree family history of social phobia (70%) and selective mutism (37%).
2. **Speech and language delays** are present in 20%–30 % (most commonly language and articulation disorders).
3. **Bilingualism.** Immigrant children who are unfamiliar with or uncomfortable in a new language may refuse to speak to strangers in their new environment; this behavior should not be misdiagnosed as selective mutism. However, a prolonged silent phase should be seen as a potential red flag when selective mutism and language delay should be considered.
4. Contrary to popular belief, **no research has associated selective mutism with abuse, neglect or trauma**.

II. **Making the diagnosis.** Initial screenings are simple, involving some observation and a few questions. The classic sign of selective mutism is that the child talks well within the home but not outside social settings.

A. **Behavioral observations.**
- Symptoms of withdrawal in unfamiliar situations, difficulty with eye contact, avoidance of social interaction, stiff body language, blank facial expression, using only gestures to communicate in the office.
- Marked contrast between selected environments and **the home situation,** where parents often report a very chatty child. Clinicians may want to view a videotape of child at home to be reassured that the child's language in a comfortable environment is normal.
- Shy children will "button up" and not speak for a few hours or days but will eventually start speaking. A shy child can function. Those with selected mutism will not speak for a prolonged period of time, causing significant and prolonged social dysfunction.

B. **History: Key clinical questions.**
- *"How was your child as an infant or toddler?"*
- *"How is he at school? Or birthday parties?"*
- *"How is he at home?"*
- *"Is there anybody in your family with selective mutism, anxiety, panic attacks, extreme shyness or other emotional issues?"*

C. **Differential diagnosis.** In the past, selective mutism was sometimes misunderstood as a strong-willed and manipulative child *refusing* to speak (as in oppositional defiant disorder), as opposed to a child conditioned by a true fear of speaking. It should be distinguished from speech disturbances that are **better accounted for by a commu-**

nication disorder such as phonological disorder or developmental language disorder. Individuals with pervasive developmental disorder or mental retardation may have problems in social communication and be unable to speak appropriately in social situations. However, in contrast, in selective mutism the child has an established capacity to speak in some social situations, e.g., typically at home.

    D. Tests.

        1. Audiogram —as with any speech and language disorder, it's always prudent to assure normal hearing.

        2. Speech and language evaluation is often indicated as 20%–30 % of children with selective mutism also have some speech and language delay. This may be very difficult to obtain as the stress of the testing situation may preclude optimal testing in which case a videotape may suffice.

III. Management.

    A. Early diagnosis and rapid referral is essential for the child with selective mutism. Children with selective mutism do not necessarily outgrow their disability. Many may start to speak a little, others spend years growing up without speaking. If these children do not learn to cope they may remain significantly impaired compared to their unaffected peers. The overall goal is to treat the anxiety rather than force the child to speak.

        1. Team approach. Family, school and therapist should work together to develop an individualized plan to **reduce anxiety, reduce pressure to speak and increase self-esteem**. Consistent, supportive relationships out side the home are the mainstay of achieving these goals.

        2. Behavioral therapy. Positive reinforcement encourages all forms of communication, nonverbal (smiling, pointing) or verbal (whispering to selected friends or adults). Desensitization offers situations where the child is able to practice speaking.

        3. Cognitive behavioral therapy can help the child work towards specific goals.

        4. Other psychological therapies such as play therapy. May allow the child to express themself without pressure and without words.

        5. Medication in combination with therapy is used in the most chronic cases. Selective serotonin reuptake inhibitors (SSRIs), most commonly fluoxetine, have been shown to have a positive effect as they lower the anxiety threshold. They are usually given for 9–12 months.

BIBLIOGRAPHY

For Parents

Selective Mutism www.selectivemutism.org
Anxiety Network www.anxietynetwork.com

For Professionals

Black B Uhde TW. Psychiatric characteristics of children with selective mutism: a pilot study. *J Am Acad Child Adolesc Psychiatry* 34:847–856, 1995.
Dow SP, et al. Practical guidelines for the assessment and treatment of selective mutism *JAACAP* 34:836–846, 1995.
Dummit ES III, Klein RG, Trancer NK, et al. Systematic assessment of 50 children with selective mutism. *J Am Acad Child Adolesc Psychiatry* 36:653–660, 1997.
Stein M (ed). Selective mutism. *J Develop & Behav Pediatrics* 22(Suppl 2):S123–S126, 2001.

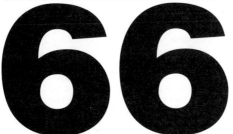

Self-Esteem and Resilience

Robert B. Brooks

I. **Description of the problem.** Self-esteem plays a significant role in virtually every sphere of a child's development and functioning. Performance in school, the quality of peer relationships, the ease and effectiveness of dealing with mistakes and failure, the motivation to persevere at tasks, and the abuse of drugs and alcohol are behaviors influenced by a child's self-esteem.

Self-esteem is also implicated strongly in whether or not a child is resilient. Resilience may be understood as **the capacity of a child to deal effectively with stress and pressure, to cope with everyday challenges, to rebound from disappointments, mistakes, trauma, and adversity, to develop clear and realistic goals, to solve problems, to interact comfortably with others, and to treat oneself and others with respect and dignity.** Given the importance of self-esteem and resilience and the number of children who are burdened by low self-esteem, it is a worthwhile goal of the primary care clinician to become knowledgeable about effective strategies to foster a child's sense of self-worth, competence, hope, and resilience.

Some clinicians have proposed that self-esteem is a product of the difference between our "ideal self," or how we would like to be and what we would like to accomplish, and how we actually see ourselves—the larger the difference, the lower our self esteem. A broader definition was offered by the California Task Force to Promote Self-Esteem and Personal and Social Responsibility, which envisioned self-esteem not only in terms of "appreciating my own worth and importance" but also "having the character to be accountable for myself and to act responsibly toward others." This definition incorporates the respect and caring we show toward others as a basic feature of self-esteem, thereby lessening the possibility that self-esteem will be confused with conceit or self-centeredness.

A. **Etiology/contributing factors.**

1. **Parent–child "goodness of fit".** The development of self-esteem and resilience is a complex process that can best be understood as occurring within the dynamic interaction between a child's inborn temperament and the environmental forces that affect the child. "Mismatches" between the style and temperament of caregivers and children may trigger anger and disappointment in both parties. In such a situation children may come to believe that they have disappointed others, that they are failures, or that others are unfair and unkind. Low self-esteem and a sense of pessimism are common outcomes unless parents are able to lessen the impact of these mismatches by understanding and appreciating their child's unique make-up and by modifying their own expectations and reactions so that they are more in concert with their child's temperament.

2. **Attribution theory.** Attribution theory is one promising framework for articulating the components of self-esteem by looking at the reasons that people offer for why they think they succeeded or failed at a task or situation. The explanations given are directly linked to an individual's self-esteem and resilience. It appears that children with high self-esteem perceive their successes as determined in large part by their own efforts, resources, and abilities (internal locus of control). These children assume realistic credit for their achievements and possess a sense of personal control over what is occurring in their lives. This feeling of personal control is one of the foundations of a resilient mindset and lifestyle.

   In contrast, children with low self-esteem often believe that their successes are the result of luck or chance and factors outside their control. Such a view lessens their confidence in being successful in the future.

   Self-esteem also plays a role in how children understand mistakes and failures in their lives. Children with high self-esteem typically believe that mistakes are experiences to learn from rather than to feel defeated by. Mistakes are attributed to factors within their power to change, such as a lack of effort on a realistically attainable goal. Children who possess this view are better equipped to deal with setbacks and, thus, are more resilient.

On the other hand, children with low self-esteem, when faced with failure, tend to believe that they cannot remedy the situation. They believe that mistakes result from situations that are not modifiable, such as a lack of ability, and this belief generates a feeling of helplessness and hopelessness. This profound sense of inadequacy makes future success less likely because these children expect to fail and begin to retreat from age-expected demands, relying instead on self-defeating coping strategies. Resilience is noticeably absent when a child's life is dominated by feelings of resignation and hopelessness.

Attribution theory has significant implications for designing interventions for reinforcing self-esteem, optimism, and resilience in children. It serves as a blueprint for asking the following questions:

- "How do we create an environment in homes and schools that maximizes the opportunity for children not only to succeed but to believe that their accomplishments are predicated in great measure on their own abilities and efforts?"
- "How do we create an environment that reinforces the belief in children that mistakes and failure often form the very foundation for learning and growth–that mistakes are not only *accepted* but *expected*?"

These are important questions to address since a feeling of being in control of and taking responsibility for one's life and dealing effectively with mistakes and setbacks are significant features of resilience.

II. **Making the diagnosis.** The signs of low self-esteem and limited resilience vary considerably. Children may display low self-esteem in situations in which they feel less than competent but not in those in which they are more successful. For instance, children with a learning disability may feel "dumb" in the classroom but may engage in sports with confidence. For some children, a sense of low self-esteem is so pervasive that there are few, if any, situations in which low self-esteem is not manifested.

With some children there is little question that their self-esteem is low or that they are not very resilient. They say such things as, "I'm dumb," "I hate how I look," "I never do anything right," "I always fail," "I'm a born loser," "I'll always be stupid."

Other children do not directly express their low self-esteem. Rather, it can be inferred from the coping strategies they use to handle stress and pressure. Children with high self-esteem use strategies for coping that are adaptive and promote growth (such as a child having difficulty mastering long division who asks for additional help from a teacher). They demonstrate a feeling of hope.

In contrast, children with low self-esteem often rely on coping behaviors that are counterproductive and intensify the child's difficulties. These self-defeating behaviors typically signal that the child is feeling vulnerable and is desperately attempting to escape from the problematic situations. Commonly used self-defeating coping behaviors are listed in Table 66-1. Although all children at some time engage in some of these behaviors, it is when these behaviors appear with regularity that a significant problem with self-esteem is suggested.

III. **Management.**
A. **Primary goals.** The strategies that follow have the greatest chance of being effective if adults convey to the child a sense of hope, caring, and support. It is well established that a basic foundation of resilience in children is the **presence of at least one adult (hopefully, several) who believes in the worth and goodness of the child**. The late psychologist Julius Segal referred to that person as a "charismatic adult," an adult from whom a child "gathers strength." Primary care clinicians, even in brief encounters with a child, can become charismatic adults for that child.

Table 66-1 Counterproductive coping strategies: signs of low self-esteem

Behavior	Example
Quitting	Ending a game before it is over to avoid losing
Avoiding	Not even trying something for fear of failure
Cheating	Copying answers from someone else on a test
Clowning around	Acting silly to minimize feeling like a failure
Controlling	Telling others what to do
Bullying	Putting others down to hide feelings of inadequacy
Denying	Minimizing the importance of a task
Rationalizing or making excuses	Blaming the teacher for failing a test

Strategies to nurture self-esteem and resilience should take into consideration the child's *islands of competence*, that is, areas that are (or have the potential to be) sources of pride and accomplishment. Caregivers have the responsibility to identify and build on these islands of competence, and, in so doing, a ripple effect may occur that prompts children to be more willing to venture forth and confront the tasks that have been problematic for them.

B. **Selected strategies for fostering self-esteem and resilience.**

1. **Developing responsibility and making a contribution.** If children are to develop a sense of ownership and commitment, it is important to provide them with opportunities for assuming responsibilities, especially those that involve helping them to feel that they are capable and are contributing in some way to their world and that they are truly making a difference. For example:

   • Asking an 8-year-old to set the table at dinner or a 4-year-old to place his clothes in the laundry bag at the end of each day—requests framed as ways of helping the family.

   • Encouraging and helping a child to write a story about his learning disability to be used to increase the understanding of others about the challenges faced by children with learning problems.

   • Asking a sixth grader with low self-esteem who enjoyed interacting with younger children to tutor first and second graders in the school or to be a babysitter.

   • Enlisting children to participate in a "Walk for Hunger" charity drive.

2. **Providing opportunities for making choices and decisions and solving problems.** An essential ingredient of high self-esteem and resilience is the belief that one has some control over the events of one's life. To reinforce this belief, adults must provide children with opportunities to make choices and decisions, and to solve problems that have an impact on their lives. These kinds of choices promote a sense of personal control and ownership. For example:

   • A clinician allowing a fearful child the choice of having his eyes or ears examined first, so that the child is provided a sense of control.

   • Parents permitting a finicky eater to select (and eventually help prepare) the dinner meal at least once a week.

   • Having a group of elementary school students interview a town selectman, a police officer, and a lawyer as part of the process to decide whether skateboards should be allowed on school grounds, especially given the possible liability issues.

   • Parents asking their children whether they wanted to be reminded 10 or 15 minutes before bedtime that soon it will be time to get ready to go to bed.

   • A teenager deciding at what time parents may remind him to take medication, should he or she forget to do so.

3. **Offering encouragement and positive feedback and helping children to feel special.** Self-esteem and resilience are reinforced when adults communicate appreciation and encouragement to children. Words and actions conveying encouragement and thanks are always welcome and energizing. They are especially important for children burdened by self-doubt. Even a seemingly small gesture of appreciation can trigger a long lasting, positive effect. For example:

   • Parents setting up a "special" 15-minute time in the evening with each of their two young children. The time can occur before each child goes to bed. The parents can highlight the importance of this time by calling it "special" and by saying that even if the telephone rings they will not respond to the call but instead will let the answering machine do so.

   • A primary care clinician sending a postcard to a child after an examination, saying how much he or she enjoyed seeing the child (as long as this is an honest sentiment).

   • Parents writing a brief note to their child commending the child for a particular accomplishment.

   • A recognition assembly in school in which student achievements and contributions are highlighted.

4. **Establishing self-discipline.** If children are to develop high self-esteem, they must also possess a comfortable sense of self-discipline, which involves the ability **to reason and to reflect on one's behavior and its impact on others**. The goal of discipline is to teach children, not to ridicule or humiliate them. If children are to take ownership for their actions and become resilient, they must be increasingly involved in the process of understanding and even contributing to the rules, guidelines, limits, and consequences that are established. Adults must maintain a delicate balance between being too rigid and too permissive. They must strive to blend warmth, nurturance, and acceptance with realistic expectations, clear-cut rules, and

logical consequences. In addition, if children are continuously misbehaving, the adults in their lives should attempt to understand why and focus on ways to prevent misbehavior from occurring in the first place. Examples of the effective use of discipline—including those that emphasize a preventive approach—are:

- Parents having difficulty getting a preschool child to bed. They yelled, but this only made matters worse. A consultation with a clinician revealed that the child was having nightmares and was frightened about going to bed. Greater empathy on the part of the parents and the use of a nightlight, as well as placing a photo of the parents next to the child's bed, significantly lessened his anxiety and misbehavior.
- Parents not permitting their child to use the bike for several days after he had taken a bike ride on a dangerous street that he was not allowed to ride on (an example of the use of logical consequences).
- Parents asking a child who bounced a ball that broke a window in the house to help pay for the repairs.

5. **Teaching children to deal with mistakes and failure.** The fear of making mistakes and feeling embarrassed is a potent obstacle to meeting challenges, taking appropriate risks, and therefore, to the achievement of positive self-esteem and resilience. Caregivers should find ways to communicate to children that mistakes go hand in glove with growing and learning. Examples of helping children to deal more effectively with mistakes include:

- Parents who avoid overreacting to their children's mistakes and who avoid remarks such as "Why don't you use your brain?" or "What a stupid thing to do!"
- Adults who share what they personally learned from mistakes and failures during their own childhood.
- A teacher who on the first day of the new school year asks students, "Who thinks they will probably make a mistake or not understand something in class this year?" Then, before any of the children can respond, the teacher raises his own hand. Acknowledging openly the fear of failure renders it less potent and less destructive and increases the child's courage to face new tasks. This courage is a major characteristic of resilient children.

BIBLIOGRAPHY

For Parents

Books

Brooks R, Goldstein S. *Raising Resilient Children: Fostering Strength, Hope, and Optimism in Your Child.* New York: Contemporary Books, 2001.
Brooks R, Goldstein S. *Nurturing Resilience in Our Children: Answers to the Most Important Parenting Questions.* New York: Contemporary Books, 2003.
Samalin N. *Loving without Spoiling and 100 Other Timeless Tips for Raising Terrific Kids.* New York: Contemporary Books, 2003.

Websites for Parents and Professionals

National PTA http://www.pta.org/parentinvolvement/helpchild/hc_IO_self_esteem.asp
Community Learning Network http://www.cln.org/themes/self_esteem.html
www.drrobertbrooks.com

For Professionals

Brooks R. *The Self-Esteem Teacher.* Circle Pines, MN: American Guidance Service, 1991.
Katz, M. *On Playing a Poor Hand Well.* New York: Norton, 1997.
Shure, M. *Raising a Thinking Child.* New York: Holt, 1994.

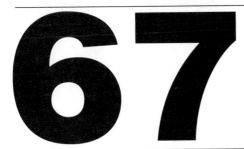

Sensory Integration Disorder

Marie E. Anzalone

I. **Description of the problem.** Sensory integration disorder (SID, also referred to as dysfunction in sensory processing disorder, or SPD) refers to problems in organizing and using sensory information from both the environment and the body. The ability to integrate or process sensory information is a temperament related process that varies in children and, if problematic, may interfere with the child's ability to participate in activities and relationships and affect learning capacities.

Dysfunction of sensory integration can be seen in three different domains.
- Problems with **sensory modulation**
  - **over responsive** to sensory input with or without sensory avoidance
  - **under responsivity** to sensory input or sensory seeking
- Problems with **discrimination or perception of sensory input**
- Problems with **motor performance** that require sensory input (dyspraxia, or postural disorders)

Underlying problems in sensory integration are often expressed clinically as **poor self-regulation of arousal, attention, affect, and action.** These symptoms may then contribute to functional difficulties in play, peer relationships, and school performance.

  A. **Epidemiology.** No empirical studies have been conducted on the incidence of sensory processing or integrative disorders. Clinicians report higher incidence of SID disorders in boys than girls. Families often report similar untreated traits in parents of identified children. In addition, SID may be present in children with varying diagnoses including autism, nonverbal learning disabilities, attention deficit hyperactivity disorder (ADHD), and developmental coordination disorder.

  B. **Etiology/contributing factors.** The etiology of sensory processing disorder is not known. It is known that children with sensory modulation disorders have atypical autonomic (both sympathetic and parasympathetic) responses to sensory challenges. It is hypothesized, but not verified, that the underlying processes contributing to SID are temperamentally related differences in the way sensory input in processed in the central nervous system. While individual temperamental differences are considered the basis of SID, the ultimate expression of that challenge is often dependent upon the children's interaction with their environments. Social environments that are responsive to the child's cues and thereby providing an optimal goodness-of-fit with the child's sensory needs and motor capacities can decrease behavioral disorganization, thus forming the theoretical basis of intervention.

II. **Making the diagnosis.**
  A. **Signs and symptoms.**
    1. **Sensory modulation disorder (SMD).** Sensory modulation is the process of **grading and regulating one's response to sensory input**. It is dependent upon:
       - The subjective interpretation of the intensity of both internal and external stimuli
       - How sensation interacts with the child's previous experiences and baseline state of arousal
       - The child's ability to organize regulated behavior.

       Table 67-1 outlines the behavioral manifestation of this self-regulation in four different types of sensory modulation disorder.
    2. **Sensory discrimination disorder** is characterized by a **deficit in perception or discrimination** in one or more sensory modalities (including vision, tactile, proprioception/kinesthesia). Poor discrimination involves:
       - Decreased perception of salient qualities of stimuli (including temporal and spatial qualities)
       - Possible co-occurrence with sensory under-responsivity or dyspraxia
       - Functional sequelae including associated learning disorders, dysgraphia, awkward gross or fine motor coordination, and limited play schemas

Table 67-1 Behavioral regulation in children with different types of sensory modulation disorder

	Sensory Over-Responsivity (SOR)	Sensory Avoidant (a subgroup of SOR)	Sensory Under-Responsivity (SUR)	Sensory Seeking
Arousal	Usually high arousal	Attempts to modulate arousal, so often (not always) appears calm	Usually decreased arousal	Arousal may be heightened, but labile
Attention	Inability to focus attention, distractible	Hyper-vigilant, since need to "scan" for sensory threats	Inattentive, has a latency to attend, lack of awareness of novelty	Poorly modulated attention
Affect	Predominantly negative affect— often in "fight or flight" state	Fearful or anxious—when older may be demanding	Restricted or flat affect—may appear sad or emotionally unavailable	Affect is variable, but may become over-excited with excess sensory input
Action	Impulsive reaction—may seem aggressive	Constrained, and often avoids developmentally appropriate exploration	Passive—may observe other children, but not engage in active peer play	Action is geared primarily to gaining sensation, may be impulsive and take excess risks

3. **Sensory-based motor disorders.** There are two different types of sensory-based motor disorders: **dyspraxia** and **postural disorders**.
   a. *Dyspraxia* is an **inability to formulate, plan, and execute unfamiliar complex motor acts**. Motor praxis occurs in three steps:
      - **Ideation** (the cognitive process of formulating a goal for action that is dependent upon perception of salient aspects of the environment)
      - **Motor planning** (the planning and sequencing of action)
      - **Execution** (the actual observed motor action)

      Children with dyspraxia may have problems in one or more of these steps. All children with dyspraxia appear **clumsy** or **accident-prone**, and tend to avoid unfamiliar gross and fine motor actions while inflexibly relying on the "over learned" activities. Children may also have difficulty initiating age-appropriate action or play schemes and prefer familiar to novel situations. When motor planning is involved, children may have poor timing, grading, and accuracy of movement, poor handwriting, inability to imitate static or dynamic postures, or exhibit general sloppiness in schoolwork. Motor planning problems may result in difficulty learning new motor tasks or generalizing a learned skill to new situations.

      Motor planning deficits are also associated with a poorly developed somatosensory-based body scheme that is characterized by a poor awareness of where the body is in space and judging where their body is in relation to objects. They tend to bump into things and/or have poorly guided movements.

      Children with dyspraxia, often aware of their difficulty in learning and performing motor actions, may have low self-esteem, a low frustration tolerance, engage in controlling behaviors, prefer sedentary or language-based activities, and prefer to play with children significantly younger or older than they are.
   b. **Postural disorders** are characterized by difficulty moving, stabilizing, and adjusting posture. It is often associated with neurological soft signs such as mild hypotonia, poor bilateral coordination, and poor equilibrium reactions. These disorders are thought to be associated with poor processing of vestibular and proprioceptive input. Postural disorders often occur in combination with sensory modulation and discrimination disorders or dyspraxia.

B. **Differential diagnosis.** SID is not a discrete medical diagnosis, but is often seen as a dimension of other diagnoses such as learning disabilities, autism, or ADHD. SID, as described in this chapter, is consistent with, and does not need to be differentiated from, a *regulatory disorder* (as outlined in the Diagnostic Classification of Mental Health and Developmental and Disorders of Infancy and Early Childhood [DC:0-3]). Sensory-based motor disorders are considered to be subtypes of developmental coordination disorder (DCD) as described in DSM-IV. Sensory modulation disorders should be differentiated from a purely *behavioral* patterns in which children exhibit undesired behaviors (e.g., hand flapping).

SID should be considered when behavior management techniques result in one behavior being extinguished, only to be replaced by another undesired behavior that provides similar sensory input. It should also be noted that a diagnosis of sensory integrative disorder should only be made when sensory preferences **interfere with the child's function;** not all stylistic differences in sensory processing are indicative of dysfunction. Finally, parents are frequently confused because different professionals label/diagnose these behaviors differently.

C. **History: Key clinical questions.**
   1. **Developmental history.** Parents of children with sensory integrative dysfunction usually report development histories that are within low normal limits. If present, delays are most often seen in gross motor area with late onset walking and limited flexibility in the generalization of new skills.
   2. **Sensory history.** The historian often reports **unusual sensory avoidances** or **craving** and concomitant behavioral disorganization in children with sensory processing disorder. These tendencies are often longstanding, even though not problematic until the children reach school age. Problematic behaviors may be inconsistent (i.e., present in the evening, but not in the morning; or present when touched, but not when the child touches).
   3. **Key clinical questions.**
      - *"Does the child have sensory preferences or avoidances in attention and learning? Are these preferences inconsistent?"*
      - *"Does the child overreact to input in particular modalities? Does the child express and appropriate range of affect in response to sensory input?"*

- *"Was the child unusually fussy, difficult to console, or easily startled as an infant?"*
- *"Did the child have difficulty regulating sleep/wake cycle—settling for sleep, staying asleep, and waking without irritability or strongly dislike baths, haircuts, or nail cutting?"*
- *"Does the child use an inappropriate amount of force when handling objects, coloring, writing, or interacting with siblings or pets?"*
- *"How does the child manage transitions and changes in daily routines? Is there a predictable time of day or type of activity when the child is most and least organized?"*
- *"Does the child need more practice than other children to learn new skills?"*
- *"Is the child clumsy, fall frequently, bump into furniture or people, or have trouble judging position of body in relation to surrounding space?"*

III. Management.

A. Evaluation. If sensory processing problems are suspected, an occupational therapy evaluation should be performed. The evaluation should include both standardized testing, as well as informal observation by a qualified specialist. Since children with sensory processing disorder often have concomitant learning or behavioral disorders, a multidisciplinary team evaluation and treatment plan may be indicated.

B. Parent education. Parents of children with sensory processing disorder need help understanding the problematic behaviors. There should be three goals for this education:
- To help parents understand their child's unique sensory profile
- To help them create a better goodness of fit between their child's needs and the sensory-motor challenges in their environment
- To encourage parents to support the child's self-esteem and social participation

Parents may need help to **understand their child's affective response to sensation** (e.g., pulling back from hugs may be due to hypersensitivity but may be interpreted as withdrawing from social contact). It is also important to share information with parents about what types of behaviors to observe after changes in routines or environment (e.g., autonomic signs, increased arousal, and more disorganization during holiday chaos).

While structure and predictability are important for some children, a sense of novelty is essential for others to encourage sensory-based exploration. The pediatric clinician, in addition to the occupational therapist, is essential in developing parental understanding and enhancing their ability to advocate for their child across contexts.

C. Intervention. Direct and indirect strategies for sensory integration disorder are usually provided by specially trained occupational therapists. The goals of the intervention should be individualized based on each child's unique sensory and motor profile. Direct intervention usually requires a specialized treatment environment to enable flexible enhancements of sensory and motor challenges, and works toward integrating improved sensory-based self-regulatory abilities into social and functional participation. Indirect strategies and consultation should be implemented to improve goodness-of-fit in school or other environments.

BIBLIOGRAPHY

For Parents

Books

Heller S. *Too Loud, Too Bright, Too Fast, Too Tight: What to Do If You Are Sensory Defensive in an Over Stimulating World.* New York: Harper Collins, 2002.

Kranowitz CS. *The Out of Sync Child: Recognizing and Coping with Sensory Integrative Dysfunction.* New York: Perigee, 1998.

Websites

Sensory Integration Network http://www.sinetwork.org

Come Unity: Children's disabilities and special needs (sensory integration) http://www.comeunity.com/disability/sensory_integration

For Professionals

Bundy AC, Lane SJ, Murray, EA (eds). *Sensory Integration: Theory and Practice (2nd ed).* Philadelphia: FA Davis Co., (2002).

Mangeot SD, Miller LJ, McIntosh DN, et al. Sensory modulation dysfunction in children with attention-deficit-hyperactivity disorder. *Dev Med Child Neurol* 43:399–406, 2001.

Williamson GG, Anzalone ME. *Sensory integration and self-regulation in infants and toddlers: Helping young children to interact with their environments.* Washington, DC: Zero-to-Three, 2001.

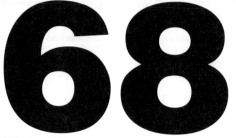

Sex and the Adolescent

Linda Grant

I. **Description of the problem.** The expression of human sexuality is the result of a complex interplay of biologic, psychological, interpersonal, and social factors—each with varying importance as the child grows up. In adolescence, the newly discovered ability to engage in sexual activity implies neither the cognitive and emotional maturity to deal with intimacy nor an understanding of its negative consequences (such as premature pregnancy and sexually transmitted diseases). It is the role of the primary care clinician to: (1) prepare the family to guide their adolescent through puberty and (2) guide the adolescent in *responsible sexual decision making.*

   A. **Epidemiology.**
       1. **Teenage pregnancy.**
           - The United States has a higher rate of teenage pregnancy than any other industrialized country.
           - There are 800,000 pregnancies in 15–19 year olds annually. Approximately half of these are carried to term; the other half are therapeutically or spontaneously terminated.
           - The rate of teen pregnancy has been decreasing over the last decade, while the number of sexually active teens is increasing.
       2. **Sexual experience.**
           - There is no one profile of adolescent sexuality. Trends in coital initiation and continuation of sexual activity reflect differing ethnic and sex-specific rates. There are also few methodically sound scientific investigations of teen sexuality, due to the controversial nature of interviewing adolescents about their sexual behavior.
           - In general, the majority of adolescents are virginal at age 15 years; by the senior year in high school, approximately 60% are coitally experienced.
           - Males consistently report earlier coital initiation than females.
           - Noncoital sexual behaviors vary by ethnic group. Studies indicate that white adolescents, in general, start with petting behaviors and move to greater intimacy in a sequential manner. Black adolescents are more likely to engage in intercourse sooner and without much initial petting behaviors.
           - Gay, lesbian, bisexual, and transgender adolescents have higher rates of attempted and completed suicide, violence victimization, substance abuse and HIV risk. Most have an awareness of their orientation by the age of 9 or 10.
       3. **Sexually transmitted diseases.**
           - The 15–24-year-old age group has a higher rate of most sexually transmitted diseases (e.g., gonorrhea, chlamydia, pelvic inflammatory disease) than any other age group.
           - 25% of 20–29 year olds who have AIDS were infected during their adolescence.

   B. **Developmental considerations.**
       1. **Dealing with body changes.** Adolescents must learn to be comfortable with their new physical identity. Puberty is a time when they come to terms with a changing body and bewildering emotions fueled by hormonal surges. The reproductive capacity, however, is present well before emotional and cognitive maturity have developed.
       2. **Developing a separate identity.** The adolescent must develop an identity that is separate from the family. Sexual behavior is often viewed as a rite of passage into adulthood and as a way to become a distinct entity from the family. As adolescents separate from the family, they develop replacement relationships with their peers.
       3. **Developing intimate relationships.** Another task of adolescence is to achieve the capacity to develop intimate and meaningful mutual relationships. Early relationships may involve physical intimacy as a means of comparison and experimentation. Later, with the addition of formal operational thinking, emotional intimacy and reciprocity can be incorporated into relationships.
       4. **Developing the ability to think abstractly.** Concrete operational thinking dominates

early and mid-adolescence. Therefore, young adolescents are incapable of fully understanding the ramifications of their actions. This, coupled with a sense of infallibility and invulnerability, heightens the risk for sexual activity. Formal operational thinking, which develops around age 15 years, allows the adolescent to generate a more appropriate decision-making tree and to develop abstract thinking on moral values.

5. **Personality characteristics.** The degree of any risk-taking behavior in adolescence is mitigated by the individual's personality profile. In general those with low self-esteem, a tolerance for deviant behavior, and a propensity for sensation-seeking are at highest risk. Those who place a high value on achievement and future orientation and who have strong religious beliefs are generally in lower-risk categories.

II. **Making the diagnosis.**

A. **History.** The key to engaging adolescents is providing a trusting, confidential, non-judgmental, and honest atmosphere. In order for adolescents to talk about their risk behaviors with the primary care clinician, they must be assured that disclosure will not compromise their relationships with their family, their friends, or the community. Adolescents often resist medical visits because they fear that the information will be shared with the parent. **It is important to establish with them that what is said will be confidential and to inform them of any qualifying parameters.** For example, when an adolescent's or another's safety is jeopardized (as in suicidal or homicidal ideation, physical or sexual abuse, and life-threatening illnesses), confidentiality may need to be breached. Informing the adolescent and his or her parent of these guidelines at the initial visit allows for a clarifying discussion of safety, communication, and trust. Clinicians should be aware of their state's statutes regarding mature and emancipated minors.

The sexual history should be part of a larger sociologic history that screens for all risk behaviors. The goal of a sexual history is to determine if there has been sexual activity and if so, the degree of health or emotional risk involved. Questioning needs to be direct and comprehensive. The clinician should make no a priori assumptions about the sexual activity, practices, or sexual orientation of any adolescent.

B. **Key clinical questions.**

1. *"Are you currently in a relationship?"*
2. *"Does this relationship include having sex?"*
3. *"What kind of protection do you use to avoid pregnancy and sexually transmitted diseases?"*
4. *"Have you ever had any sexually transmitted disease?"*
5. *"How many partners have you had?"*
6. *"How old were you when you first had intercourse?"*
7. *"What made you decide to have sex?"*
8. *"Has anyone ever forced you to have sex?"*
9. *"Have you ever been pregnant? What happened to the pregnancy?"* or *"Have you ever fathered a child?"*
10. *"Have you ever had sex with someone of the same sex?"*
11. *"Have you ever had rectal or oral sex?"*
12. *"Is sex an enjoyable experience for you?"*
13. *"Tell me what you know about AIDS."*
14. *"What do you know about the different methods of birth control?"*
15. *"How do you feel about not being sexually active?"*

C. **Physical examination.**

1. **Pelvic examination.** Sexually active adolescents should seek preventative health care to address risks and screen for sexually transmitted diseases. However, new guidelines suggest that adolescents do not need cervical cancer screening until three years after coital initiation or the age of 21. Before that time, the need to perform a pelvic exam will depend on the gynecological symptoms, history and the availability of newer urine tests for sexually transmitted diseases.
    - There continues to be some debate as to whether to initiate a pelvic examination in an adolescent who is *not* sexually active. Variables to consider include the patient's request, the nature of the gynecologic complaint, and the gynecologic versus chronologic age of the adolescent. For the young, virginal adolescent with a gynecologic complaint, external visualization and bimanual rectal palpation and/or pelvic ultrasound may be adequate.
    - The development of a positive attitude toward pelvic examinations begins with the first. It is helpful to have the adolescent as involved as possible so that she feels in control of the process. For example, she can be asked if she wants to look

at her cervix and external genitalia in a hand-held mirror. She should also be told that the examination will be stopped if she feels pain, and she should describe any discomfort. Each step should be anticipated so that there are no surprises.

- As the examination proceeds, the clinician should continue a relaxing and empowering dialogue, such as: "In order to see your cervix, the opening into your uterus, I need you to relax your muscles as much as possible. By taking deep breaths and focusing on relaxing your muscles, your vagina will open wider and the exam will be more comfortable."

2. **Male genitalia examination.** The male examination may be anxiety provoking for the adolescent, especially when the practitioner is female (and vice versa for females, i.e., the pelvic examination performed by a male). Explanations and demonstrations of testicular self-examination as well as reassurance of normality help to relieve the anxiety. The male should be examined while standing, and it is helpful and educational to describe anatomic findings as a diversion during the examination. It is not necessary to comment on an erection unless the adolescent seems particularly embarrassed by it. The normality of the examination should always be stressed.

D. Tests. If an adolescent is sexually active, there should be routine screening for sexually transmitted diseases (STDs). In females this means at least yearly testing for gonorrhea and chlamydia. (However, screening intervals should take into account the epidemiology of the community.) Rectal and pharyngeal gonococcal cultures should be performed if there is a history of oral or rectal sex and rectal chlamydia screening in males who have receptive intercourse. A PAP smear should be performed annually. Males can be screened for asymptomatic STDs using urine dipstick testing for leukocyte esterase in areas of high STD prevalence. Both males and females should have syphilis serology testing. Adolescents should be aware of and have access to confidential and anonymous human immunodeficiency virus testing.

III. Management.

A. Anticipatory guidance. Anticipatory guidance about sexual issues should be a part of routine health care maintenance throughout childhood (Table 68-1) and adolescence (Table 68-2). Thoughtful, knowledgeable, and developmentally appropriate parental guidance as well as preparation of young children allow for a more natural dialogue about sexual issues at puberty.

B. Addressing adolescent sexuality.

1. **Primary goals.** The primary goals are to promote a healthy sexual attitude, to decrease sexual risk behaviors, and to assist parents in dealing with their child's sexuality.

2. **Developmental level.** Throughout adolescence, the progression of cognitive and emotional development influences sexual practices. A 13-year-old deals with sexuality in a different way than does a 19-year-old. The older teenager may better understand the repercussions of unprotected sex, be less dominated by the need for romantic spontaneity, and may begin to examine differential benefits and risks of various birth control methods. The younger teenager tends to be dominated more by immediate gratification, spontaneity, and peer approval. Male-oriented methods of contraception (e.g., withdrawal and condoms) tend to be more popular with the younger age group, while middle adolescents opt for pharmacologic management, whether oral, transdermal, or injectable. As adolescents mature, they develop comfort with their own bodies and a better ability to assess a situation and employ methods such as the diaphragm or the vaginal ring. The challenge is to interest adolescents in using condoms, in addition to whatever other method of birth control they may use.

3. **Empowerment.** Whether it is "saying no" or requesting that a partner use a condom, all adolescents need to hear that it is their right with whom, when, and how they express their sexuality. The clinician should help them understand that sex should never be something that is "done" to them. The practitioner can role-play situations to assist these concepts. For example, he or she can strategize empowered constructive responses to typical lines, such as "It doesn't feel as good with a rubber" or "If you really loved me you'd do it with me," or "What? You're still a virgin! I can't believe it!"

4. **Sexuality and a partner.** Involving a partner in the visit can help to facilitate joint sexual decision making and may improve compliance with safer sexual practices. Males often have no understanding of the nature of a pelvic examination. Observation of the examination can be a powerful reinforcer of mutual sexual responsibility.

5. **Promoting condoms.** If an adolescent is sexually active, condom use should be promoted at every opportunity, no matter what the nature of the office visit is.

6. **Abstinence as a healthy choice.** An adolescent needs to hear that abstaining from sexual activity is normal and is becoming increasingly common, and that

Table 68-1 Preadolescent sexuality anticipatory guidance

Age	Sexuality issues and development	Parental concerns	Areas of anticipatory guidance
Prenatal	Fetuses have been shown to suck their fingers in utero	"I don't care if it's a boy or girl as long as it's healthy" "If it's a boy, what about circumcision?" "Should I breast feed?"	Sex stereotyping: expectations for male–female differences in behavior are present even before birth. Awareness of this allows for later dialogue about expressions of individuality. Discussing circumcision provides an introduction to discussing sexually related topics. Breast-feeding discussions help emphasize importance of body contact. It is also important to stress importance of paternal body contact, cuddling, stroking.
2 wk	Temperament	"When I change the baby, his wee-wee stands up. Am I stimulating him too much?"	Use appropriate genitalia names (*penis, vagina, clitoris*) during the examination. This facilitates discussions as child ages. Infants and children enjoy and respond to touch but not with the same sexual/erotic context as adults. It is unlikely that normal touching is ever overstimulating at this age.
2 mo	Bonding	"I feel sexually aroused when I nurse." "My wife and I don't have a relationship like we used to."	Parents (both father and mother) may have erotic sensations and dreams about their child, especially in the first few months. This is normal. (Acting on one's fantasies with a child is not.) The postpartum period is often a stressful time in a previously happy relationship. The clinician may be the only medical provider involved with the family at this point and can help the parents recognize and deal with the changes a new baby brings, including changes in sexual activity.
4–6 mo	Genital play initiation Body exploration	"My son plays with his penis when I change his diaper."	Exploration of the body (toes, fingers, genitalia) is a normal aspect of human development. Self-pleasuring (thumb sucking, genital manipulation) is a natural extension of this. Masturbation continues throughout life. Start discussions early.
9–12 mo	Avoidance of stigmatization	"I'm afraid to let my daughter go without a diaper at the beach because she plays with herself."	As with other social behaviors (e.g., eating, play) sexuality and its expression must be shaped into a social context. This is a process that starts at this age and proceeds gradually to ages 3–4 yr. Shame, doubt, and confusion result from inappropriate expectations.
12–15 mo	Sex-stereotyped play	"I bought my son a doll, but he only wants to play with trucks."	Most parents would like their daughters to achieve to their abilities and sons to be empathetic and caring. Responding to the child's individuality rather than trying to alter sex-specific behaviors is the appropriate path to this goal.

(continued)

Table 68-1 Preadolescent sexuality anticipatory guidance *(continued)*

Age	Sexuality issues and development	Parental concerns	Areas of anticipatory guidance
18 mo	Toilet training	"I want her out of diapers before this baby is born."	Toilet training should be initiated on the child's schedule of readiness, not the parents'.
2–3 yr	Anatomical comparisons	"He's asking questions. What should I say?"	Simple but accurate explanations are best. If a child wants to know more and if the answer is straightforward, he will generally ask more. Pregnancy is a fascination; sibling births provide opportunities to discuss reproduction as well as feelings. Toddlers are very much aware of the anatomical similarities with the same-sex parent and the contrasts with the opposite-sex parent. They identify their concept of gender role in this manner.
	Relationships	"My son saw my husband and I having sex. Is that bad for him?"	If intercourse is explained as a way that mothers and fathers have of showing affection and love, there is no psychological trauma for the child who interrupts his parents *in flagrante delicto*. Parents should initiate discussions of privacy and closed doors.
3–4 yr	Family flirtation	"My daughter flirts with my husband. Is this normal?"	Family members are the child's source of learning about human relationships. This is a time of magical thinking when children imagine marrying their opposite-sex parent. At this time children can begin to understand parental love for each other as different from a parent's love for a child.
	Sex play with peers	"I found my 4-year-old daughter with the 4-year-old neighbor boy without any clothes."	Sex play between children of the same or opposite sexes continues through childhood without harm, as long as adults remain calm when they discover their children in these games. Children at this age can begin to understand the difference between such play with same-age children and such play with adults or older children.
4–6 yr	Sexual appropriateness	"When can I teach my child about good and bad touching?"	Children at this age can understand that their bodies are their own, that sex play between adults and children is not appropriate, that children have a right to say "no" to an adult's touching if it makes them feel funny or uncomfortable or if they don't understand what's happening.
	Modesty	"My son and daughter share a room. Is this a problem?"	The beginnings of privacy were taught with early body exploration. No matter how relaxed a child's family has been about bodies, the child's natural modesty at this age should be respected.

(continued)

Table 68-1 Preadolescent sexuality anticipatory guidance (*continued*)

Age	Sexuality issues and development	Parental concerns	Areas of anticipatory guidance
6–10 yr	Intimacy	"I've taken showers with my daughter since she was an infant. Should I stop this?"	Each family needs to decide what they are comfortable with and to discuss it. As long as feelings can be discussed openly, there should be no conflict or feelings of rejection if parent–child bathing is discontinued. There are many other comfortable ways for families to show affection.
			Children and parents sometimes find it comfortable to acknowledge that fantasies are common and are not a problem unless acted upon.
	Fantasy versus reality	"My 9-year-old son seems to have a crush on a 14-year-old neighbor boy. I'm concerned he might be gay."	Same-sex crushes are a normal part of development for both males and females and help consolidate gender identity. Discussion helps both child and parent appreciate normal development. Most who will continue with same-sex experiences recognize their homosexuality at this age.
	Out-of-home influences increase	"I won't let him watch the Playboy channel on cable so he goes next door and watches it."	Media influences are so pervasive that isolated censorship generally does not work. Open discussion of sexual themes in movies, magazines, and songs can help parents open conversations about attitudes that they are not comfortable with and allows their children to express their viewpoints.
	Sex education	"When should I be having the 'birds and the bees' talk?"	Puberty is occurring at an earlier age. The average 8-year-old is developmentally able to understand simple explanations about sexual activity. Parents should be encouraged to initiate this discussion.

Table 68-2 Anticipatory guidance for adolescent sexuality

Age	Sexual areas of concern	Risk factors	Anticipatory guidance
Early adolescence, early puberty: 10–12 yr	Pubertal changes	Self-image	Gynecomastia is normal in adolescent males as is breast asynchrony in females. Such body disproportions distort adolescents' image of themselves.
		Hormonal influences	Early maturers, particularly females, need special guidance to avoid low self-esteem and premature sexual advances.
			Masturbation is a normal behavior that relieves sexual tension. Fantasies are normal while masturbating. Masturbation is a choice—teens can choose to do it or not.
	Children with developmental disabilities		Issues of sexuality are as important to children and adolescents with disabilities as they are to other children and adolescents. Providing clinical supervision to children and adolescents with disabilities includes helping them understand their changing, maturing bodies and the choices available to them.
Late puberty: 12–14 yr	Initiation of sexual activity without intimacy	Concrete thought. Cannot perceive long-range implications of current actions	Discussions of sexual choices should emphasize that it is all right to say "no"; discussions regarding contraceptive use need to emphasize more immediate as well as long-term benefits (e.g., in addition to pregnancy prevention, oral contraceptives may relieve dysmenorrhea).
Mid-adolescence: 14–17 yr	Intimacy related to sexual romanticism rather than genuine commitment	Looks to peer group for support as he separates from family	Parents should be encouraged to continue sexual dialogue begun in latency. They should know their own values (what sex is for; who it is for; what makes it enjoyable; what makes it exploitive). Parental values should be shared with opinions, rather than judgments. Parents should respect teens' decisions.
	Sporadic or absent use of birth control; sexual experimentation	Formal operational thinking, variably applied	Teens begin to understand future implications of current actions; they know that use of birth control will protect from unwanted pregnancy, condoms will protect from sexually transmitted diseases. Adolescents at this age may believe that oral sex is not as big a deal as sexual intercourse and is safe.
		Risk taking and sense of omnipotence	Risk taking should be discussed. Once a young woman risks unprotected intercourse without becoming pregnant, she is likely to risk it again. Other risk behaviors such as drunk driving and drug use may have a negative interactive effect on sexual decision making.
Late adolescence: 17–21 yr	Intimacy involves commitment	Family conflicts resolving as independence established	Teen begins to plan for future, including marriage and family.
		Comfort with bodies and gender identity	Relationships involve a mutual reciprocity. Counseling involves understanding of female sexual response, couple discussions of feelings.

Adapted from Grant L, Efistratios D. Adolescent sexuality. *Pediatr Clin North Am* 35:1988.

masturbation and noncoital petting are acceptable ways to relieve sexual tensions safely.

7. **Contraceptive choices.** What might work for one adolescent may not work for another, irrespective of developmental level. The best contraceptive is one that will be used; the adolescent is often the best judge of which method will work best for him or her.

8. **"Teachable moments" in daily life.** Broadcast and written media offer frequent examples of sexual subject matter. News events cover stories on sexual assault and controversies over gay and lesbian issues. Rock stars use explicit language in their lyrics, and actors have explicit love scenes. Parents and clinicians should be encouraged to use these examples to initiate conversations with their children and patients around these experiences.

9. **Advertising in the waiting room.** Adolescents may need an impetus to begin discussions of sexual issues. Availability of factual sexual information in the waiting room (e.g., posters, pamphlets, books, or fact sheets) will alert the adolescent that it is acceptable to raise these issues.

10. **School-based teaching.** School systems have become increasingly active in dealing with many adolescent behavioral issues, including sexuality. Condom availability and distribution programs, for example, have been incorporated into some health programs and have been shown to support sexual responsibility. The pediatric practitioner is in an ideal position to advocate for these services in his or her school system and help dispel the myths that open discussions of sexuality contribute to sexual risk taking.

IV. **Clinical pearls and pitfalls.**
- A clinician must come to terms with his or her own sexuality. A clinician who is uncomfortable with gender issues or explicit sexual questions cannot effectively counsel. A practitioner who is unwilling to discuss sexuality issues objectively should have appropriate referral sources so that patients are not denied information. Alternatively, this practitioner should not see adolescent patients.
- Teenagers need guidance, not directives. A practitioner should express his or her opinions in a nonjudgmental way and allow adolescents the legitimacy of their own opinions.
- Do not assume that all sexual relationships are heterosexual. Providing literature in the waiting room on gay, lesbian, and bisexual health issues signals that the practitioner is comfortable in discussing same-sex experiences.
- The parent–practitioner relationship needs to be renegotiated prior to puberty so that parents understand confidentiality issues. Practitioners and parents should be partners in educating about sexuality.
- Sexuality is not a joking matter. Too often, adults deal with their own discomfort about sex by making jokes. Discussions with adolescents should always be serious but not somber.

BIBLIOGRAPHY

For Parents and Adolescents

Books

Bell R. *Changing Bodies, Changing Lives. Expanded Third Edition. A Book for Teens on Sex and Relationships.* New York: Random House, 1998.

Harris R. *It's Perfectly Normal: Changing Bodies, Growing Up, Sex and Sexual Health.* Cambridge, MA: Candlewick Press, 1996.

Websites

SIECUS (Sexuality, information and education council of the United States), excellent resources for accurate information for both parents and teens; includes numerous websites.www.siecus.org

For Professionals

Grunbaum J, Kann L, Kinchen S, et al. Youth risk Surveillance (YRBS)–United States, 2001. *Morbidity Mortality Weekly Report* 51(SS-4):1–64, 2002.

Hoff T, Greene L, Davis J. *National Survey of Adolescents and Young Adults: Sexual Health, Knowledge, Attitudes and Experiences.* Menlo Park, CA: Henty Kaiser Family Foundation, 2003.

American Academy of Pediatrics. Sexuality education of children and adolescents with developmental problems; American Academy of Pediatrics Policy Statement: *Pediatrics* 97(2):275–227, 1996.

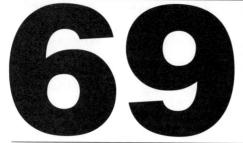

Sexual Abuse

Deborah Madansky
Christine Barron
Carole Jenny

I. **Description of the problem.** Sexual abuse is defined as the **engagement of a child in sexual contact or activities that the child cannot comprehend, for which the child is developmentally unprepared and cannot give informed consent, and/or that violate societal, legal, and social taboos.** The activity occurs for the **gratification of the older individual** and may include forms of anal, genital, and oral contact to or by the child, and exhibitionism, voyeurism, or using the child for the production of pornography. Force is often not involved, but coercion or threats may be.

A. **Epidemiology.**
   - The true prevalence is unknown since most cases go unreported. In retrospective surveys of adults, about **25% of women and 15% of men** report sexual contact with an adult during childhood or adolescence.
   - 40% of reported cases of child abuse and neglect involve sexual abuse.
   - 75% of reported victims are female, but there is evidence that male victims are less likely to report.
   - Male perpetrators are more common.
   - The vast majority of perpetrators are known to the child.
   - Sexual abuse crosses all socioeconomic, ethnic, and racial lines.

B. **Contributing factors.** Children at higher risk are those with a diminished capacity to resist or disclose, such as preverbal, developmentally delayed, or physically handicapped children, and children in dysfunctional or reconstituted families.

II. **Making the diagnosis.**

A. **Presentations of child sexual abuse.**
   1. **Acute assault.** A child presenting within 72 hours of an assault should be referred to an emergency room, or child protection programs when available, where forensic specimens may be collected.
   2. **In the pediatric office.**
      a. The child is **referred by protective services or law enforcement** for a medical evaluation as part of an investigation.
      b. The child is **referred by a family member** who is aware of or suspects sexual abuse.
      c. The child is **seen for a routine examination** or medical and behavioral complaint where the differential diagnosis includes sexual abuse.

B. **Signs and symptoms.**
   1. **Specific indicators.**
      a. Genital or rectal pain, bleeding, trauma, or infection.
      b. Sexually transmitted diseases (Table 69-1).
      c. Developmentally inappropriate sexual behavior in young children, such as engagement in intercourse, oral sex, or sexual coercion.
   2. **Behavioral indicators** are nonspecific and similar to symptoms due to other stressors. They are not indicative of specifically sexual abuse.
      a. Fears and phobias, especially of circumstances similar to the abuse.
      b. Nightmares and other sleep disturbances.
      c. Appetite disturbance or eating disorders.
      d. Enuresis or encopresis.
      e. Change in behavior, attitude, or school performance.
      f. Depression, withdrawal, or suicidality.
      g. Excessive anger, aggression, or running away.
      h. Promiscuous behavior or substance abuse.
   3. Some children may have **posttraumatic stress disorder**, whose diagnostic criteria include having the following symptoms for at least 1 month's duration:
      a. **Reexperiencing the traumatic event,** such as in recurrent dreams, flashback memories, or repetitive traumatic play.

Table 69-1 Implications of commonly encountered sexually transmitted diseases for the diagnosis and reporting of sexual abuse of prepubertal infants and children

STD confirmed	Sexual abuse	Suggested action
Gonorrhea[a]	Certain	Report[b]
Syphilis[a]	Certain	Report
Chlamydia[a]	Probable[c]	Report
Condylomata acuminatum[a]	Probable	Report
Trichomonas vaginalis	Probable	Report
Herpes 1 (genital)	Possible	Report[d]
Herpes 2	Probable	Report
Bacterial vaginosis	Uncertain	Medical follow-up
Candida albicans	Unlikely	Medical follow-up

[a]If not perinatally acquired.
[b]To agency mandated in community to receive reports of suspected sexual abuse.
[c]Culture only reliable diagnostic method.
[d]Unless there is a clear history of autoinoculation.
Reprinted with permission from the American Academy of Pediatrics. Committee on Child Abuse and Neglect. Guidelines for the evaluation of sexual abuse of children. *Pediatrics* 87(2):254–260, 1991.

    b. Persistent avoidance of certain stimuli or numbing of general responses.
    c. Persistent symptoms of increased arousal, such as difficulty falling or staying asleep, irritability or angry outbursts, difficulty concentrating, hypervigilance, exaggerated startle, or physiologic reactivity to a memory of the event.
C. History.
    1. The **parent or guardian** should be interviewed alone regarding his or her concerns, the child's disclosures or complaints, and a review of the child's medical, developmental, emotional, and behavioral status. The clinician should ask specifically about:
        a. The child's disclosures.
        b. Content of sexual play with peers, adults, or dolls.
        c. Masturbation or genital fondling.
        d. Genital complaints or symptoms.
        e. Toileting difficulties.
        f. Sleep disturbances (difficulty falling asleep, night waking, nightmares).
        g. Behavioral difficulties or changes.
        h. School performance.
    2. The **child** should be interviewed, unless he or she has already been interviewed or is too young or unwilling to talk. Follow this sequence.
        a. Interview the child alone, and record the child's statements. (The parent may be the perpetrator, or even if not, children often are uncomfortable speaking to a parent.)
        b. Sit at eye level and take time to establish rapport with neutral topics (e.g., ask about the child's living situation, pets, school, favorite activities, etc.).
        c. Gear the discussion to the child's developmental level, and use his or her own terms for body parts. (For young children line drawings may be helpful.)
        d. Introduce the topic of possible sexual abuse in a general way, such as
          • *"Is there anything that you feel uncomfortable about that you would like to talk about?"* or *"I know you have had to leave your family and are now in a foster home. Can you tell me how that happened?"*
          • If these opening questions do not result in a spontaneous account, inquire more specifically, *"Has anyone touched you or bothered you in a way that made you feel uncomfortable?"* or *"Lots of children come to see me because someone touched them in a way they didn't like. Did that ever happen to you?"* If the child says, *"Yes,"* then ask, *"What happened?"*
          • Use **nonleading questions**, such as what, who, where, and when. Avoid any demonstration of emotion, pressure, or correction of the child. Have a "then what happened/tell me more" approach.
        e. Be aware that **disclosures may take place during the physical examination** as the affected body parts are examined.
        f. Document what the child says verbatim in the record. Videotaped interviews are usually conducted by protective services or law enforcement and are probably unwise in the pediatric office.
        g. Reassure the child that it was okay to tell you, and whatever happened was not his or her fault.

D. Physical examination. Do a complete physical examination. This allows a familiar context for the child, opportunities for further rapport, and screening for other problems.
   1. **Genital examination.**
      a. **Be aware of examination positions** (supine frogleg, prone knee-chest, lithotomy) and techniques (labial separation, labial traction).
      b. **Use a good light source with magnification,** such as an otoscope head, handheld or headpiece lens, magnifying fluorescent light, or colposcope.
      c. **Be aware of genital anatomy and normal developmental variations.**
         (1) All girls are born with a hymen.
         (2) Newborn hymens are fleshy and redundant secondary to maternal estrogen effect.
         (3) Prepubertal hymens have thinner tissue.
         (4) Pubertal hymens are thickened and petaled from renewal of the estrogen effect.
      d. **Be aware of normal anatomic variations.**
         (1) Most hymens fit into one of five categories: crescentic (posterior rim), circumferential (annular), fimbriated (redundant), sleevelike, or septate.
         (2) Nontraumatic variations include periurethral and perihymenal bands, small hymenal mounds adjacent to vaginal ridges, perineal midline raphe, and hymenal flaps.
      e. **Be aware of abnormal findings not due to sexual abuse** (straddle injuries, genital hemangiomas, lichen sclerosis, urethral caruncles, urethral prolapse).
      f. **Prepare the child** prior to the examination with an explanation of the examination.
      g. **Boys** should receive a careful inspection of the penis, urethral meatus, scrotum, and surrounding skin.
      h. Prepubertal girls require a careful inspection of the vulva, unless internal trauma is suspected (which requires a pelvic exam under anesthesia). Pubertal girls require a complete pelvic with a speculum.
      i. **Genital findings consistent with sexual abuse:**
         (1) **Acute:** lacerations, abrasions, ecchymoses, edema.
         (2) **Chronic:** scarring of hymen or other genital structures; absent hymen, attenuated hymen, distorted hymen, or U- or V-shaped indentations in posterior or lateral portions of the hymen
   2. **Anal examination.**
      a. Be aware of **normal anal anatomy and variations**, including smooth areas at 6 and 12 o'clock (diastasis ani), erythema, midline skin tags, increased pigmentation, venous congestion, anal dilation with feces in the rectum.
      b. **Findings consistent with sexual abuse.**
         (1) **Acute:** lacerations, edema, abrasions, ecchymoses, fissures that come out past the anal verge.
         (2) **Chronic:** scars, dilation 20 mm or more without rectal feces, altered anal contour.
E. Laboratory tests.
   1. When indicated by the history or physical findings, culture for **gonorrhea** in the throat, anus, and vagina/urethra, and *Chlamydia* in the vagina and anus.
   2. **Serologic tests for syphilis and human immunodeficiency virus** (**HIV**) should be performed if the history warrants (taking into account of the incubation periods: up to 3 months for syphilis; up to 6 months for HIV).
   3. **Symptomatic children** should be investigated for other genital infections, such as trichomonas, herpes, condyloma acuminata, *Gardnerella vaginalis*, and *Candida.*
   4. Consider a **urinalysis** and **urine culture.**
   5. Consider a **pregnancy test** for pubertal girls.
III. Management.
A. Primary goals. The goals of management are to provide medical treatment for injuries or infections, arrange for psychosocial support for the child and family, and protect the child from further abuse by reporting to child protective services(Table 69-2).
B. Ongoing role of the practitioner.
   1. **Help guide the family toward healing.**
      a. **Provide or arrange crisis intervention counseling.**
      b. **Alert the family to their possible behavioral and emotional reactions,** especially if the family constellation is disrupted.
      c. **Encourage a sense of physical security for the child after the disclosure;** reassure children who were threatened with harm that there is no danger.

Table 69-2 Guidelines for making the decision to report sexual abuse of children

| History | Data available | | | Response | |
	Physical	Laboratory		Level of concern about sexual abuse	Action
None	Normal examination	None		None	None
Behavioral changes	Normal examination	None		Low (worry)	± Report*; follow closely (possible mental health referral)
None	Nonspecific findings	None		Low (worry)	± Report*; follow closely
Nonspecific history by child or history by parent only	Nonspecific findings	None		Possible (suspect)	± Report*; follow closely
None	Specific findings	None		Probable	Report
Clear statement	Normal examination	None		Probable	Report
Clear statement	Specific findings	None		Probable	Report
None	Normal examination, nonspecific or specific findings	Positive culture for gonorrhea; positive serologic test for syphilis; presence of semen, sperm, acid phosphatase		Definite	Report
Behavioral changes	Nonspecific changes	Other sexually transmitted diseases		Probable	Report

*A report may or may not be indicated. The decision to report should be based on discussion with local or regional experts and/or child protective services agencies.
Reprinted with permission from the American Academy of Pediatrics Committee on Child Abuse and Neglect. Guidelines for the evaluation of sexual abuse of children. *Pediatrics* 87(2): 254–260, 1991.

    d. Parents should neither try to make children forget nor pry into details, but rather be open to children's negative or positive expressions about the experience.

    e. Help parents avoid overprotection and maintain normal routines, physical affection, and limit setting whenever possible.

    f. Help parents remember the needs of the rest of the family and themselves.

  2. Monitor the child and family adjustments over time. As the victim enters each succeeding developmental stage, new questions and feelings may arise.

  3. Be aware of local resources, such as parent groups, offender treatment, victim witness advocates, and children's groups available to the family.

C. Criteria for referral.

  1. A clinician who does not have sufficient evidence to report to child protective services but is still concerned should refer to an experienced mental health provider for a full sexual abuse evaluation.

  2. A clinician who cannot conduct a complete medical evaluation (or if the initial evaluation raises questions) should refer to a pediatric specialist in sexual abuse.

  3. All sexually abused children should be referred to an experienced mental health provider to evaluate the need for ongoing treatment. Even children without overt symptoms may harbor negative or confused feelings that may be revealed only in the context of a full evaluation.

IV. Clinical pearls and pitfalls.

- Rely on the history for the diagnosis; most sexually abused children have no physical findings. This is because they were fondled, engaged in oral sex, or had minor injuries that healed quickly. Even hymenal tears can heal without a trace. A normal examination neither rules out nor confirms the possibility of sexual abuse or prior penetration.
- Take the child's statements and behavior seriously. The incidence of genital complaints is higher than the incidence of genital findings in sexually abused children.
- Children who imitate adult sex acts or molest other children are highly suspect. (Normal sex play among peers is, "You show me yours, and I'll show you mine.")
- Make sure the parent(s) have adequate support; the child's adjustment is related to family adjustment.
- Sexually abused children may feel like "damaged goods" and need reassurance that their bodies are fine. Even if there is damage, the clinician can still honestly say that something is healed or will heal quickly.

BIBLIOGRAPHY

For Parents

Crow P, Butler J. *Helping Children Recover from Sexual Abuse: A Guide for Parents.* Portland, OR: Emanuel Hospital and Health Center, 1991.

MacFarlane K. *Please, No, Not My Child–Coping with Sexual Abuse of Your Preschool Child.* Los Angeles: Children's Institute International, 1983.

For Children

For Preschoolers

Freeman L. *It's My Body.* Seattle: Parenting Press, 1987.

For School-Aged Children

My Very Own Book About Me. Spokane, WA: Rape Crisis Resource Library, 1982.

For Adolescents

Davis L. *The Courage to Heal Workbook.* New York: Harper & Row, 1990.

For Professionals

American Academy of Pediatrics. Committee on Child Abuse and Neglect. Guidelines for the evaluation of sexual abuse of children. *Pediatrics* 87(2):254–260, 1991.

Botash AS. *Evaluating Child Sexual Abuse: Education Manual for Medical Professionals.* Baltimore: The Johns Hopkins University Press, 2000.

Chadwick DL, et al. *Color Atlas of Child Sexual Abuse.* Chicago: Year Book Medical Publishers, 1989.

Heger A, Emans SJ (eds). *Evaluation of the Sexually Abused Child.* New York: Oxford University Press, 1992.

Jones DPH, McQuiston M. *Interviewing the Sexually Abused Child.* Denver: C. Henry Kempe Center for the Prevention and Treatment of Child Abuse and Neglect, 1986.

Reece RM (ed). *Child Abuse Medical Diagnosis and Management.* Baltimore: Williams & Wilkins, 1996.

70 Shyness

Jonathan M. Cheek

I. **Description of the problem.** Shyness is the tendency to feel tense, worried, or awkward during social interactions, especially with unfamiliar people. This definition reflects three categories of shyness symptoms: **somatic anxiety**, **cognitive anxiety**, and **observable behavior**.

A. **Epidemiology.**
- Although transient situational shyness is virtually universal, about 33%–45% of school-aged children and adults in the United States label themselves as shy.
- There is a developmental peak for shyness during adolescence, when 60% of the girls and 50% of the boys in seventh and eighth grades identify themselves as shy.
- Less than 50% of the children who first became shy during later childhood and early adolescence still consider themselves to be shy by age 21.
- 75% of college students who say they were shy in early childhood continue to identify themselves as shy persons.

B. **Clinical features.** *In early childhood*, shyness is usually manifested as the relative absence or inhibition of normally expected social behaviors. The child appears excessively quiet, with diminished social participation. For shy children, the normal peaks of stranger anxiety (9 months) and separation anxiety (18 months) do not fade away. *In later childhood and early adolescence*, the cognitive symptoms of shyness, such as painful self-consciousness and anxious self-preoccupation, begin to become a significant component of this personality syndrome.

Longitudinal research indicates that shyness that continues into adulthood can create significant barriers to satisfaction in love, work, recreation, and friendship. Shy adults tend to be more lonely and less happy than those who are not shy. Childhood shyness does not, however, predict psychopathology in adulthood and should be considered part of the normal range of individual differences in personality and social behavior.

C. **Etiology.**
1. **Temperament.** Shyness is one of the few temperamental traits whose precursors in infancy are often clear. About 15%–20% of infants typically respond to a new situation or stimulus (e.g., an unfamiliar toy, person, or place) by withdrawing and becoming either emotionally subdued or upset (crying, fussing, and fretting). It has been speculated that this pattern of inhibition to novelty is related to a lower threshold for arousal in sites in the amygdala. Infants with this highly reactive temperament in the first year of life are more likely to be wary or fearful of strangers at the end of the second year and are also more likely to be described as shy by their kindergarten teachers.
2. **Transactional model.** Behavioral inhibition in infancy does not lead invariably to childhood shyness. Parents who are sensitive to the nature of their inhibited child's temperament, who take an active role in helping the child to develop relationships with playmates, and who facilitate involvement in school activities appear to ameliorate the impact of shyness on the child's subsequent social adjustment. Childhood shyness is a joint product of temperament and socialization experiences within and outside the family.
3. **Late-onset shyness.** Many of the children who first become troubled by shyness between the ages of 8 and 14 years do not have the temperamental predisposition for behavioral inhibition. **Late-developing shyness is usually caused by adjustment problems in adolescent social development**. The bodily changes of puberty, the newly acquired cognitive ability to think abstractly about the self and the environment, and the new demands and opportunities resulting from changing social roles combine to make adolescents feel intensely self-conscious and socially awkward.

The inability of some adolescents to outgrow late-developing shyness has been linked to several factors. Research on the timing of puberty indicates that early-maturing girls and late-maturing boys suffer more severe social adjustment problems with their peers. Moving to a new neighborhood or school can disrupt the development of social skills, which are most easily practiced in safe and familiar surroundings. Shy adolescents need to experience positive social relationships in order to develop a healthy level of self-esteem. If parents, siblings, teachers, or peers tease and embarrass the shy adolescent, they may develop the self-image of being an unworthy and unlikable person.

Sex role socialization puts different pressures on adolescent girls and boys. Teenage girls experience more symptoms of self-conscious shyness, such as doubts about their attractiveness and worries about what others think of them, whereas teenage boys tend to be more troubled by behavioral symptoms of shyness because the traditional male role requires initiative and assertiveness in social life.

II. Recognizing the issue.
  A. **Signs and symptoms**. The child's visit to a primary care clinician is itself a prototypical shyness-eliciting situation, so signs of fearfulness and inhibition should be easily detectable.
  B. **Differential diagnosis.** Some people prefer to spend time alone rather than with others but also feel comfortable when they are in social settings. Such people are nonanxious introverts, who may be unsociable but not shy. The opposite of shyness is social self-confidence, not extroversion. The problem for truly shy people is that their anxiety prevents them from participating in social life when they want to or need to.
  C. **History: Key clinical questions.**
     1. *"Is your child usually shy and withdrawn in new situations and when meeting new people?"* An affirmative answer rules out the possibilities that the child is just nervous about the visit or is just in a sensitive mood on that particular day.
     2. *"Are you worried that your child is too shy to make friends or to do well in school?"* Answers that indicate severe anxiety reactions, phobias, or withdrawal similar to mild forms of autism are red flags for more severe pathology. Some parents, particularly those who are somewhat shy yet have adapted well themselves, will label their child as shy but not see it as a problem. They are often sufficiently sensitive to the issue that no further intervention may be necessary.
     3. *"Do you feel disappointed or embarrassed that your child can't seem to be more outgoing or adventuresome?"* Research suggests that an affirmative answer indicates the potential for significant long-term adjustment problems for shy children. For example, the feelings of disappointment in some fathers that their shy sons are not "masculine" enough can be a particularly painful problem. It is important for the parents of a shy child to understand the nature of the temperament and to help their child develop an individual pathway, rather than attempting to enforce a personal or cultural ideal that will never be a good fit for the shy child.

III. Management.
  A. **Advice to parents.** The goals of intervention in this case are essentially proactive and preventative in nature: helping the shy child to achieve better adjustment in his/her current and future social life. It is worth noting that retrospective interviews with painfully shy adults frequently contain complaints that doctors and teachers had ignored their childhood shyness. They expressed the wish that some adult had become an ally or advocate by validating their problem and persuading their parents to help them deal more effectively with their shyness at an early age.
     1. **Do not overprotect or overindulge.** Allow the shy child to experience moderate amounts of challenge, frustration, and stress rather than rushing to soothe away every sign of anxiety. With emotional support from parents and gradual exposure to new objects, people, and places, the child will learn to cope with their own special sensitivity to novelty. *Gently and consistently nudge (but do not push) the child to continue gaining experience with new things.*
     2. **Respect the shy temperament.** Talk with the child about feeling nervous or afraid. Once the reality of these negative feelings has been acknowledged, encourage the child to talk about what can be gained from trying a new experience in spite of being afraid (an example from the parent's own childhood might be particularly helpful). Progress is usually slow because shy feelings may remain even after a particular shy behavior has been overcome. *Sympathy, patience, and persistence are needed.*
     3. **Help the child deal with teasing about being shy.** Shy children are highly sensitive to embarrassment and need extra comfort when they have been the victim of teasing. They also need more support and encouragement to develop positive self-esteem than do children who are not shy.

4. **Help the child to build friendships.** Inviting one or two playmates over to the house lets the child experience the security of being on home territory. Sometimes a shy child will do better when playing with children who are slightly younger.
5. **Talk to teachers.** The child's teacher can be an important ally, but teachers sometimes overlook the shy child or incorrectly assume that excessive quietness indicates lack of interest or lack of intelligence.
6. **Prepare the child for new experiences.** Take the child to visit a new school or classroom before school starts. Help the child rehearse (e.g., by practicing for show-and-tell or an oral book report). **Role-play anticipated anxieties**, such as what a party or the first day of summer camp will be like.
7. **Find appropriate activities.** Help the child get involved in a club or after-school activity that can expand social contacts with others who share similar interests and enthusiasms. Be careful not to impose what you would like, or wish you had done as a child, onto a child who has different likes and dislikes.

B. **Advice to the shy child.** Shy children usually appreciate being made to feel that their problems of social anxiety are understood sympathetically by an adult and that they are not alone in experiencing these feelings. It is important not to minimize the significance of shyness but rather to emphasize to the child the increased enjoyment of social rewards that can be obtained if he begins to participate more actively in social life. Acknowledge that the shy child may always feel a bit anxious inside but emphasize that the anxiety is not nearly as visible to other children or adults as the child thinks it is. By focusing on what others are saying or doing a shy child can practice being less self-focused and self-critical.

IV. **When to refer.** If the parents of a child troubled by shyness appear to lack confidence in their ability to implement the advice, it may be appropriate to suggest a referral to a mental health professional. Children who appear particularly silent or withdrawn should be screened for social phobia, selective mutism, and Asperger's syndrome.

BIBLIOGRAPHY

For Parents

Books

Carducci BJ. *The Shyness Breakthrough: A No-Stress Plan to Help Your Shy Child Warm Up, Open Up, and Join the Fun.* Emmaus, PA: Rodale, 2003.
Zimbardo PG, Radl SL. *The Shy Child: Overcoming and Preventing Shyness from Infancy to Adulthood.* Cambridge, MA: Malor Books, 1999.

Websites

The Shyness Clinic www.shyness.com
Anxiety Disorders Association of America www.adaa.org

For Professionals

Beidel DC, Turner SM. *Shy Children, Phobic Adults: Nature and Treatment of Social Phobia.* Washington, DC: American Psychological Association, 1998.
Cheek JM, Krasnoperova EN. Varieties of shyness in adolescence and adulthood. In LA Schmidt, J Schulkin, eds. *Extreme Fear, Shyness, and Social Phobia: Origins, Biological Mechanisms, and Clinical Outcomes.* New York: Oxford University Press, 1999.
Crozier WR, ed. *Shyness: Development, Consolidation, and Change.* London: Routledge, 2001.

71 Sleep Problems

Judith A. Owens

I. Description of the problem.

A. Sleep problems constitute one of the most frequent parental complaints in pediatric practice.

- Childhood *sleeplessness,* insufficient or disturbed sleep, in its many forms, clearly is a common parental concern.
- In contrast, the relationship between **sleepiness** and its many manifestations is less frequently recognized by parents, but is nonetheless a significant clinical concern. A wealth of empirical evidence from several lines of research clearly indicates that children and adolescents experience significant daytime sleepiness as a result of inadequate or disturbed sleep, and that significant performance impairments and mood dysfunction, as well as behavior, academic, and health problems in childhood, are associated with that daytime sleepiness.

B. Epidemiology.

1. 25% of all children experience a sleep problem at some point during childhood, ranging from short-term situational difficulties in falling asleep, to night wakings, to more chronic and persistent sleep disorders.

2. Although many sleep problems in infants and children are transient and self-limited, the common wisdom that children "grow out of" sleep problems is not an accurate perception. Certain intrinsic and extrinsic risk factors (e.g., difficult temperament, maternal depression, family stress) may predispose a given child to develop a more chronic sleep disturbance.

3. Sleep problems are a **significant source of distress** for families they may be, for example, a primary reason for caregiver stress in families with children who have chronic medical illnesses or severe neurodevelopment delays.

4. The impact of childhood sleep problems is intensified by their direct relationship to **the quality and quantity of parents' sleep,** particularly if disrupted sleep results in parental daytime fatigue and mood disturbances, which impact negatively on the quality of parenting.

5. Vulnerable populations, such as children who are at high risk for developmental and behavioral problems because of poverty, parental substance abuse and mental illness, or violence in the home, may be even more likely to experience "double jeopardy" as a result of sleep problems.

C. Etiology/contributing factors.

1. **Child variables** include temperament and behavioral style, individual variations in circadian preference, cognitive and language **delays**, and the presence of comorbid medical and psychiatric conditions.

2. **Parental variables:** include parenting and discipline styles, parents' education level and knowledge of child development, mental health issues such as maternal depression, family stress, and quality and quantity of parents' sleep.

3. **Environmental variables** include the physical environment (space, noise, perceived environmental threats to safety, room and bed sharing, televisions in the bedroom), family composition (number, ages, and health status of siblings and extended family members), and lifestyle issues (parental work status, competing priorities for time).

4. **Cultural and family context:** for example, cosleeping of infants and parents is a common and accepted practice in many ethnic groups (including African Americans, Hispanics, and Southeast Asians) both in their counties of origin and in the United States. Therefore, the developmental goal of independent "self-soothing" in infants at bedtime and after night wakings may not be shared by all families.

5. **Specific medical conditions** that may have an increased risk of sleep problems include
   - Asthma and allergies
   - Headaches
   - Neurologic disorders and rheumatologic conditions

- Children with anxiety and affective disorders are particularly vulnerable to sleep problems. Studies of children with major depressive disorder, for example, have reported a prevalence of insomnia of up to 75%, and sleep onset delay in 1/3 of depressed adolescents. Use of psychotropic medications in these children may have significant negative effects on sleep.
- Significant sleep problems occur in 30%–80% of children with severe mental retardation and in at least 50% of children with less severe cognitive impairment. Similar estimates in children with autism/pervasive developmental delay are in the 50%–70% range.

II. Making the diagnosis.
A. Sleep physiology.
1. **The framework or architecture of sleep** is based upon recognition of two distinct sleep stages. These stages are defined by distinct polysomnographic (or "overnight sleep study") features of EEG patterns, eye movement, and muscle tone.
   - **REM sleep** (rapid eye movement or "dream" sleep). REM sleep (20%–25% of total) is characterized by high levels of cortical activity and low or absent muscle tone.
   - **Non–REM sleep** (75%–80% of sleep in healthy young adults). Non–REM sleep is further divided into:
     - **Stage 1** sleep (2%–5%) which occurs at the sleep-wake transition and is often referred to as "light sleep"
     - **Stage 2** sleep (45%–55%) which is usually considered the initiation of "true" sleep and is characterized by bursts of rhythmic rapid EEG activity and high amplitude slow wave spikes
     - **Stages 3 and 4** sleep (3%–23%) which are otherwise known as "deep" sleep, "slow wave sleep", or "delta sleep", during which the highest arousal threshold (most difficult to awaken) also occurs
2. **Cycling of stages.**
   - Non–REM and REM sleep alternate throughout the night in cycles of about 90–110 minutes in adults (50 minutes in infancy and gradually lengthening through childhood to adult levels).
   - Brief arousals normally followed by a rapid return to sleep often occur at the end of each sleep cycle (4–6 times per night in adults; 7–10 times per night in infants).
   - The relative proportion of REM and non–REM sleep per cycle changes across the night, such that slow wave sleep predominates in the first third of the night and REM sleep in the last third.
3. **Two process sleep system**. Sleep and wakefulness are regulated by two basic highly coupled processes operating simultaneously:
   - The **homeostatic process**, which primarily regulates the length and depth of sleep. The homeostatic "pressure" for sleep builds as time awake increases in duration.
   - **Endogenous circadian rhythms** ("biological time clocks") which influence the internal organization of sleep, and the timing and duration of daily sleep/wake cycles
   - **Circadian rhythms** (which govern many other physiologic systems in addition to sleep wake cycles) are also synchronized to the 24 hour day cycle by environmental cues, the most powerful of which is the light-dark cycle which influences melatonin secretion by the pineal gland
4. **Duration of sleep.**
   a. **Newborns.**
   - Newborns sleep approximately 16–20 hours per day, in 1–4 hour sleep periods, followed by 1–2 hour awake periods.
   - Sleep/wake cycles are largely dependent upon hunger and satiety. Sleep amounts during the day approximately equal the amount of nighttime sleep.
   b. **Infants (0–12 months).**
   - Infants generally sleep a total of about 14–15 hours at 4 months and 13–14 hours total at 6 months.
   - Sleep periods last about 3–4 hours during the first 3 months, and extend to 6–8 hours at 4–6 months.
   - By 9 months, 70%–80% **"sleep through the night"** (*sleep consolidation*).
   - **Day/night differentiation** develops between 6–12 weeks and nocturnal sleep periods become increasingly longer.
   - The ability to **regulate sleep or control internal states of arousal in order to fall asleep** at bedtime and to fall back asleep during the night, begins to develop in the first 12 weeks of life.

- Most infants nap between 2 and 4 hours divided as 2 naps/day.
- Issues of attachment and social interaction also play an important role in shaping sleep behaviors in infants. Transitional objects such as a pacifier or a blanket and bedtime routines become more important as infancy progresses.

   c. Toddlers (12–36 months).
- Toddlers sleep about 12 hours per 24 hours.
- Most give up a second nap by 18 months and generally nap 1.5 to 3.5 hours as 1 nap/day.
- The peak of separation anxiety at 9–18 months is often associated with increased night wakings.

   d. Preschoolers (3–5 years).
- Total sleep duration is about 11–12 hours/night.
- Most children give up napping by 5 years.
- Difficulties falling asleep and night wakings (15%–30%) are still common in this age group, in many cases coexisting in the same child.

   e. Middle childhood (6–12 years).
- Total sleep duration is approximately 10–11 hr/night.
- Although it was previously believed that sleep problems are rare in middle childhood, recent studies have reported a high prevalence of significant parent-reported sleep problems in this age group.

   f. Adolescents (12–18 years).
- Adolescents require just over 9 hr/night. However, a number of studies have suggested that the average adolescent actually *gets* about 7 hours of sleep.

B. Etiology.
- **Behavioral insomnia of childhood (difficulty initiating and/or maintaining sleep).** "Insomnia" is a symptom and not a diagnosis. The causes of insomnia are varied, and range from the medical (i.e., drug-related, pain-induced, associated with primary sleep disorders such as obstructive sleep apnea) to the behavioral (i.e., associated with poor sleep hygiene or sleep onset association disorder) and are often a combination of these factors. The most common causes of adolescent insomia are listed next.

   1. Sleep onset association disorder. The child has learned to fall asleep only under certain conditions or associations, such as being rocked or fed, and does not develop the ability to self-soothe. During the night, when the child experiences the type of brief arousal that normally occurs at the end of a sleep cycle (7–10 times per night) or awakens for other reasons, he is not able to get back to sleep without those same conditions being present. Thus, the problem is one of prolonged night waking resulting in insufficient sleep.

   2. Limit setting sleep disorder. Characterized by difficulty falling asleep and bedtime resistance ("curtain calls") rather than night wakings. Most commonly, this disorder develops from a parent's inability or unwillingness to set consistent bedtime rules and enforce a regular bedtime, often exacerbated by the child's oppositional behavior. In some cases, however, the child's resistance at bedtime is due to an underlying problem in falling asleep caused by other factors (e.g., medical conditions such as asthma or medication use, a sleep disorder such as restless legs, or anxiety) or a mismatch between the child's intrinsic circadian rhythm ("night owl") and parental expectations.

   3. Psychophysiologic insomnia (difficulty initiating and/or maintaining sleep) is more common in older children and adolescents. In this disorder, the individual develops conditioned anxiety around falling or staying asleep, usually in combination with poor sleep habits, which leads to heightened arousal and further compromises the ability to sleep.

   4. Sleep anxiety. Nighttime fears are common, and typically both normal and benign. Parental anxiety and family conflict may also play a role in exacerbating nighttime fears in children by increasing the level of emotional arousal in the child. Anxiety around sleep is characterized by fearful behaviors, such as crying, clinging, and leaving the bedroom to seek parental reassurance (at bedtime or in the middle of the night), and bedtime resistance, including refusal to go to bed, frequent "curtain calls", or requiring a parent to be present at bedtime. Some children may also experience frequent nightmares as part of the anxiety picture.

C. Differential diagnosis.
   1. Insufficient sleep and inadequate sleep hygiene. The resulting chronic sleep deprivation impacts on daytime functioning and causes excessive daytime sleepiness, which can be manifested in a number of ways in children and adolescents: falling

asleep at unintended times, overactivity, and behavior problems. Inadequate sleep hygiene includes practices that increase arousal and practices that are inconsistent with sleep organization.

    a. Practices that increase arousal include caffeine intake, evening television viewing, and bright light in the bedroom during the night or in the early morning.

    b. Practices that are inconsistent with sleep organization include napping late in the day, a disorganized sleep-wake cycle, and excessive time in bed in comparison to time asleep.

  2. Circadian issues may also play a role in some cases of bedtime struggles. When a relatively early bedtime coincides with the normal late-day circadian-mediated surge in alertness ("circadian nadir"), a child may have significantly more difficulty settling and this can result in bedtime resistance. Children with an "owl" circadian preference for later sleep onset and wake times also tend to have a later circadian nadir and are thus particularly likely to have a settling problem if bedtime is set too early.

  3. Bedtime struggles may be the result of a more global problem with **noncompliance,** including **oppositional defiant disorder (ODD)** or may be a feature of a more pervasive psychiatric problem.

  4. Primarily medically based sleep problems such as **obstructive sleep apnea and restless legs/periodic limb movements** may present with bedtime resistance and/or night wakings and disturbed sleep.

D. History: Key clinical questions. The clinical evaluation of a child presenting with a sleep problem involves a **careful medical and developmental history** to assess for potential medical causes of sleep disturbances, such as allergies, concomitant medications, and acute or chronic pain conditions.

  1. Current **sleep patterns**, including usual sleep duration and sleep/wake schedule, are often best assessed with a sleep diary, in which parents record daily sleep behaviors for an extended period.

  2. A review of **sleep habits**, such as bedtime routines, daily caffeine intake, and the sleeping environment (temperature, noise level, etc.) may reveal environmental factors that contribute to the sleep problems.

  3. Use of additional diagnostic tools such as **polysomnographic evaluation** are seldom warranted for routine evaluation of pediatric insomnia, but may be appropriate if organic sleep disorders, such as obstructive sleep apnea or periodic limb movements, are suspected.

III. Management. Successful treatment of pediatric sleep problems is highly dependent upon identification of parental concerns, clarification of mutually acceptable treatment goals, active exploration of opportunities and obstacles, and ongoing communication of issues and concerns. Hypnotic medications are rarely needed.

A. Sleep onset association disorder. The treatment approach to sleep onset association disorder typically involves a program of withdrawal of parental assistance at sleep onset and during the night (**systematic ignoring**).

  1. In older infants, the introduction of more appropriate sleep associations which will be readily available to the child during the night (**transitional objects** such as a blanket or toy) in addition to **positive reinforcement** (e.g., stickers for remaining in bed) are often beneficial. The goal is to allow the infant or child to develop skills in self-soothing during the night, as well as at bedtime.

  2. Graduated extinction is a more gradual process of weaning the child from dependence upon parental presence that utilizes periodic "checks" by the parents at successively longer time intervals during the sleep-wake transition. Parents must be consistent in applying behavioral programs to avoid inadvertent intermittent reinforcement of night wakings; they should also be forewarned that crying behavior frequently temporarily escalates at the beginning of treatment (**"post-extinction burst"**).

B. Limit setting sleep disorder. Successful treatment of limit setting sleep disorder generally involves a combination of:

- Decreased parental attention for bedtime-delaying behavior.
- Establishment of bedtime routines.
- Positive reinforcement (eg, sticker charts) for appropriate behavior at bedtime.
- Older children may benefit from being taught relaxation techniques to help themselves fall asleep more readily.

C. Psychophysiologic insomnia. Treatment usually involves educating the adolescent about **principles of sleep hygiene** (e.g., regular sleep-wake schedule, avoidance of stimulants like caffeine and nicotine, bedtime routine), instructing them to **use the bed for sleep only** and to get out of bed if unable to fall asleep (**stimulus control**), restricting time-in-bed to the actual time asleep (sleep restriction), and teaching **relaxation techniques to reduce anxiety**.

D. **Sleep anxiety.** In general, strategies aimed at younger children more often involve parental reassurance, while older children typically benefit from an approach that includes teaching and positive reinforcement for independent coping skills.

- Use of security objects should be encouraged, as they can be comforting to the child
- Television shows and movies that may be frightening or overstimulating, particularly just before bedtime, should be avoided. Also, televisions should be kept out of the bedroom.
- Many children may benefit from learning relaxation strategies, such as deep breathing or visual imagery, which can help a child relax at bedtime and fall asleep more easily.

IV. **Clinical pearls and pitfalls.**

- Because multiple sleep problems may co-exist in the same child, it is always important to assess for additional nocturnal symptoms that may be indicative of a medically based sleep disorder, such as obstructive sleep apnea (loud snoring, choking/gasping, sweating) or periodic limb movements (restless sleep, repetitive kicking movements), even if the presenting complaint appears behaviorally based.
- All children presenting to pediatric clinicians with learning, attention, behavioral, or emotional concerns, especially attention deficit hyperactivity disorder (ADHD), should be carefully assessed for underlying or comorbid sleep disorders as part of the routine evaluation. There is considerable overlap between the diagnostic features of ADHD (inattention, hyperactivity, impulsivity) and neurobehavioral deficits associated with any significant sleep problems in children. A number of primary sleep disorders, including Obstructive Sleep Apnea (OSA) and Restless Legs/Periodic Limb Movements (RLS/PLMD), frequently include ADHD-like symptoms as part of their clinical presentation.
- Because parents of older children and adolescents, in particular, may not be aware of any existing sleep difficulties, it is also important to directly question the patient about sleep issues as well.

V. **When to refer.** Referral to a sleep specialist for diagnosis and/or treatment should be considered under circumstances in which children or adolescents with persistent or severe bedtime issues do not respond to simple behavioral measures or for whom the sleep problems are extremely disruptive.

BIBLIOGRAPHY

For Parents

Books

Cohen G, ed. *American Academy of Pediatrics Guide to Your Child's Sleep*. New York: Villard, 1999.

Ferber R. *Solve Your Child's Sleep Problems*. New York: Simon & Schuster, 1985.

Mindell J. *Sleeping Through the Night: How Infants, Toddlers, and Their Parents Can Get a Good Night's Sleep*. New York: Harper Collins, 1997.

Websites

National Sleep Foundation www.sleepfoundation.org
American Academy of Sleep Medicine www.aasmnet.org

For Professionals

Kryger M, Roth T, Dement W. *Principles and Practices of Sleep Medicine*. Philadelphia: Saunders, 2000.

Mindell J, Owens J. *A Clinical Guide to Pediatric Sleep: Diagnosis and Management of Sleep Problems in Children and Adolescents*. Philadelphia: Lippincott Williams & Wilkins, 2003.

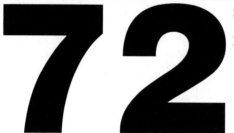

Speech-Sound Disorders

Rebecca McCauley

I. **Description of the problem.** Speech-sound system, or articulation, disorders consist of a *delay or difference in speech-sound acquisition, resulting in speech that is difficult to understand or sounds immature.* Many children with these disorders are at risk for social-emotional and learning difficulties because of their poor speech or because of associated speech and language problems. When severe, these disorders may be identified as "developmental apraxia of speech," "developmental verbal dyspraxia," or most recently "childhood apraxia of speech."

A. **Epidemiology.** Speech-sound disorders have a prevalence of 5% in the school-aged population and 10% in younger children, making it one of the most frequently identified communication disorders.
- Increased risk in boys.
- Increased risk in children with mental retardation.
- A significant number of children with a history of unintelligibility will experience academic difficulties through high school. Some will have negative academic and job prospects thereafter, especially those who also have identified language problems
- Whereas almost all children will outgrow this disorder by adolescence, its academic and social-emotional consequences nonetheless make identification and treatment an important goal. In addition, a small number of these children will exhibit mild distortion errors that will affect their speech into adulthood.

B. **Familial transmission/genetics.** A familial basis for severe forms of speech-sound disorder has recently been suggested. Family histories of children with this disorder are often positive for other speech and language disorders and for dyslexia.

C. **Etiology/contributing factors.**
1. **Organic.** Early recurrent periods of otitis media with effusion are an important risk factor in about one third of children with speech-sound disorders. There is little evidence that an abnormally short lingual frenulum ("tongue-tied") affects articulation and ambiguous evidence for the role of infantile swallow (tongue thrust) in the disorder.
2. **Developmental.** Diagnosis before age 3 is difficult because young children are highly variable in their speech-sound productions and in their cooperation with structured tasks. However, infrequent vocalizations or feeding or swallowing problems may indicate oromotor problems that can predispose the child to speech-sound disorders.

II. **Making the diagnosis.**
A. **Signs and symptoms.** (See Table 72-1.)
B. **Differential diagnosis.** Conditions resulting in delayed speech-sound development include oral anomalies (e.g., submucous cleft palate), hearing impairment, frank neurologic conditions associated with dyspraxia or dysarthria, and mental retardation. Co-occurrence with language disorders is quite common and the frequency of co-occurrence with voice disorders and with stuttering also appears to be elevated.
C. **History: Key clinical questions.**
1. *"How well do you and others understand your child's speech, compared to the speech of other children his or her age?"* Reduced intelligibility compared to peers is a strong indicator of a speech-sound disorder.
2. *"Has your child's speech changed much during the past 6 months?"* For children up to age 5 years, any response suggesting little change over time is a cause for concern.
3. *"How do you and others respond to your child's poor speech? How does your child respond to any negative reactions?"* Teasing, frequent corrections, or requests to repeat can make the child frustrated or shy and withdrawn. Spontaneous and frequent use of informal signs and gestures by the child is facilitative, but may suggest compensation for speech motor planning difficulties.
4. *"Does your child have a history of problems with feeding or swallowing?"* This question

Table 72-1 Signs and symptoms of speech-sound disorders

Any age	Speech is more difficult to understand than that of peers
	Teasing by others about speech (e.g., about a lisp)
	Shyness about speaking or excessive frustration when not understood
2 years or older	Intelligibility less than 50%
	Use of only 4–5 consonants (e.g., sounds represented by the letters *p, b, w, y, m*) and a limited number of vowels
	Consistent errors in the use of the sounds represented by the letters *p, b, m, n, h, w,* or any vowel sounds
	Consonants at the beginning of words are omitted (e.g., "ow" for "cow")
	One sound is used in the place of many others (e.g., *p* is used when *f, v, t, or k* is expected)
	The sounds *k* or *g* is used when *t* or *d* is expected (e.g., "ko" for "toe")
3 years or older	Intelligibility less than 75%
3½ years or older	Consistent errors in the use of the sounds *f, v, k, g,* or *y* (e.g., "wu" for "you")
	Consistent errors that assume the following patterns:
	Consonants at the ends of words are omitted
	The sounds *t* or *d* is used when *k* or *g* is expected
4 years or older	Intelligibility less than 100%
5½ years or older	Errors on two or more speech-sounds that are obvious enough to call attention to the child's speech

addresses the possibility of developmental dysarthria as part of differential diagnosis.

    5. *"Do you ever think your child has day-to-day fluctuations or problems in hearing?"* This question addresses the potential for chronic hearing impairment, as well as the issue of fluctuating hearing loss related to otitis media.

  D. Physical examination. The physical examination can help rule out significant oral anomalies and frank neurologic abnormalities, and provide information about the child's middle ear status.

  E. Tests. A certified speech-language pathologist can perform testing necessary for confirmation of speech-sound disorder.

III. Management.

  A. Primary goals. The primary care clinician's principal goals in speech-sound disorders are appropriate referral as well as management of middle ear status.

  B. Criteria for referral. Refer to a speech-language pathologist if the child's speech demonstrates any of the signs or symptoms in Table 72-1. Speech-language pathologists in public school systems assess and treat children with communication disorders—regardless of age. Even very young children at risk for speech-sound system disorders may benefit from early efforts to stimulate vocal production and language development.

IV. Clinical pearls and pitfalls.

  • Remember the guidelines regarding intelligibility (Table 72-1): A stranger should be able to understand about 50% of what a 2-year-old says, 75% of what a 3-year-old says, and 100% of what a 4-year-old says.

  • Tantrums or indications of extreme frustration from a child over age 3 years because of the parent's inability to understand the child's speech suggest a significant problem in speech development.

  • To avoid judging the child in terms of their own speech dialect, clinicians should ask parents to gauge how well the child is understood compared to peers.

  • Delays in referral not only can deprive the child of early treatment but can also result in increased parent-child conflict.

BIBLIOGRAPHY

For Professionals

Caruso A, Strand E. *Clinical Management of Motor Speech Disorders in Children.* New York: Thieme, 1999.

McCauley R. Description and classification of child speech disorders. In Kent RD, ed., *MIT Encyclopedia of Communication Disorders.* Cambridge, MA: MIT Press, 2004;

Websites

Apraxia, for parents and professionals on severe speech sound system disorders in children, including childhood apraxia of speech. www.apraxia-kids.org

American Speech-Language-Hearing Association, an information page prepared by the organization responsible for credentializing speech-language pathologists. http://www.kidsource.com/ASHA/articulation.html

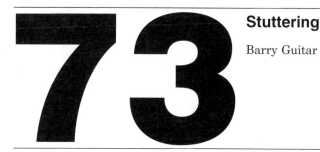

Stuttering

Barry Guitar

I. **Description of the problem.** Stuttering is a disruption of speech, characterized by repetitions, prolongations, and/or complete blockages. These may be accompanied by physical struggle, frustration and fear of speaking. The term *disfluency* is often used synonymously with *stuttering,* but it also may refer to the hesitations common in the speech of normal children learning to talk.

A. **Epidemiology.**
- The prevalence of stuttering is 1% among school-aged children, slightly lower in adults, and slightly higher in preschool children. The incidence is 5%.
- The difference between prevalence and incidence figures reflects the tendency for children who stutter to recover, usually before puberty.
- The male-female ratio among preschool children is about 2:1 and rises to 4:1 in adulthood, suggesting that females are more likely to recover.

B. **Familial transmission/genetics.** Parents who stutter are more likely to have children who stutter; this is especially so for women who stutter. A multifactorial (polygenic) model has been suggested to account for the transmission.

C. **Etiology/contributing factors.**
1. **Environmental.** A home or school environment that places high demands on a child's performance can contribute to stuttering. Examples of demands include pressure to speak more rapidly, articulately, or with more advanced language than the child is able or pressure to succeed socially, academically, or athletically. Stuttering may also be exacerbated by stressful but normal life events such as the birth of a sibling, separation from a parent, or a family move.
2. **Organic/transactional.** Predispositions to stuttering include an inherited or acquired difficulty in speech motor coordination and a temperament which reacts to stress with excess muscular tension and effort.
3. **Developmental.** Stuttering usually appears between 18 months and 5 years. In most children, early symptoms will resolve (*transient disfluency*). In others, the signs and symptoms may worsen from easy repetitions with minimal awareness to rapid and physically tense repetitions with evidence of frustration to blockages of speech, accompanying struggle behaviors, and avoidance of words and speaking situations. Onset of stuttering after age 5 may be associated with emotional trauma; in these cases stuttering is often associated with tight closure and squeezing in the larynx.

II. **Making the diagnosis.**

A. **Signs and symptoms/differential diagnosis.** (See Table 73-1.)

B. **History: Key clinical questions.**
1. *"How long have you been aware of your child's stuttering?"* If the child has stuttered for more than 6 months, suspect a potential chronic problem, particularly if it has not decreased in frequency or severity since onset.
2. *"How have the disfluencies changed since they began?"* If there has been an increase in effort, emotion, or avoidance associated with stuttering, it is worsening.
3. *"What is your child's stuttering like at its worst?"* Many children who stutter will not stutter in the clinician's office; it is important to have the parents describe the signs and symptoms which have caused them concern.
4. *"Is the child bothered by their stuttering?"* If so, the child will soon react to their stuttering with physical tension and struggle and should be referred.

C. **Tests.** Ask the child several direct questions (e.g., name, age, address) that must be answered without substitution or circumlocution. This is likely to elicit disfluency or avoidance if child is a stutterer.

III. **Management.**

A. **Primary goals.** The family must understand that the child is doing the best that they can with their speech and will only get worse if the family criticizes. Rather, the family should find ways to reduce stress and to verbalize their acceptance to the child.

Table 73-1 Signs and symptoms of normal disfluency and stuttering

	Normal Disfluency	Mild Stuttering	Severe Stuttering
Speech Behavior	Occasional brief repetitions of sounds, syllables or short words (li-like this).	Frequent long repetitions of sounds, syllables, or short words (li-li-li-like this). Occasional prolongations of sounds,	Very frequent and often very long repetitions of sounds, syllables or short words. Frequent sound prolongations and blockages.
Other Behavior	Occasional pauses, hesitations or fillers. Changing of words or thoughts.	Repetitions and prolongations associated with blinking, looking away, and physical tension around mouth.	More evidence of struggle, including pitch rise in voice. Extra words used as "starters"
When Most Noticeable	Comes and goes when child is excited, tired, sick, talking to inattentive listeners.	Comes and goes in similar situations but is more often present than absent.	Present in most speaking situations. More consistent.
Child's Reaction	Usually none apparent.	May show little concern or some frustration and embarrassment.	Embarrassment, shame and fear of speaking. Lack of eye contact when speaking.
Parent's Reaction	None to a great deal.	Some concern, but not a great deal.	Considerable degree of concern
Referral Decision	Refer only if parents quite concerned.	Refer if continues for 6 to 8 weeks or if parental concern justifies it.	Refer as soon as possible.

B. Information for family.
  1. It should be emphasized to the parents that *they did not cause the problem*.
  2. The etiology may be slight differences in brain organization which favors some skills (e.g., drawing or music) but creates more hesitancy in speech, especially during childhood.
  3. The onset of stuttering may be associated with a spurt in speech and language development or an increase in stress, but most frequently onset occurs in normal circumstances.
  4. Parents should know that if the child is frustrated by their stuttering, **the parents should occasionally acknowledge it in an accepting, encouraging way**. Parents can also assure the child that if he or she would like help with it, there are professionals who can help.
C. Initial treatment strategies.
  1. As much as possible, **parents should talk with their child in a slow, relaxed manner**, using short sentences and frequent pauses to promote fluency.
  2. **A brief period should be set aside each day at a regular time when one parent can interact alone with child.** The parent should use a slow speech rate and follow the child's lead in choosing topics of conversation and play activities. The aim is to give the child a sense of being the center of attention for a brief period.
  3. **The family should institute turn-taking in competitive speaking situations,** such as dinner table conversations.
  4. **Parents should occasionally make a comment expressing empathy,** such as "Lots of kids get stuck on their words sometimes. I know it makes talking hard, but it's ok and you can take as long as you like."
  5. **Attempts should be made to slow down the pace of life in the home,** including the pace of conversations. After the child says something, parents should pause for a second or two before responding.

D. Criteria for referral.
1. The child is stuttering with physical tension and is showing concern or frustration. The child should be referred immediately.
2. If initial strategies have been tried for a month without appreciable lessening of the stuttering, referral should be made.
3. Referral should be made to a speech-language pathologist certified by the American Speech-Language-Healing Association, preferably one who specializes in stuttering. (The Stuttering Foundation of America site contains a referral list of experienced clinicians.)

IV. Clinical pearls and pitfalls.
- Most parents blame themselves. Reassure them that they didn't cause their child's stuttering, but they can play a big part in their child's ability to cope with it.
- Most children will outgrow stuttering, especially if parents can reduce psychosocial pressures and increase acceptance of the child as he is now.
- Parental attitudes that put a high premium on completely fluent speech probably interfere with recovery.
- Effective programs for preschoolers who stutter are intensive, involve the parents, and use behavior therapy to teach fluent speech. Intervention in the preschool years can eliminate stuttering.
- Effective treatments for school age children help the child speak in a more natural way, with less effort and struggle, but do not aim for perfection.
- Transient stuttering is sometimes associated with allergies or with the use of some medications, such as Ritilan.

Stuttering Foundation of America P.O. Box 11749 Memphis, TN 38111 1-800-992-9392
National Stuttering Project 2151 Irving Street, Suite #208 San Francisco, CA 94122-1609 1-800-364-1677
Conture E. *Stuttering and Your Child: Questions and Answers.* Memphis, TN: Stuttering Foundation of America, 2002.
Guitar B, Guitar C. *Stuttering and the Preschool Child – Help for Families [Videotape].* Memphis, TN: Stuttering Foundation of America, 2001.
Stuttering Foundation. This site contains a referral list of experienced clinicians for every state and for other countries; an online store contains many inexpensive books and videos; and information for parents and professionals, as well as links to other sites. www.stutteringhelp.org
Stuttering Home Page. This site contains excellent information about stuttering as well as support and discussion groups for parents, children, and teens. www.mankato.msus.edu/dept/comdis/kuster2/welcome.html
National Stuttering Association. This site is run by a national organization of people who stutter and has information about support groups around the world and about NSA's annual conference. www.nsastutter.org
Guitar B, Conture E. *The Child Who Stutters: To the Pediatrician.* Memphis, TN: Stuttering Foundation of America (2001).
Guitar B. *Stuttering: An Integrated Approach to Its Nature and Treatment (2nd ed).* Baltimore: Williams & Wilkins, 1998.

74

Substance Abuse in Adolescence

John R. Knight

I. **Description of the problem.** The use of alcohol and drugs by adolescents is a major national problem:
- Alcohol use is associated with the leading causes of death among US teenagers, including unintentional injuries (e.g., motor vehicle crashes), homicides, and suicides.
- Greater than 30% of all deaths from injuries can be directly linked to alcohol.
- Substance use is also associated with a wide range of nonlethal but serious health problems, including school failure, respiratory diseases, and high-risk sexual behaviors associated with HIV infection.
- Early age of first use of alcohol and drugs increases the risk of developing a substance use disorder during later life.
- The age of first use among US teens has fallen.

A. **Epidemiology.**
- According to the Monitoring the Future Study, 77% of adolescents have begun to drink, 58% have gotten drunk, 51% have tried an illicit drug, and 28% have tried an illicit drug other than cannabis by the time they reach senior year in high school.
- Because of relatively high prevalence, experimentation with alcohol or cannabis or getting drunk once can arguably be considered developmentally normative behaviors. However, recurrent drunkenness, recurrent cannabis use, or any use of drugs other than cannabis are not normative behaviors and healthcare providers should always consider them serious risks.
- During recent years, adolescents have increasingly reported misuse of prescription drugs, including psychostimulant medications used to treat attention deficit hyperactivity disorder (ADHD) as well as oral opioid analgesics.
- Misuse of alcohol and drugs is found among all demographic subgroups, with higher risk associated with being male, white, and from middle to upper socioeconomic status families.
- Despite common stereotypes, drug use may be less prevalent among inner city minority students compared to their white suburban counterparts.
- Rises in prevalence of use of specific illicit drugs can be predicted by two factors: an increase in the perceived availability of the drug and a decrease in the perceived risk of harm associated with use of the drug.

B. **Etiology/contributing factors.**
1. Substance use during adolescence is associated with a variety of risk and protective factors, which may be characteristic of the individual, family, or community.
   a. **Individual risk factors** include male gender, school failure, ADHD and learning disability, other co-occurring mental disorders (e.g., depression, conduct disorder), nonconformity, and low religiousness.
   b. **Family factors** include genetic risks, a parent or sibling who is actively abusing alcohol or drugs, and parent-child conflict.
   c. **Community risks** include increased availability and substance using peers.
   d. **Individual protective factors** include high self-esteem, internal locus of control, and school achievement.
   e. **Family protective factors** include frequent communication about alcohol and drug use, good parental modeling, and eating meals together regularly as a family.
   f. **Community protective factors** include use of evidence-based prevention programs, availability of after school programs and mentoring, and low density of alcohol outlets.
2. Substance use disorders (i.e., alcohol/drug abuse or dependence) have a **multifactorial etiology**, including interactions between genetic predisposition, environmental exposures during childhood, and personal choice.
   a. Twin and adoption studies have shown that alcoholism has strong genetic deter-

minants, and recent genomic studies have shown that a number of specific genes are likely involved.

  b. Exposure to parental heavy drinking, especially during adolescence, is also associated with higher risk of substance abuse.

  c. Recent animal studies suggest that early nicotine use may independently increase the risk of substance abuse by altering the dopaminergic pathways within the brain's reward system.

II. Making the diagnosis.

  A. Signs and symptoms. A myriad of behaviors—some obvious, some subtle—may signal a substance abuse problem, including: odor of alcohol on breath; appearance of obvious intoxication; dilated pupils (stimulants, cocaine); volatile odor on person or clothes (inhalants); constricted pupils (alcohol, opioids, sedatives); change in school performance, dress, and friends; drug or drug paraphernalia found in room, car or clothes; moodiness or sudden mood swings (either depression or euphoria); diluted or missing alcohol from parent's home supply; stealing, lying, or missing money, including unexplained withdrawals from a bank account.

  B. History.

  1. Screening. As part of a routine history, every adolescent should be asked about use of alcohol and drugs. *"Have you ever tried alcohol? Have you ever tried marijuana? Have you ever tried any other drug?"* A yes answer to any of these questions should be followed by a structured substance abuse screening tool. One such screen is the CRAFFT test, which consists of six, orally administered yes/no questions that are easy to score (each "yes" answer = 1). A CRAFFT total score of two or higher has sensitivity of 80% and specificity 86% for identifying a diagnosis of substance abuse or dependence.

CRAFFT*

C	"Have you ever ridden in a CAR driven by someone (including yourself) who was 'high' or had been using alcohol or drugs?"
R	"Do you ever use alcohol or drugs to RELAX, feel better about yourself, or fit in?"
A	"Do you ever use alcohol or drugs while you are by yourself, ALONE?"
F	"Do you ever FORGET things you did while using alcohol or drugs?"
F	"Do your family or FRIENDS ever tell you that you should cut down on your drinking or drug use?"
T	"Have you ever gotten into TROUBLE while you were using alcohol or drugs?"

*CRAFFT screen reprinted with permission from the Center for Adolescent Substance Abuse Research at Children's Hospital Boston.

  2. Assessment. A positive CRAFFT should be followed by a more comprehensive alcohol and drug use history, including **age of first use, current pattern of use** (quantity and frequency), and **impact on physical and emotional health, school and family,** and other negative consequences from use (e.g., legal problems). Taking a substance use history begins the process of therapeutic intervention. Helpful questions include

  • *"What's the worst thing that ever happened to you while you were using alcohol or drugs?"*

  • *"Have you ever regretted something that happened when you were drinking or drugging?"*

  • *"Do your parents know about your alcohol and drug use? If so, how do they feel about it? If not, how do you think they would feel about it?"*

  • *"Do you have any younger brothers or sisters? What do (or would) they think about your alcohol and drug use?"*

  • The assessment should also include a screening for co-occurring mental disorders and parent/sibling alcohol and drug use.

  C. Other diagnostic procedures.

  1. Physical findings. A physical examination should be performed, but is unlikely to yield significant findings in the absence of acute intoxication. Check vital signs and pupil size. Hypertension, tachycardia, and dilated pupils may suggest either acute intoxication (amphetamines, cocaine, MDMA) or withdrawal (opioids). Inflammation or erosions of the nasal septum may suggest insufflation ("snorting") of drugs, but can also result from common upper respiratory infections or digital excoriation. Auscultation of the lungs may reveal wheezing in those who smoke drugs. Abdominal tenderness may occasionally be found in heavy drinkers. Examination of the skin should be performed, but venous scarring from intravenous drug use is uncommon in adolescents.

2. **Drug testing.** Laboratory testing for alcohol or drugs of abuse should not be performed on a conscious adolescent without their knowledge and consent. Clinicians should consult with a toxicologist before ordering drug screens to minimize the risks of false negatives. The window of detection for most drugs of abuse is no more than 24 hours, with the notable exception of cannabis which for heavy users may be detectable in the urine up to several weeks after the last episode of use. Taking a good history, with reasonable assurance of confidentiality, is often more informative than laboratory testing. However, properly conducted laboratory testing may be a useful therapeutic adjunct for drug using adolescents who are receiving treatment and/or motivated to stop using.

III. **Management.**
  A. **Assess the level of severity of use.** A developmental model of substance use follows the following progression:
    1. **Experimentation:** first use of psychoactive substance, most commonly alcohol, marijuana or inhalants
    2. **Non-problematic use:** regular pattern of use, regardless of frequency, usually with peers and without negative consequences
    3. **Problem use:** adverse consequences first appear (e.g., decline in school performance, suspension, accident, injury, arguments with parents or peers)
    4. **Abuse:** defined by 1 or more of 4 criteria occurring repeatedly over the course of the past 12 months, but not meeting criteria for diagnosis of dependence:
      a. Substance-related problems at school, work, or home
      b. Use of substance in hazardous situations (e.g., driving a car)
      c. Substance-related legal problems
      d. Continued use despite problems or arguments with friends or family
    5. **Dependence:** defined by meeting any 3 of 7 criteria during the past 12 months:
      a. Tolerance
      b. Withdrawal (may be either physiological or psychological)
      c. Using more of substance of for longer periods of time than intended
      d. Unsuccessful attempts to quit or cut down use of substance
      e. Spending a great deal of time obtaining, using, or recovering from effects of the substance
      f. Giving up important activities because of substance use
      g. Continued use of substance despite medical or social problems caused by the substance
  B. **Assess the level of motivation to change.** Prochaska and DiClemente have described readiness to change along a continuum that includes **precontemplation, contemplation, preparation, action, maintenance, and relapse.** Many adolescents will be at precontemplation (e.g., "I don't have a problem.") or contemplation (e.g., "I don't think I have a problem" or "I'm not sure I really want to change.").
    1. For those at *precontemplation*, the best strategy is to list the problems and risks that you elicited while taking the history and express your concern. This will introduce doubt and may lead to *contemplation.*
    2. For those at *contemplation*, the best strategy is to elicit the pros and cons of substance use (*"What do you like about your substance use? What don't you like about it?"*), discuss the pros and cons of change (*"Who do you think would be proud of you if you stop using alcohol/drugs?"*), and try to tip the balance in favor of change (*"It sounds like you may be interested in stopping, at least for a while."*)
  C. **Deliver a therapeutic intervention.** Stage specific therapeutic office strategies include:
    1. **Provide positive reinforcement for those who are abstinent.**
    2. For those at the stages of experimentation and nonproblematic use, it is most productive to focus on **risk reduction**. For example, the clinician may initiate a discussion of the serious risks associated with drinking and driving, or riding with an intoxicated driver, and suggest strategies for safe transportation home following events where alcohol or drugs are present.
    3. For those at the stages of problematic use or abuse, **office-based brief interventions** have been shown to be effective among adults. However, less is known about the effectiveness of these strategies among adolescents and among those who use drugs. Most brief interventions include the following steps:
      • **Feedback:** Deliver feedback on the risks and/or negative consequences of substance use.

- **Education:** Explain how substance use can lead to consequences that are relevant to the adolescent (i.e., immediate rather than long-term consequences).
- **Recommendation:** Recommend that the adolescent completely stop all use of alcohol and drugs for a specified time period (e.g., 3 months).
- **Negotiation:** If your recommendation is declined, attempt to elicit some commitment to change. For example, try to have your patient commit to stopping drugs (if he refuses to stop drinking), or cutting back use of alcohol or drugs.
- **Agreement:** Secure a specific, concrete agreement. Ask for a brief written contract that both of you will sign that specifies the change and the time period.
- **Follow-up:** Make an appointment for a follow-up meeting to monitor success (or need for more intensive treatment) and consider use of laboratory testing to verify abstinence.

D. **Referral.** Some adolescents, such as those with alcohol/drug dependence or co-occurring mental disorders, will require more directive intervention, parental involvement and referral to intensive treatment. Healthcare providers should be familiar with treatment resources in their own communities. Whenever possible, refer adolescents to programs that are limited to adolescents or have staff specifically trained in counseling adolescents. However, adolescent specific treatment is uncommon in many communities. Effective treatment programs should offer treatment for co-occurring disorders and include parents in treatment.
   1. **Outpatient treatment** may include:
      a. **Behavioral therapies:** individual, group, or family counseling. Cognitive behavioral therapy and multisystemic family therapy appear promising.
      b. **Pharmacotherapies:** These are seldom used in adolescents. Naltrexone appears promising for relapse prevention among adults with alcohol disorders. Methadone and buprenorphine are effective for treatment of opioid dependence.
      c. **12-step fellowships** (e.g., Alcoholics Anonymous). Adolescents may need an adult guide or temporary sponsor to make attendance at AA groups meaningful.
   2. **Inpatient treatment** may include:
      a. **Detoxification:** 2–3 days of medical treatment for physiological withdrawal symptoms, indicated only for acute management of alcohol, sedative-hypnotic, benzodiazepine, or opioid dependence.
      b. **Rehabilitation:** 2–3 weeks of intensive behavioral therapy, usually including individual and group counseling, psychoeducational sessions, family therapy, and introduction to 12-step fellowships.
      c. **Long-term residential treatment:** These include residential schools, therapeutic communities, and halfway houses. Most offer 3–12 months closely supervised aftercare (i.e., following completion of a detoxification and/or rehabilitation program), which includes weekly counseling and group therapy, behavioral management strategies, and required attendance at school and/or work.
      d. **Unproven programs:** Some families may choose to send their teenaged children to wilderness programs or so-called boot camps, which have not been scientifically evaluated.

IV. **Clinical pearls and pitfalls.**
- Many adolescents who abuse substances are also depressed. Provide treatment for substance abuse and depression *simultaneously* when they co-occur. Treatment of either one alone is unlikely to be successful.
- Children with untreated ADHD are at increased risk of abusing substances during adolescence. However, appropriate treatment with psychostimulant medication does not increase this risk, and several studies suggest that it is protective. Nonetheless, as a precaution, parents of adolescents with ADHD should retain control of the prescription bottle.
- Treatment of chronic severe pain with opioid analgesics seldom causes addiction in individuals who do not have pre-existing substance abuse or some other mental disorder. Chronic use of opioid analgesics leads to development of physiological tolerance and withdrawal, but these two alone do not define an addictive disorder. *Physiological dependence* on opioid analgesics should not be confused with a *drug dependence* diagnosis.

BIBLIOGRAPHY

For Parents

Publications

Keeping Your Kids Drug Free, a how-to guide for parents and caregivers. http://store.health.org/catalog/ProductDetails.aspx?ProductID = 16061

Keeping Youth Drug Free http://store.health.org/catalog/ProductDetails.aspx?ProductID = 14602
Treating Teens: A Guide to Adolescent Drug Programs. Washington, DC: Drug Strategies, 2003.
   Can be ordered at: http://www.drugstrategies.org/pubs.html#teen

Websites for Parents

A Family Guide to Keeping Youth Mentally Health and Drug Free http://family.samhsa.gov/
Mothers Against Drunk Driving www.madd.org
Parents: The Anti-Drug www.theantidrug.com/
Partnership for a Drug Free America www.drugfreeamerica.org

Websites for Adolescents

Students Against Destructive Decisions http://saddonline.com
Check Yourself http://www.checkyourself.com/main.html
NIDA for Teens (National Institute on Drug Abuse) http://www.teens.drugabuse.gov/
What's Driving You? http://www.whatsdrivingyou.org/

For Professionals

Publications

American Academy of Pediatrics. Tobacco, alcohol, and other drugs: The role of the pediatrician
   in prevention and management of substance abuse. *Pediatrics;* 1998 101(1):125–128.
Levy S, Knight JR. Office management of substance use. *Adolescent Health Update;*15(3):1–9,
   2003.
Schydlower M (ed). *Substance Abuse: A Guide for Health Professionals (2nd ed).* Elk Grove Village,
   IL: American Academy of Pediatrics, 2002.

Websites

National Clearinghouse for Alcohol and Drug Information (includes a special section for health
   professionals) www.health.org
National Institute on Drug Abuse www.nida.nih.gov
National Institute on Alcohol Abuse and Alcoholism http://niaaa.nih.org

75

Suicide

Karen Norberg

I. **Description of the problem.** Because suicidal ideation is so common, primary care clinicians need to know how to distinguish those at greatest risk for suicide or serious injury, from among the large number of adolescents with suicidal thoughts or self-injurious actions who have a benign prognosis. Emergency clinicians need to know how to provide acute treatment for the suicidal patient, and behavioral pediatricians may be asked to provide consultation to educational and public health agencies about appropriate and inappropriate strategies for suicide prevention.

- **Completed suicide** refers to a self-directed action that results in death.
- **Suicide attempt** or **suicide gesture** refers to intentional behavior that the child believes might result in self-harm (whether or not this assessment is medically realistic and whether or not the intention actually includes death).
- **Suicidal ideation** refers to self-reported thoughts about self-harm (not necessarily accompanied by action).

A. **Epidemiology.**
  - Suicide is currently the third leading cause of death among 15–24-year-olds in the United States.
  - In 2001, about 19% of adolescents in the US reported having serious thoughts of suicide and 8.8% reported making a self-injury attempt within the past 12 months.
  - In the US, about 1% of adolescent suicide gestures that come to medical attention are lethal.
  - In 2001, the rate of completed suicides was 9.9 /100,000 among young adults aged 15–24 years and 0.7 /100,000 among children aged 5–14 years. These rates reflect a small decline starting in 1995, after a steady increase over the previous three decades.
  - School-aged children report suicidal thoughts as often as adolescents, but the likelihood of actual self-harm increases with age.
  - In the US, adolescent girls are almost 2 times more likely to attempt suicide as boys, but adolescent boys are more than 5 times more likely to complete suicide.

B. **Contributing factors.** The most important known risk factors for completed suicide among adolescents, given an attempt, are listed in Table 75-1. Mood disorders (juvenile onset major depression, bipolar disorder, and panic disorder), sexual abuse, and early onset substance abuse are the most important risk factors for serious self-injury among both boys and girls. Others include:
  1. **Life stresses/social communication.**
     a. Suicide attempts are most often precipitated by **crises** for which the child or adolescent fears rejection (e.g., arguments with girlfriend or boyfriend, school failure, legal problems, identification of gay sexual orientation).
     b. Most attempts have a **strong communicative intent,** expressing a wish to change a situation or relationship or to show anger.
  2. **Developmental.**
     a. Completed suicide in children **under age 10 years** is rare; however, children as young as age 4 or 5 years may make a potentially serious gesture (e.g., wrapping a cord around the neck, running into traffic) during which they may specifically state a wish to die.
     b. Children **over age 10 years** have a generally realistic understanding of what might be harmful or lethal.
  3. **Biological.**
     a. **Serotonin hypothesis.** Many studies have implicated disturbances of norepinephrine and serotonin regulation in persons who have attempted or completed suicide, and in persons with traits or conditions that have been associated with an increase in the risk of suicide, including major depression, panic disorder, and

Table 75-1 Risk factors predicting greater lethality of suicide attempts in children and adolescents

Demographics
Male>>female
Older teen>>younger
Family history of suicide increases risk
Lethality ofintent
Stated intensity of wish for death
Specific, realistically lethal plan
Rescue/discovery was not expected
History of previous suicide attempt, especially recently
Method
Higher lethality: guns, hanging, use of motor vehicle, jumping from a great height
Lower lethality: overdose, wrist cutting, attempted suffocation
Concurrent problems
Alcohol intoxication (increases impulsivity)
Major depression
Bipolar disorder
Panic disorder
Posttraumatic stress disorder
Psychosis
History of impulsive aggression towards others
Social environment, trauma
Rejection, lack of support from family
Recent loss or disappointment
Current legal problem
Past history of sexual victimization, other trauma or abuse
Behavioral contagion; exposure to suicidal behavior in relative or acquaintance
Shame, reluctance to discuss problems

impulsive aggression. In particular, there is evidence of reduction of serotonin or its metabolite, 5-HIAA, in the brainstem of victims of suicide, regardless of diagnostic category.

   b. **Physiological stress system.** Acute stress activates the glucocorticoid system, and adaptations of the hypothalamic-pituitary-adrenal (HPA) axis to chronic stress have been implicated in the relationship between early socioenvironmental stress, and later psychopathology. There may be a reciprocal relationship between the serotonergic system and the HPA axis, with the chronic stress of adverse rearing leading to low levels of central serotonin responsivity in primates and humans.

   c. **Genetics of suicide.** There is now evidence for a genetic liability for suicidal behavior from two sources: 1) genetic liability for mood disorders or other established psychiatric syndromes, and 2) genetic liability for impulsive aggression. Candidate gene studies implicate polymorphisms in genes regulating the serotonergic pathway in both cases.

4. **Social and physical environment.**

   a. **"Contagion."** Suicide and suicide attempts may appear in clusters, especially in circumstances that dramatize or intensify the effects of a suicide gesture as an attempt to communicate. Publicizing a real or fictional suicide in newspapers or on television, for example, has been reported to increase the suicide rate by 7%–10% among adolescents and young adults.

   b. **Lethality of opportunity.** Access to lethal methods may affect the rate of completed suicide. For example, the increased lethality of gestures among older adolescents may be related to their increased access to alcohol, motor vehicles, and guns.

II. **Assessing the risk.** Among adolescents who complete suicide, about half have had a known history of depression, alcohol abuse, psychosis, or previous suicide attempt. Most adolescents who succeed in suicide have given some sign or warning shortly before the event—a note, a gesture, or a verbal statement to someone important to them—that in retrospect might have offered an opportunity for intervention. In general, **all suicide gestures and suicidal ideation should be immediately evaluated by a mental health profes-**

sional. The primary care clinician can serve the adolescent as a known and trusted professional in the initial assessment of the situation.

   A. **Interview with the child.** If possible, the interview with the child or adolescent should take place in a quiet, private area, without interruptions. Details of the interview depend on the urgency of the situation and the developmental level of the child. See Table 75-2 for suggested questions. Issues to be explored include:

      1. Severity of intent at time of attempt
      2. Circumstances of injury (if any)
      3. Precipitating events
      4. Past history, presence of risk and protective factors
      5. Present mental status, severity of suicidal intent

   B. **Interview with parents.** Information should be gathered from as many other informants as possible. Although care must be taken to protect the confidentiality of the adolescent, and to attend to conflicts of interest between child and parent that may have contributed to the present crisis, it is ethical and almost always necessary to communicate with

---

Table 75-2 Questions for assessing suicide intent in children

Present episode
"Can you tell me what happened? What happened next?"
"Did you [try to/want to] hurt yourself?"
"How did you [plan to] hurt yourself?"
"Was anyone else nearby at the time? Expected?"
"Had you been drinking or using other drugs?"

Motivation: death
"What did you think would happen if you tried to hurt yourself?"
"What did you want to have happen?"
"Did you think you would die? Get hurt badly?"
"Have you ever tried to hurt yourself before? What happened?"

Concepts of death
"What do you think happens when a person dies? Do you believe in life after death?"
"What did you think would happen if you died?"
"Have you known anyone who has died? Who? How did they die?"
"Do you have a wish to join them in death?"
"Have you pictured what your funeral would be like? Who would be sad?"

Motivation: communication
"Why did you want to hurt yourself?"
"Did you want to frighten someone?"
"Did you want to get even with someone?"
"Did you wish someone would rescue you?"
"Did you hear voices telling you to hurt yourself?"
"Did you change your mind afterward? How do you feel now?"

Motivation: family, school stresses
"Do you feel very sad or upset about anything?"
"Has anything upsetting happened that you have had trouble telling someone about?"
"Did you or do you feel that your family does not care about you?"
"Have you had a fight with someone important to you?"
"Do you have difficulty in school? Do you worry about school?"
"Do you get into fights at school? Do other kids tease you?"
"Do your parents punish you a lot? Do you argue with your parents?"
"Do your parents fight with each other?"
"Have you been separated from your parents? When?"
"Has anyone important left or stopped seeing you? Who?"
"Is anyone in your family sick? Who?"
"Is anyone else in your family sad or upset? Who?"

Motivation: hopelessness and depression
"Have you been thinking about death for a long time?"
"Do you often blame yourself for things?"
"Do you cry a lot? Do you prefer to stay by yourself?"
"Do you have trouble paying attention in school?"
"Do you have trouble sleeping or eating? Do you feel tired a lot?"
"Do you feel that things are likely to get better?"

Table 75-3 Criteria for referral of suicidal children or adolescents

Refer for hospitalization if
The child has made a medically significant gesture.
The child expresses a strong intent to harm himself, verbally or through ongoing behavior.
The child is uncommunicative or unwilling to give convincing reassurances of safety.
The child has evidence of psychosis or other abnormal mental status impairing judgement or
impulse control.
Hospitalization may not be required if
Strong social supports and supervision are available.
The gesture was not medically serious.
The gesture seems to have accomplished its communicative intent.
The patient no longer expresses suicidal wishes
Follow-up treatment is available.

the family, even against an adolescent's wishes, in a life-endangering situation. Issues
to be explored include:
1. **The family's knowledge of current stresses in the patient's life.**
2. **The family's attitude toward the patient** (supportive or devaluing?) and the status
of ongoing conflicts between parent and child.
3. **Any parental or family history of suicide, alcoholism, drug abuse, depression, or
family violence.**
4. **The willingness of the family to seek help for the patient.**
C. **Behavioral observations.** The child's behavior may give clues about the presence of
depression or anxiety. Emotional expressiveness and general cooperation may indicate
the child's desire for help and may provide clues about the dependability of the child's
promises not to hurt themselves in the future.
III. **Management.** Any child or adolescent who has made a gesture of intentional self-harm or
who is expressing a strong wish to hurt themselves should be seen by a mental health
professional for consultation.Table 75-3 lists criteria for hospitalization.
A. **Primary goals.** The primary goals of acute management of suicidal behavior are:
1. The provision of physical safety.
2. The establishment of a relationship with the suicidal patient and with the family, and
the use of this relationship to encourage the importance of follow-up and treatment.
3. The initial identification of underlying problems, in order to make the most appropriate referrals.
4. Long-term goals may include changes in family patterns of communication, and
cognitive and/or pharmacological treatment of underlying mood disorder or substance abuse.
B. **Medication.**
1. Lithium has been shown to reduce the rate of both suicides and suicide attempts in
adults with bipolar disorder, above and beyond its effect in the stabilization of depressed or manic mood states. Studies are underway to evaluate the effectiveness
of lithium prophylaxis in suicidal patients with other kinds of disorders. It is not
yet known whether other mood stabilizers, used in bipolar disorder, have a similar
effect.
2. Antidepressant medications may be indicated and can prove helpful in some cases
in reducing symptoms of depression, suicidal ideation and suicide attempts. Children
and adolescents on any psychotherapeutic medication should be closely monitored
to insure that new suicidal ideation is noted.
C. **Psychotherapy.** Cognitive-behavioral therapy, interpersonal therapy, dialectical behavioral therapy, psychodynamic therapy, and family therapy are all options.
D. **Ongoing safety.**
- **Advise** parents to **prevent access to means** of self-injury by securing or removing
firearms and lethal medications from the home.
- **Warn** parents and child about **disinhibiting** effects of alcohol and drugs.
- Check that there will be a **supportive person** at home with the patient.
- Check that a **follow-up appointment** or contact has been made available.

BIBLIOGRAPHY

American Academy of Child and Adolescent Psychiatry. Practice parameter for the assessment
and treatment of children and adolescents with suicidal behavior. *J Am Acad Child Adolesc
Psychiatry;*40(7 Suppl):24S– 51S, 2001.

Centers for Disease Control and Prevention factsheet http://www.cdc.gov/nccdphp/dash/yrbs/pdf-factsheets/suicide.pdf.

GoldsmithSK, PellmarTC, KleinmanAM, et al (eds). *Reducing Suicide: A National Imperative.*Washington, DC: National Academies Press, 2002.

KhanA, KhanS, KoltsR, and Brown WA.Suicide rates in clinical trials of SSRIs, other antidepressants, and placebo: Analysis of FDA reports. *Am J Psychiatry;*160(4):790– 792, 2003.

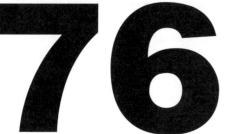

Temper Tantrums
Robert Needlman

I. **Description of the problem.** Behaviors comprising temper tantrums include crying, yelling, shouting, pushing, pulling, hitting, throwing things, stamping, stiffening, dropping to the floor, and running away. Tantrums typically begin with shows of anger (e.g., yelling or hitting), then progress to signs of distress or sadness (e.g. crying and attempts to gain proximity to the parent). Most tantrums last less than 5 minutes; the briefest ones tend to begin with stamping or dropping to the ground. Frequent, prolonged tantrums often elicit concern, anger, and guilt in parents and may indicate serious emotional disturbance with poor long-term prognosis.

A. **Epidemiology.**
- 50%–80% of 2–3-year-old children have tantrums at least weekly.
- 20% have at least daily tantrums.
- 60% of 2-year-olds with frequent tantrums will continue to have them at age 3 years. Of these, 60% will continue at age 4 years.
- The prevalence of explosive "tempers" remains approximately 5% throughout childhood.
- Severe tantrums are often accompanied by other significant behavioral problems, such as disturbed sleep or overactivity.
- Tantrum frequency is not related to gender or social class.
- There is no known genetic or familial predisposition.

B. **Etiology/contributing factors.**
1. **Normal development.** In toddlers, tantrums arise when normal drives for autonomy conflict with parental prohibitions or limited competence. Toddlers typically lack the ability to regulate frustration through self-directed speech or to communicate emotional upset verbally. Tantrums may be reinforced either by parental compliance or, paradoxically, by the intense negative attention they elicit.
2. **Medical problems.** Consider (among others) recurrent upper respiratory illnesses or otitis; respiratory or GI allergies; eczema; endocrine disorders (particularly androgen excess); obstructive sleep apnea; other sleep disturbance; hospitalization; invasive medical procedures; certain medications (e.g., most anticonvulsants, many antihistamines.)
3. **Disabilities.** Consider autism spectrum disorders (PDD, etc.); mental retardation; attention deficit hyperactivity disorder (ADHD); traumatic brain injury (especially frontal lobe); unrecognized deafness or visual impairment.
4. **Temperament.** Predisposing traits include high intensity and activity; persistence; predominantly negative mood; low sensory threshold; and high sensitivity to novel stimuli. Irregular timing of sleep and hunger make it difficult for parents to anticipate the child's needs.
5. **Environment.** Physical factors include overcrowding; limited access to outdoor play; and non-childproofed homes that make frequent parental prohibitions necessary. Social factors include martial stress and verbal or physical violence; tensions arising from siblings or grandparents with behavioral problems or medical illness; parental depression, and alcohol and/or drug abuse.
6. **Parenting.** Contributors include corporal punishment or abuse; inconsistent limit setting; over-permissiveness; intrusiveness; failure to recognize stressors (e.g., frightening movies or even the TV news); and unrealistic expectations for self-control or delay of gratification.

II. **Recognizing the issue.**
A. **Signs and symptoms.** Features of problem tantrums include:
1. A high degree of parental concern, anger, guilt, or sadness. Tantrums are a problem if parents think they are.
2. Parents are unable to identify positive things about the child, seeing the child as antagonistic and controlling. Such complaints may signal a toxic parent-child relationship.

3. Child age less than 12 months or greater than 48 months. Tantrums, if present, tend to be mild and infrequent in these age ranges.
4. Tantrums that occur more than 3 times a day, or last 15 minutes or longer. Frequent, prolonged tantrums are associated with multiple behavior problems, e.g., problems with sleeping, eating, or peer interactions.
5. Tantrums in school. Children typically "pull it together" in front of peers; tantrums in school may be due to social, academic, or emotional problems.
- B. **History: Key clinical questions.**
  1. *"What exactly happened the last time your child had a tantrum? What set it off? What did your child do first? How did you respond? Was that a typical episode?"* Try to get a play-by-play account of a recent episode. Focus on the ABCs: antecedents, behaviors, and consequences. Look for triggers (hunger, tiredness, sources of frustration); unintentional reinforcement (e.g., increased attention); and delayed consequences, such as special treats the parents may offer to atone for their own feelings of anger.
  2. *"What feelings do our child's tantrums bring out in you?"* If parents report extreme anger, shame, or guilt, these feelings need to be addressed for intervention to succeed.
  3. *"How often do tantrums result in your child's getting what he or she wants?"* When parents occasionally give in to tantrums in order to get them to stop, they inadvertently teach the child to carry on for increasingly longer periods. Behaviors maintained by intermittent reinforcement are particularly resistant to extinction.
  4. *"What do other adults in the family say about the tantrums? How do they respond? How do they say you should respond?"* Family dynamics often plays a role in maintaining tantrums. If tantrums occur more frequently with, say, the mother, it may be that she is more ambivalent about limit setting; or the other parent may be subtly undercutting her authority, e.g., by acting overly solicitous to the child after a tantrum.
  5. *"Does your child have other behavior problems, such as overactivity, aggressiveness, food refusal, difficulty separating from you, or sleep problems?"* A pattern of multiple behavior problems suggests the need for a more comprehensive psychological evaluation. Consider the possibility of developmental delay as well.
  6. *"When your child is happy, how does the child show it? Are all emotions expressed intensely? Does your child tend to stick with a challenge until he or she masters it?"* In the absence of other concerning features, long, loud tantrums in an intense, persistent child may be normal.
  7. *"How was your pregnancy with this child? What about the delivery, newborn period, first year of life, etc.? Any significant illnesses or injury?"* Past medical history may point to an episode in which the parent feared the child might die, and made an unspoken promise to make the child's life perfect, if only the child would survive. Such episodes may trigger the vulnerable child syndrome, which typically includes severe tantrums.
- C. **Office evaluation.**
  1. **Physical examination.** Look for signs of allergies, recurrent otitis, dental caries (a source of pain), scars suggestive of abuse, evidence of endocrinopathy (e.g., genital enlargement, striae).
  2. **Observations.** Crayons and paper may elicit themes of anger or threat (e.g., a burning house, a shark that eats everything up), indicating that the child understands that gaining some control over such feelings is the purpose of the visit. Provision of a few age-appropriate toys allows observation of the child's play skills, (an indication of cognitive development) and the child's response to the request to clean up.
  3. **Written data and tests.** A tantrum log, listing the antecedents, behaviors, and consequences of each tantrum, as well as the times of onset and resolution, can help you identify patterns, and document improvement with therapy. A standardized parent-report instrument (e.g., the Pediatric Symptom Checklist), can detect relevant patterns of behavior, and may suggest the presence of more significant problems.

III. **Management.**
- A. **Primary goals.**
  1. **Clarify the diagnosis.** Differentiate between tantrums due to developmentally appropriate stresses or challenges of temperament (parents' and/or child's), and tantrums due to underlying delays, disorders, or family dysfunction.
  2. **Address contributing factors.** For example, refer for speech and language therapy; adjust medications for asthma or allergies; advocate for improved housing; refer parents for marital counseling or treatment of depression.
  3. **Educate parents.** Reduce parental distress by correcting unrealistic expectations and

fears, and explaining the developmental forces driving the tantrums; help parents to problem solve (e.g., providing a small snack before going to the grocery store.)

B. **Specific strategies.**
1. **Childproof the home.** Reducing hazards and temptations minimizes how often the child must hear "no"; nonetheless, there will be plenty of opportunities for the child to learn to accept limits.
2. **Allow choices.** Children comply better when they feel in control. For a young child, it's best to offer two alternatives, both acceptable (e.g., red shirt or blue shirt.) Small children need to make small choices.
3. **Provide routines.** Predictability increases a small child's sense of control, reducing frustrations.
4. **Adjust to temperament.** A very active child needs space to run around; a slow-to-warm-up child needs time to adjust to new situations and people; a highly persistent child may need 5- and 1-minute warnings to prepare to end a pleasurable activity.
5. **Pick battles and win them.** Parents often say "no" when they really mean, "I'd rather you didn't." If the issue really isn't worth a fight, the parents are apt to reverse themselves in the face of a tantrum. For such issues, it's better for parents to state their preference ("I'd rather you didn't have a cookie right now"), offer alternatives ("How about a carrot stick?), or simply say "yes" right off the bat. When parents do say "no," they should mean it, and stick to their guns. "No" needs to be absolute and nonnegotiable.
6. **Ignore when possible.** Specific instructions for ignoring may include, "Stand 5 feet away. Keep doing whatever you were doing. Do not speak to your child, or speak in a neutral tone of voice." When ignoring is first instituted, tantrums may get worse for several days. With young children, parents may need to stay in the same room so the child does not become scared, in addition to being upset.
7. **Prevent harm.** The parent may have to move the child to a rug or away from hard furniture. A child intent on hurting himself or anyone else needs to be stopped, even if that means physical restraint. Parents should not allow a child to hit, pinch, or bite them.
8. **Use helpful language.** How parents talk about a child's tantrums matters. Tantrums are about "losing control" rather than "being bad." It isn't helpful to dwell in detail on tantrums past, but it may help to remind a child to "Tell me when you're mad; use your words." Parents can make up stories about children who are furious but triumph by controlling themselves, or stories about how they (the parents) have needed to take three deep breaths to avoid "losing it."
9. **Celebrate successes.** Parents need to pay attention whenever their child uses words to express frustration or to protest a perceived injustice. A warm "good job!" and a hug powerfully reinforce the child's accomplishment.

C. **Criteria for referral.** The following features should suggest referral for sub-specialist care for tantrums.
1. **Developmental disability.** Severe tantrums arising in the context of mental retardation, autism spectrum disorders, deafness, or other developmental disabilities may benefit from intensive behavioral approaches.
2. **Emotional disturbance.** Consider referral to child psychology if you identify significant trauma (e.g., the child witnessed domestic violence or endured a traumatic separation), if the child expresses violent themes in play or drawings (e.g., repeated play about people burning up) or acts out in disturbed ways (e.g., fire-setting, tormenting pets). Parental depression or other mental health issues, traumatic or recurrent hospitalization, or presence of a sibling with special healthcare needs, may also signal the need for psychological intervention.
3. **Failure to improve.** In the absence of any more specific indications, failure for tantrums to show improvement after two or three visits may trigger referral for more extensive evaluation and protracted management.

BIBLIOGRAPHY

For Parents

Ginott H. *Between Parent and Child.* New York: Macmilan, 1965. (Still one of the best guides for talking with children, giving clear messages and effective feedback.)

Lieberman A. *The Emotional Life of the Toddler.* New York: Free Press, 1993. (A remarkably clear, insightful, readable explanation of toddlers and their feelings.)

Turecki S, Tonner L. *The Difficult Child.* New York: Bantam Doubleday, 1989. (Practical and sensitive advice, with an emphasis on temperament as a major determinant of children's behavior.)

Websites

Iowa State University–University Extension http://www.extension.iastate.edu/Publications/PM1529J.pdf

KidsHealth http://kidshealth.org/parent/emotions/behavior/tantrums.html

For Professionals

Goodenough F. *Anger in Young Children.* Minneapolis: University of Minnesota Press, 1931. (A classic monograph.)

Needlman R, Stevenson J, Zuckerman B. Psychosocial correlates of severe temper tantrums. *J Dev Behav Pediatr;*12:77–83, 1991. (An analysis of a large, community-based sample.)

Potegal M, Davidson RJ. Temper tantrums in young children: 1. Behavioral composition. *J Dev Behav Pediatr;* 24: 140–147, 2003. (A detailed description of the phenomenology of tantrums.)

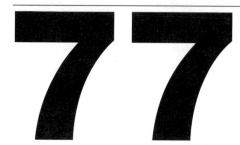

Temperamentally Difficult Children

Stanley Turecki

I. **Description of the problem.** A "difficult child" is a normal young child whose innate temperament makes them hard to raise. Inherent in this definition is a view of normality that is broad: children are different and do not have to be average in order to be normal. For a child to be considered temperamentally difficult, a basic criterion has to be met: the child's constitutionally determined personality traits—their very nature—must cause significant problems in child rearing.

A. **Epidemiology.**
- About 15% of young children are temperamentally difficult according to this definition.
- Difficult children are not all alike. Some are impulsive, distractible, and highly active; others are shy and clingy. Some throw loud tantrums; others whine and complain. Some can hit, kick, or even bite; others are verbally defiant. Some are unpredictable in their eating or sleeping habits; others are sensitive to noise, textures, or tastes. Most difficult children have trouble dealing with transition and change, and almost all are strong-willed and extremely stubborn.
- Highly active, impulsive, difficult children are more likely to be boys. All other temperamentally difficult traits are as likely to be seen in girls as in boys.
- There is no correlation with birth order, intelligence, or socioeconomic status.

B. **Etiology.**
- Temperament refers to dimensions of personality that are largely constitutional in origin. Genetic factors definitely contribute. Pregnancy and delivery complications may be somewhat more common in the histories of difficult children. Some of these children are allergic, with a propensity to develop ear infections. Uneven language and learning skills development are not uncommon. Many difficult children are intelligent but socially immature. All of these factors suggest a biologic basis for a difficult temperament.

C. **The concept of temperament.** Temperament is the *how* of behavior, rather than the *why* (motivation) or the *what* (ability). For example, three equally motivated and able children may approach a homework assignment quite differently, depending on their behavioral style. One will begin on time and work steadily to completion, the second will delay and procrastinate but then work very persistently, and the third will jump in immediately and quickly lose patience. Inherent in the temperamental perspective is a broad view of normality and a bias towards seeing atypical behavior as different rather than abnormal.

Temperament may also be defined as the behavioral expression, evident early in life, of those dimensions of personality that are constitutional in origin. Family, twin and adoption studies point to a 50% multigenetic heritability. The stability of temperament is detectable at 18 months, substantial at 3 years and most evident in middle childhood. As development proceeds, temperamental qualities are neither rigidly fixed nor completely malleable—like cartilage rather than bone or muscle. A range exists for each category. Table 77-1 lists the categories of temperament.

1. **The child and the environment: A transactional model.** The concept of a difficult temperament should always be combined with that of *goodness of fit*—the match or compatibility between a child and their environment. Behavior that presents a problem to one family may be readily accepted by another. For example, a child's idiosyncratic and strongly held tastes in clothing and food would only trouble a fashion- and nutrition-conscious parent. The context of the behavior is always important. A highly active boy who has some problems with self-control and concentration, if placed in a class of (25 children (of whom another 5 are "challenging") with one somewhat inexperienced teacher, would undoubtedly meet all the criteria for attention deficit hyperactivity disorder (ADHD). However, if the following year he is in

Table 77-1 Categories of temperament

Trait	Description	Easy	Difficult
Activity level	General statement about level of motor activity; actual amount of physical motion during play, eating, sleep etc.	Low to moderate	Very active, restless, fidgity; always into things; makes you tired; "ran before they walked"; easily overstimulated; gets wild or "revved up"; impulsive, loses control, can be aggressive, hates to be confined
Self control	Ability to delay action or demands	Good, patient	Poor, impulsive
Concentration	Ability to maintain focus in the face of distractions	Good, stays with task	Poor, distractible, has trouble concentrating and paying attention especially if not really interested; doesn't listen, tunes you out; daydreams, forgets instructions
Intensity	Energy level of responses; how forcefully or loudly reactions are expressed, whether positive or negative	Low, mild, low-keyed	High, loud, forceful whether miserable, angry or happy
Regularity	Predictability of physical functions such as appetite, sleep-wake cycle, and elimination	Regular, predictable	Irregular, erratic, can't tell when they'll be hungry or tired; has conflicts over meals and bedtime; wakes up at night, moods are changeable; has good or bad days for no obvious reason
Persistence	Single-mindedness, "stick-to-it-iveness"; may be positive (focused when involved) or negative (stubborn and doesn't give up	Low, easily diverted	High, stubborn, won't give up, goes on and on nagging, whining or negotiating if wants something; gets "locked in"; has long tantrums
Sensory threshold	Sensitivity to physical stimuli—sound, light, smell, taste, touch, pain, temperature	High, unbothered	Low, physically sensitive, "sensitive"—physically not emotionally; highly aware of color, light, appearance, texture, sound, smell, taste or temperature; "creative" but with strong and unusual preferences that can be embarrassing; clothes have to feel and look right; picky eater; refuses to dress warmly when weather is cold
Initial response	Characteristic initial reaction to new persons or new situations	Approach, goes forward	Withdrawal, holds back, doesn't like new situations; may tantrum if forced to go forward
Adaptability	Tolerance of change; ease with which gets used to new or altered situations	Good, flexible	Poor, rigid, has trouble with change of activity or routine; inflexible, very particular, notices minor changes; can want the same food or clothes over and over
Predominant mood	General quality of mood; basic disposition	Positive, cheerful	Negative, serious or cranky; doesn't show pleasure openly; not a "sunny" disposition

a class of 15 children with a high ratio of girls to boys and the teacher has an assistant, the child would still be a handful but a clinical diagnosis of disorder would be inappropriate.

2. Difficult children are, above all, **hard to understand**. Their behavior confuses and upsets the most experienced parent or teacher. The tried-and-true methods of child rearing simply do not work, so that effective discipline is replaced by inconsistency, power struggles, excessive punishment, or overindulgence. Parents will say that "nothing works" or that the child controls the family. A vicious cycle develops wherein the child's trying behavior and the erratic overreactions of the parent augment each other.

The primary caregiver of such a difficult child (usually the mother) may also be bewildered, overinvolved, and exhausted. She may feel guilty, inadequate, and victimized. Often such children are somewhat easier with their fathers, who may become increasingly critical of the mothers. Marital strain is common. A fragile but potentially viable marriage may be ruptured by the stress of a difficult child. In addition, individual vulnerabilities of adult personality may be accentuated, resulting in parental syndromes of anxiety, depression, or substance abuse. The siblings are often expected to behave in an excessively adult manner and their needs can be neglected as the household increasingly revolves around the difficult child. The child is also affected by the vicious cycle. Behavior problems are accentuated and secondary manifestations, such as fears and feelings of being "bad" are quite often evident.

II. **Making the diagnosis.** A pathology-oriented model is limiting and often counterproductive. There is no "difficult child syndrome," just as there is not a definitive "test for ADHD." Much more valid in dealing with problem behaviors in young children is a **model that focuses on individual differences and goodness of fit**. The aim is to describe the child's behavior, temperamental profile, and strengths, as well as areas of vulnerability.

A. **History.** Questioning the parent about the manifestations of a child's difficult temperament and its impact on the family is the key to identification. The clinician should inquire about the parents' approach to discipline, the child's school functioning, and the presence of secondary manifestations, such as fearfulness, nightmares, excessive anger, and emotional oversensitivity. Impaired self-image is seen in poorly managed difficult children.

B. **Temperamental questionnaire.** These may be used as part of well-child examinations or to determine areas of difficulty with a view to temperament based parent guidance. Research-based questionnaires tend to be lengthy with 75–100 parent responses. It is often acceptable for a busy primary care provider to devise their own brief questionnaire, provided it is used as an aid in conjunction with other information and not as a "diagnostic instrument."

C. **Behavioral observations.** Some problem behaviors are readily apparent in the office visit: impulsivity, hyperactivity, disruptiveness, clinging and withdrawal, tantrums, aggressiveness, or undue sensitivity to pain. However, a child may be stubborn, irregular, negative and cranky, intense, sensitive to light and taste, or poorly adaptable. When a parent reports such "nonvisible" difficult behavior that is not apparent during the office visit, the clinician should not assume that the parent is inventing or causing the problem.

D. **Differential diagnosis.** A difficult temperament is evident from an early age and is relatively stable and consistent over time. A child, 3 years or older, whose behavior has become difficult may be going through a developmental stage or reacting to stress. An example is a youngster who begins to misbehave after parents separate. When does the clinical picture go beyond a very difficult temperament and become indicative of a psychiatric disorder? The distinction is not only problematic but it is actually often irrelevant to treatment decisions. A "brain disorder", such as ADHD, is essentially a behavioral syndrome based on descriptive criteria subject to some extent observer bias. There is no "test" for ADHD. While it is now generally accepted that ADHD is neurobiologically based, the same can be said for temperament. Adopting a continuum based, rather than a categorical approach to diagnosis allows a clinician much greater flexibility.

III. **Management: The role of the pediatric clinician—helping the child and family.** The difficult child's adjustment can be greatly enhanced by the ongoing involvement of the primary care clinician. The central therapeutic goals are to improve the compatibility between a child and the significant persons in their life, relieve the child's suffering and improve adaptation.

A. **General issues.**

1. **Erroneous perceptions can be corrected.** The parents of very difficult children invariably feel victimized and often assume that the child's behavior is intentional. Parents need to understand that their children are not enemies who are "out to get them." Seeing the problem behavior as temperamentally determined rather than willful disobedience allows the parent to deal with it far more neutrally. Many parents are confused and made anxious by pressures to have their child "diagnosed" and placed on medication.
2. **The caregivers need support and understanding**, especially when the child's behavior is very difficult at home but unremarkable at school or in the clinician's office.
3. **Practical advice can be offered** on issues such as school selection and communication with teachers. The parents may need guidance on how to share responsibility more evenly, how to deal with other family members, and how to respond to the often plentiful advice offered from several quarters that tends to make parents (particularly single parents) feel defensive and inadequate.

B. **Principles of adult authority.** The fundamental goal for the parents of a difficult child is to replace the power struggles, frustration, and wear-and-tear of an ineffective disciplinary system with an educated, rational, kind, accepting, yet firm attitude of adult authority. Inevitably, habitual patterns of negative interaction have developed. It is the parents' job to initiate the necessary changes to improve the fit between their child-rearing style and expectations and their child's temperament. In order to begin the process, a key shift in attitude is needed. It should be clear to everyone that the parents are in charge. Certainly the child's opinion should be solicited when appropriate, but the ultimate decision lies with the parents. The model is that of the excellent supervisor at work: approachable, supportive, clear in expectations, and very much in charge. Key ingredients of this model are:

1. **Strategic planning and planned discussions.** The automatic, often excessively punitive, reactions to the child's behavior must be replaced with a system that emphasizes structure and predictability. Decisions about rules, new procedures or routines, and consequences should be made privately by the adults and then presented to the child. Such a planned discussion always takes place away from the heat of the moment. The child is calmly, clearly, and deliberately told what will be expected from now on. Both parents, if possible, should be present at such a meeting. The attitude is kind but serious. The parents should be concise and avoid moralizing, lest they lose the child's attention. The child should be viewed to some extent as a junior collaborator in the planning to improve the family atmosphere and input elicited. At the end of a planned discussion, the child needs to repeat the key points to make sure they understood them and is then encouraged to "do your best." Asking a young child, at a calm time, to try hard to meet a specific and reasonable expectation is a very powerful statement. Generally planned discussions can be used with children as young as age 3 years.
2. **Active acceptance.** The parent makes the deliberate choice, based on understanding their child and the child's temperament, to accept the youngster for the person they truly are, vulnerabilities as well as strengths. The practical consequence of this conscious decision is that parental expectations become more consistent with the genuine capacities of the child.
3. **Rational punishment.** Going hand in hand with planned discussions is the clear, firm enforcement of consequences for unacceptable behaviors that are within the child's control and important enough to warrant taking a stand. In a typical vicious cycle, a mother may find herself punishing and saying "no" repeatedly, but no parent can possibly be effective in such circumstances. Most difficult children need less punishment, rather than more, and this can be achieved through consistency, structure, and routines in everyday life.

   The important first step for parents is to recognize and address major unacceptable behaviors and ignore the myriad minor irritations that take place every day with a very difficult child. Whenever possible punishment should contain a natural consequence. For example, a child who continues to act too roughly with the family pet should be prohibited contact for a day— rather than being given a time-out. Ideally, a punishment should be administered briefly and without anger. Its main objective is to show the child that the parents are serious about stopping the behavior. Simplicity and predictability are important; a variety of punishments are unnecessary. With a younger child, parents can show seriousness by facial expression, direct action and tone of voice.

C. **Management strategies.** Management, as distinct from punishment, is used when the adult decides that the misbehavior is temperamentally based; the child, in effect, "can't help it." The parent's attitude, while still firm, is much more sympathetic and kind. The basic message is "I understand what's happening. I know you can't really control yourself, and I am going to help you with this." Sometimes behavior falls into a gray area, where it is not clear whether it is deliberate. In such instances, it is best for the parent to make the emotionally generous decision and help rather than punish the child.

Management suggestions designed to promote the child's success can be geared to particular temperamental characteristics. Strategies should be explained to the youngster during a planned discussion.

1. **The impulsive child.** A child who is easily excited can lose control in an overly stimulating environment and misbehave or become aggressive. The most common mistake parents and teachers make is to wait for the youngster to strike out and then lecture or punish, instead of intervening early.

   If the child is easily excited, it is important to recognize the signs of escalation—for example, moving more rapidly, talking in a louder voice, or laughing excessively. The adult should try to step in before the child gets out of hand. This technique is called **early intervention.** Some youngsters can be distracted. Others need a **time-out** (not as punishment, but as a cool-down period away from the action). A parent can say, "You're getting too excited. Let's do something quiet until you calm down."

2. **The highly active child.** High-energy children can become restless when they are confined to the dinner table or a classroom seat. They may begin to fidget or have difficulty paying attention. This behavior can be managed once the adults in charge **recognize the signs.** A restless youngster can be permitted to leave the dinner table and walk around between courses; a sympathetic teacher could ask the child to run an errand. Building vigorous physical activity into their daily routine is also helpful.

3. **The irregular child.** Most people fall easily into a regular rhythm of sleeping and eating, but some are naturally irregular. Battles can result when parents insist that a child who is not hungry must eat or that a youngster who is not tired must sleep. One strategy is to **differentiate between bedtime and sleep time, mealtime and eating time**. It is reasonable to require a child to be in bed by a certain hour or to join parents and siblings at dinner. However, parents should not force a youngster to sleep when he is not tired, or to eat when he is not hungry. To avoid overburdening the family chef, a child with an irregular appetite can be taught to fix simple snacks, such as fruit, cold cereal, or yogurt.

4. **The poorly focused child.** Some children are easily distracted by their environment or even by their own thoughts. As a result, they appear to not "listen" or, if they miss instructions, to be willfully disobedient. Parents and teachers can manage the problem by **making eye contact** in a friendly way before giving such a child directions. Instructions should be kept brief and simple. Set up, with the child, a system of reminders. Begin to teach organizational skills early.

5. **The child who resists change.** Some youngsters have difficulty with transitions. A poorly adaptable or shy child may be distressed by anything new. Other children focus so intently that they are locked into one activity and refuse to move to another. When they are asked to shift gears, they may cling, have a tantrum, or otherwise react negatively. If the issue is poor adaptability, parents can help by **preparing the child for change.** Even a simple warning, such as, "Finish playing with your trains, because we have to go shopping in 10 minutes," can be effective.

6. **The shy child.** Shy children require time and sympathetic understanding. A parent might say, "I know it's hard for you to get accustomed to new things, so I won't leave until you're used to being here." At the same time encourage a time-limited trial of an activity the youngster has previously shown he enjoys.

7. **The stubborn child.** Persistent, stubborn children can be extremely frustrating for parents and teachers. With these children, adults can take a stand early and terminate the confrontation. This technique is called **bringing it to an end.** A parent should not try to reason with a stubborn expert negotiator. Instead, the discussion should be ended. However, it is common for parents of a stubborn child to engage in a constant battle of wills and say "no" all the time. They should be encouraged to say "yes" more often, especially when the issue at hand is not really important.

8. **The finicky child.** Certain children are particular because they have heightened sensitivity to touch, taste, smell, sound, temperature, and colors (not necessarily all of these). Parents may get into arguments because a youngster insists on wearing the same comfortable green corduroy pants day after day or refuses to eat the inexpensive brand of frozen pizza that the rest of the family enjoys. Parents should be advised

to **respect a child's preferences** when possible and to seek compromises that avoid unnecessary power struggles.

9. **The cranky child.** Parents can be distressed and angered by a child who is generally negative, somber, or pessimistic. Treats that would delight most children scarcely rate a smile from this youngster. The harder the parent tries (and fails) to make the child happy, the greater the tension becomes. A suggestion for parents is to **accept the child's nature** and not to expect a level of enthusiasm that they cannot give. The parent should not feel guilty; the child's negative mood is not the parent's fault.

D. **The use of medication.** If one aims for the relief of suffering rather than the cure of illness, target symptoms can be greatly reduced by the judicious and often temporary use of psychotropic medications. According to this view, the use of a stimulant would be completely appropriate for the balance of the school year in the child described earlier who was in an unfortunate but unavoidable classroom situation. A referral to the parent's provider may be appropriate for the parent who is tense and caught up in the "vicious cycle."

E. **Criteria for referral.** The decision to refer to a mental health professional is often determined by the primary care clinician's interest in behavioral issues, expertise in parent guidance, and time availability. Assuming the presence of all these, a referral would still be needed in the case of an extremely difficult child, when the vicious cycle of ineffective discipline is longstanding, or when a clinical syndrome is suspected or can be identified in the child or other family members.

BIBLIOGRAPHY

For Parents

Books

Brazelton T. *Touchpoints.* Reading, MA: Addison-Wesley, 1992.
Carey WB. *Understanding Your Child's Temperament.* New York: MacMillan, 1997.
Chess S, Thomas A. *Know Your Child.* New York: Basic Books, 1987.
Turecki S. *The Difficult Child.* New York: Bantam, 1989.

Websites

About Our Kids http://www.aboutourkids.org/articles/parentingstyles.html

For Professionals

Carey WB, McDevitt S. *Coping with Children's Temperament.* New York: Basic Books, 1995.
Chess S, Thomas A. *Temperament in Clinical Practice.* New York: The Guilford Press, 1986.
Kagan J. *The Nature of the Child.* New York: Basic Books, 1984.
Thomas A, Chess S. *Temperament and Development.* New York: Brunner-Mazel, 1977.
Turecki S. *The Emotional Problems of Normal Children.* New York: Bantam, 1994.

78 Thumb Sucking

Stephanie Blenner

I. **Description of the problem.** Most infants engage in nonnutritive sucking. They may use fingers, toes, a pacifier, or other object as a means of self-soothing. In some children this behavior persists into early or middle childhood.

A. **Epidemiology.**
- Seen in the fetus as early as 18 weeks.
- 80% of infants suck their fingers or toes.
- 30%–45% of preschool children and 5%–20% of children over age 5 continue to engage in thumb sucking.
- Most long-term thumb sucking begins prior to age 9 months.
- Slightly more prevalent in girls than boys.
- More common in children of higher socioeconomic status.
- 30%–55% of children who suck their thumb or fingers also have an attachment object, such as a blanket, toy, or their own hair.

B. **Etiology.** Some believe thumb sucking is a learned habit. Others, especially psychoanalysts, believe thumb sucking is an expression of infantile drives and can reflect emotional disturbance if it persists beyond infancy. Most view thumb sucking as a means of self-comforting. It may help relieve stress and calm a child in face of environmental challenges. Thumb sucking is often seen when a child is falling asleep, tired, bored, hungry, or anxious.

C. **Negative sequelae.**

1. **Dental.** The most common consequences of thumb sucking are dental, in particular malocclusion of both primary and permanent dentition. It may also lead to temporomandibular problems, anterior overbite, posterior crossbite, atypical root resorption, mucosal trauma, narrowing of the maxillary arch, and abnormal facial growth. The risk is highest among children who suck continuously and persist beyond age 4.

2. **Digit abnormalities.** With chronic thumb sucking, a digital hyperextension deformity can occur that may require surgical correction. Callous formation, paronychia, irritant eczema, and herpetic whitlow are also seen.

3. **Psychological effects.** Thumb sucking can contribute to impaired parental and peer relationships. It is often viewed as immature and socially undesirable. Parents and peers may criticize, tease, or punish the child for engaging in thumb sucking. These reactions may, in turn, adversely affect a child's self-esteem.

4. **Accidental poisoning.** Children who thumb suck are at increased risk of accidental poisoning (e.g., lead poisoning).

II. **Making the diagnosis.** Thumb sucking becomes a problem at any age when it interferes with normal developmental achievements, physical health, social interactions, or self-esteem.

A. **Physical examination.** Examination may reveal a wrinkled, red digit with or without callous formation. Oral examination should be performed looking for malocclusion or other dental complications.

III. **Management.**

A. **Primary goals.** The goals of treating thumb sucking are to prevent dental complications and potential adverse effects on the child's social interactions and self-esteem. In general, targeted intervention is not necessary until after age 4 when adverse sequelae become more common. Most children will spontaneously stop thumb sucking as they develop other self-regulatory strategies.

B. **Treatment strategies.**

1. **Identify triggers and reinforcers.** Emotional and situational triggers should be identified. Thumb sucking often occurs at particular times of day, during certain activities, or accompanying specific emotional states. Some children only thumb suck while

twirling their hair or holding a blanket. As a child gets older, thumb sucking may provide secondary gain through attention paid to the behavior.

2. **Empower the child.** For successful treatment, the child must be actively involved, cooperative and motivated to stop. Parents should be counseled not to use threats or punishment as these may increase resistance, paradoxically prolonging the behavior. Parents should remain patient and provide support without criticism. They need to realize it is the child's, not their, task to overcome the habit.

3. **Interventions.**

   a. **Prior to age 4 years.** Thumb sucking is normal if it does not interfere with social or developmental functioning. The behavior should be ignored and given no special attention lest it accrue secondary gain. When thumb sucking is noted, the child should be distracted without mentioning the behavior. The child should be praised when not sucking their thumb.

   b. **After age 4 years.** If thumb sucking is persistent and problematic, several behavior modification and habit reversal techniques can be used:

      (1) **Gentle reminders** such as a chart or calendar the child uses to keep track of progress.

      (2) **Rewards** such as stickers, treats, extra story time, or special outings with parents for specified periods without thumb sucking.

      (3) **Praise** given when the child is not thumb sucking.

      (4) **Modifying associations** by changing the bedtime routine for a child who sucks while falling asleep or encouraging giving up attachment objects, like a blanket used while sucking.

      (5) **Changing the habit from pleasurable to obligatory.** A specific time (10–15 minutes) and place is set aside each day during which the child is required to suck their thumb. For some children, thumb sucking then loses its appeal.

      (6) **Replacing** thumb sucking with a socially acceptable habit that occupies the thumb, such as squeezing a foam ball or holding the thumb with the other hand.

      (7) **A bitter liquid** (available over the counter) is consistently applied to the thumb morning, night, and each time the child is known to thumb suck. If after 1 week, the child does not thumb suck, the morning application is discontinued. After another week passes with no thumb sucking, the nighttime application is stopped. Should thumb sucking recur the full application schedule is resumed. This approach is useful with children who want to stop but put their thumb in their mouth without thinking. It should be emphasized the liquid is a reminder to help the child stop, not a punishment.

      (8) If thumb sucking occurs at night, **thumb splints, gloves, or socks** can be tried. An elastic bandage can be wrapped around a straightened elbow. When the child raises hand to mouth, gentle pressure is exerted reminding the child not to thumb suck. The child should be responsible for putting on the glove or bandage at bedtime and should not be reminded.

      (9) **Referral to a pediatric dentist** for placement of an intraoral device may be considered with a motivated child who has been unsuccessful using other measures. A palatal bar or crib interferes with placement of the thumb in the palatal vault. It may be appropriate for the older child developing malocclusion as a consequence of thumb sucking.

IV. **Clinical pearls and pitfalls.**

   • Do not worry about thumb sucking until a child is at least age 4 years.

   • Keep the child actively involved in management and treatment choice.

   • Ensure the solution is not worse than the problem and doesn't become the focus of parent–child interactions.

BIBLIOGRAPHY

For Parents

Mayer CA. *My Thumb and I: A Proven Approach to Stop a Thumb or Finger Sucking Habit, For Ages 6-10.* Chicago: Chicago Spectrum Press, 1997.

Van Norman RM. *Helping the Thumb-Sucking Child: A Practical Guide for Parents.* Vonore, TN: Avery Pub. Group, 1999.

For Children

Ages 4 to 8

Dionne W. *Little Thumb*. Grenta, LA: Pelican Pub Co, 2001.
Heitler, S. *David Decides About Thumbsucking*. Denver, CO: Reading Matters, 1996.
Sonnenschein H. *Harold's Hideaway Thumb*. New York: Simon & Schuster Books for Young Readers, 1991.

Ages 6 to 10

Mayer CA. *My Thumb and I: A Proven Approach to Stop a Thumb or Finger Sucking Habit, For Ages 6-10*. Chicago: Chicago Spectrum Press, 1997.

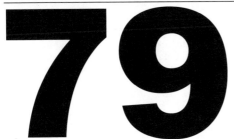

Tics and Tourette Syndrome

Adrian Sandler

I. Description of the problem.

A. Definitional issues.

1. Tourette syndrome (TS).

- TS is a disorder with multiple motor and vocal tics (not necessarily concurrently) lasting for a period of at least 1 year, in which the individual is never tic-free more than 3 consecutive months.
- The tics may change in nature and severity, and are associated with distress or impairment in function.
- Onset is before age 18 years, with peak onset around 5 to 8 years.
- Although there is wide variability in symptoms and clinical course, there is a tendency for severity to peak around 8 to 11 years, with improvement or even resolution during puberty.

2. The tic disorder spectrum.

- *Transient tic disorders* include single or multiple motor and/or vocal tics, lasting at least 4 weeks up to 12 months.
- Most transient tics are simple rather than complex and they do not usually cause great distress. A child with complex and distressing motor and vocal tics lasting a few months may be at risk for developing TS.
- *Chronic tic disorders* are single or multiple motor *or* vocal tics that last more than a year. It is thought that these disorders share the same pathogenesis and occur on a spectrum.

B. Epidemiology.

1. Prevalence of tic disorder spectrum.

- Simple tics are very common in childhood. The 3-month prevalence is 4.3% in boys and 2.7% in girls.
- 6%–13% of all children will experience a transient tic at some time during childhood.
- The childhood incidence of chronic tic disorder is around 1%–2%, with approximately 3:1 ratio of boys to girls.
- In contrast, TS is much less common, around 5–10/10,000. Neither race nor socioeconomic status is strongly related to risk of tic disorders.

2. Comorbidity of TS with obsessive-compulsive disorder (OCD) and attention deficit hyperactivity disorder (ADHD).

- More than 50% of children with TS have extensive obsessions and/or compulsions; 40% meet criteria for OCD.
- More than 20% of all children with any tic disorder have OCD and 18% of children with OCD also have a concurrent tic disorder.
- Many children with TS have clinical depression or anxiety.

3. Comorbidity with ADHD is more controversial, and data vary because of clinic referral bias.

- Most studies show that around 8%–27% of children with TS also have ADHD, but most children with TS show impulsive behavior.

C. Etiology/contributing factors.

1. The genetics of tic disorders and TS.

The precise etiology is not known. Twin studies show fairly high heritability, but there are clearly nongenetic factors influencing phenotypic expression. A single autosomal dominant gene with incomplete penetrance is likely, but linkage studies have not identified a strong candidate region. Other lines of evidence suggest several vulnerability genes plus environmental stressors causing increased fetal sensitivity in regions of the developing brain. Similar genetic and non-genetic factors appear to be operating in OCD.

2. The neurobiology of tic disorders and TS.

Specific cortico-striato-thalamo-cortical circuits have been implicated because of their role in initiating and inhibiting psychomotor activity and in harm detection/avoidance. There is evidence of reduced globus pallidus volume in TS and imbalance between excitatory and inhibitory neurotransmitters. Cortical disinhibition may be related to hypersensitivity of dopamine D2 striatal receptors.

II. Making the diagnosis.

A. Signs and symptoms.

1. **What is a tic?** Tics are more easily recognized than precisely defined. They can be described as rapid, coordinated, isolated fragments of normal motor or vocal behaviors. Tics can be easily mimicked and sometimes are confused with normal behavior. Motor tics are typically brief clonic movements of eyes, face, neck and shoulders, with eye blinking, facial grimacing and head jerking the most common. Vocal or phonic tics may commonly include repetitive throat clearing, grunting or barking.

   Tics may be described in terms of location, number, frequency and duration. They may also be characterized by their intensity, forcefulness and complexity. Whereas tics are most commonly *simple* (brief and meaningless), they may be *complex* (longer and more elaborate). A few specific terms have been used to describe particular recognizable kinds of tic, such as *palilalia* (repeating others), *coprolalia* (uttering obscenities), and *copropraxia* (making obscene gestures).

   Individuals with tics describe premonitory sensory urges, a "feeling of pressure", a kind of "itch" articulated by children as young as 7 years. These distracting urges may contribute to attentional problems. Tics are often not entirely involuntary, and may be experienced as intentional surrender to virtually irresistible sensory urges, usually accompanied by a fleeting and incomplete sense of relief.

2. **Differential diagnosis: What isn't a tic?** Children with allergies often have recurrent throat clearing and sniffing, but tics are more repetitive and less variable. Habits such as hair twirling, nose touching, skin picking and other self-soothing behaviors also lack the repetitive uniformity of tics. Brief epileptic seizures and movement disorders (such as chorea, athetosis, dystonia and myoclonic jerks) are more clearly abnormal movement patterns than tics. There is no definitive test for tics and so there are gray areas between habits and simple tics and between the compulsions of OCD and complex tics.

3. **Evaluation of tic disorders.** Evaluation of tic disorders includes detailed medical and developmental history, child interview and careful neurologic examination. It is important to ask the child and family about the time course of tics, relationship to medication use, and possible exacerbating factors. The child's subjective experience of the tics and their social or emotional consequences should be explored. Specific inquiry about recent or previous streptococcal exposures or infections should be made. The history should include screening questions regarding OCD, ADHD, learning problems and depression. In addition, the pediatric provider should take a family history regarding tic disorders and these associated conditions.

   Physical and neurological examination is important to rule out other movement disorders. Other than tics, children with TS usually have a normal examination. Many children effectively suppress tics during the clinic visit, and the absence of tics does not preclude a diagnosis of tic disorders. Neurodevelopmental examination can be helpful in eliciting soft signs (such as choreiform twitches) and providing opportunities to observe attention deficits and other processing problems. Also, many children begin to have tics when stressed in this way.

   There are **no specific diagnostic tests**. EEG and imaging studies are not routinely indicated. Standardized rating scales and checklists may be very helpful regarding ADHD symptoms and general functional impairment at home and school. Other self-report or clinician-rated measures of tics and obsessive compulsive symptoms may be useful both for clinical and research purposes.

B. Pediatric autoimmune neuropsychiatric disorders associated with group A streptococcus (PANDAS).
Some children appear susceptible to the abrupt onset of tics, compulsions, emotional lability and anxiety during or following streptococcal pharyngitis. This condition may be episodic and recurrences are common. Children usually (but not always) have clinical evidence of tonsillopharyngitis. AntiDNAase B titers are very high. The condition generally responds to antibiotics. PANDAS are closely related to Sydenham chorea of rheumatic fever. Circumstantial evidence suggests antineuronal antibodies are affecting basal ganglia function. If there are clinical indications, including sudden onset of symptoms or known exposure to streptococcus, most clinicians obtain streptococcal culture, ASO titers and antiDNAase B. If there is confirmation of streptococcal infection, treatment with penicillin often leads to improvement in tics and obsessive compulsive symptoms.

III. **Management.**
  A. **Treatment goals and modalities.** The goals of management of tic disorders are to **minimize stress, social isolation and functional impairment.** Education and demystification for the affected child, his/her family and school personnel help to promote support and tolerance, reinforcing the message that the tics are involuntary. Brief supportive family counseling is helpful in achieving these goals, and some children may benefit from individual psychotherapy.
  1. **Habit reversal psychotherapy** involves increasing the individual's awareness of the tics and establishing a competing response, although effectiveness in TS is not well established. Cognitive behavior therapy involving repeated exposures and response prevention is of benefit in OCD, sometimes enhancing medication response or allowing responders to discontinue medications. Relaxation and self-hypnosis may be useful adjunct treatments in tic disorders and TS.
  2. **Pharmacotherapy** is the cornerstone of treatment of tic disorders, but tics should not be treated too aggressively if they are not causing major functional impairment. The presence, scope and severity of comorbid diagnoses (ADHD, OCD, depression) should be assessed in planning pharmacotherapy.
      a. **Alpha-2 norepinephrine agonists.** Clonidine and guanfacine may be useful first line medications in tic disorders and Tourette syndrome. These agents tend to decrease hyperactivity, impulsivity, hyperarousal, exaggerated stress responses and aggression in addition to decreasing tics. An adequate trial may be 2 months. Sedation is the major side effect, especially for clonidine.
      b. **Stimulant therapy in children with ADHD and tic disorders.** In children with ADHD and tics, the alpha agonists are not likely to be effective in improving attentional problems. A combination of stimulant plus alpha agonist may be necessary. In children with tic disorders, a trial of stimulant therapy may increase tics in one third, have no effect in one third, and lead to improvement in tics in one third. The combination of methylphenidate and clonidine in children with Tourette syndrome and ADHD was more effective than either medication alone. Although this combination appears to be safe and well tolerated, four case reports of sudden death raise caution regarding preexisting cardiac problems and emphasize the need for EKG monitoring.
      c. **Other medications in tic disorders.** The selective serotonin reuptake inhibitors (SSRIs) are of proven effectiveness in the treatment of OCD, and they may also help to decrease complex tics and compulsions in children with tics and TS. In children with TS, OCD and ADHD, a combination of SSRI and stimulant may be helpful. Children with tic disorders and ADHD who have side effects on stimulants may respond to tricyclic antidepressants or atomoxetine.
        • In children with serologic evidence of recent streptococcal infection and a clinical presentation consistent with PANDAS, a course of penicillin may be helpful.
        • Nicotine patches and swipes have been used to treat severe tics resistant to other treatments but are associated with nausea and other side effects.
        • **Neuroleptics** such as haloperidol and pimozide can be quite effective in treating severe tic disorders. Pimozide may have fewer extrapyramidal side effects but can cause QT prolongation. Risperidone, a potent D2 antagonist, has proven effectiveness in short-term clinical trials in children and adults with TS, and pilot data with other atypical antipsychotics are encouraging.
IV. **Clinical pearls and pitfalls.**
    • Demystification is critical: this is very largely an involuntary condition, and it is important for family members and teachers not to aggravate the situation by calling attention to the tics.
    • Tics should not be treated too aggressively unless they are causing major stress, social rejection or other functional impairments.
    • The presence of tics is not a contraindication to the use of stimulants in children with ADHD.
    • Think of PANDAS when there is a sudden and dramatic increase in tic frequency/severity or the emergence of obsessive compulsive symptoms.

BIBLIOGRAPHY

For Parents

Books

Chansky TE. *Freeing Your Child From Obsessive-Compulsive Disorder. A Powerful, Practical Program for Parents of Children and Adolescents.* New York: Crown Publishers, 2000.

Dornbush MP, Pruitt SK. *Teaching The Tiger: A Handbook for Individuals Involved in the Education of Students with Attention Deficit Disorders, Tourette Syndrome or Obsessive-Compulsive Disorder.* Duarte, CA: Hope Press, 1995.

Haerle T. *Children with Tourette Syndrome: A Parent's Guide.* Rockville, MD: Woodbine, 2003.

Websites

OC Foundation www.ocfoundation.org

Tourette Syndrome Assocation www.tsa-usa.org

For Professionals

Leckman JF, Cohen DJ (eds). *Tourette's Syndrome – Tics, Obsessions, Compulsions: Developmental Psychopathology and Clinical Care.* New York: Wiley, 1999.

Leckman JF, Zhang H, Vitale A, et al. Course of tic severity in Tourette syndrome: the first two decades. *Pediatrics;*102:14–19, 1998.

Tourette Syndrome Study Group. Treatment of ADHD in children with tics: a randomized controlled trial. *Neurology;*58:527–536, 2002.

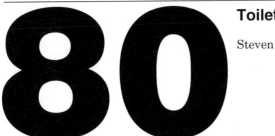

Toilet Training

Steven Parker

I. **Description of the problem.** Toilet training is one of the great developmental challenges of early childhood. After 2 years of glorious indifference to social niceties regarding the process of excretion, in Selma Fraiberg's phrase: "The missionaries arrive ··· bearing culture to the joyful savage." Armed with Dr. Spock rather than the Bible, the adults try to cajole the skeptical child into making a dramatic developmental leap without clear benefits. It is a difficult sales pitch and is best attempted only after the child exhibits developmental readiness to understand and master the complex physiologic and psychological tasks of toilet training (Table 80-1). This "child-centered" approach, described by Brazelton in 1962, is the most commonly used in the United States and almost always effective. However, for situations in which immediate results are needed, the motivated parent can attempt the "toilet training in less than a day method".

A. **Epidemiology.**
   - In the United States, 26% of children achieve daytime continence by age 24 months, 85% by age 30 months, and 98% by age 36 months.
   - Nighttime continence usually occurs within a few months after daytime control is achieved.
   - The average time to successful toilet training is 3 months.
   - Girls are usually faster than boys in achieving control.

II. **Management.** Suggestions for parents on toilet training strategies are set out in Table 80-2.

A. **Information for parents.** The issue of toilet training is best discussed as part of anticipatory guidance at the 15–18 month visit. A number of key principles should be discussed with the parents:

   1. **There is usually no hurry or benefit to early toilet training.** Although the process can be initiated in response to outside pressures (e.g., daycare requirements), there are good reasons to try to wait until the child is developmentally prepared.
   2. Like most other developmental challenges of childhood, **it is best to empower the child to take responsibility for achieving continence.** Since control of stool and urine will be achieved sooner or later, the most important outcome of toilet training is a boost in the child's self-esteem at mastering the task. It is a long-term goal that should never be sacrificed to the short-term strategies to achieve continence.
   3. **Toilet training is not a contest; it proceeds by fits and starts with successes and frequent relapses; if the timing is wrong, it can always be postponed.** Say to parents: "I guarantee that your child will not walk off to kindergarten wearing a diaper."
   4. **The parents should not transmit a sense of disgust toward the stool but treat it as a wonderful gift from the child.**

B. **Resistance to toilet training.** Some children resist toilet training, even if the parental technique is impeccable. The primary care clinician can make these suggestions to the parents:

   1. **Do not fight, punish, shame, or nag under any circumstances.** Be sympathetic and try to understand the resistance from the child's point of view.
   2. **Discontinue training for a few weeks or months if the child is emphatically negative.**
   3. **Continue discussions with the child** about toilet training and emphasize the maturity demonstrated by such behavior.
   4. **Encourage the child to imitate parents and siblings** by inviting the child into the bathroom.
   5. **Read potty training books or view potty training videos together.**
   6. **Remind the child that it is their responsibility for this task,** not yours.
   7. **Encourage the child to change their own diapers.** Remind the child how "yucky" it feels to walk around with a wet or soiled diaper.

Table 80-1 Signs of developmental readiness for toilet training

Language skills
Able to follow two-step independent commands (e.g., "Take off your pants and go to the bathroom")
Uses two-word phrases (e.g., "bye-bye poop," "go potty")
Cognitive skills
Imitates actions of caregivers (e.g., sweeps the floor)
Understands cause and effect (i.e., is capable of understanding the reasons for mastering the actions involved in toilet training)
Emotional skills
Desires to please parents/caregivers by complying with their requests
Shows diminishing oppositional behaviors and power struggles
Shows drive for independence and autonomy in self-care activities (e.g., insists on feeding self, tries to take off own clothes)
Evinces pride and possessiveness toward belongings ("*my* car" and eventually "*my* poop")
Motor skills
Can ambulate with ease
Is capable of pulling pants off independently
Can sit still for 5 min. without help
Can somewhat control urinary/anal sphincter (e.g., urinates large amounts sporadically, rather than constant wetting)
Body awareness
Shows awareness of wet or soiled diaper
Manifests signs of urge to void or defecate (e.g., facial expression, goes off into a corner)

Table 80-2 Ten steps to successful toilet training

1.	Buy a potty chair, and place it in a conspicuous, convenient place. Tell the child, "This is your potty chair. This is where you will [use child's terms for urination and defecation]." Be sure to stress what a special and wonderful chair it is.
2.	Allow the child to get used to the chair by sitting on it, fully clothed, for about 5 minutes a couple of times a day for about a week. Try to choose times that the child is more likely to have a bowel movement (e.g., after meals). Never force the child to sit on it.
3.	Encourage the child to watch parents or siblings use the bathroom. Explain, "This is where we go potty." Let the child watch the excreta being flushed down the toilet and wave "bye-bye" to it (skip this if the flushing frightens the child).
4.	Have the child sit on the potty with the diapers off. Do not urge or expect results, but if it happens, praise the child. Move the potty chair progressively closer and finally into the bathroom.
5.	With the child, throw the stool from the soiled diaper into the potty. Tell the child that this is where the stool and urine should go. Then take the pail and dump the stool down the toilet. Wave "bye-bye poop" with the child.
6.	Ask the child during the day, "Do you have to go potty?" to keep attention on bodily sensations. Observe the child for signs of impending urination or defecation. Say: "Let's take off your pants and go potty." Assist the child in disrobing and going to the potty chair. Sit for as long as the child wants. Praise success, but do not criticize failure ("Oh, you don't want to go. Okay. Maybe next time").
7.	Reinforce positive features of potty training to child (e.g., "just like a big boy," "just like Mommy does," "You did it by yourself!"), and praise successes as they occur.
8.	Once a semiconsistent pattern of avoiding stooling on the potty is established, ask the child if they want to give up the diaper "like a big boy or girl" during the day. If yes, make a show of throwing them all away in the garbage and wave "bye-bye" to them. Admire the child for putting on training "big boy or girl" pants.
9.	Once training is well established, try an over-the-toilet-seat chair.
10.	Nighttime continence may take a few months to acquire after daytime dryness is achieved. There is usually no special strategy needed; simply ask your child when they would like to try training pants in the night.

8. **Matter-of-factly ask the child at the first sign of impending defecation if the child wants to use the potty.**
9. **If the child appears afraid of painful stools, add prune juice or fiber to the diet to ensure soft stools.** Postpone potty training until fear of defecation subsides.
10. **Discuss what rewards the child would like in response to successful toilet training.** Try star charts to reinforce successful attempts.
11. Take the child to settings where other children their age are successfully potty trained.
12. **If the child is obstinately recalcitrant, is clearly capable of mastering the task, is developmentally and emotionally healthy, is more than age 3 years, and the lack of training is a significant problem for the family,** have a solemn ceremony of throwing away the diapers, announce that the child is an official big boy or girl now, give encouragement to "do your best," and allow maturational urges to overtake autonomy issues.

BIBLIOGRAPHY

For Parents

Books

Azrin NF, Foxx RM. *Toilet Training in Less Than a Day.* New York: Simon & Shuster, 1974
Brazelton TB, Sparrow J. *Toilet Training the Brazelton Way.* Cambridge, MA: Da Capo Press, 2003.

Websites

Medem Network
   http://www.medem.com/MedLB/article_detaillb.cfm?article_ID = ZZZR6LONH4C&
   sub_cat   109
Parent Soup
   http://www.parentsoup.com/toddlers/potty/articles/0,,262585_260941,00.html

For Professionals

Brazelton TB. A child-oriented approach to toilet training. *Pediatrics;*29:121–128, 1962.
Michel RS. Toilet training. *Pediatr Rev;*20(7):240–245, 1999.
Schum TR, Kolb TM, McAuliffe TL, et al. Sequential acquisition of toilet-training skills: a descriptive study of gender and age differences in normal children. *Pediatrics;*109(3):E48, 2002.
Stadtler AC, Gorski PA, Brazelton TB. Toilet training methods, clinical interventions, and recommendations. American Academy of Pediatrics. *Pediatrics* 1103(6 Pt 2):1359–1368, 1999.

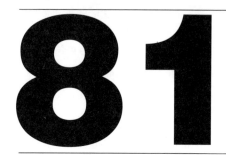

Unpopular Children

Melvin D. Levine

I. **Description of the problem.** Chronic rejection by peers condemns a child to a life of isolation, extreme self-doubt, and perpetual anxiety. The unpopular schoolchild is susceptible to daily embarrassment through both passive and active exclusion by classmates. Such a child must endure the inevitable painful refrain, "Sorry, this seat is saved." In many cases exclusionary comments and actions may be augmented by bullying and verbal abuse. It is regrettably true that many of the most popular children are able to boost their status among peers by being especially creative and demonstrative in their predatory acts against unpopular children. The victim's imposed isolation and constant fear of further humiliation is likely to take its toll on development and behavior.

A. **Contributing factors.** There are multiple pathways that may culminate in a state of unpopularity during the school years. In many instances, more than one factor may predispose a child to peer rejection. The following are among the common predisposing factors:

1. **Intrinsic social cognitive dysfunction,** such as a "learning disability," impairing social awareness, practice, and skill. Social cognitive dysfunction, probably the most common source of unpopularity, may mediate or interact with other factors to yield unpopularity in a child. Table 81-1 contains 18 of the most important subcomponents of social cognitive dysfunction. A clinician assessing a patient's social cognition can make use of such a list to pinpoint a child's troubles in specific subcomponents. This process may ultimately provide a basis for coaching the child in the social domain.

2. **Attention deficits.** Traits such as impulsivity, insatiability, and verbal disinhibition associated with attentional dysfunction engender unpopularity.

3. **Physical unattractiveness.** Children whose physical appearance is somehow displeasing to their peers have been shown to be vulnerable to social isolation.

4. **Poor gross motor skills.** Inferior athletic abilities may potentiate unpopularity.

5. **Language disability.** Children with expressive language problems may not be able to use verbal communication to control relationships and keep pace with the banter and lingo of peers.

6. **Autism and autism-like conditions.** Children who show signs of autism (including very mild forms, such as Asperger syndrome) display varying degrees of social cognitive dysfunction, which commonly incites peer rejection.

7. **Shyness.** Some youngsters who are chronically shy in their temperament and therefore avoid social contact may fail to gain the experience needed in the quest for popularity.

8. **Poor coping skills.** A lack of adaptability and problem-solving skills may cause some children to react to daily stresses and conflicts with maladaptive behaviors, such as aggression. Such behaviors alienate others and promote rejection by classmates.

9. **Eccentricity.** Children who are nonconformists or have unusual interests, speech patterns, tastes, or values may be rejected by their more conventional peers who feel more comfortable with close replicas of themselves and harbor fears of contamination with "weirdness." Thus, a child who loves to learn about spiders or enjoys listening to Handel oratorios may be ostracized by more conventional classmates.

10. **Family patterns.** There exist self-contained families that do not value generalized popularity, or the family unit itself remains isolated either voluntarily or of necessity (perhaps due to genetic social cognitive dysfunctions).

B. **Secondary phenomena.** The clinical picture of an unpopular child is likely to be complicated by a chain of secondary phenomena, which may include extreme anxiety (or even depression), low self-esteem, and a repertoire of maladaptive defense tactics, such as excessive and inappropriate clowning, extreme controlling behaviors, or outright withdrawal. Often these children seek relationships with adults or with much younger

Table 81-1 Social cognitive dysfunction: the troubled subcomponents

Subcomponent	Description
Weak greeting skills	Trouble initiating a social contact with a peer skillfully
Poor social predicting	Trouble estimating peer reactions before acting/talking
Deficient self-marketing	Trouble projecting an image acceptable to peers
Problematic conflict resolution	Trouble settling social disputes without aggression
Reduced affective matching	Trouble sensing and fitting in with others' moods
Social self-monitoring failure	Trouble knowing when one is in social trouble
Low reciprocity	Trouble sharing and trouble supporting/reinforcing others
Misguided timing/staging	Trouble knowing how to nurture a relationship over time
Poor verbalization of feelings	Trouble using language to communicate true feelings
Inaccurate inference of feelings	Trouble reading others' feelings through language
Failure of code switching	Trouble matching language style to current audience
Lingo dysfluency	Trouble using the parlance of peers credibly
Poorly regulated humor	Trouble using humor effectively for current context/audience
Inappropriate topic choice/maintenance	Trouble knowing what to talk about and for how long
Weak requesting skill	Trouble knowing how to ask for something inoffensively
Poor social memory	Trouble learning from previous social experience
Assertiveness gaps	Trouble exerting right level of influence over group actions
Social discomfort	Trouble feeling relaxed while relating to peers

children because they are unable to form alliances within their own age group. In some cases, school phobic behaviors or somatic symptoms may be encountered. Finally, it is not unusual for children who experience social difficulties at school to become aggressive, oppositional, and/or excessively demanding and dependent at home.

II. **Making the diagnosis.** Unpopular children merit careful clinical assessment. Their social difficulties may in fact represent the tip of an iceberg with respect to behavioral and developmental health. The causal factors and potential complications of unpopularity need to be sought through direct history taking, direct observations of the child's image and manner of relating, physical and neurodevelopmental examinations, and reports from teachers. Especially difficult cases may necessitate investigation by a multidisciplinary team.

Information can be gathered from several sources to detect the presence of subcomponents of social cognitive dysfunction listed in Table 81-1.

The unpopular child should be interviewed alone to elicit their perspective. Nonthreatening questions may be posed to acquire insight into traumatic social scenarios at school. The most common interpersonal "hot spots" are the bus stop, the school bus, the playground, the bathroom, the gymnasium, and the area around lockers. Children can often recreate vividly the stressful scenes that unfold daily against these backdrops. The patient should be reassured that many other children have such difficulties and that it is safe and important to talk about them with an adult.

III. **Management.** The management of the unpopular child must take into consideration the multiplicity of factors operating to engender peer rejection. Associated neurodevelopmental problems (such as a language disability or an attention deficit) require appropriate treatment. The complications, such as somatic symptoms or depression, also demand targeted intervention. In addition, the child's individual social cognitive dysfunction must be addressed. Some possible management approaches to deal directly with a child's unpopularity are summarized below.

A. **Explain the social skill problems carefully to the child.** These may require multiple sessions; not all affected children can process such information readily.

B. **Have the parent of the child who needs social improvement accompany that child to an activity with other children.** Then, during a calm and private interlude, the parent can discuss the social interactions (especially the *faux pas* and transgressions) that occurred.

C. **Help the child locate one or two companions with whom to relate and begin to build skills.** It can be helpful if such peers share interests and perhaps some traits with the unpopular child.

D. **Inform the classroom teacher or building principal if a child is victimized by peer**

abuse in school. It is the school's responsibility to make every effort to contain this activity. A strongly worded note from a primary health care provider may be vital in such cases.

E. **Help the rejected child to develop skills, hobbies, or areas of expertise that can enhance self-esteem and be impressive to other children.** The management of such a child should always include the diligent quest for and development of such specialties. Ideally, such pursuits should have the potential for generating collaborative activities with other children.

F. **Never force these children into potentially embarrassing situations before their peers.** For example, an unpopular child with poor gross motor skills needs some protection from humiliation in physical education classes.

G. **Manage any family problems or medical conditions** through counseling, specific therapies (e.g., language intervention or help with motor skills), and/or medication (e.g., for attention deficits or depression).

H. **Identify social skills training programs within schools and in clinical settings.** Clinicians should be aware of local resources that offer social skills training to youngsters with social cognitive deficits. Most commonly this training makes use of specific curricula that are used in small group settings in a school or in the community.

I. **Reassure these children that it is appropriate for them to be themselves, that they need not act and talk like everyone else in school, that there is true heroism in individuality.** Clinicians, teachers, and parents need to tread the fine line between helping with social skills and coercing a child into blind conformity with peer pressures, expectations, and models.

BIBLIOGRAPHY

For Parents and Children

Books

Levine MD. *All Kinds of Minds.* Cambridge, MA: Educators Publishing Service, 1993.
Levine MD. *Educational Care.* Cambridge, MA: Educators Publishing Service, 1994.
Levine MD. *Keeping a Head in School.* Cambridge, MA: Educators Publishing Service, 1990.
Osman B. *No One to Play With: The Social Side of Learning Disabilities.* New York: Random House, 1982.

Websites for Parents and Professionals

All Kinds of Minds http://www.allkindsofminds.org/index.aspx

For Professionals

Asher SR, Coie JD (eds). *Peer Rejection in Childhood.* Cambridge, MA: Cambridge Press, 1990.
Cartledge G, Milburn JF (eds). *Teaching Social Skills to Children.* New York: Pergamon Press, 1980.
Coleman WL, Lindsay RL. Interpersonal disabilities: Social skill deficits in older children and adolescents: Their description, assessment, and management. *Pediatr Clin North Am* 1992;39(3): 551–568.
McTear MF, Conti-Ramsden G. *Pragmatic Disability in Childhood.* San Diego: Singular Publishing Group, 1992.

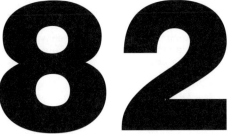

Violent Youth

Peter Stringham

I. **Description of the problem.** Parents are anxiously searching for sensible advice to keep their children safe in what they perceive to be an increasingly violent world. Pediatric practitioners can suggest behaviors that will increase nonviolent problem solving skills in their patients.

A. **Epidemiology.**
- The murder rate of men ages 15–24 years in the United States is 1/5,000 (compared to 1/80,000 in England and 1/200,000 in Japan).
- Murder is the second leading cause of death (after auto accidents) in this age group.
- The lifetime risk for being murdered in the United States is 1 in 450 for white females, 1 in 164 for African American females, 1 in 117 for white males and 1 in 28 for African American males.
- The rate of assaults outnumber fatalities by a ratio of more than 100.
- Adolescents' victimization rates are almost twice the rates for adults 25–34 years old (74/1,000 vs 38/1,000/year).
- For adolescents in dating relationships, rates are between 32%–50% for females using violence and between 20%–32% for males. Three percent of female college students admit to injuring their boyfriends; 7% of males admit to injuring their girlfriends.
- There are 50 million handguns now in circulation in the United States.

B. **Etiology/contributing factors.**
1. **Environmental.** A host of environmental factors have been shown to contribute to violent behaviors in children and adults:
   - A cold, inconsistent child rearing style
   - The experience of child abuse
   - Excessive corporal punishment
   - Witnessing violence in the home and community
   - Viewing media violence
   - Coping with socioeconomic disadvantage
   - The use of alcohol and other drugs
   - Equally important, the presence of a gun can turn a violent impulse into a lethal event

2. **Developmental.**
   - Constant exposure to environmental violence in an infant and young child can create a **disconnected, hypervigilant style of relating** to adults and peers.
   - Witnessing violence in the home neighborhood and television may teach children that the 'best' way to solve conflict is through violence.
   - Some parents actively teach their children to use violence to resolve conflicts.
   - Violent individuals tend to believe that violence is the *preferred* way to handle most conflict. They tend to experience the world as harsh and interpret ambiguous situations as laden with hostility. They view people as either victims or bullies and have few nonviolent strategies for resolving potentially violent conflicts. Many have an impulsive style of acting when assessing the situation or the consequences of their actions.
   - Nonviolent teenagers experience the world as a neutral or positive place. They believe themselves to be of high value and think even potentially violent opponents are of high value. In a potentially violent conflict they are not impulsive; they ask questions of their opponents, state their own positions, and offer to work out compromises. Their response to conflict is respectful, deliberate and not impulsive.

II. **Making the diagnosis.**
A. **History: Key clinical questions.** The goal of the history is to assess the risk that the child is or will become violent. As in other aspects of clinical care, the best way to determine the risk for violence is to ask directly about violence in the home, disciplinary

techniques, violent encounters in the community and personal behaviors and attitudes. Clinical judgment must be exercised in pursuing these lines of questions; there is no need to ask all the question at each visit or for every patient.

1. **For parents.**
   a. **Spousal abuse.**
      - *"How do you and the baby's father get along? How often to you have yelling or screaming fights? How about pushing or shoving fights?"* If answers are negative, no other questions are necessary. At subsequent visits the clinician can inquire about how the couple is getting along. An alternate question for some immigrant families might be, *"Is this a respectful relationship?"*
      - *"Any injuries? What was it about? Tell me about your worst fight. Tell me about your last fight. Are you afraid? Are you safe now? Do you know what to do if you are not safe? Is there a gun in the house?"*
   b. **Gun in the house**
      - *"Is there a gun in any place where your child spends time? What kind? What is it for? Is it loaded? Is it locked up?"*
   c. **Discipline**
      - *"How do you correct the child if the child slaps or bites?* [For an older child] *How do you correct your children if they misbehave?"*
   d. **Attitudes toward violence**
      - *"If a child tries to pick on your child what do you think your child should do?"*
   e. **Street fighting**
      - *"How many fights has your child had in the last year? What were they about? What did you do about it?"*
2. **For older children and teenagers: The FIGHTS pneumonic can be used:**
   F–Fights
   "How many pushing or shoving fights have you had in the last year?"
   "What were they about? How do you usually get out of a fight?"
   I–Injuries
   "Was anyone injured in any of these fights?"
   G–Guns
   "Is there a gun in your home? Do you ever carry a weapon for self-protection?"
   H–Home
   "Has anyone hit you at home in the last year?"
   T–Threats
   "Have you ever been threatened with a weapon?"
   S–Sexual Violence
   "Have you ever had a pushing or shoving fight with a child of the opposite sex? Have you ever been forced to have sex against your will?"

III. **Management.**
   A. **Primary goals.**
      1. To teach beliefs and skills that enhance the child's ability to respond to stress and perceived threats in a nonaggressive way.
      2. To help parents and patients incorporate nonviolent behavior as an integral part of their self-image.
      3. To decrease the environmental factors that increase violence.
   B. **Initial treatment strategies.**
      1. **Spousal abuse.** Pediatric clinicians need basic skills for treating spousal abuse because medical people may be the only adults outside the family who have any contact with a coerced or battered parent.
         a. **Small risk.** A parent tells of physical fights in the past, but none now, and they state that they have no fear, but that sometimes their partner tells them who their friends can be and where they can go. The parent might be considered at low risk for spousal abuse. Advocate that coercion be stopped and that fighting be discussed with the spouse. Try to see if the parent could say to their partner, "If you are upset and tell me you are upset, I will try to help you. If you attack me verbally or in any other way I will put a lot of distance between us—emotionally or physically". The parent may need other counseling.
         b. **Moderate risk.** A parent describes some physical fighting, but no injuries. The parent denies fear and says they are safe. The fights are not initiated by the parent who tries to placate the partner. The clinician can come down strongly on the side on nonviolence: "This worries me a lot" or "You do not deserve to be hit" or "This may be getting out of control. Are you safe now? Do you know what to do if you don't feel safe" The clinician can give the telephone number of a domestic

violence hotline and attempt to refer for counseling specifically to discuss the violence and abuse. If the clinician has excellent rapport with the abuser, sometimes the abuser can be engaged in a discussion of the dangers of losing love in a coercive relationship.

    c. **Large risk.** A parent describes injuries from beatings, fear, a gun in the home, serious threats to themselves or the children. The family should not leave the office until the clinician feels they are 'safe.' Other professionals will need to be involved. The clinician should not intervene with the abusing partner as this may cause more harm. The police might need to be involved.

2. Promoting nonviolent discipline.

    a. Ask about disciplinary techniques at the 10-month visit and suggest to parents: *"Your child will soon be getting into everything. While curiosity is essential, there are some things a child should not do. I recommend that a major rule in your house be 'No hurting anyone.' They cannot hurt themselves or anyone else. If they hit you might be able to stop it by just saying 'no' and redirecting them toward another activity. Sometimes you may need to go further and use a 'time-out.' We don't recommend hitting. It is confusing to a child when you say he should not hurt and then hit him yourself."* (See other methods of discipline in Chapter 13)

    b. If a parent prefers corporal punishment or slaps a child in your office the clinician should not shame the parent. Behavior change comes from an alliance between practitioner and parents. "I agree with you that discipline is very important. Children who do not know what is right can grow up insecure. There are some new ways to correct poor behavior that seem to work better, or as well as hitting and I can tell you about them."

3. Teenagers with street violence. All the described interventions are in the office, but they can be adapted to larger groups and to the community. Clinicians should try to involve parents, schools, and community leaders to promote nonviolence as the norm in the larger community. Don't promote coercion or fear in this effort, i.e, don't conduct a "war on violence."

    a. **Lowest risk.** A teenager with no or few nonserious fights, knows how to get out of a fight, does well in school, and does not have other high-risk adolescent behaviors. Teach the 6 steps to getting out of a fight (Table 82-1). If they say these strategies won't work, ask teenagers what would work for them.

       For young children as well teenager as you might say:

- *"I see a lot of older kids around here and most of them don't fight with anybody. In addition most of those kids are not wimps. I've asked kids who don't get picked on and who don't fight how they do it and they have told me ways to be safe on the streets, and I will tell you what they said. First they say to have a good attitude. The good attitude is that they treat everyone like they are a cousin. You might have a cousin who is upset and really making you mad, but you probably are going to treat your cousin with respect and try not to fight him. With your cousin you try to find out what they are upset about and ask, 'Why are you doing this?' If you did something wrong you can apologize. If you didn't do anything wrong or if they are misunderstanding you can say, 'It isn't that way.' The kids that don't fight with anyone, treat everyone even those people they don't know like they are a cousin. They treat them with respect."*

Table 82-1 Steps for getting out of a fight

1. Treat everyone you meet like they are a cousin: If you have an attitude that everyone is worthy of respect, like they are a cousin, when they are in a conflict with you, you probably can resolve the conflict without a fight. Everyone has a decent side.
2. Try to find out why the other person is upset. If you did something wrong you can apologize and try to make it right. If you didn't do anything wrong you can say that. All the time you talk to the decent side of the person.
3. Leave if you feel fear. Fear is designed to protect you.
4. Leave if you think you will lose your temper. You cannot think straight if you are angry.
5. Sometimes you have to walk away. If a kid is high, or just too upset, staying and talking won't work. It takes a bigger person to walk away from a fight.
6. Get help. Some conflicts are too big for you to handle alone. If you feel you someone is being a bully, you may need to find another person to help resolve conflict the conflict nonviolently.

- *"These kids tell me that there are some times when you should definitely walk away from a fight. You should get away the best you can if you feel fear. What would you do if you saw a tiger running down the street toward you? You would run. If you really feel afraid, don't ignore that feeling. We are designed to survive if we pay attention to our fear. If you are ever in a situation and you begin to feel afraid, you may be noticing something very dangerous even if you cannot put it into words. If you feel afraid, trust your body and leave. If someone asks you why you left, you may not know, but you are better off if you trust your "feelings."*

- Another time you should leave a potential fight is if you feel you are going to lose your temper. Do you think a kid can think well if they have lost their temper? Most kids can't. If it is a serious conflict you need to think clearly and carefully. You can say, *"I am beginning to lose my temper. I have to leave. I'll talk to you about this later when we have calmed down."*

- *"Most of the time you are not afraid and don't lose your temper so you can handle conflicts, by treating a kid like your cousin. You try to figure out what is wrong. If you did something wrong you can apologize and offer to make it right. If you didn't do anything wrong you can say that. You might be able to explain your side of it. When you are talking, don't get too close to a kid who is upset. Sometimes an angry kid gets afraid of you and if you crowd the kid, they may hit you because they get afraid. So give an upset kid space."*

- *"Often talking works, but sometimes talking does not work. If a kid is high on drugs or alcohol, or if a kid is too upset, they cannot listen to you. In those situations you can just leave the best way you can. It is very easy to fight. It takes a big hearted person to walk away from a fight. If the kid was drunk or high, they probably won't remember why they wanted to fight. If the kid was just upset, sometimes they appreciate that you didn't make them fight."*

- *"If a kid is being a bully, pushing you or other people around, you may not be able to handle this alone without fighting. In that case, walk away and fine some other person like a trusted adult to resolve the conflict nonviolently."*

- *"Does this fit with your personality? What things work for you?"*

  b. Moderate risk. A teenager in a few fights who says they would never walk away from a fight. No weapon carrying, no major injuries, doing okay in school and not many other high risk behaviors. You might say:

  - *"Your examination shows that you are strong and well, but you told me that you have been in a few fights and that you would never walk away from a fight. That worries me. Not many, but a few, kids around here carry weapons and you should not have to walk around in fear of these few kids. There are some things teenagers around here do to keep themselves safe. They go pretty much everywhere and are afraid of no one, because they know how to not fight with everyone."*

  c. High risk. A teenager in many fights, who has dropped out of school, is involved with other high-risk behaviors, likes to fight, may be in a violent gang, may carry a weapon.

  (1) Express your concern or worry about their behavior.

  (2) Discuss how they might handle their own frustration or depression better. Identify who they can talk to, teach meditation.

  (3) Present dilemmas that show they can handle some situations nonviolently:

  - *"Your best friend's aunt is in the hospital. You really feel sorry for your friend and would like to help him out, but he begins to yell at you, 'You and your family always looked down on me. You always thought you were better than me. Let's step outside and settle this right now!'* You don't want to hurt them, what could you do?" After the child struggles through a solution show them how they used nonviolence to solve the problem. Suggest that the same techniques that work with a friend can work with a stranger.

4. Address weapon carrying. *"You told me that sometimes you carry a gun to feel safe. Have you told anyone about this? Do you think teenagers keep secrets well? So your friends might have told other kids and many people might know about this. What might happen if a kid had a genuine disagreement with you and needed to discuss it, but they worried that the disagreement might turn into a fight? Do you think they might bring a weapon or have friends bring weapons? Wouldn't that make you less safe? I think teenagers are safer if they have a reputation for settling conflicts by talking about it calmly."*

5. **Try to teach a deliberate, nonimpulsive approaches to ambiguous situations**. *"When most guys are approached by a guy who wants to fight they ask themselves, 'Why is this guy trying to fight me? Is he upset? Is he high? Have I caused this in any way?' Then they ask 'Is he armed?' and then they ask, 'If I wanted to calm him down, what could I do?' After they have answered all those questions they decide whether or not to fight."*

6. **Help them with their depression, unemployment, alcoholism or other problems** and try to refer them to a program that will help address all their needs.

7. If there is a history of violence towards a girlfriend, keep approval of the patient while expressing disapproval of the poor behavior. *"Has your significant other begun to fear you yet? Most will say 'no.' That is really lucky, because if you ever get to the point where your partner fears you then love will surely die. You deserve support, respect, and love. You can only get that when you are in a relationship with someone who treats you like a best friend. That means you treat them like a best friend. Fear poisons all love relationships."*

BIBLIOGRAPHY

For Parents

Websites

The National Youth Violence Prevention Resource Center
  http://www.safeyouth.org/scripts/parents/index.asp
EuroWRC Resource Center/YOUTH VIOLENCE
  http://www.eurowrc.org/07.web_sites/05.links.htm

For Professionals

Publications

American Psychological Association. *Violence and Youth: Psychology's Response: Volume 1 Summary Report of the American Psychological Association Commission on Violence and Youth.* Washington, DC: American Psychological Association, 1993.

Hennes H, Calhoun A (eds). Violence among children and adolescents. *Pediatr Clin N Am* 1998; 45:2.

Prothrow-Stith D. *Deadly Consequences: How Violence Is Destroying Our Teenage Population and a Plan to Begin Solving the Problem.* New York: Harper Collins, 1991.

Websites

Youth Violence: A Report of the Surgeon General
  http://www.surgeongeneral.gov/library/youthviolence/report.html
National Library of Medicine/Youth Violence Prevention Resources
  http://www.nlm.nih.gov/pubs/cbm/youthviolence.html
CDC/*Best Practices of Youth Violence Prevention: A Sourcebook for Community Action*
http://www.cdc.gov/ncipc/dvp/bestpractices.htm

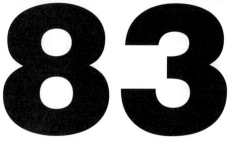

Visual Impairment

Michael E. Msall

I. **Description of the problem. Legal blindness** is defined as **central visual acuity in the best eye with corrective lenses of 20/200 or worse, or a restriction in the visual field so that the widest diameter of vision subtends an angle of 20 degrees.**
   - The term "legal blindness" is a misnomer as approximately 75% of individuals with legal blindness have some residual visual function. In addition, the majority of adults with legal blindness can read large print.
   - For children with vision worse than 20/400, ophthalmologists use functional descriptors such the child's ability to count fingers or detect hand motion, nearby large objects, the direction of a light source or its presence.
   - Students can be classified as "educationally visually impaired" if their corrected vision is 20/70 or worse.
   The World Health Organization (WHO) classifies visual disability into five categories described in Table 83-1.
   A. **Epidemiology.** The epidemiology of severe visual impairment is changing. Both laser surgery for severe threshold retinopathy of prematurity and advances in the prevention of congenital, perinatal, and postnatal infections have substantially decreased their contributions to visual and multiple disabilities.
      - Current estimates of the prevalence of blindness is **approximately 6 per 1000**.
      - Congenital blindness occurs with a frequency of 30 per 100,000.
      - The US does not keep a registry for children with severe visual disability, but 50,000 children are considered visually impaired by school systems, of which 20,000 require Braille as a reading medium.
      - Children with combined deafness and blindness number 500 per year and include 10,000 children birth to age 21 years.
      - Worldwide there are 1.5 million children who are legally blind. In developing countries, the major contributors to visual disability include gonoccal ophthalmia neonatorum, trachoma, vitamin A deficiency, and measles.
   B. **Etiology.**
      1. Table 83-2 describes the major known etiologies of severe visual impairment in childhood. The timing of these etiologies is prenatal in 43%, perinatal in 27%, postnatal in 8%, and unknown in 22%.
      2. Several **multiple malformation syndromes** include ocular findings: chromosomopathies, CHARGE association, Lowe syndrome (mental retardation, cataracts, renal tubular dysfunction), neurocutaneous disorders (tuberous sclerosis, optic gliomas in neurofibromatosis-1), metabolic disorders (homocystinuria), and neurodegenerative disorders (leukodystrophies and optic atrophy, gangliosidosis and cherry red macula, Batten disease) involve ocular findings.
      3. Many syndromes affect **both vision and hearing**. These include Alport, Usher, Cockayne, Stickler, and Refsun syndromes as well as congenital infections, lysosomal storage disease, and leukodystrophies.
      4. **Postnatal causes** of blindness account for 8%–11% of all childhood blindness. Etiologies include infections, trauma, complicated hydrocephalus, retinoblastoma, craniopharngioma, demyelinating diseases, and leukemia with CNS involvement,

Table 83-1 WHO classification of visual disability

Category 1	Visually Impaired	20/60–20/200
Category 2	Severe Visual Impairment	20/200–20/400
Category 3	Blind	20/400–20/2400
Category 4	Blind	<20/2400 and light perception
Category 5	Blind	No light perception

Table 83-2 Major known etiologies of severe visual impairment

Retina	Optic Nerve	Lens	Posteriorvisual pathways
Severe retinopathy of prematurity	Optic nerve atrophy	Cataract	Periventricular leukomalacia
Retinitis pigmentosa	Optic nerve hypoplasia	Corneal dystrophies	Occipital malformations
Toxoplasmosis, rubella	Leber's congenital amaurosis	Galactosemia	Occipital infarction
Rubella	Leber's opticneuropathy	Mucopolysacc-haridosis	Meningitis/encephalitis

5. **Blindness and associated developmental disabilities.** More than 50% of children with visual disability—especially those with cortical visual impairment—have additional major disorders including cerebral palsy, cognitive-adaptive developmental disability, autistic spectrum disorders, recurrent seizures, hearing impairments, and learning disabilities.

C. **Developmental aspects of vision.** Pupillary light reactions and lid closure to bright light are present at 30 weeks gestation. Brief visual fixation is present at birth including brief saccades to a moving person, moving face, and dangling ring. At birth, acuity has been assessed as approximately 20/400 by optokinetic nystagmus, forced preferential looking, and visual evoked potentials (VEP)

II. **Making the diagnosis:**

A. **Clinical presentation.** Infants with visual impairment typically present in 1 of 3 clinical scenarios.

1. **Parents are concerned that their child is not seeing.** At 6–10 weeks, the child is not smiling reciprocally and does not follow faces or rings (but does have a normal papillary response, red reflex, and intact globe). These children either have cortical visual impairment (CVI), delayed visual maturation (DVM), or evolving developmental disability. Both CVI and DVM have high rates of motor, cognitive, and communicative disability. However, functional visual recovery occurs in DVM. In CVI, some visual improvement may occur but low vision is a common sequelae. In children with severe evolving developmental disability the children stare and are inattentive because of disorders of nonvisual higher cortical function impacting on learning, perception, communicating, and social skills.

2. **The child presents in infancy with nystagmus, sluggish pupils, and visual inattention.** Ophthalmologic findings reveal anterior segment or optic nerve disorders such as cataract, corneal opacities, glaucoma, and microphthalmia. The posterior segment abnormalities include colobomas of the optic nerve or retina, optic nerve hypoplasia or atrophy, retinal dystrophy, retinopathy of prematurity, or retinoblastoma.

3. **The infant shows visual inattention, nystagmus, and variable pupillary responses.** Ophthalmological evaluation reveals a normal globe and intact red reflex. Strabismus may be present electoretinogram (ERG) testing is most helpful in revealing the nature of these disorders.

B. **Physical exam.**

1. **Neonatal period.**
   • Careful observation of the shape and size of the eye and the position of the pupil.
   • Response of the pupil to light and the presence of the red reflex. The ability of the infant to track a human face or patterned card visually for 30–60 degrees horizontally.

2. **Infancy and early childhood.**
   • Conjugate gaze should be achieved by 6–12 weeks. Eyes that do not see well tend to deviate or drift, and this along with nystagmus may be the first indication of poor vision.
   • Pupillary responses, an intact red reflex and the ability child to track 360 degrees are indicators of globally adequate vision.

C. **Acuity testing.** By age 3 years, many children can cooperate with visual screening. The Allen Card and Multiple E, and HOTV cards have proved to be the most specific and sensitive measures of visual acuity in preschool children. Any questions concerning

vision should be referred to an ophthalmologist, who can provide a comprehensive evaluation.
  D. **Developmental assessment of blind children.**
    1. **Cognitive development.** A key area to monitor in children with severe visual impairment is communicative milestones. Children who are blind and who do not have associated neurological abnormalities achieve developmental milestones at a slower pace but should not be considered motor or cognitively disabled. The slower developmental milestones are the result of different experiences of nonverbal skills, motor exploration, and understanding spatial relations of objects. For example, the infant is unable to see details of facial expression, lip movements, gestures, object position in space, use of utensils, indoor and outdoor activities. As a result, different and supplemental tactile, verbal, and orientation experience are required to help the child construct knowledge of both immediate and distant environments.
    2. **Motor development.** There are often differences in the learning of gross motor and hand skills. In one study, the median age of sitting steadily was 8 months, pulling to stand was 13 months, walking alone was 15 months, and walking across a room was 19 months.
III. **Management.**
  A. **Primary goals.** The responsibility of the primary care clinician is to interpret and facilitate the infant's behavior and development, to facilitate the family's adaptation to and understanding of the child with blindness, to coordinate the diagnostic evaluation, and to understand their child's strengths, challenges, and ways of learning. In addition referral to early intervention programs, supplemental social security income(SSI), visual aides, parent groups, family supports, and advocacy may be indicated.
  B. **Emotional support.** The typical emotional response of a family is to grieve the loss of the expected sighted child. It is the clinician's task to support parents through the stages of normal grieving and to allow them to express their sadness and anger. While most grief reactions lead to an adaptive accommodation to the child's blindness, some parents do not transcend their grief and become chronically depressed and emotionally unavailable to the infant. This is a devastating experience for any child, and especially so for the blind child. Identification of parental depression and appropriate counseling and referral may be necessary.
  C. Several **model curricula for blind infants** are available to early intervention teams:
    • **Auditory-tactile paired cues** to stimulate interactions. Parents are taught to recognize infant's tactile gestures to communicate basic needs.
    • **Joffee program** is a home-based model for orientation and mobility. Parents learn how to enrich their home environment by auditory toys that are brightly colored and have tactual cues, interactive paired verbal and tactile activities, singing, guided touch, and describing daily activities.
    • **Erwin parent-centered approach** in which parents are trained to teach toddlers how to ask questions, describe objects by using modifiers (e.g. hot, warm, and cold water), and to use personal social labels in speech.
    • **Klein's Parent and Toddler Training** emphasizes social responsiveness. Six target areas are involved, including early childhood development, social development, family reactions, behavior management, enhancing infant development, family communication, and problem solving.
  D. **Developmental interventions.** Guidelines for developmental interventions with blind children are listed in Table 83-3.
    1. **Infant.** Mobility and orientation should be the early ingredients of any program. Touching, labeling, smelling, and exploring toys and objects encourage the infant to learn about their surroundings and prepare them for preschool education.
    2. **Preschoolers.** Preschoolers without associated significant handicaps can attend a regular, well-structured program with extensive consultation from a teacher of the visually handicapped. The curriculum must be rich in sensory experiences, including objects that can be manipulated and audio programs that will expand the child's knowledge of the world.
    3. **School age.** An individualized curriculum is essential. The school-aged child without significant associated handicapping conditions should participate in regular community-based classroom activities that will prepare them for higher education, as well as for independent living.
       Braille continues to be the mainstay of nonvisual communication. The use of records and tapes presents significant adjuncts to reading. Such instruments as the opticon, which converts the printed word into a form that can be felt with the finger, hold a great deal of promise.

Table 83-3 Methods of facilitating the development of the infant who is blind

Developmental skill	Activity
Affective	Supplemental carrying, touching, hugging, comforting
Fine and gross motor (awareness of body image)	Putting bells on extremities; encourage reaching on sound cues; exposing to textured surfaces; placing objects in the infant's hand
Language	Labeling objects, activities; consistently responding to utterances
Cognitive	Searching for objects with sound, smell; touching and labeling objects
Feeding	Providing early exposure to textured foods and self-feeding
Personal and social behavior	Facilitating self-quieting behavior, encouraging self-help skills

E. **Orientation and mobility skills (peripatology).** Training in mobility is a key component of early intervention, teaching the child **orientation** (recognizing their present position and space, the destination, and the route they will travel.) and **mobility** (the technique for safely and efficiently traveling to a predetermined destination). These skills can later be enhanced with the use of a guide dog or electronic travel aids.

BIBLIOGRAPHY

For Parents

Books

Fraiberg S. *Insights from the Blind.* New York: Basic Books, 1977.
Holbrook C. *Children with Visual Impairments – A Parent's Guide.* Bethesda, MD: Woodbine House Inc, 1996.

Websites

American Foundation for the Blind www.afb.org
Blind Childrens Center, educational booklets and videos in English and Spanish www.blindcn-tr.org.
National association for parents of children with visual impairments www.spedex.com
National Library Services for Blind and Physically Handicapped www.loc.gov/nls/

For Professionals

Capute AJ, Accardo PJ. *Developmental Disabilities in Infancy and Childhood.* Baltimore, MD: Paul H Brookes, 1996.
Wolraich M. *Disorders of Development and Learning.* Hamilton, Ont.: BC Decker Inc., 2003.

84

Witness to Violence

Betsy McAlister Groves

I. **Description of the problem.** Children who witness violence in their communities or in the home are often hidden victims. Although it has been well established that children who are the *victims* of violence (e.g., child abuse and sexual abuse) suffer severe and long-lasting consequences, there is now ample evidence that *witnessing* violence is also damaging to children. Because their scars are emotional and not physical, the primary care clinician may not fully appreciate their distress and miss an opportunity to provide needed interventions.

   A. **Epidemiology.**

   1. **Community and international violence.**
      - In one study, more than a third of school-aged children in New Orleans had witnessed severe violence; 40% had seen a dead body.
      - In a study of inner-city children under the age of 6 who attended clinics at Boston City Hospital, 10% had seen a knifing or shooting.
      - Many children of refugee/immigrant parents have experienced the trauma of war or political violence in their country of origin.

   2. **Domestic violence.**
      - At least 3 million children in the United States witness domestic violence every year.
      - Children age 5 and younger are disproportionately represented in households with domestic violence.

   B. **Etiology.**

   1. Research in the past decade has shown that children of all ages may be adversely affected by violence in their environments and that young children are especially vulnerable. Children may experience overwhelming terror, helplessness, and fear, even if they are not immediately in danger. Studies suggest that preschoolers are most vulnerable to threats that involve the safety (or perceived safety) of their caregivers.

II. **Making the diagnosis.**

   A. **Symptoms.** Children may develop symptoms of posttraumatic stress disorder (PTSD) (Table 84-1). Although young children may not fully meet these criteria, certain behavioral changes are commonly associated with exposure to trauma, sleep disturbances, aggressive behavior, new fears, and increased anxiety about separations from caretakers.

   B. **History: Key clinical questions.** It is important for the primary care clinician to inquire about violence in the lives of all children. Questions may be prefaced by a statement that assures the family members that they are not being singled out for this line of questioning and that the clinician considers the topic of violence to be within the scope of problems to be addressed in a medical visit. By doing so, the clinician has communicated that violence and exposure to violence are a risk to the child's well-being and are a legitimate focus of concern during the clinical visit.

   1. *"I know that there is a lot of violence in our world these days. I have begun to ask all of my patients about their experiences with violence. I would like to ask you a few questions."*
      - *"Are you ever worried about your child's safety?"*
      - *"Has your child seen frightening things?"*
      - *"What does your child watch on television? Are you concerned about what your child is watching on television?"*
      - *"Has your child witnessed violence on the streets or in the neighborhood?"*
      - *"Has your child witnessed violence in the home?"*

   2. If there are disclosures of witnessing violence, the following questions will explore how the child may have been affected.
      - *"What happened? What did the child see or hear?"*

Table 84-1 Symptoms of posttraumatic stress disorder

Numbing of responsiveness to the outside world
Constriction of emotions
Reduced involvement with play
Dissociative states
Foreshortened view of the future
Intrusive recollections of the traumatic event
Flashbacks or intrusive recollections
Reenactment through play
Avoidance of traumatic cues
Difficulties with concentration
Autonomic disturbances
Hyperarousal, hyperalertness
Sleep disturbances
Distractibility

The clinician should elicit the story from both the child and the parent. It is preferable to hear the child's story first and, if possible, separately. Children's accounts of traumatic events give important clues about how they viewed the event, how they perceive their role, and what kind of meaning they make of the event. Since children frequently misunderstand or misperceive a sequence of events, the child's account provides important information about how to correct misperceptions.

- [To the child] *"When and how often do you think about what happened? Do thoughts come to you while you are in school? What do you do when these thoughts occur?"*
- [To the parent] *"Are there sleep difficulties? What kind? Nightmares? Difficulties sleeping alone?"*
- *"Does the child seem less interested in play or school? Does the child worry more?"*
- *"What behavioral changes have you observed in the child? Is the child fearful of being apart from you or other caretakers?"*

III. **Management.**

A. **Counseling the parents.** Intervention is much more difficult if the child is living with ongoing domestic violence. Maximizing safety may be a difficult task because the mother may have few options in terms of leaving the batterer. In cases of domestic violence, it is necessary to help the woman assess the safety of her children and herself. This discussion should convey the clinician's concern about the impact of violence on the child and mother. The clinician should help to formulate a plan the mother can use in the event of future violence, including the telephone numbers of the local domestic violence hotline and battered women's shelter. A referral to a battered women's support service should be encouraged. Regardless of the type of violence that the child has been exposed to, the primary care clinician should include the following components of parent guidance in their intervention with the parents.

1. A careful **review** of the facts and details of the violent event.
2. **Information** about the expectable symptoms and behaviors associated with witnessing violence.
3. **Assistance** in restoring a sense of stability to the family in order to enhance the child's feelings of safety (e.g., by establishing consistent routines, assistance in accessing concrete supports such as housing, benefits).
4. **Strategies** to encourage the child to express feelings about the event (e.g., verbally, through drawings or play).
5. **Assurance** that it is not a forbidden topic for discussion. It is helpful to the child to be able to talk about it within the family. Without overfocusing on the incident, parents can communicate their willingness to talk to the child about what has happened.

B. **Counseling the child.** For some children the process of telling their story in detail is in itself therapeutic. The child has a chance to reflect on the event, to try out new coping strategies, and to receive empathic and supportive feedback. By asking sensitive and detailed questions, the clinician models for the parents how to talk to children about frightening or unpleasant events. Thus, the primary care clinician's role with the child is to:

1. Review the facts and details of the traumatic event and help the child accurately understand what has happened.

2. Give the child a forum to share worries, fears, and anxieties and to help the child accommodate to the trauma.

3. Schedule a follow-up appointment within 2–3 weeks of the initial session. This is particularly important in cases involving domestic violence.

C. **Criteria for referral.** The child or family should be referred for mental health intervention in the following circumstances:

- The child's symptoms have persisted for more than 3 months.
- The trauma was particularly violent or involved the loss of a parent or caretaker.
- The caretakers are unable to be empathetically attuned to the child.
- The child is in an unsafe environment.
- Referral should be made to mental health specialists familiar with treating children who have experienced trauma. If the case involves domestic violence, the clinician should also have experience with the particular dynamics of these families. Specialized treatment for these children may include psychological debriefing through play therapy, behavioral/cognitive strategies to decrease sensitivity to traumatic reminders, and pharmacological interventions.

BIBLIOGRAPHY

For Parents

Books

Groves BM. *Children Who See Too Much: Lessons from the Child Witness to Violence Project.* Boston: Beacon Press, 2002.

Monahon C. *Children and Trauma: A Parent's Guide to Helping Children Heal.* New York: Lexington Books, 1993.

Websites

Child Witness to Violence Project www.childwitnesstoviolence.org
National Center for Children Exposed to Violence www.nccev.org
The Child Trauma Academy www.ChildTrauma.org

For Professionals

Groves B, Zuckerman B, Marans S, Cohen DJ. Silent victims: Children who witness violence. *JAMA* 1993;269(2):262–264.

Groves BM, Augustyn M, Lee D, Sawires P. *Identifying and Responding to Domestic Violence: Consensus Recommendations for Child and Adolescent Health.* San Francisco: Family Violence Prevention Fund, 2002. (Can be downloaded at www.endabuse.org.)

Osofsky JD (ed). *Children, Youth and Violence: The Search for Solutions.* New York: The Guilford Press, 1997:124–148.

Pfefferbaum B. Post-traumatic disorder in children: A review of the past ten years. *J Amer Acad Child Adolesc Psychiatry* 1997;36(11):1503–1511.

Scheeringa MS, Zeanah CH. Symptom expression and trauma variables in children under 48 months of age. *Infant Mental Health Journal* 1995;16(4):259–269.

Family Issues

85

Adoption
Nancy Roizen

I. **Description.**
   A. **Epidemiology.**
   - Approximately 2% of the population is adopted—52% by nonrelatives and 48% by relatives.
   - For parents adopting because of infertility, the rate of conception after adopting is 8%–14%.
   - The outcome of adoptions are considered good to excellent in 70%, unclear in 20%, and bad in 10%.
     - In 3% of adoptions, problems lead to discontinuation of the adoption.
     - In special-needs adoption, discontinuation occurs in 11%–14%.
   - Placement with one or two parents is equally successful.
   - In general, the younger the child is at the time of adoption, the more successful is the adoption.
   - Adoption should be considered a risk factor for mental health disorders such as conduct disorder, antisocial personality, and drug abuse.

II. **Primary care clinician's role: information gathering.**
   A. **Preadoption.** During the preadoption process, the clinician should attempt to obtain information from the birth parents and medical records. Adopted children are somewhat more likely than the general population to have attention deficit hyperactivity disorder, fetal alcohol syndrome, mental retardation, or congenital malformations. The clinician should specifically ask about a family history and look for indications of their presence in the child. The clinician should also try to obtain details about the birth parents' appearance, interests and talents, and the reason for placing the child for adoption; information that the adoptee may want later in adolescence.
   B. **Postadoption.** Studies indicate that almost all adoptions have transitional problems. Parents have had idealized expectations about the child's behaviors that may not be realized. For instance, the adoptive parents may think that the child is too cuddly (or not cuddly enough), eats too much (or not enough), or does not signal needs clearly. The clinician should plan a follow-up visit within days rather than weeks of the adoption, and keep close and frequent contact with the adoptive parents to monitor the goodness of fit between parental expectations and child behavior.
   C. **Older adoptee.** For the older adoptee, the clinician should seek additional information on the history and quality of the child's social attachments, history of adverse experiences (such as abuse, deprivation, neglect, rejections, and separations) and educational experience (including quantity, quality, and potential special needs).

III. **Management.**
   A. **When to tell the child he is adopted.** The age at which parents should tell the adoptee about the adoption is somewhat controversial. The goal is that the adoptee remembers always knowing that they were adopted. This can be accomplished by it being known from the date of adoption. If the parents elect to wait until the child is older, they should know the importance of the child's learning of the adoption from the adoptive parents. To learn of adoption from someone else can cause an irreparable breach of trust. The clinician should strongly encourage parents to tell the child early, when he is an egocentric preschooler (age 3 or 4 or earlier). Following disclosure at the preschool age, most parents report a positive reaction from their child, and the adoption is clearly an acceptable topic of conversation from then on.
   B. **How to tell the child he is adopted.** The adoption story should be explained at the child's developmental level and include the following elements.
      1. The adoptive parent's motivation for adoption.
      2. Acknowledgment of the important role of the birth parents in the creation of the child.
      3. The information that the child was conceived, grew inside the birth mother, and was born just like all other children.

4. A suggestion that the decision of the birth parents to place him or her for adoption was in no way the fault of the child.
5. Acknowledgement that there are happy and sad feelings associated with adoption.
6. A statement of the adoptive parents' love for the child and how happy they are that he joined their family.
7. The specifics of each adoption story will vary according to the circumstances.
   - The adoption story might be something like, "*We could not make a baby ourselves so we decided to adopt. You were made by another man and woman, your birth parents, and born to your mother, just like all other children. But, your birth parents could not take care of a baby, so we adopted you. We're sure that they were sad that you were separated from them. You came to live with us, and we're happy we're a family.*"

C. **Sequence of developmental issues.** The adoptee's understanding of adoption changes as he develops. At different ages, the child will focus on different issues and need access to different information to answer questions (Table 85-1).
   1. During the **preschool** age, children are interested in the facts of how they were born and came to be part of their families. A picture book that depicts the story can be very helpful.
   2. Around **age 7–11 years**, the child begins to appreciate the uniqueness and implication of his or her adoptive status. The child's questions, however, may be viewed by the adoptive parents as a potential rejection. The clinician needs to reassure them that the emergence of the child's questioning is part of the normal development sequence and may herald even tougher questions. Children at this age may imagine their birth parents to be richer, more famous, and otherwise more attractive than their adoptive parents. For this reason, many adoptive parents share letters from and pictures of the birth parents with the child. If the birth parents are known to the child (but not as his or her birth parents) the elementary school years are an opportune time to reveal this information to the child.
   3. In the **early adolescent search for identity**, the adoptee may begin to seek more specific information about the birth parents. Teenagers master the task of developing an identity by discovering how they are different from every other human being and how connected they are to "their people". Having more than two parents makes this task more complicated. If little is known about the birth parents, the adolescent may create an idealized picture of them.
   4. In the **late adolescent period**, the adoptee may muse about marriage and children and become even more interested in the biologic and medical status of the birth parents. Concerns about family illnesses such as insanity may surface. Adolescents, with rare exceptions, should have all the available information about their origins to help them make sense of their life.

D. **Adoptee's questions about birth parents.** As the child asks more probing questions about the birth mother and why she did not keep him or her, the answers should afford the opportunity to develop a positive attitude about her. In a discussion of this issue, a parent could say, "Your mother chose adoption because she felt unprepared to raise

Table 85-1 Issues of adoption at different ages

Preschool
"Where did I come from?"
Life and death issues
Generally accepting of being adopted
School age (7-11 years)
"Why was I adopted when most people aren't?"
Worried that their value as a person is less because they are adopted
Concerns about being different
Aware that they have lost someone who played an extremely important role in their life
Imagines both parents as rich, famous, and more attractive than adoptive parents
Adolescence
Task of developing an identity and discovering how they are different and how they are connected to "their people"
Concerns about family illness such as insanity and talents, and physical appearance of birth family
Interest in meeting birth parents

a child, any child, at that time." The adoptive parent could go on to explain that the birth mother felt unprepared for reasons related to a lack of money, maturity, and resources. The adoptive parent should never imply that the reason for the adoption had anything to do with something the child did.

Often there is little information available about the birth father. As the child realizes that there most certainly was a father involved, the child also realizes that he or she, too, has been abandoned by the father. An adoptive parent could say to the child, "Your birth father was most likely overwhelmed by the situation and thought that he was not entitled to be more involved. He probably thinks about you and wonders about how you are doing." As with discussions about the birth mother, the child should be encouraged to think positively about the birth father.

In some cases, the birth parents had problems, such as alcoholism, drug abuse, child abuse, or mental illness, which led to the adoption. These circumstances need to be discussed and explained in an understanding way, such as: "Your parents needed help but did not know how to ask for it. So their problem with alcoholism was a signal that they needed help and needed someone else to care for their child."

E. Outsiders and adoption. People may ask personal questions about an adopted child out of curiosity or because the child looks different from the adoptive parents. Parents should never hide the fact that a child is adopted but always respect the child's right to privacy with regard to the details about the birth parents and the circumstances of the adoption. Private details about the birth might include genetic and social history or details that have not yet been shared with the child. One way to respond to such questions would be to say, "I don't want to go into all those details because I think it should be our child's choice when he or she is older as to what information will be shared."

In the early elementary school years, the adoptee may be teased about being adopted. When this happens, the child needs to tell a sympathetic and supportive adult and be helped to develop a reply. The child needs to tell what happened and how he or she felt, responded, and would like to respond if it happened again. For instance the child could be coached to say, "Yeah, I'm adopted, So what? So were Presidents Ford and Reagan!"

F. Searching for the birth parents. Some adolescents express an interest in meeting their birth parents; others may only be interested in knowing certain information (such as what they look like). About **40% of adoptees seek the identity of their birth parents** or seek to locate and meet them. Studies show that following reunions with birth parents, the majority of adoptees have shown more positive relationships with their adoptive parents. The adolescent adoptee should be encouraged to postpone the search until young adulthood, when he or she may have the maturity and experience to put the adoption in proper and healthy perspective. Searching is time consuming and energy draining, and it may be confusing to try to establish relationships with biologic parents while trying to become independent of adoptive ones.

G. Special-needs adoptees. Special-needs or hard-to-place adoptees include certain minorities, children older than age 6 years, children with a chronic illness or a psychological problem, or children who must be adopted with a sibling. Discontinuation of the adoption is more likely if the child is older, if the child has made many moves, and if there is another child in the home (especially if the child is of the same age). Some special-needs children have been enormously deprived, and the behaviors caused by deprivation make special demands on a family. In pre-adoptive counseling, the clinician should explore the adoptive parents' readiness to assume the extra effort and time demanded in adopting a child with special needs.

H. Transracial or mixed racial adoption. The American Academy of Pediatrics recommends that a child be placed with a family of the same racial and cultural background whenever possible. However, minorities are over represented in the group of children available for adoption. In 1970, 35% of African American adoptees were adopted by white families. By age 3 years, children are aware of differences in skin color and, by age 4 years, they are aware of racial groupings. Since every child needs a positive sense of racial and ethnic identity, adoptive parents have a responsibility to acquaint the child with his or her heritage and to integrate aspects of the child' heritage into the family's life (e.g., celebrating the holidays of the child's ethnic origin, making foods from the child's country of origin). Although various minority groups have long opposed adoption of minority children by parents of a different racial background, the long-term follow-up studies of African American children adopted by white parents do not show evidence of undue difficulties.

I. Open adoption. "Open adoption" is the continuum of options that enables birth parents and adoptive parents to have information about and communication with one another before and after placement of the child or at both times. One advantage is the ready source of information available as the child feels a need for it. The practice of open adoption has not been well researched and the long-term effects on the child are not known. Initial data indicates that open adoption is associated with positive attitudes in the adoptive mother toward the biological mother.

J. **International adoption.** In the 1990s, international adoptions increased to about 10,000 a year. Ninety percent of the children come from Asia, South America, and Eastern Europe. Perhaps as many as 60% of the children come with infectious diseases such as hepatitis, cytomegalovirus, intestinal pathogens, tuberculosis, syphilis, and HIV. Other diseases to be considered include hemoglobinopathies. Many of the children exhibit developmental delays and growth retardation. All medical records must be scrutinized and laboratory tests should be repeated if there is any question as sometimes documentation, even the date of birth, may be inaccurate.

BIBLIOGRAPHY

For Parents

Books

Hopkins-Best M. *Toddler Adoption: The Weaver's Craft.* Indianapolis: Perspectives, 1997.
Melina LR. *Making Sense of Adoption: A Parent's Guide.* New York: Harper & Row, 1989.

Websites

U.S. Department of State Office of Children's Issues http://travel.state.gov/adopt.html
The Joint Council on International Children's Services, site on most recent issues. www.jcics.org

Organizations

National Adoption Center, information on adoption by local area.
1-800-TOADOPT
www.adopt.org
Adoptive Families of America
3333 Highway Loon
Minneapolis MN 55422
612-722-5362

For Professionals

Barnett ED, Miller LC. International adoption: the pediatrician's role. *Contemporary Peds* 13: 29–46, 1996.
Borchers D and Committee on Early Childhood, Adoption, and Dependent Care. Families and adoption: The pediatrician's role in supporting communication. *Pediatrics* 112(6):1437–1441, 2003.
Committee on Infectious Diseases, American Academy of Pediatrics. Medical evaluation of internationally adopted children for infectious diseases. *2003 Red Book: Report of the Committee on Infectious Diseases (26th ed).* Elk Grove Village, IL: American Academy of Pediatrics, 2003, pp. 173–180.
American Academy of Pediatrics. Coparent or second-parent adoption by same-sex parents. *Pediatrics* 109(2):339–340, 2002.

Bereavement and Loss

Benjamin S. Siegel
Maria Trozzi

I. **Description of the problem.** It is estimated that 5% of all children will experience the death of a parent by age 15 years, and 40% of junior and senior high school students have experienced the death of a friend or an acquaintance their age.

A. **Coping with loss.** The task of children who experience a great loss is to attempt to understand what happened and why the death occurred, to mourn the lost person in their own way and at their level of cognition and affective development, and to construct an enduring inner reality of that lost person and the lost relationship.

Long-term mental health outcomes of bereaved children are influenced by:
- The age at which death takes place.
- The person who has died (parent, sibling, friend, or relative).
- The nature of the relationship between that person and the child.
- The nature of the death (illness, suicide, SIDS, AIDS, murder, accident; was it witnessed by the child).
- The child's history of losses.

It is useful to divide childhood into four major age categories to understand the child's knowledge of and emotional reaction to death and loss (Table 86-1).

B. **Communication issues.** Most adults in our culture feel uncomfortable talking with children about death. Death is viewed as outside the normal cycle of life, something to be fought against and to be denied. This attitude is problematic when the adults who are most needed by children are in the midst of their own mourning and grief, so that their grief intensifies when their children question them or discuss the death. Other times, adults may wish to protect children from emotional distress by denying the loss altogether. Well-meaning adults may use euphemisms to explain about death, such as "going to sleep," which may be confusing to children and make them afraid to go to sleep or fearful when a loved one is sleeping.
- Adults must help children to come to terms with difficult questions: "What is death? Can it happen to me? Can it happen to some other loved one? Am I responsible for the death? Who will take care of me now? Why did the person die? Where is the dead person now? Why won't the dead person come back?"

II. **Role of the primary care clinician.** The primary care clinician, especially one who has had a long-term relationship with the patient and family, is in an excellent position to provide initial counseling and appropriate referral (Table 86-2). Competence in this area requires not only the willingness to explore these issues with families but also an honest appraisal of one's own thoughts and feelings about the meaning of death.

III. **Management.** The most important goal for the provider is to help the parents address their thoughts and feelings about the loss and to encourage them to be emotionally available to their children. The provider should encourage the adult caretakers to communicate with the children and remember that accommodation and adaptation to the death of a loved one are a continual process, often lasting a lifetime. Children confront the loss at each stage of development as they gain a greater understanding of the world and themselves, and they experience new feelings at each stage of development. Since it is a developmental process, children grieve *longer* than adults, as they apparently re-grieve at each developmental stage. Providers need to remind parents of this phenomenon. Nurturing and support over time by family and friends are the best healing experiences for the bereaved child.

A. **Very young children (to age 2 years).**
1. **Encourage parenting figures to provide consistent care in a familiar environment** since children at this age react to death primarily with feelings of separation and loss.
2. **Familiar toys, appropriate transitional objects, and consistent caretaking are crucial.** Frequently, family members are involved in their own grief and have little energy to spend with the infant or toddler. A close relative or even a babysitter well

Table 86-1 Cognitive and Affective Stages of Grief and Loss

Age	Cognitive understanding	Emotional/affective	Potential symptoms
Young children less than age 3	Death is separation abandonment, change	Feelings of loss	Sadness
			Fearfulness
			Poor feeding
			Sleep problems
			Irriitability
			Developmental delay
			Regression
			Increased ciying
Preschool (3–6 yr)	Realization that death exists	Guilt (I am responsible	Delayed grief
Preoperational (prelogical)	Reversibility of death (3–5)	Shame	Enuresis
Magical thinking	Death equals sorrow of others	Fear of punishment because of my thoughts, feelings, and actions	Encopresis
Fantasies	Death is temporary	Fear of catching whatever caused the death	Sleep Disturbances
Causation of thought*	Death is catching	Fear of other loved one dying	Nightmares
Egocentric	Fear that sleep = death	Anger at loved one	Temper tantrums
	Loving someone is dangerous	Denial	Hyperactivities
	Dead people still eat and breathe		Loss of control of behavior
School age (6–11 yr)	Death is permanent	Anger, sadness	
Concrete operations (logical)	Death will not happen to me	Guilt	
Problem solving	Biologic understanding of death	Some fear of retribution	Somatic complaints
	Death is universal	Denial	Resistance to going to school
	Dead people do not think, feel		Decreased school performance
	Dead people can sometimes look alive		Inattention, fighting, daydreaming, failure to complete work
			Acting-out behavior
Adolescence (12 + yr)	Death an an inevitable universal process	Strong denial of death	Delinquency
Formal operations (abstract logical)	Death as irreversible	Anger	Drug and alcohol abuse
	Death can happen to me	Guilt	Somatic complaints
	Idealization of dead person	Sadness	Depression
		Embarrassment	Suicide ideation
		Wanting to join loved one	Sexual acting out
			School failure

*The idea that one's thoughts or wishes can cause something to happen.

Table 86-2 Role of primary care provider

To acknowledge one's own feelings of sadness and loss.
To demystify and explain the reasons for death at a level the child can understand.
To encourage the child to ask questions and explore his fear and fantasies.
To encourage the child to see the body of the person who has died if the child and adults feel comfortable, and to participate in the religious or cultural rituals of grief and mourning as practiced by the family.
To explore hidden feelings and memories of the dead person.
To explain to parents different stages of cognitive and affective development of children and anticipate specific kinds of grief reactions.
To deal with and accept any of the displaced anger family members may have. To monitor the grief reaction and refer for mental health consultation when appropriate.
To support the child and family over time.
To consult with the school or other community institutions as appropriate.

known to the child could be engaged to provide the support of which others may be incapable.

B. Preschool (ages 3–6).
1. **The child's understanding.** Since children at this age are egocentric, they believe they may have caused the death. It is important to emphasize that the loved one really has died, that they did not cause the death, and that they will be taken care of. Often children at this age appear not to acknowledge the death. However, their behavior often belies this, as their grief is often expressed through aggressive, mischievous behavior. Sometimes the pain of the loss is simply too great for children to comprehend, and they behave as if nothing has happened. Or they become angry with whomever brought the bad news or angry with family members because they were not strong enough to prevent the death.
2. **Explanations.** Because children at this age believe that death is reversible they may ask such questions as, "When is Daddy coming home?" or questions of bodily functioning, such as, "If Grandma is in the coffin underground, won't she get cold?" or "How will she breathe if she is all covered up?" These questions may be upsetting for grieving adults, who need to be encouraged to be quite direct and honest: "He is dead. We will never see him again. We are all very sad." "I will try to answer your questions and would like to know what you think or feel when someone dies. I also want you to know that you will be taken care of at all times." Sometimes referring to a dead pet (if that had been in the child's experience) is a useful way to link the child's past lost to the present. Reading selected stories can also be useful.
3. **Participation in rituals.** The child's participation in rituals can be helpful, *assuming* that the child is able to understand a concrete explanation of the event; e.g., the wake, sitting Shiva, the funeral, a visit to the graveside. The adult should ask the child what he is curious about, as well as what concerns he may have in order to uncover fantasies prior to the child's participation. Children should be accompanied by an empathetic adult who is well known to them and emotionally available to meet their needs. The direct experience about what happens at funerals prevents unrealistic fears and fantasies from developing and enhances long-term adaptation. If a child does not wish to go to the funeral or is overwhelmed by the crowd and the communal grief reaction, special times may be established for later visitation to the funeral home or gravesite. If children choose not to participate, a clear, concrete description of what happened should be provided.

C. School age (ages 6–12 years)
1. **The child's understanding.** At this age children can understand biologic functioning. Adults should be encouraged to give more information about the reasons for the death (e.g., "His body stopped working completely," or "Her heart stopped," or "The lungs no longer worked," or "He died of cancer").
2. **Explanations.** Honesty, even about suicide or homicide, usually facilitates long-term adaptation. Explanations regarding what will remain the same, and what will be different as a result of this death, can be particularly useful. Some children may require more detailed explanations, regarding both the death as well as what will happen to the person's body after death. Let the child lead the discussion. Questions such as "What do you know?" or "Tell me what you think happened," are helpful.
3. **Grieving.** Parents should be encouraged to acknowledge their emotions to their chil-

dren and give their children permission to express their own feelings. Grieving of parents and children may be dyssynchronous. The child's grief reaction may appear just at the time that adults are getting over the acute mourning stage.

    4. **Participation in rituals.** Children at this age should be encouraged to participate in all formal events, such as funeral services, burial services, memorial services, and other rituals dictated by religion or culture. The child needs an empathic person present and should not be forced to participate if he does not wish to.

  D. **Adolescence.**

    1. **The adolescent's understanding.** Adolescents understand death as adults do; however, they are new to the philosophical "why's" involved in any death. Although they have a mature understanding of death, they fantasize about their own immortality and may engage in risk-taking behavior, as though they are invincible to death. Many choose to create their own rituals with their peers in addition to/instead of participating in traditional rituals.

    2. **Adolescents can sometimes harbor guilt** that they may have been responsible for the death.

    3. Peer relationships are very strong and **adolescents often prefer to be with their friends** rather than family members. The death of a peer may shatter their fantasies of immortality and their grief reaction often appears excessive to adults. Denial of their feeling from adults in their lives may prolong their grief reaction.

    4. **Sometimes they develop idealized images of the loved one, occasionally want to "join" the loved one**, and have thoughts of suicide. Although suicidal ideation is a common symptom in bereaved adolescents, it is rare for adolescents actually to attempt suicide.

  E. **School.** The school is a natural environment for groups of children to face the death of a teacher or classmate. Trained teachers, who already know the students, have an increased capacity to assist them with the tasks of mourning: understanding, grieving, commemorating, and moving on. The school itself naturally creates a safe, structured environment for teachers to model their own grief response, normalize individual grief reactions, particularly when the death is stigmatic, and assist students who choose to informally commemorate through activities; such as planting a tree, drawing pictures, making a memory book, talking about the "friend" who dies. As school resumes its regular activities, counselors should be sensitive to those youngsters who require a professional referral. When a youngster returns to school after a death in his family, his teacher should be informed so that she can facilitate the child's return. Again, the classroom setting provides an inclusive environment for strengthening and mastering the coping skills required to face future losses.

IV. **Criteria for referral.** In order to help the child and the family, time needs to be set aside to address many of the issues mentioned. Some primary care providers feel that their role is to obtain a history and to refer to a mental health provider. Others, especially if there has been an ongoing relationship and they enjoy the role of counseling and education, can use that relationship to address immediate issues of grief and follow the child and family through the grief process. After the initial consultation at the time of the death, a 2–4 week and 4–6 month follow-up consultation are appropriate. A mental health referral is advisable when the provider feels uncomfortable by the feelings or generated during the consultation. Other reasonable criteria include distress for more than 6 months; intense, inconsolable grief; and poor functioning at home, in school, or with peers.

BIBLIOGRAPHY

For Children

Books for Ages 3–6(Preschool)

Brown L, Brown M. *When Dinosaurs Die: A Guide to Understanding Death.* Boston: Little, Brown, 1996.

Brown M. *The Dead Bird.* New York: Dell, 1939.

Bryan M, Ingpen R. *Lifetimes: The Beautiful Way to Explain Death to Children.* New York: Bantam Books, 1983.

Clifton L. *Everett Anderson's Goodbye.* New York: Holt, 1983.

Cohen M. *Jim's Dog Muffins.* New York: Greenwillow, 1984.

Cohn J. *I Have a Friend Named Peter.* New York: William Morrow, 1987.

De Paola T. *Nana Upstairs and Nana Downstairs.* Penguin Books, 1978.

Johnston T. *Day of the Dead.* New York: Harcourt, Inc., 1997.

Kohlenberg S. *Sammy's Mommy Has Cancer.* New York: Imagination Press, 1993.

Lanton S. *Daddy's Chair*. Rockville, MD: Kar-Ben Copies, 1991.
Rogers F. *When a Pet Dies*. New York: Putnam & Sons, 1988.
Thomas P. *I Miss You (A First Look at Death)*. New York: Barrons, 2000.
Vigna J. *Saying Goodbye to Daddy*. Morton Grove, Ill.: Albert Whitman and Co., 1991.
Viorst J. *The Tenth Good Thing About Barney*. New York: Atheneum, 1971.
Wilhelm H. *I'll always Love You*. New York: Crown Publishers, 1985.
Wintrop E. *Promises*. New York: Clarion Books, 2000.

Books for Ages 6–9

(Many of the above books are also appropriate)
Alexander A. *A Mural for Mamita*. Omaha, NE: Centering Corp., 2002.
Alexander A. *Sunflowers & Rainbows for Tia – Saying Good-bye to Daddy*. Omaha, NE: Centering Corp., 1999.
Bahr M. *If Nathan Were Here*. Grand Rapids, MI: Eerdman Books, 2000.
Egger B. *Marianne's Grandmother*. New York: E.P. Dutton, 1978.
Girard L. *Alex, the Kid with AIDS*. Morton Grove, Ill.: Albert Whitman and Co., 1991.
Jukes M. *Blackberries in the Dark*. New York: Knopf, 1985.
Machenski M. *Some of the Pieces*. Boston: Little, Brown, 1991.
Miles M. *Annie and the Old One*. Boston: Little, Brown, 1971.
Powell S. *Geranium Morning*. Minneapolis: Carol Rhoda Books, 1990.
Schwiebert P, DeKlyen C. *Tear Soup*. Portland, OR: Grief Watch, 1999.
Sims A. *Am I Still a Sister?* Albquerque, N.M.: Big A and Co., 1986.
Tiffault B. *A Quilt for Elisabeth*. Omaha, NE: Centering Corp., 1992.
White EB. *Charlotte's Web*. New York: Harper, 1952.

Books for Ages 9–12 (Preadolescents)

Aub K. *Children Are Survivors Too*. Boca Raton, FL: Grief Education Enterprises, 1995.
Baur MD. *On My Honor*. New York: Bantam Doubleday, 1986.
Creech S. *Walk Two Moons by*. New York: Harper Collins, 1994.
Krementz J. *How It Feels When A Parent Dies*. New York: Knopf, 1983.
Krementz J. *How It Feels When Parents Divorce*. New York: Knopf, 1988.
Lowry L. *A Summer to Die*. New York: Bantam, 1970.
Mann P. *There Are Two Kinds of Terrible*. New York: Avon, 1979.
Park B. *Mick Harte Was Here*. New York: Scholastic Inc., 1995.
Paterson K. *Bridge to Terebithia*. New York: Harper and Row, 1977.
Smith D. *A Taste of Blackberries*. New York: Crowell, 1973.

Books for Ages 13+ (Adolescents)

Agee J. *A Death in the Family*. New York: Grosset & Dunlap, 1938.
Blume J. *Tiger Eyes*. New York: Macmillan, 1981.
Dower L. *I Will Remember You*. New York: Scholastic Inc., 2001.
Fitzgerald H. *The Grieving Teen*. New York: Simon & Schuster, 2000.
Gravelle K. *Teenagers Face to Face with Bereavement*. New York: Messner, 1989.
Grollman E, Malikow M. *Living When a Young Friend Commits Suicide*. Boston: Beacon Press, 1999.
Grollman E. *Straight Talk About Death for Teenagers*. Boston: Beacon Press, 1993.
Guest J. *Ordinary People*. New York: Ballentine Books, 1976.
LeShan E. *Learning to Say Good-Bye When a Parent Dies*. New York: Macmillan, 1975.
Richter E. *Losing Someone You Love: When a Brother or Sister Dies*. New York: Putnam, 1986.
Scrivani M. *When Death Walks In*. Omaha, NE: Centering Corp., 1991.
Shakespeare W. *Romeo and Juliet*. *[Various editions.]*

For Parents and Adults

Gravelle K. *Teenagers: Face to Face With Bereavement*. Messner: New York. 1989.
Grollman E (ed). *Bereaved Children and Teens*. Beacon Press: Boston, 1995.
Grollman EA. *Talking about Death. A Dialogue Between Parents and Child (3rd ed)*. Boston: Beacon Press, 1990.
Kubler-Ross E. *On Children and Death*. New York: Macmillan, 1983.
Rando T. *How To Go On Living When Someone You Love Has Died*. New York: Bantam Books, 1991.

Ross EK. *On Children and Death, (Reprint edition)* New York: Scribner 1997.

Trozzi M. *Talking With Children About Loss.* New York: Penguin Putnam, 1999.

For Professionals

Committee on Psychosocial Aspects of Child and Family Health. The pediatrician and childhood bereavement. *Pediatrics* 89:516–518, 1992.

Siegel B. Helping children cope with death. *Amer Fam Physician* 31:175, 1985.

Trozzi M, Massimini K. *Talking with Children About Loss: Words, Strategies and Wisdom to Help Children Cope with Death, Divorce and Other Difficult Times.* New York: Penguin Putnam, 1999.

Websites

Centering Corporation www.centering.org

Connect For Kids www.connectforkids.org

Crisis, Grief, and Healing (links to hundreds of online resources) www.webhealing.com

The Good Grief Program of Boston Medical Center
   http://www.bmc.org/pediatrics/special/GoodGrief/overview.html

Grief Watch www.griefwatch.com

87

Child Care

Laura A. Jana

I. **Description of the problem.** With increasing numbers of families consisting of single- or dual-working parents and more women entering the workforce, spending time in the care of someone other than a parent is now a fact of life for a majority of today's children. Child care has become the second largest expense for many families, surpassed only by housing. The sheer amount of time spent by today's children in child care, coupled with the growing body of research suggesting that early childhood experiences play a significant role in shaping future life outcomes, has led to an increasing need for children's health professionals' involvement in early education and care-related issues.

A. **Epidemiology.**
- Over 20 million families in the United States have either a single working parent or two working parents and, as a result, rely on some form of nonparental child care.
- 6.7 million children under the age of 3 years have working mothers and 73% of these children are cared for by someone other than a parent.

B. **Types of care.** The term "child care" has come to represent a wide variety of options, all of which involve nonparental supervision. There are for-profit and nonprofit, faith-based and nondenominational, company-based or employer-supported/affiliated, private and public. Most permutations of which fall into the following major categories:

1. **Home-based care.** This category includes care either in the home of the child or in another residential facility (typically that of the caregiver). It encompasses care provided by relatives and nonrelatives.
   a. **In-home care.** This type of care involves a caregiver, such as babysitter or nanny, coming to the child's home. Such an arrangement can be costly, but often offers children the familiarity of their home environment, as well as added convenience and flexibility for parents.
   b. **Family-based care.** Family child care is care provided in someone else's home. According to the National Association for Family Child Care (NAFCC), there are approximately 1 million family child care providers providing care for 4 million children in the United States. For regulation purposes, family-based care is subcategorized into small (less than 7 children) and large (7 or more children). Many parents are attracted to the home-like atmosphere and the potential for close bonding with a single child care provider that family-based care offers. Family-based care may offer more flexibility in hours and be less expensive than center-based, but can also be less reliable when the caregiver becomes ill or goes on vacation. Quality, although regulated by the state, also tends to be far more variable.
2. **Center-based care.** Center-based care is a broad category that generally refers to care provided in a nonresidential facility. For regulation purposes it also includes residential-based facilities that serve more than 12 children. Common examples include nursery schools, child care centers, preschools, pre-kindergarten programs, church-based centers, and Head Start programs. While generally open year-round and allowing children the opportunity to interact with a greater number of peers, centers tend to be less flexible, more expensive, and in some instances offer less opportunity for close bonding with caregivers due to large class sizes, changing classrooms, and high staff turnover. In 1999, a majority (60%) of the 3–5 year olds in child care were enrolled in some form of center-based care.
3. **School-age care.** Included in this category are before- and after-school programs, and vacation programs. School-age care settings include both school-based facilities and other locations. They offer an alternative to unsupervised after-school time and provide children with the opportunity to interact with peers, but they introduce added cost, their structure can be quite variable, and not all programs are regulated.

C. **Ratios, licensure, and accreditation**
1. **Ratios.** Ratios refer to the number of children per caregiver. Although not a guaran-

Table 87-1 Recommended child-to-adult ratio and group size for large family child home care and centers

Age	Child-to-staff ratio	Maximum group size
Birth–12 mo	3:1	6
13–30 mo	4:1	8
31–35 mo	5:1	10
3 year olds	7:1	14
4–5 year olds	8:1	16
6–8 year olds	10:1	20
9–12 year olds	12:1	24

American Public Health Association and American Academy of Pediatrics. *Caring for Our Children: Guidelines for Out-of-Home Child Care Programs, a Collaborative Project.* Copyright 2002 by the American Public Health Association, the American Academy of Pediatrics, and The National Resource Center for Health and Safety in Child Care.
Note: Group size refers to number of children in a room or other well-defined space.

tee of quality, lower child to staff ratios (as well as total group size) have been deemed to be very important indicators in the setting of national standards (Table 87-1).

2. **Licensure.** Regulated by state agencies, licensure of childcare programs and certification of childcare providers can vary significantly from state to state. Criteria for licensure typically include standards relating to child to staff ratios, staff qualifications and training, supervision and discipline, administration of medication, emergency planning, and hand washing and diapering procedures. In some states, certain types of care (such as faith-based, school-age, or summer programs) may be exempt.

3. **Accreditation.** Some childcare programs voluntarily undergo a process of accreditation to demonstrate their commitment to and delivery of quality child care above and beyond what is required for licensure. Accreditation offers parents and caregivers a useful way to assess quality, and the process of attaining and maintaining accreditation may actually improve quality of care and increase professionalism. There are almost 8,000 programs currently accredited by the National Association for Early Childhood Education (NAEYC). Once approved, accreditation is granted for five years. Organizations such as the National Association for Family Child Care (NAFCC) have also developed quality standards for family care accreditation.

II. **Role of the clinician.**

A. **Parental support and guidance.** A 1999 AAP survey of pediatric clinicians found that while 79% felt they should be involved in childcare decisions made by families in their care, only 32% offered parents resources and information on the subject. Pediatric clinicians should be willing and able to discuss a family's childcare options and arrangements, address any concerns that might arise, and offer guidance on how to find safe, affordable, child care that is developmentally, educationally, and nutritionally sound. The following is a sample list of some of the key questions clinicians can recommend parents ask in their search for quality child care:

1. *"Is it a stimulating and nurturing environment?"* Clinicians can reiterate to parents that they must feel comfortable that the caregiver(s) they choose is caring and able to provide a nurturing environment. Parents should be encouraged to ask about licensure and accreditation, the training and experience of the staff, the rate of turnover, and references. Additionally, parents should look for childcare programs that exceed ratio requirements, that are structured so that children can bond with a single or with only a few primary caregivers, that have established routines that still allow for appropriate exploration, adequate time, space, and supplies for age appropriate play, and use defined discipline techniques with which the parents are comfortable. Recommendations—whether from a childcare referral agency, other parents, or a clinician—can also be quite valuable.

2. *"Is it safe?"* Thousands of children each year are injured while in child care. Having studied the prevalence of potential safety hazards in child care, the Consumer Product Safety Commission recommends that parents assess for several specific areas of risk, including:
   - Infant sleep position, i.e., sleep on their backs
   - Cribs safety and without any soft bedding, pillows, or comforters
   - Play area safety—looking specifically for surfacing made of safe materials and well maintained

- Windows and blinds should be safely secured
- Safety gates properly installed and used

3. *"Does it fit the family's financial and scheduling limitations?"* The quality of childcare programs is quite often directly correlated with expense, and parents should consider how much they are willing and/or able to pay. Location and accessibility factor into many parents' selection, and scheduling considerations should also be taken into account—asking about earliest drop-off and latest pick-up times, vacation time and holidays (as well as whether or not parents must pay for them), summer-time program schedules, and part-time options.

B. Provide health consultation. In some states, the affiliation of childcare programs with a health consultant is mandated. By establishing relationships with childcare providers, either informally or in the role of an official health consultant, pediatric providers can help improve and insure the health, safety, and quality of care. Childcare providers and the families whose children are in their care can benefit from such basic contributions as the dissemination of accurate health and medical information, the administration of commonly used medications, principles of first aid, safety and injury prevention, and discussion of special care plans for children with special health needs.

C. Advocacy. Clinician involvement at the local, state, or national level can help effect change in areas such as access to quality care and the establishment and/or enforcement of healthy and safe standards of care.

III. Common issues in child care.

A. Communicable diseases. Childcare attendance has been implicated as a cause of more frequent illnesses in early childhood. Pediatric providers can counsel parents and providers on the prevalence, methods of prevention, and appropriate management of commonplace childhood. "Universal precautions" with good hygiene and infection control measures—particularly as it pertains to diaper-changing, hand-washing, and food handling— should be reinforced for childcare providers. Written explanations or instructions regarding specific illnesses and medication administration are helpful to childcare providers as well as parents.

B. Behavioral. Behavioral issues rank high on the list of concerns for both parents of children in child care and their childcare providers.

1. Separation. The introduction of young children to new settings and/or unfamiliar caregivers can cause separation challenges that vary considerably in duration and extent. Clinicians can help families transition their children into child care by routinely discussing age-appropriate handling of separation, such as allowing adequate time for children to transition, facilitating bonding with a single caregiver, establishing predictable times of parental departure and return, and the establishment of well-defined routines.

2. Aggression. Aggression, typically in the form of hitting and/or biting, is a common challenge for both providers and parents of young children in child care. Pediatric providers can educate parents and providers on reasonable expectations for play, sharing, and communicating between young children, potential causes of such behavior, and recommend methods of age-appropriate management/discipline.

C. Long-term outcome. Recently there has been increasing research and debate on the developmental implications on childcare, particularly focusing on quality, duration and time of initiation. No clear guidelines have emerged to date but providers should be aware of the controversy to address parental questions and concerns.

BIBLIOGRAPHY

For Parents

Choosing Child Care: What's Best for Your Family. American Academy of Pediatrics, Pamphlet ID#: HE0028, 1997.
Child Care Safety Checklist for Parents and Child Care Providers. Document #242, U.S. Consumer Product Safety Commission www.cpsc.gov/cpscpub/pubs/childcare.org
Zero to Three: Choosing Quality Child Care http://www.zerotothree.org/choose_care.html
National Resource Center for Health and Safety in Child Care http://nrc.uchsc.edu/
National Association for the Education of Young Children www.naeyc.org

For Professionals

Caring for Our Children: National Health and Safety Performance Standards: Guidelines for Out-of-Home Child Care Programs (2nd ed), 2002. Available at: http://nrc.uchsc.edu/CFOC/index.html

The Pediatrician's Role in Promoting Health and Safety in Child Care. AAP Bookstore, ID#: MA0175, 2001.

Moving Kids Safely in Child Care. 2002. An American Academy of Pediatrics/The National Resource Center for Health and Safety resource serving as the first national occupant protection curriculum for childcare providers and administrators. www.healthychildcare.org

National Child Care Information Center www.nccic.org

NICHD Study http://www.nichd.nih.gov/od/secc/pubs.htm

88

Cultural Competence

Lee M. Pachter

I. **Description of the issue.** A cultural group is a **collective of individuals who share common beliefs, values, attitudes, and behaviors**. Individuals may consider themselves members of many different cultures based on ethnic heritage, occupation, lifestyle, or any other grouping to which the individual feels connected—and has a shared identity. With this perspective every clinical interaction may be considered "cross-cultural"—between the culture of "medicine" and the culture of "patients." We, as healthcare providers, enter into the doctor–patient relationship with our own set of values, beliefs, and assumptions. As the cultural distance between individuals increases—as when traditional beliefs and practices of a family may be discordant with the mainstream biomedical view—it becomes crucial to find ways to bridge the gap between the two belief systems.

Ethnocultural beliefs and practices regarding childrearing and child behavior and development are based on a group's adaptation to specific environmental, economic, social, and family contexts. These beliefs and practices have formed over many years and many generations and although they change over time, they do so at varying rates and degrees. They are often reinforced by older family members, as well as recollections of parents when they were growing up.

A. **Culture versus class and minority status.** In many industrialized countries, individuals from minority cultural groups are often over-represented in low socioeconomic categories. The effects of (1) **traditional cultural beliefs**, (2) **poverty and access to material goods**, and (3) **being a minority** are distinct but often interlinked. The clinician needs to be aware of these distinctions and try to tease out whether any clinical issues that come up may be in part related to any or all of these three separate but interrelated issues.

B. **Intracultural variability.** *There is as much variability in beliefs and practices within cultural groups as between cultural groups.* Any one individual's approach to parenting and child development is an amalgamation of personal beliefs, past experiences, media and expert influence, *and* traditional cultural beliefs (as well as other factors). Nonetheless, it is important to have a general understanding of traditional beliefs and practices as a background and a starting point for discussion and communication.

C. **Cultural change.** One source of intracultural variability is the effect of **acculturation,** or the changes that take place over time in individuals and groups due to continuous contact with other cultures and living environments. Modern theories of acculturation stress that it is not a unidirectional process; individuals do not acculturate "from" a traditional culture "to" the host culture. Instead, the process is one better described at becoming "bicultural" or "multicultural." Individuals retain certain aspects of their traditional cultural views while at the same time incorporating beliefs and values of other groups, as well as the general majority culture and environment. Cultural change occurs in areas such as traditional practices, ethnic pride, self-identity, and language use. Not all of these dimensions change at the same pace or with the same influence.

II. **Ways that culture affects child behavior and development.**

A. **Parenting practices and beliefs about childrearing.** For example, norms regarding sleeping arrangements (e.g., co-sleeping), discipline practices, infant and child feeding practices, parental interactions with teachers and the role of the parent in a child's education, specific parenting roles of the father and mother, and discussions about topics such as sexuality all may be influenced by traditional beliefs and practices.

B. **Family composition/structure.** In some cultural traditions different structures may be the norm, such as the extended family or fictive kin (e.g., godparents or nonrelated cousins).

C. **Culturally normative values.** A major aspect of child development includes the learning of acceptable and "normal" behaviors, values, and ideals. This includes the foundations of beliefs which may not be specific to parenting or child development, but nonetheless create the milieu in which children live, grow, and learn. They comprise the "models" of behavior to which children are taught to conform. Styles of communication and interaction among individuals, for example, are in part culturally constructed. Some cultures put high value on an interactive style that is warm and personal, while others prefer styles that are more reserved during communication and interaction. Sometimes the style of interaction is based on the relative social position of the individuals involved, and different cultures have different "rules" to do this.

The value system that underlies proper personal behavior is in part culturally mediated as well. For example, some cultures put a high value on individualism (e.g., independence, self-confidence), whereas other cultures put a higher value on the attainment of social competencies based on collectivism (e.g., interdependence, respectfulness). Acceptable physical distance between individuals in different social settings, physical touch, and eye contact are other examples of belief systems which are in part culturally mediated.

- **D. Perceptions about normal child behavior.** The Victorian concept of "children should be seen but not heard" is an example of one such culturally derived model of child behavior. A physically active child may be seen as "a problem" in one system and "naturally inquisitive" in another. A quiet child may be seen as "slow, dull, or unmotivated" in one context, but "quiet and respectful" in another. These different expectations about child behavior may become an issue as the growing child begins spending time in multiple settings (such as at home, at school, and in the community) where the cultural beliefs may clash.

- **E. Perception about normal child development.** Studies have shown differences in both perceptions and expectations. The Digo people in Kenya believe that infants are ready to learn developmental tasks such as toilet training at a very early age. They begin training in the first month, and have some degree of bowel and bladder control by 4–6 months of age. This is accomplished by maternal sensitivity to the infant's cues, positioning the infant to facilitate elimination, and behavior modification.

  In a more recent study from the United States, parents from four different ethnocultural groups (African American, West Indian/Caribbean, Puerto Rican, and European American) were asked about their beliefs regarding the ages at which infants and children were able to attain specific developmental milestones. While most of the responses from all the groups were within what would be considered appropriate range of developmental expectations, there were group differences, even after controlling for other variables such as socioeconomic status, education, and maternal age. The greatest differences were found in the person and social domains of development. Specific differences (for example, in tasks such as sleeping throughout the night, or age at which an infant could be fed from a spoon) could be explained by either difference in core cultural values, childrearing practices, or the physical environment of family life.

  In all of the above examples, culture is but one of many factors which moderate child development and behavior. It is important to remember that other variables such as the physical environment, socioeconomic conditions, and intergroup relationships have important effects. It is also necessary to recognize that cultural beliefs and practices are not static but are constantly changing as a result of interaction with other groups and differing living contexts.

III. Clinical approaches.

- **A. Screening/testing.** *Most questionnaires and instruments used to assess behavior and development were created and tested on white, middleclass children.* Although they may have "face validity" for use in minority children, be aware that differences in cultural beliefs and practices, perceptions of normal and abnormal behavior, and even scoring style differences need to be taken into account when evaluating responses. Translations of questionnaires are helpful for limited English proficient families, but **mere translation does not guarantee crosscultural conceptual or measurement equivalency.** Clinicians who use screening and diagnostic surveys often in their practice should try to choose instruments that have some data on validity and reliability for diverse populations.

- **B. Health beliefs history.** A health beliefs history is a way of getting the perspective of the patient or family regarding the clinical issue at hand. By inquiring into the parent's "ethnotheories" about children, one may be able to ascertain whether the specific clinical issue is being viewed by the parent as problematic or not. What might be considered "a problem" from the clinical standpoint may not be a problem from the perspective of the parent.

- **C. Key clinical questions.** Examples of questions eliciting the patient's or family's perspective
  - *"Do you think that this behavior is a problem? Why (or why not)?"*

- *"What is most concerning to you about this?"* (Sometimes the issues that's most important for the family is not the same as the issue that's most important from the clinical standpoint.)
- *"Why does he or she have this problem?"* (You may get to some beliefs about causation that need to be addressed before intervention)
- *"How should a __-year-old act?"* (This may also uncover attitudes and knowledge about child behavior and development that will need follow-up education.)
- *"What problems does it create for your child?"*
- *"Are there other people who you've spoken with, and have they given you opinions and ideas about it?"* (Other family members may have strong opinions and influences.)
- *"Sometimes there are ways of treating problems that doctors don't know about. They might be effective. Have you tried anything yet to help solve this?"* (Approach alternative treatments and practices in a nonjudgmental fashion.)
- *"What do you expect from the treatment?"*

D. **Clinical communication.** The goal of a culturally informed approach to clinical pediatrics is to try to **gain an understanding of the patient or families understanding of a clinical issue.** Often, children present either because the parents are concerned about a problem with the child's development or behavior, or because another agent (usually the school or childcare) has identified a potential issue. Be aware that families from different cultural backgrounds may interpret child behavior and development with different underlying frameworks.

1. The **Awareness-Assessment-Negotiation** approach may help work through cultural and individual differences in the clinical setting. This approach recommends:
   - The clinician become *aware* of any general beliefs and practices concerning parenting and child behavior/development in the groups commonly seen in a particular practice. This information only provides a general orientation that should not be used in clinical practice until validated by the direct discussion with particular families.
   - In the *assessment* phase, assess the likelihood that a particular family subscribes to the beliefs and practices, keeping in mind the importance of intracultural diversity.
   - If there are discrepancies between parent-held beliefs and practices and biomedical/clinical point of view, attempt to *negotiate* between models. Negotiation allows a common ground to be created which acknowledges and respects the family's views and beliefs and builds upon them whenever possible. Incorporate family-held beliefs into patient education, and culturally acceptable treatments into the care plan whenever possible. It may be helpful to include other individuals such as grandparents, godparents, or other identified family support in the plan. When modifications to the family's beliefs or practices are necessary, do it in an open way that allows for discussion and feedback. Recognize that behavioral change usually does not occur in a brief 15–30 minute visit, but laying the groundwork for an ongoing relationship which includes bidirectional and respectful communication may result in such a change over time.

BIBLIOGRAPHY

For Parents

Beal AC, Villarosa L, Abner A. *The Black Parenting Book.* New York: Broadway, 1999.
Comer JP, Poussaint AF. *Raising Black Children.* New York: Plume. 1992.
Rodriguez G. *Raising Nuestros Ninos: Bring Up Latino Children in a Bicultural World.* New York: Fireside, 1999.

For Professionals

Garcia Coll C, Lamberty G, Jenkins R, et al. An integrative model for the study of developmental competencies in minority children. *Child Development* 67(5):1891–1914, 1996.
Pachter LM, Harwood R. Culture and child behavior and psychosocial development. *J Dev Behav Pediatr* 17:191–198, 1996.
Pachter LM, Dworkin PH. Maternal expectations about normal child development in 4 cultural groups. *Arch Pediatr Adolesc Med* 151:1144–1150, 1997.
National Center for Cultural Competence http://gucchd.georgetown.edu//nccc/

Divorce

Margot Kaplan-Sanoff

I. **Description of the problem.** Divorce is not a single event. Rather **divorce is a process** that begins in an unhappy marriage, extends through the separation, and continues into the new life. Long before a marriage ends, children have begun the process of coping with the parental coldness and hostility that leads to or is the consequence of an unraveling relationship between their parents. It has been said that "it is not divorce per se that makes kids crazy but the craziness of divorcing parents that disrupts the orderly process of their children" (Hetherington, 1989).

A. **Incidence.**
- Approximately 50% of all marriages end in divorce, usually within the first 7 years of marriage.
- 85% of parents who divorce remarry, and 40% of these new marriages also end in divorce.

B. **Stages of divorce for the parents.** In many divorcing families, each parent is in a different stage of the process. Often one parent is ready to let go of the relationship while another is still holding on. For parents, the timeline for moving through the stages is thought to be 1 year for every 5 years of marriage.

1. **Holding on.** In this first stage, one or both parents are in denial, looking backwards to determine what went wrong. Even 12–18 months after filing for divorce, parents feel angry, guilty, humiliated that the marriage didn't last, depressed, anxious, and afraid to move forward, often with little energy to attend to their children.
2. **Letting go.** This stage brings an acceptance of the loss of the relationship, with parents feeling relief, exhilaration and grief at the ending of the marriage, often without much emotional availability for their children.
3. **Starting over.** Parents in this stage are ready to take risks and find a new identity as a single person. They tend to be future oriented and quite enthusiastic as they try out new lifestyles and begin dating.
4. **Building a new life.** This final stage represents stabilization for families as they begin to feel "back-to-normal".

C. **Emotional tasks for children during the divorce.** The basic task for children is to integrate, without psychic damage, the loss of the parenting relationship and the change in their social status. Children need to perceive events as being under their control, even though the divorce was not their decision. They need to avoid constructing a view of divorce and its consequences as random and one in which they view themselves as the hapless targets of external forces.

Thus, the tasks for the children are to:

1. **Understand the divorce.** Children must understand the immediate changes that the divorce brings and sort out their fantasies and fears from the reality of the divorce. They may respond with blaming, sadness, anger, guilt, and/or anxiety to the separation and decision to divorce. How children are told about the divorce and the way the family separates in part determines the nature of the postdivorce year. Children may blame themselves for the divorce and try to be the "perfect child" in hopes of reuniting the family.
2. **Strategically withdrawal.** Children need to get on with their own lives and to have permission to remain children by continuing to join extracurricular activities, such as sports or art programs. Very young children are unable to avoid the anger and hostility of the divorce, whereas older school age children and adolescents often simply escape from the house.
3. **Cope with loss.** In a divorce children often lose daily contact with one of their parents and they lose the family into which they were born. Other loses and changes for many children include a decrease in financial resources, a move to a new neighborhood, school, and peer group.

   4. Deal with anger. Although divorce is a voluntary action for at least one of the adults in the marriage, it is an event completely out of the control of the children who feel cheated out of family experiences and exposed in front of peers.

II. Factors which affect children's adjustment to divorce.

   A. Temperament. Children with difficult temperaments may receive more negative attention and become the object that distracts the family from the real issue of conflict—the divorce.

   B. Developmental level. As Table 89-1 shows, the age and developmental level of the child at the time of the divorce greatly affects their response to the event.

   C. Predivorce developmental achievements. Although we cannot predict what developmental progress children *might* have made had their parents stayed together, their achievements prior to the divorce continue to impact their abilities postdivorce.

   D. History of previous loss. For children who may have experienced earlier losses such as the death of a grandparent or pet or the loss of a beloved childcare provider prior to the divorce, the new loss experienced as a result of the divorce will trigger memories of old losses.

   E. Gender. Consistently, **boys have been found to be more disrupted by divorce.** Boys often receive less positive support and nurturance, and are viewed more negatively,

Table 89-1 Responses of child to parent's divorce within the first year

Developmental status	Child's response	Primary care clinician's role
Preschool	Regressive behavior	Encourage stable, predictable meal and bedtime routines
	Sleep disturbance	Develop consistent patterns of joining and separating from child
	Tantrums	Continue contact with noncustodial parent
	Aggressive behavior	Provide reassurance
	Bowel and bladder difficulties	
	Clinging	
	Fears of abandonment	
Younger school age	Sadness	Empathize with child's feelings
	Fearfulness	Provide regular opportunities for child to talk
	Loyalty conflicts	Support child's continuing relationship with both parents
	Attempts to determine responsibility for divorce	Offer reassurance
	Hopes for family reconciliation	
	Declining school performance	
Older school age/ prepubertal	Grief, intense anger	Express interest in and availability to the child
	Declining school performance	Support child's school and peer involvement
	Disrupted peer relationships	Provide clear acknowledgment and support for child's working through feelings on the divorce
	Attempts to clarify responsibility for the divorce	
	Caretaking of a parent	
Adolescence	Depression	Provide opportunities for discussion
	Anger	
	Premature emancipation	
	Increase in adolescent acting out	
	Sleeper effects, particularly in females	

Adapted from Wallerstein JS. Separation, divorce, and remarriage. In: Levine MD, Carey WB, Crocker AC (eds), *Developmental-Behavioral Pediatrics* (2nd ed). Philadelphia: Saunders, 1992.

particularly by their mothers, which then exacerbates their acting out, dependency and immature behaviors. Girls, on the other hand, tend to be more compliant immediately following the divorce, but experience "sleeper effects" 5–10 years later as they begin to confront the commitment, intimacy, and loyalty demands of young adulthood.

F. **Extent of parental hostilities before and after the divorce.** The prime determinant of adverse outcomes for children, regardless of age or gender, is ongoing parental hostility. Parents involved in a conflictual relationship are less emotionally available and less effective disciplinarians to their children.

G. **Level of economic stress.** For many women, divorce brings a dramatic change in their financial security. They may have to return to school or work, work longer hours, and/or move to a less expensive home and neighborhood, necessitating more changes in the children's lives.

H. **Emotional stability of the custodial parent.** Although both parents may experience emotional lability, depression, emotional dependence or disengagement with their children, overindulgence, the excitement of a new active social life or the risk for alcohol or substance abuse, it is the custodial parent upon whom the child relies to create a stable, familiar environment.

I. **Stability of visitation.** Seeing where the noncustodial parent lives can help a child create a new image of family, whereas inconsistent visitation offers children no such relief from their anxiety and fear of abandonment.

J. **Support systems.** Children who can access social supports outside the home, especially a consistent, empathic relationship with another family member, supportive adult, friend or sibling are better able to manage their anxieties and anger about the divorce. Many schools offer support groups for divorcing children within the structure of the school day.

III. **Management.**

L. **Help families develop a plan.** Helping parents develop a plan for how to tell the children is invaluable. Children who experienced the most precipitous regressions were those children who had been given no explanation for the separation or for their father's departure. Children need to be reassured clearly and repeatedly that "*divorce is a grown-up problem*" and that they were not responsible for the breakup of the marriage. They need to be reassured about what will stay the same for them and what will change. Help parents to determine whatever was steady in their child's life and problem solve with them about how to try to keep that aspect intact. Use trigger questions to ask each parent about discipline problems and changes in the child's sleep patterns to generate information about each one's style of parenting and their level of concern about the child's behavior.

B. **Advise parents to inform their child's clinicians and teachers about the divorce.** Both parents should sign a "consent to treat" form so that medical decisions can be made quickly if necessary. Ask parents if they each want to receive copies of medical reports. Suggest that they each request in writing to receive school reports and notices so they can be equally informed about their children's progress.

C. **Maintain structure and organization.** All children have difficulty exerting self-control and organizing their lives when their family arrangement is changing; they need more external control and structure during the stress of a divorce. Regardless of the custodial parent's feelings about the other parent, continuity of the child's relationships with both parents should be promoted.

D. **Answer children's concerns.** Parents should be informed that when children ask questions about the divorce, they should try to give truthful answers, even if they need to omit certain information. One technique to help parents is to have them acknowledge the child's wish for reconciliation while making it clear that the request will not happen—-"You really wish that Daddy and Mommy would live together again in this house. That won't happen, but you will see Daddy in his new house every weekend". Reassure parents that it is expected that children will feel sad and that they should give their children permission to grieve and to cry, regardless of their age and gender.

E. **Avoid conflictual interactions around the children.** Watching parents argue without a positive resolution is particularly difficult for children. They bear the guilt of thinking they are the reason for the conflict. Encourage parents to seek mediation and/or therapy to help them resolve their conflicts without the children needing to witness their anger.

F. **Should we stay together for the sake of the children?** Although there is never a good time for a family to divorce, growing up in a family in which there is an "emotional divorce" characterized by high levels of tension and low levels of warmth between parents, parents who discredit each other, where one parent aligns with the children to form a coalition against the other parent, or where the child manipulates the parents, is also not in the best interests of the child. Staying together for the children places an enormous burden on the children to fill the emotional void between the parents.

BIBLIOGRAPHY

For Children

Blackstone-Ford J. *My Parents Are Divorced Too: A Book for Kids by Kids.* New York: Magination, 1998. (Ages 9–12)

Brown KB, Brown M. *Dinosaurs Divorce: A Guide for Changing Families.* Boston: Little, Brown, 1986. (Ages 3–7)

Rogers F. *Let's Talk About Divorce.* New York: Putnam, 1996. (Ages 3–7)

Swan-Jackson A. *When Your Parents Split Up ⋯ How to Keep Yourself Together.* New York: Price Stern Sloan, 1998. (Ages 9–13)

Thomas P. *My Family's Changing.* Happauge, NY: Barron's Education Series, 1999. (Ages 3–8)

For Parents

Books

Gardner RA. *The Parents Book about Divorce (rev. ed).* New York: Bantam, 1991.

Lewis J, Sammons W. *Don't Divorce Your Children: Parents and Children Talk about Divorce.* Chicago: Contemporary Books, 1999.

Teyber E. *Helping Children Cope with Divorce.* New York: Lexington Books, 1992.

Websites

Divorce and Children www.divorceandchildren.com

DivorceInfo http://www.divorceinfo.com/children.htm

Divorce Magazine http://www.divorcemag.com/cgi-bin/redirNoYesState.cgi?/cgi-bin/show.cgi?template = choosestate&article = children;/cgi-bin/show.cgi?template = children

For Professionals

Publications

Hetherington EM. Marital transitions: A child's perspective. Special issue: Children and their development: Knowledge base, research agenda, and social policy application. *Amer Psychol* 44(2): 303– 312, 1989.

Lewis J, Sammons W. *Don't Divorce Your Children: Parents and Children Talk about Divorce.* Chicago: Contemporary Books, 1999.

Wallerstein JS, Blakeslee S. *Second Chances: Men, Women, and Children: A Decade after Divorce.* New York: Ticknor & Fields, 1989.

Websites

American Academy of Child and Adolescent Psychiatry http://www.aacap.org/publications/factsfam/divorce.htm

Divorce Source http://www.divorcesource.com/info/children/children.shtml

Dying Children

David J. Schonfeld
Melvin Lewis

I. **Description of the problem.** When a child is dying, the child and the family need reassurance, support, and guidance. The primary care provider who has a supportive and ongoing relationship with the child and the family is in a unique position to provide them with that support throughout this difficult period. Some general principles to consider in providing care to dying children and their families are presented in Table 90-1.

II. **Issues in helping the dying child.**

A. **Healthcare providers must attend to the immediate physical needs of these children.** It is crucial to relieve pain and suffering and to assure the children that adults are always available. Children should be told by both the parents and the healthcare providers, "We want you to tell us whenever anything is bothering you. I will always be here (or be able to be reached) anytime you want me. We will all do our best to make sure that you feel as comfortable as possible."

B. **Children at different developmental stages have different conceptual understandings of the meaning of death,** which will affect their ability to understand and adjust to their impending death(see Chapter 86). Children with a terminal illness usually do appreciate the seriousness of their illness and may develop a precocious understanding of death and their personal mortality.

C. **Many parents and clinicians are uncomfortable when children openly acknowledge an awareness of their impending death.** Children often feel that it is their task to provide emotional support to their parents and to carry on the mutual pretense that they are unaware of their health status. This conspiracy of silence isolates the child from available supports. Most children, in fact, fear the *process* of dying more than death itself.

D. **To the extent possible, children should be informed about their health status.** Children often turn to members of the healthcare team to ask questions, directly or indirectly, about their illness and impending death. Children who are dying may also directly ask family members and staff, "Am I going to die?" Adults should initially clarify the motivation for such questions: Is the child seeking reassurance that all efforts will be made to minimize pain, that parents and family members will remain available, or that every reasonable effort will be made to treat the underlying illness? Is the child merely attempting to determine the seriousness of his illness? Once the motivation for the question is identified, the adult family member or healthcare provider can provide the necessary reassurances or information. Prohibitions on informing children about their condition force parents and professionals to lie, thereby jeopardizing a caregiving relationship built on mutual trust and respect. The principles to consider in informing children about a terminal illness or impending death are summarized in Table 90-2.

E. **Facilitating discussion about children's concerns often involves projective techniques,** such as play or picture drawing. Many children choose not to discuss their impending death directly. It is rarely necessary (or appropriate) to confront children with the reality that they are dying after they have been appropriately informed. Instead, clinicians should remain available and offer indirect outlets for addressing the child's concerns. Children will avail themselves of these opportunities when, and if, they are ready.

F. **Clinicians are often anxious that they will not know what to say to a child who is dying.** The goal of counseling children who are dying is not to take away their sadness or to find the "right" answers to all their questions. Rather, it is to listen to their concerns, to accept and empathize with their strong emotions, to offer support, and to assist them in finding their own coping techniques (e.g., "Some children find it helpful to talk to others about what is worrying them; other children prefer to draw pictures or keep a diary. Whatever you decide to do is fine. I'm always available to talk with you about your feelings, or just to sit and talk about something else."). In many cases,

Table 90-1 General principles for practitioners in the care of dying children and their families

Physical context
Minimize physical discomfort and symptoms.
Optimize pain management.
Emotional context
Provide an opportunity for the expression and sharing of personal feelings and concerns for both the children and their families in an accepting atmosphere.
Tolerate unpleasant affect (e.g., sadness, anger, despair).
Social context
Facilitate communication among members of the healthcare team and the children and their families.
Encourage active participation of the children and their families in the treatment decisions and the management of the illness.
Personal context
Treat each child and family member as a unique individual.
Attempt to form a personal relationship with the child and the family.
Acknowledge your own feelings as a healthcare provider and establish a mechanism(s) to meet your personal needs.

the best approach is to talk about a topic of interest to the child or merely to sit quietly and hold the child's hand.

G. **Children must be allowed, even encouraged, to continue to have hope and to go on with their lives.** These children should be regarded less as children who are dying and more as individuals living with a serious and/or life-threatening condition. The goal must be to optimize the quality of their remaining life, not merely to prolong its duration. Important routines should be continued with as little disruption as possible, such as allowing them to attend school or to do schoolwork in the hospital. Although regressive behavior may be normative and appropriate at times of stress, excessively regressive behavior (e.g., a 6-year-old who begins biting staff) should be addressed supportively but firmly, often employing a behavioral management approach developed by the treatment team and family.

H. **Many children and adolescents feel guilty and ashamed about their illness.** Children who rely on magical thinking and egocentrism to explain the cause of illness may assume that terminal illness and death are the result of some perceived wrongdoing ("immanent justice"). Children need to be reassured frequently that they are not responsible for their illness.

I. **To the extent possible, children should be informed about and participate in the decisions regarding their health care.** Older children and adolescents may possess the intellectual and emotional maturity to allow them to play a significant role regarding critical and difficult decisions (e.g., whether to discontinue aggressive treatment). All

Table 90-2 Principles involved in informing children about a terminal illness or impending death

Inform the child over time, in a series of conversations. During the initial conversation, it is important to convey that the child has a serious illness.
If the child asks directly if he or she is going to die, initially explore the reason for the question and the child's concerns (e.g., "Are you afraid that you might die?" "What are you worried about?"). Do not provide false reassurances ("No, don't worry, you're going to be okay."), but always try to maintain hope ("Some children with your sickness have died, but we're going to do everything we can to try and help you get better").
Focus initial discussions on the immediate and near future. Young children have a limited future perspective. Dying "soon" to them may mean minutes, hours, or days, not months or years.
Answer questions directly, but do not overwhelm the child with unnecessary details.
Assess the child's understanding by asking him or her to explain back to you what you have discussed.
Reassure the child of the lack of personal responsibility or guilt. For this reason, avoid the use of the term *bad* in the description of the illness (e.g., "You have a bad sickness").

children need to be aware of the nature and rationale of planned treatments and should be active participants in the treatment process, even if they are able to make only seemingly minor decisions (e.g., whether they should take the pill with juice or with soda).

III. **Issues in helping the parents.**

A. **Parents faced with the impending death of their child may demonstrate shock, denial, anxiety, depression, or anger.** Almost any reaction can be seen; there is no "correct" way to deal with the death of a child. Additionally, parents may alternate among these emotional states without demonstrating any clear pattern of progression.

B. **The response of family members to the death may be affected by the duration of the illness.** Anticipatory grieving allows family members to experience graduated feelings of loss while the child is still alive. In the setting of open communication, many families will take advantage of this time to resolve conflicts with the dying child and to express love. Clinicians should appreciate that other families may approach this impending loss with a different coping style and may not choose to engage in this form of leave-taking behavior.

C. **Members of the family may proceed with anticipatory grieving at different rates.** Conflicts may result when one family member's course of grieving is not synchronous with that of another member of the family. Primary care clinicians can help families to identify when someone (either a member of the family or healthcare team) has abandoned the child after having prematurely reached resignation and acceptance of the child's death.

D. **As part of anticipatory grieving, family members and healthcare professionals may wish for the death of a seriously ill child.** This wish may result in excessive guilt and cause the individual to compensate by becoming overly protective or indulgent with the dying child. The healthcare provider can assist parents with such comments as: *"Many parents of children who have been critically ill for a prolonged period sometimes find themselves wishing their child would just die quickly. This is a common and normal feeling, even for parents who love their children dearly".*

E. **Family members should be allowed, even encouraged, to continue to have hope and to go on with their lives.** While the desire for second opinions should be honored, excessive searches for cures that compromise the health of the child or the financial well-being of the family should be discouraged. Parents must be actively assured that they have done everything reasonable to ensure the highest quality of care for their child and that they have no reason to feel guilty.

F. **To the extent possible, parents should be informed about and participate actively in decisions regarding their child's care. The healthcare providers must provide families with clear professional recommendations and be willing to discuss alternate options, when appropriate options exist.** When families are faced, for example, with the difficult decision of whether to continue aggressive therapy when little hope of cure remains, the clinician must provide information on the likelihood of success and the anticipated morbidity associated with the treatment process. Palliative and supportive care should always remain available, even if children and their families choose a management plan that is not the preferred option of the provider. For terminal children maintained on life support at the time of death, the clinician should elicit and honor the parents' wishes about the timing of termination of life support. Care should be taken so that parents do not infer that they are being asked about whether to allow their child to die.

G. **Sudden or unexpected death requires an immediate recognition of the loss.** In this setting, families often initially use denial to cope. Family members should be allowed additional time to hold or be with the child's body in a quiet and private area of the hospital and should be given an opportunity to express their shock, disbelief, and anger before further and more detailed explanations of the cause of death are provided.

H. **Support systems for families of dying children are often hospital based and frequently withdrawn at the time of the child's death.** Providers should remain available to families after the death has occurred and should help the family establish ties, prior to the death, with community-based support systems, such as parent groups, clergy, and counseling services. Hospital support networks should not become an additional loss coincident with the death of the child.

I. **At the time of the child's death, parents and other family members should be offered assistance with immediate and pragmatic needs.** Such diverse needs include ensuring safe transportation home for grieving family members at the time of the death, making funeral and burial arrangements, and deciding how to notify family members and friends. Families should be given an appointment for a follow-up meeting (often 2–6 weeks after the death; earlier if necessary) to answer remaining questions about the illness and death (e.g., to review the autopsy report) and to inquire about adjustment of family members. Time can also be arranged to meet later with the siblings either individually or with their parents.

  J. Families in grief may feel immobilized and incapable of making even simple decisions. Complex and emotionally laden decisions such as those regarding autopsy or organ donation may seem especially overwhelming at this time. When death is anticipated, the primary care provider may suggest that family members consider their personal feelings about such decisions before the fact. In sudden and unanticipated deaths, families may need a period of time (1–2 hours) to adjust to the reality of the loss before such questions are asked.

IV. Issues in helping the siblings.

  A. The needs of the siblings are often neglected when a child in the family is dying. Parents have limited reserves of energy, time, and money and strained emotional and psychological resources. Providers must ensure that outreach is provided to siblings to meet their needs.

  B. The siblings should be included in receiving information about the child's health status and treatment plan and should participate to some extent in the provision of care for the ill child. Young children may be given simple tasks such as bringing and opening mail, watering plants in the room, or bringing toys to a child in bed. Parents must be careful not to overburden the siblings, especially the older children and adolescents, with unreasonable chores or responsibilities. Siblings should be encouraged to maintain their peer groups and continue involvement in activities outside the family.

  C. Siblings respond to the death with the same diversity of emotional responses seen in adults. They may be angry at the child who has died or experience guilt over having survived. Primary care clinicians need to monitor how families reorganize after the death of a child, so that siblings are not scapegoated or the focus of projected defenses. For example, parents who continue to feel guilty about their child's death may overprotect the surviving siblings and interfere with normative attempts to achieve independence.

V. Helping the healthcare providers.

  A. Healthcare providers must understand their personal feelings about death in order to be effective in providing support to others. Often this will involve some introspection about one's own losses and an awareness of the impact of the deaths of their patients on their professional and personal lives.

  B. Providers must extend the same quality of care to themselves as they would offer to patients. The death of a patient is one of the most stressful personal and professional experiences faced by healthcare providers. It triggers a similar, albeit less intense, grief response as would a personal loss. Permission and tolerance for professionals to discuss and have their personal needs met regarding bereavement (e.g., for support or reassurance of lack of personal responsibility for a patient death) is necessary. Psychosocial rounds (especially in intensive care settings), retreats, and other support services dealing directly with providers' responses to patient death are important aspects of professional development.

  C. All members of the healthcare team should be involved in important decisions regarding the care provided to a dying child. Conflicts that arise when one or more members of the team disagree on the appropriateness of care being provided can seriously undermine clinical care. For example, physicians who avoid clarifying do-not-resuscitate orders with the family of a dying child may place the nursing staff in the uncomfortable position of having to initiate resuscitation efforts when the death occurs. House staff forced to continue treatment that they feel is not in the best interest of the child or family may be angry if they were not involved in the decision. Often staff differences are best resolved through team meetings.

  D. Primary care providers should avail themselves of the expertise and skills of members of related disciplines, such as the clergy, child life, nursing, psychiatry, psychology, and social work when responding to the needs of the child and family members, as well as their own personal needs.

BIBLIOGRAPHY

For Parents

Organizations

Candlelighters Childhood Cancer Foundation. For information and referral for parents, families, and professionals working with children with cancer.
P.O. Box 498

Kensington, MD 20895-0498
1-800-366-2223
www.candlelighters.org
Children's Hospice International. For information and referral regarding local hospice care and
bereavement counseling services.
901 North Pitt St., Suite 230
Alexandria VA 22314
1-800-24-CHILD
www.chionline.org
Compassionate Friends. For referral to a self-help group for families who have experienced the
death of a child.
P.O. Box 3696
Oak Brook IL 60522-3696
1-877-969-0010
www.compassionatefriends.org
National SIDS/Infant Death Resource Center. For information and referral for parents who have
lost an infant to sudden infant death syndrome.
2070 Chain Bridge Road, Suite 450
Vienna, VA 22182
1-866-866-7437
www.sidscenter.org

For Professionals

Publications

Adams D, Deveau E. When a brother or sister is dying of cancer: The vulnerability of the adolescent
sibling. *Death Stud* 11:279–295, 1987
Greenham D, Lohmann R. Children facing death: Recurring patterns of adaptation. *Health Social
Work* 7(2):89–94, 1982.
Lewis M, Lewis D, Schonfeld D. Dying and death in childhood and adolescence. In Lewis M (ed),
Child and Adolescent Psychiatry: A Comprehensive Textbook (2nd ed). Baltimore: Williams &
Wilkins, 1996, pp. 1066–1073.
Schonfeld D. Talking with children about death. *J Pediatr Health Care* 7:269–274, 1993.

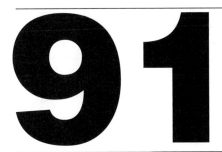

Foster Care

Moira Szilagyi

I. **Description of the problem.** Foster care **is government subsidized and regulated temporary care for children who have been removed from their families for reasons of abuse and neglect**. The goals of foster care are the health, safety and permanent caretaking for children. The main types of care are family foster care, placement with relatives (kinship care) and residential group care. For brevity, the term *foster care* will be used for all three.

   A. **Epidemiology. (See Table 91-1.)**

   B. **Contributory factors.** Children entering foster care have typically endured multiple and chronic adverse life experiences, including abuse and neglect, inconsistent and chaotic parenting from multiple caregivers, severe emotional and financial deprivation, and limited access to appropriate services. Removal from their families and all that is familiar is often a traumatizing event and the uncertainty inherent in the foster care system may further erode a child's sense of well being. The impact of foster care on individual children depends on their personal strengths and coping skills, prior life experiences, developmental abilities and the availability of protective environmental factors.

II. **Identifying problems.**

   A. **General issues.**

      1. The periodicity schedule of the American Academy of Pediatrics for child health supervision may need to be adjusted to reflect the more intensive support and monitoring necessary because of the many junctures in foster care that may adversely affect a child's health and well being.

      2. Intensive healthcare management to guarantee access to an appropriate array of developmental, mental health, medical and dental services is essential to good health outcomes for children in foster care.

      3. The single greatest health need of children in foster care is for mental health services and support.

   B. **Specific issues.** Health practitioners should consider children in foster care as a population with special health care needs.

      1. **Primary pediatric care.** Children in foster care should have a "medical home". Primary care practitioners should address the adjustment of the child to the foster care placement, emotional and behavioral issues, school functioning, and the capacities of all the child's families to meet the child's needs. Clear communication and collaboration with the other professionals involved in the child's care is essential. Frequent follow-up visits and a high index of suspicion for emotional and psychological problems are fundamental to providing appropriate health care for this population.

         Children in foster care may have to deal with issues of separation and loss, and may feel unloved or abandoned by their parents or experience anger, anxiety and depression. It may help children to describe their parents as *unable,* rather than *unwilling,* to care for them. Children with a history of maltreatment may have extreme behaviors and difficulty trusting others. Clinicians can play a valuable role by supporting and educating foster parents and engaging the child in a consistent and caring manner during more frequent office visits.

      2. **Transitions in foster care.** Placement changes, sibling separation or reunion, changes in visitation patterns, the termination of parental rights are but a few of the instances during which children in foster care need special support. The primary care practitioner can advocate for appropriate preparation for the child to facilitate these transitions and provide anticipatory guidance to the foster parent about ways to support the child. The clinician should emphasize the need for abundant patience, affection, consistency and nurturance during these difficult junctures.

      3. **Screening questions for foster parents to assess how the transition is progressing include:**

        • *"How do you think your child is doing? How does this child fit in with your family?"*

Table 91-1 Dimensions of foster care

Relevance
542,000 children are in foster care (an increase of 90% since 1982); 130,000 freed for adoption,
about half of whom are in pre-adoptive placement
Types of care
72% in regular (including kinship) care
18% in group or residential care
8% in other arrangements
Age of foster children
4% infants
24% ages 1–5 years
24% ages 6–10 years
41% teenagers
Race; ethnicity of foster children
37% white, non-Hispanic
38% African American, non-Hispanic
17% Latino
6% Other

- *"Are there some behaviors you're worried about?"*
- *"What has it been like for others in your home since your foster child moved in?"*
- *"How are you coping?"*
- *"Have there been any other significant changes in your family?"*

4. **The child's view of being in care.** Depending on a child's maturity and expressive abilities, it may be possible to ascertain directly how he or she perceives foster care. Useful questions, without the caregiver present, include
   - *"What is it like for you living in this home?"*
   - *"What do you like best? Least?"*
   - *"How do you get along with the people in your new home?"*
   - *"What would you like to change?"*
   - *"Do you feel loved and cared for where you are living?"*

5. **Visitation with parents.** Visits with birth parents can evoke strong, ambivalent emotions and difficult behaviors in children. Practitioners should encourage foster parents to maintain a positive view of the birth parents, at least, in front of the child. For example, foster families should help the child prepare for visits and rehearse their response to potentially difficult situations. Occasionally, the clinician may need to recommend a change in visitation that is clearly stressful to a child; for example, the clinician might recommend that the child only go for a visit if the parent calls ahead if there has been repeated failure by the parent to show up for visits. The practitioner has to be careful to avoid simplistic explanations for children's responses to visits (e.g., interpreting aggressive behavior after a visit as reflecting a child's negative feelings toward his or her parents when, it fact, it is due to the anxiety of separating from them).

6. **Discipline in substitute care.** Foster caregivers are not allowed to use corporal punishment for children placed in their care. Practitioners can explain a child's behavior and offer constructive disciplinary alternatives (e.g., time-outs, withholding privileges, point systems to earn privileges etc.). Understanding a foster caregiver's parenting skills and abilities is fundamental to offering them parenting advice (e.g., "How do you cope when your child is acting this way?")

7. **Abuse and neglect in substitute care.** Abuse and neglect occasionally occur in substitute care. Primary care clinicians need to remain alert to the physical and behavioral markers of maltreatment and assess whether these resulted from abuse or neglect prior to or during placement. Weight loss or poor weight gain in a young child is often the first sign of a neglectful foster care placement.

8. **Discontinuous health care.** Children in foster are have had frequent changes in health care providers or inadequate access to health care. Health information is often sparse or unavailable and the primary care clinician should be mindful of gathering and maintaining medical documentation that will be useful to future clinicians. Communication with child welfare professionals about health information is crucial to appropriate permanency planning for children in foster care.

9. **Support for substitute caregivers.** Many children in foster care have serious prob-

lems, especially emotional and behavioral, that their foster parents and caseworkers are not equipped to manage. Primary care clinicians can help through more frequent visits for education, emotional support, and counseling. Many foster parent groups have newsletters for which some practitioners write a column on health issues. Timely referral to appropriate mental health, developmental and home health services may stabilize a foster care placement for a child. The clinician can offer foster parents support and respect by expressing admiration for their parenting skills, and the stability and consistency they are providing children in their care.

10. **Involvement with birthparents.** Birth parents retain legal custody of their children unless they have been freed for adoption. Consent and confidentiality issues are complex in foster care and the clinician should clarify who has the capacity to consent for a given child with the foster care agency. Involvement of the birth parent in the health care of their child is encouraged when deemed appropriate by the agency.

11. **Support for caseworkers.** Casework staff are often overwhelmed, undertrained, and underpaid. As the case managers for children in foster care, caseworkers are mandated to work with the birth family toward reunification while ensuring the health, safety, and well being of children. Often, the latter involves the development of an alternative permanency plan. Clinicians can help casework staff by maintaining clear and open lines of communication, providing useful clinical information and acknowledging their efforts (e.g., "You're really making a big difference in his life by finding all the services he needs.")

12. **Children preparing for independence.** In almost every state, children in foster care are expected to assume increased responsibility for themselves as they reach age 18 years. Since very few have the experience to manage independently, this raises complex ethical and practical issues. The clinician can suggest measures to prepare the adolescent for independent living. (Materials to assist caregivers and youth in this task are available from the National Foster Care Resource Center.) Ideally, the pediatric clinician will continue caring for the young adult or make a referral to another healthcare provider.

BIBLIOGRAPHY

For Parents

Organizations

American Professional Society on the Abuse of Children www.apsac.org
Child Welfare League of America
440 First Street, NW,
Washington DC 20001-2085
202-638-2952
www.cwla.org
Committee on Early Childhood, Adoption, and Dependent Care, American Academy of Pediatrics
141 Northwest Point Boulevard
P.O. Box 927
Elk Grove Village, IL 60009-0927
1-800-433-9016.
www.aap.org
National Foster Parent Association
2606 Badger Lane
Madison WI 53713-2115
608-274-9111.
http://nfpainc.org

For Parents

Publications

American Academy of Pediatrics; Committee on Early Childhood, Adoption and Dependent Care. Developmental issues for young children in foster care. *Pediatrics* 106:1145–1150, 2000.
Task Force on Health Care for Children in Foster Care. *Fostering Health: Health Care for Children in Foster Care.* Lake Success, NY: American Academy of Pediatrics, District II, NYS, 2000.
Child Welfare League of America. *Standards for Health Care Services for Children in Out-of-Home Care.* Washington, DC: Child Welfare League of America, 1988.

Dubowitz H, et al. The physical health of children in kinship care. *Am J Dis Child* 146:603–610, 1992.

Simms M, Dubowitz H, Szilagyi M. Health care needs of children in the foster care system. *Pediatrics* 106:909–918, 2000.

Websites

The Future of Children http://www.futureofchildren.org/pubs-info2825/pubs-info.htm?doc_id = 209538

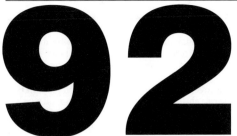

Gay and Lesbian Parents

Ellen C. Perrin

I. Description of the issue.

A. Epidemiology.

- Up to 9 million children in the United States under the age of 18 have one or both parent(s) who is/are lesbian or gay. Until recently most children with a lesbian and/or gay parent were conceived in the context of a heterosexual relationship. A parent (or both parents) of a heterosexual couple may recognize, acknowledge and/or disclose his/her homosexuality, after which some parents divorce and others continue to live as a couple. Increasing social acceptance of diversity in sexual orientation has allowed more gay men and lesbians to form committed intimate relationships and to become parents as a couple. Most of the same considerations that exist for heterosexual couples when they consider having children also face lesbians and gay men: concerns about time, finances, how children will affect their relationship, their own and their children's health, and their ability to manage their new parenting roles.

- Lesbians and gay men undertaking parenthood face additional challenges, including deciding whether to conceive or adopt a child, obtaining donor sperm or arranging for a surrogate mother (if conceiving), finding an accepting adoption agency (if adopting), making legally binding arrangements regarding future parental relationships, creating a substantive role for the nonbiologic or nonadoptive parent, and confronting emotional pain and restrictions imposed by heterosexism and discriminatory regulations.

- Most lesbians who conceive a child do so using alternative insemination with sperm either from a completely anonymous donor, from a donor who has agreed to be identifiable when the child becomes an adult, or from a fully known donor (e.g., a friend or a relative of the nonconceiving partner). Lesbians also can become parents by fostering or adopting children, as can gay men. These opportunities are increasingly available, though local legal statutes in some states and countries may still impose limitations. A growing number of gay men have chosen to become fathers through the assistance of a surrogate mother who bears their child. Others have made agreements to participate as sperm donors in the conception of a child (commonly with a lesbian couple), and arranged to have variable levels of involvement with the child.

- When a lesbian or a gay man becomes a parent through alternative insemination, surrogacy, or adoption, the biologic or adoptive parent is recognized legally as having full and more or less absolute parental rights. Despite the biologic or adoptive parent's partner functioning as a co-parent, he/she has no formal legal rights with respect to the child unless he/she formally adopts the child. Such co-parent (or second-parent) adoption has important psychological and legal benefits.

B. Psychological adjustment and parenting attitudes of parents.
Empirical evidence obtained over the last three decades reveals few differences between lesbian and heterosexual parents' self-esteem, psychological adjustment, attitudes toward child rearing, anxiety, depression, social support, and parenting stress. Much less is known about gay fathers and their children since, to date, no research has investigated children born into families headed by a gay couple.

C. Children's gender identity and sexual orientation.
The gender identity of preadolescent children raised by lesbian mothers or gay fathers has been found repeatedly to be consistent with their biologic sex. No differences have been found in the toy, game, activity, dress, or friendship preferences of prepubertal boys or girls who had lesbian mothers, compared with those who had heterosexual mothers. Limited longitudinal research suggests that adult men and women whose parents are heterosexual are as likely to identify themselves as gay or lesbian as are adults who had a homosexual parent. Young adults who had homosexual parents have more often reported feelings of attraction toward someone of the same sex and were slightly more likely to consider the possibility of having a same-sex partner.

D. Children's emotional and social development.
Because historically most children whose parents are gay or lesbian experienced the divorce of their biologic parents, de-

scriptions of their subsequent psychological development has to be understood in that context. Whether they are subsequently raised by one or both separated parents and whether a stepparent has joined either of the biologic parents are also important factors for children.

- A considerable body of research reveals that children of divorced lesbian mothers grow up in ways that are very similar to children of divorced heterosexual mothers. Several studies comparing children after divorce whose mothers were lesbian versus heterosexual have failed to document any differences in personality, peer group relationships, self-esteem, behavioral difficulties, academic success, or the quality of family relationships. Adult children of divorced lesbian mothers have recalled more teasing by peers during childhood than have adult children of divorced heterosexual parents, but also report satisfaction with their friendships and social relationships.
- Children born to and raised by lesbian couples also appear to develop normally. Ratings by their mothers and teachers have demonstrated good social competence and self-esteem, and the prevalence and types of behavioral difficulties they demonstrate are comparable to population norms. Some reports suggest that these children may be less aggressive and more tolerant of diversity. Children in one study whose lesbian parents reported greater relationship satisfaction, more egalitarian division of household and paid labor, and more regular contact with grandparents and other relatives were rated by parents and teachers to be better adjusted and to have fewer behavioral problems.
- Although gay and lesbian parents may not, despite their best efforts, be able to protect their children fully from the effects of stigmatization and discrimination, parents' sexual orientation is not a variable that, in itself, appears to predict their ability to provide a home environment that supports children's development. Overall it appears that children are more powerfully influenced by their own biology, family processes and relationships than by family structure.

E. Legal issues. As long as the permanence and full legal status of marriage are not possible for gay and lesbian parents in the United States, it is important for gay and lesbian parents to consider obtaining "power of attorney" for their children and/or seeking full parental rights for both parents via co-parent adoption. Decisions about custody and visitation for children whose parents are separating should be made independent of either parent's sexual orientation.

II. Pediatric management.

A. The office context. The pediatric office settings should be welcoming to families of diverse constellations. Posters, books, and magazines, and relevant information on the bulletin board can signal to gay and lesbian parents and their children that families like theirs are welcome. The language on office handouts and forms should be checked to eliminate heterosexist bias (e.g., be sure they have spaces for "parent", not "mother" and "father"). Signs and policies should emphasize confidentiality and a respect for diversity, and a policy of "zero tolerance" regarding homophobic jokes and comments.

B. Clinical care.
1. Health care for children whose parents are gay or lesbian differs little from health care that is appropriate for all children. Just as for all children, both parents should be invited to prepare for and to participate in healthcare visits. Discussions about family and peer relationships are always an important part of health supervision. Parents and children should be invited to discuss their family's structure and functioning, including any concerns they may have about it. Parents are wise to build social relationships with other families in which the parents are gay or lesbian, as it is helpful for children of all ages to know others in similar circumstances. Information about helpful reading materials as well as about national and local groups of families in which one or both parents is/are gay or lesbian may be welcomed.
2. In addition to the developmental tasks and challenges that all children face, children growing up in a family in which one or both parents is/are gay face some predictably challenging transitions.
   - Gay and lesbian parents have to consider how they wish to respond when their child around *3 to 4 years of age* begins to be interested and curious about her/his social/biological origins. Of prime importance to children of this age is security and permanence.
   - For many parents, the impact of *social stigma* is of paramount importance, especially as their *5- or 6-year-old* child ventures out into school life. Parents should exercise some caution with regard to passing on their worry to their children, who may have an easier time introducing themselves and their families than their parents fear.
   - In *early to middle adolescence* children are likely to be particularly concerned about

their own heritage and family history. In most circumstances at this stage it is helpful for parents to be fully open about the history of the child's conception and family background.

- During *later adolescence* all children are exploring their own sexuality and romantic attractions. Teenagers who have grown up in a family that includes one or more gay parents may find that unique assets and impediments coexist in this process as compared to their peers who have heterosexual parents.

3. **Coping with stigma.** Parents may need some encouragement and/or advice regarding how to help their child(ren) recognize, discuss, and cope with stigmatization or embarrassment that arise as a result of their parent(s)' sexual orientation or their family constellation. Pediatric providers may be able to help parents to identify strategies to help their children to manage painful encounters with homophobia. It is often helpful for children to be prepared for such experiences in advance, and to know how to respond to some predictable questions from curious peers. These strategies may change as children grow up and should be reassessed and discussed repeatedly.

Adolescents may find their parents' sexual orientation of more concern, and discussion with a professional may be helpful in order to make the home environment comfortable for teenagers and their friends. Older children may not reveal their feelings of marginalization or embarrassment about their homosexual parent(s), in part out of a concern that knowledge of their stigmatization might be hurtful to the parent(s).

- In order to prepare children, parents have to make difficult and complex decisions about disclosure. How freely are they willing to allow their child to describe their family? Are there risks to the child or the parents? Can they give children guidelines about "selective secrecy" and help them to understand how to make good decisions about disclosure? If the community is supportive, full disclosure to schools and other organizations and individuals important in children's lives will be easiest for children. Parents of older children and adolescents can be helpful by describing their own encounters with homophobia and the strategies they have used to counteract it.

4. **Discussing the family's history.** Parents may ask for assistance in initiating discussions about the child's original family or about her/his conception. Reading children's books together may help parents to explain the process of their becoming a family. If children are preoccupied or worried about the absent parent or donor or if the relationship between divorced parents is strained, a short series of meetings with a family therapist may be helpful in ensuring open communication among family members and support for the child(ren).

5. **Information control.** Many parents are comfortable in letting healthcare providers know about their sexual orientation and family constellation, but for others this may represent too great a risk. Before recording this information in the office chart, parents should be asked their preference. It is especially important in referring a child to a specialist to be sure what information about the family constellation the child and parents wish to have shared.

C. **Beyond the office walls.** Health professionals can help to support parent groups and/or groups for children whose parents are gay or lesbian, advise schools and libraries, provide information and advocacy to local and national legislators, and facilitate education via the public media and through professional organizations. They should encourage their local school and community libraries to have available a wide variety of books for children from preschool through adolescence that describe families in which the parents are gay or lesbian. An annotated list of selected books for children and adults can be found in Perrin (2002) listed in the bibliography.

As advisers to schools, health care professionals have an opportunity to advocate for presentations of the diversity of family structures and to address issues related to sexuality and sexual orientation at every age level from kindergarten through high school. Explicit statements by health professionals and evidence of their acceptance of a broad range of sexual orientation and behavior carries an important message to counteract the pervasive stigma that surrounds homosexuality.

BIBLIOGRAPHY

For Parents

Organizations

Gay, Lesbian, and Straight Education Network (GLSEN)
121 West 27th Street, Suite 804

New York, NY 10001
www.glsen.org

Children of Lesbian and Gays Everywhere (COLAGE)
2300 Market Street, Box 165
San Francisco, CA 94114
415-861-5437

COLAGE@COLAGE.org
www.COLAGE.org

Family Pride Coalition (formerly Gay and Lesbian Parents Coalition)
P.O. Box 34337
San Diego, CA 92163
619-296-0199
pride@familypride.org
www.familypride.org

Human Rights Campaign *FamilyNet*
1640 Rhode Island Ave., NW
Washington, DC 20036-3278
202-628-4160
familynet@hrc.org

Books

For Parents

Benkov L. *Reinventing the Family: Lesbian and Gay Parents.* New York. Crown Trade Paperbacks, 1994.
Clunis DM. *The Lesbian Parenting Book; A Guide to Creating Families and Raising Children.* Seattle, Wash.: Seal Feminist Publications; 1995.
Glazer DF, Drescher J. *Gay and Lesbian Parenting.* New York: Haworth Press; 2001.
Martin A. *The Lesbian and Gay Parenting Handbook: Creating and Raising Our Families.* New York: Harper Collins, 1993.

For Professionals

American Academy of Pediatrics Policy Statement. Co-parent or Second Parent Adoption by Same-sex Parents. *Pediatrics* 109(2):339– 344, 2002.
Perrin EC. *Sexual Orientation in Child and Adolescent Health Care.* New York: Kluwer/Plenum Academic Press, 2002.
Schorzman C, Gold M. Gay and lesbian parenting in "Homosexuality in Child Health Care". *Curr Problems Pediatr Adolesc Health Care* 2004, in press.
Tasker F. Lesbian mothers, gay fathers, and their children. *J Devel Behav Pediatr* 2004, in press.

93

Screening for Maternal Depression

Prachi Shah

I. **Description of the problem.** Depression and depressive disorders are among the most prevalent mental health problems in the United States. For women ages 15–44, depression is the leading cause of disease burden worldwide. The effects of maternal depression on child development are well documented. Children of depressed parents are at risk for developing significant psychological, social, learning, and behavioral problems. The mechanisms by which maternal depression affects child development are multifactorial, and may be related to a transaction between genetics, parent–child interactions, parenting behaviors, and child characteristics. Maternal mental health issues often go undetected, and pediatric clinicians are in an optimal position to screen and to refer mothers at risk for further evaluation and treatment.

A. **Epidemiology.**
- Estimates of maternal depressive symptoms in a variety of pediatric practice settings has ranged from 12%–47%.
- The point prevalence for maternal depression is 4.5%–9.3%, with a lifetime risk of 20%–25%.
- Increased rates of depression are seen in families with several young children or with a child with a chronic illness in the household.
- Higher rates of depression are associated with living in the inner city, lower socioeconomic status, immigrant status, poor marital relationships, drug and alcohol usage, and lower levels of education.
- Postpartum depression has a reported incidence of 8%–15%.

B. **Classification of mood disorders.**
1. **Depression (or major depressive disorder)** is defined by the following DSM-IV criteria: Five (or more) of the following symptoms have been present during the same 2-week period and represent a change from previous functioning and at least one of the symptoms is either (1) depressed mood or (2) loss of interest or pleasure.
   - Significant weight loss when not dieting, or weight gain or decrease or increase in appetite nearly every day.
   - Insomnia or hypersomnia nearly every day.
   - Guilt (excessive or inappropriate) or feelings of worthlessness nearly every day.
   - Energy loss or fatigue nearly every day.
   - Concentration diminished or indecisiveness, nearly every day (either by subjective account or as observed by others).
   - Agitation (psychomotor) or retardation nearly every day.
   - Pleasure lost (anhedonia) in all, or almost all, activities most of the day, nearly every day as indicated by either subjective account or observation made by others.
   - Suicidal ideation or recurrent thoughts of death without a specific plan, or a suicide attempt or a specific plan for committing suicide.
2. **Postpartum mood disorders.**
   a. **Postpartum blues** is experienced by 40%–80% of new mothers, and is characterized by rapid mood swings, emotional lability, anxiety, decreased concentration, and sleeping difficulties which occur within the first 2–3 days of delivery and which **resolve by 2 weeks postpartum**. If symptoms persist more than 2 weeks, a diagnosis other than postpartum blues must be considered.
   b. **Postpartum psychosis.** Prevalence: 0.1%–0.2%, and is characterized by severe sleeping disturbances, rapid mood swings, anxiety, delusions, hallucinations, racing thoughts, rapid speech, and thoughts of suicide or infanticide
   c. **Postpartum depression.** Prevalence: 8%–15% and is characterized by sleep disturbances, changes in appetite, profound lack of energy, anxiety, anger, guilt, feeling overwhelmed, sense of being unable to care for baby, or feelings of inade-

quacy. For a diagnosis of postpartum depression, depressive symptoms must occur **within 4 weeks of childbirth**.

C. **The mother with depression.** The symptoms of depression interfere with effective parenting. Mothers with depression may have increased negative and intrusive behaviors. They may have emotional disengagement, lack of responsivity to a child's cues, lack of warmth, irritability and aggression, which can lead to an insecure pattern of attachment between mother and child. They may use increased punitive attitudes and criticism and have inaccurate expectations of child development. They are more likely to use ineffective discipline techniques with their children and exhibit more negative appraisals of their children's behavior. They often have lower level of confidence in their caregiving abilities.

D. **Children of mothers with depression** may demonstrate numerous physiologic and behavioral characteristics of dysregulation, including
   1. **Infants**
      - More drowsiness, irregular sleeping, more fussiness
      - Increased levels of stress hormones (norepinephrine, cortisol)
      - Greater difficulty in soothing
   2. **Toddlers**
      - Decreased exploratory behaviors
      - Lower Bayley mental and motor scores
   3. **Children**
      - Increased behavior problems
      - Educational difficulties: impaired cognitive and linguistic development
      - Increased vulnerability to psychiatric disorders later on
   4. **Adolescents**
      - Increased risk of depression, substance abuse, and conduct disorder
   5. **Gender**
      - Boys of depressed parents often exhibit more externalizing behaviors (aggression and oppositionality)
      - Girls of depressed parents often exhibit more internalizing behaviors (anxiety and depression)

II. **Screening for maternal depression in primary care.** Because mood disorders are so pervasive and so frequently overlooked, routine use of screening should be considered. Formal screening tools exist to assess for the presence of depressive symptomatology, but a brief 2-question screener has a similar detection for maternal depression as longer questionnaires.
   - *"During the last 2 weeks have you often been bothered by feeling down, depressed or hopeless?"*
   - *"During the last 2 weeks, have you been bothered by having little interest or pleasure in activities?"*
   - Follow-up questions can address other somatic symptoms such as changes in sleep, appetite, or activity levels. *"Has your depression made it hard for you to do your work, take care of things at home, or get along with other people?"*

III. **Treatment/interventions for suspected depression.**
   A. **The role of the pediatric clinician.** Pediatric clinicians are in a unique position to discuss family issues, probe for depressive symptoms, and possible triggers, and counsel families about the effects of depression on the child's health and well being. The pediatric clinician is also poised to provide support, comfort, and help to a mother who is suffering and vulnerable.
      1. **Give the problem a name.** *"I can tell you are having a very hard time and are not feeling like yourself. This is more than the normal adjustment to a new baby, I think you are depressed. I see this in a lot of moms. There are things we can do together to make you feel better."*
      2. **Explore the mother's perception of the problem.** *"How do you feel about what I just said? What do you think might be going on?"*
      3. **Provide emotional support and reassurance.** Inquire as to her fears, e.g., about her ability as a parent, her thoughts and feeling about her baby, including permission and space to express thoughts and feelings that she may consider "taboo".
      4. Acknowledge that the child is also experiencing the mother's depression, and that you will work with her and the child to help the child understand and cope.
      5. It may also be important to help the school-aged and adolescent children know that they did not cause mother's depression, but that their mother has a medical condition for which she needs treatment.
   B. **Initial treatment strategies.** Caregivers with unremitting depressive symptoms should be referred to a mental health provider for further evaluation and treatment. Treatment may include a trial of antidepressants as well as psychotherapy.

1. **Reassure you too will follow-up.** This is not a referral that will severe your relationship.
2. **Reassure her (if possible) about her child.** "Despite how you are feeling, your child is doing very well. We want to nip this depression in the bud before it does cause your child any problems."

BIBLIOGRAPHY

For Parents

Beardslee W. Out of the darkened room: when a parent is depressed, protecting the children and strengthening the family. 2002. Available at: http://www.parenthood.com/articles. html?article_id = 4002

For Professionals

Health Finder http://www.teachmorelovemore.org/frame.asp?newlink = http://www.healthfinder. gov/news/newsstory.asp?docID = 517225&return = /EarlyCareEduDetails.asp

94

Sibling Rivalry

Robert Needlman

I. **Description of the problem.** The child psychiatrist Donald Winnicott once said that with the birth of a younger sibling, the child "discovers hatred." Jealousy between siblings can spoil otherwise pleasant family time, generating parental upset, anger, and guilt. Sibling rivalry does not stop at feelings. Verbal aggression and physical fighting occur far more often between siblings than unrelated peers. Severe sibling conflict may reflect a larger pattern of aggressive, out of control behavior. On the positive side, cooperative play, negotiation, and nonviolent arguments between siblings teach important life skills. Putting up with siblings can teach children how to control their emotions and get along. Filial solidarity often provides life-long social support.

   A. **Epidemiology.** Following the birth of a sibling, some degree of upset and behavioral regression (e.g., bedwetting) is almost universal. One-third of children also show developmental gains after a sibling's birth, such as increased self-care and language sophistication.

     • Among younger siblings, struggles over objects; hitting or pushing; and teasing, name calling, and verbal threats have been measured to occur an average of 8 times per hour (the rate decreases with age)

     • Older siblings are more likely to engage in verbal (as opposed to physical) antagonism. However, in most surveys, the frequency of positive sibling interactions is greater still.

     • School-age children have reported sibling conflict 91% of the time. In one study, 40% of children had hit a sibling with an object. Violent acts were reported for 49%–68% of siblings, with boy–girl pairs having the most and girl–girl pairs the least.

     • Among adults surveyed, 71% recalled having rivalrous feelings with siblings. Often, these feelings persisted into adulthood.

   B. **Etiology/contributing factors.**

     1. **Loss of exclusive relationship.** Children with the closest relationships to their mothers may show the greatest upset after the birth of a sibling. In contrast, a close relationship with the father may be protective.

     2. **Spacing of siblings.** Siblings spaced about 2 years apart may experience the most intense rivalries, perhaps because the older child must deal with increased separation from the mother at a time when separation is particularly difficult. Twins, by contrast, seem less prone to rivalry, as do children born 3 or more years apart.

     3. **Immaturity.** Sibling relationships involve living in close proximity and sharing resources of space, materials and food, and parental attention. Very few young children have the mature social skills—such as perspective-taking and verbal negotiation—required to manage such an intimate relationship without travail.

     4. **Role uncertainty.** Older children are often required to take leadership or managerial roles, vis-à-vis their younger siblings. At other times, children are expected to play together as equals, with no identified boss. For many children, moving back and forth between these quite different relationships is confusing and difficult, resulting in conflict.

     5. **Favoritism and fairness.** Parental favoritism—real or perceived—exacerbates sibling conflicts, while a belief in parental fairness reduces jealousy. Fairness cannot be based on strict equality. Different children need different rules, rights, and responsibilities. They also evoke different emotional responses from their parents, based on concordance or discordance of temperament and on accidents of timing (e.g., being born during a period of economic hardship, or being the only boy after a string of girls.)

II. **Making the diagnosis.**

   A. **Signs and symptoms.** Sibling conflicts may be brought up as the chief complaint or they may be unmentioned causes or a complicating factor in other clinical situations, such as concerns about aggression or school failure. Consider sibling rivalry and jealousy when caring for a child with special healthcare needs. Withdrawn behavior in response to a sibling's birth (in contrast to the usual willful misbehavior) may signal serious psychological strain.

B. History: Key clinical questions.

1. [To the child] *"Tell me about your brother(s) and sister(s)."* Most children find this a nonthreatening question. You can also invite the child to draw a picture of everyone in the family ("functional family drawing"), then ask about each sibling: things they do together for fun, things they do that are irritating; things that often lead to fights. Focus on temperament: How are the temperaments of the children similar or clashing?

2. [To the child] *"What usually happens when you and ··· fight?"* To get past the "he's always picking on me" kind of generalizations, try to focus on specific, recent events. Elicit a play-by-play account, focusing on the antecedents, behaviors, and consequences (ABCs). What were the children doing before the conflict began? How did it start? What did the parent do? How did it end? Was it typical?

3. [To the parent] *"How have you handled sibling fights in the past?"* Before offering advice, it's helpful to know what a parent has already tried, and how the parent has conceptualized the problem.

4. *"Tell me about the children in the family."* Listen for type casting ("my touchy one; my peacemaker") stereotyping ("She's always the first to get into an argument") and siblings with special problems or accomplishments.

5. *"Do the children have separate bedrooms, separate places for personal belonging, and individual time with parents?"* Conflicts may be greater in families in which privacy and personal possessions are not respected. Individual special time is another highly valued commodity that can become a focus of contention.

6. *"How did your child respond to the birth of his younger siblings?"* Jealousy may not have arisen until after several weeks, when it became clear the new baby was staying, or until the baby became more interactive (around age 4 months), or began to walk and to take the older child's toys. Inquire about each of these developmental stages.

7. *"Tell me the history of your family, from the start."* You need to understand where the identified child fits within the history of the family: when the child was born, were the parents beginning careers or fighting to make ends meet? What was life like in the family with the addition of each child? External changes—e.g., a big promotion, move to a larger or smaller home, death of a grandparent—can greatly affect a child's experience growing up, and can lead to jealousy and conflict.

8. *"In your family, how are arguments usually settled?"* Sibling conflicts tend to be more violent in the context of marital tension and hostility. Children may fight in response to built-up anger and tension, or in order to draw attention away from simmering marital conflicts. Where sibling conflict is part of a larger pattern of hostility, whole family intervention may be necessary.

III. Management.

A. Primary goals.

1. **Insight.** Parents who can recognize in themselves and their children the very strong forces that drive sibling conflicts, may respond with greater empathy, less anger, and more firmness. Present the following scenario to the parents: "Imagine your partner comes home tonight and announces: "I have decided to bring this other new wonderful husband/wife to live with us. Isn't that great! She will take a lot of my attention and I want you to be nice to him/her. Hey, don't worry, I still love you as much as I always have." How do think you would feel about that?"

2. **Reasonable expectations.** Parents need reasonable expectations for sibling coexistence. Some degree of rivalry or conflict may be inevitable, particularly for siblings who are temperamentally incompatible. Drawing attention to the positive aspects of the relationship (e.g., loyalty) may help. It may *not* be reasonable to expect older siblings to take on a supervisory or custodial role if the maturity is lacking or the behavior of the younger sibling is challenging.

3. **Appropriate intervention.** With younger children in particular, parents need to step in often to prevent physical harm. Young siblings left to their own devices fight more. Older siblings may be better able to work out their differences on their own. A parent who always comes in on the side of one child (the identified victim) may be inadvertently fueling future attacks. Parents should intervene *as much as they have to*, but no more.

B. **Specific strategies.**

1. **Help an older sibling play a helpful role.** With a new baby in the house, a toddler (male or female) may benefit from having a baby doll to take care of (or drop head first). It may help to model ways for the parent to involve the older child, such as saying, "The baby is crying! What do you think? Should we try getting a new diaper?"

2. **Avoid comparisons and labeling.** Sensitize parents to listen for typecasting statements ("my problem child"), and avoid making them. Even positive roles, such as "my good listener" or "my little helper" can lead the child to misbehave in order to escape from the label, or can imply to the other children that they are not expected to listen or help.

3. **Explain differential treatment.** Parents should explain that everyone in the family is different and everyone needs different things. Children don't get the *same* thing, but they each get what they need. It helps to refer to fairness: "I pay attention to you when you need me, but right now your sister needs my attention."

4. **Settle disputes according to explicitly stated principles.** The perception of parental unfairness fuels sibling resentment. To demonstrate fairness, parents need to set forth principles, and refer to them when making their judgments. For example, it's a good principle that every child has the right to privacy in his or her own room or space; siblings have to go away, if asked.

5. **Separate young children.** For siblings, playing together is a privilege, not a right. Parents need to step in fairly early, before fights escalate, and separate the combatants. This may mean time-outs for both children, in chairs in opposite corners, or in separate rooms.

6. **Challenge the victim–aggressor roles.** While it is true that an older child may consistently dominate a younger sibling, it's often the case that the "innocent victim" is actually needling the other sibling to the point of explosion, after which the "innocent" one enjoys the sympathy of a loving parent while watching the rival being punished.

C. **Follow-up/backup strategies.** Repeated visits may help to reinforce new patterns of parenting. In particular, after parents limit their intervention, sibling conflicts may temporarily increase. It may be helpful to have parents role play management strategies (e.g., praising a child's behavior without commenting on the general goodness of the child, or making covert sibling comparisons.) The following features should suggest referral for sub-specialist care:

1. **Multiproblem children.** When sibling conflict is part of a larger constellation of dysfunction—e.g., oppositionality or aggression toward parents or teachers, aggression against nonsibling peers, school failure—sibling conflicts are unlikely to resolve without attention to the whole picture.

2. **Multiproblem families.** Family anger, violence, parental distance, or threatened separation may be best addressed through family therapy, which may also strengthen the sibling relationships.

3. **Physical abuse.** A pattern of actual injury inflicted by one sibling against another signals a family emergency. The inability of the parents to recognize the behavior and stop it cold is a mark of significant dysfunction. The risk to both the aggressor and the victim is very high. Intensive intervention is called for.

BIBLIOGRAPHY

For Parents

Books

Faber A, Mazlish E. *Siblings Without Rivalry: How to Help Your Children Live Together So You Can Live Too.* New York: Avon Books, 1998. (An excellent guide designed to help parents understand their children's behavior and make the necessary changes in their own. It presents sound principles using wonderfully clear examples. The cartoon scenarios are particularly helpful.)

Reit S. *Sibling Rivalry.* New York: Ballantine Books, 1985. (A good review of the subject, written for parents, full of useful information.)

Websites

Family Resource http://www.familyresource.com/parenting/34/339/
Kids Health http://kidshealth.org/parent/emotions/feelings/sibling_rivalry.html
PBS Kids http://pbskids.org/itsmylife/family/sibrivalry/
www.drspock.com

For Professionals

Dunn J. *Sisters and Brothers*. Cambridge, MA: Harvard University Press, 1985. (Dunn has carried out some of the best and most relevant longitudinal research on siblings, well summarized here.)

Newman J. Conflict and friendship in sibling relationships: A review. *Child Study Journal* 24(2): 119–152, 1994. (A thorough review of decades of studies.)

95

Single Parents

J. Lane Tanner

I. **Description of the issue.** A variety of family reconfigurations have become prevalent over the past two decades, but no change has been more dramatic than the shift toward families headed by a single parent. While single-parent status does not represent a problem in itself, single-parent families as a group are significantly more strapped for personal, social, and economic resources, and are more likely to have experienced significant losses and change. This chapter is intended to alert the clinician to the stressors and special needs that commonly confront the single-parent family.

A. **Demographics.**
- At least 50% of U.S. children born in the last two decades will spend a substantial period of time living in a home headed by a single parent or guardian.
- Between 1970 and 2000, the numbers of American children living in single mother homes has more than doubled, from 12%–26%, while those living with single fathers has increased from 1%–5% of all children during the same interval.
- Dramatic variations exist in the proportion of families headed by single parents according to race, with the 1996 census showing 22% of white children, 57% of African American children, and 32% of Hispanic children living with single parents.
- 86% of children in one-parent families live with the mother.
- Single-parent status is the result of parental divorce (37%), a never-married single parent (36%), parental separation (23%), and parental death (4%).

B. **Problems of single-parent families.**
1. **Limitations of available resources.**
   a. **Money.** With 34% of mother-only families living below national poverty levels, the clinician is increasingly obliged to inquire regarding the family's financial resources, the parent's employment status, and the family's dependency on contributions from others.
   b. **Time.** Single parents who are employed are likely to feel that they are continually in a race to provide adequate time to the family, the job, and the endless details of daily life, from groceries to taxes. Unpredictable events, such as an important school activity, a household emergency, or a child's illness, further intrude on this tightly stretched schedule.
   c. **Physical and emotional energy.** In addition to providing the tangible goods and supplies needed by the family, the single parent is called on to provide almost 100% of the emotional support and sustenance for the children. Alone, this parent must shoulder the responsibility for decisions, great and small, that shape their lives.
2. **Network of social support.** Mapping the sources of social support for the single parent requires an awareness of the availability of those sources and the frequency with which the parent actually uses them. Are there other adults (relatives, friend, lover) living in the home? Are they emotionally or responsibly involved with the family? Who is dependent on whom? Are there other people who are emotionally close to the parent who can offer understanding and support? What about institutions (such as the school, workplace, church, or clinic) that can provide support for both parent and child?
3. **Major life events, losses, or transitions.** Single-parent status is often born out of crisis (e.g., separation or divorce or the partner's death). These events may also bring a cascade of secondary losses, which may include changes in the family home, the child's school, friends, or community. Grief, anger, guilt, and depression regularly follow the trauma of such changes. The subsequent transitional period is likely to be disorganized and tumultuous until a realignment of schedule, roles, expectations, and feelings can permit a new and stabilized family life. Such events may have very different meanings for the child than for the parent. For example, divorce and the loss of the family home may bring desired independence and relief for the parent but

an unmitigated sense of loss for the child. The clinician must assess these differential meanings and be aware of the time course of adaptation displayed by each family member.

4. **Shifts in relational dynamics.** Family dynamics are substantially different when children are oriented to a single parent as the sole authority and provider, and when the parent has only the children as main companions at home.

C. **Common clinical issues.** As with other risk factors, single-parent status by itself confers no predictable condition on the child. The following clinical issues are thus presented as common concerns and in no way specifically or universally apply to single-parent families.

1. **The single parent who feels off-balance and uncertain regarding parenting and child management.** While self-doubt in parenting is surely felt by all parents from time to time, single parents are even more susceptible. The parent seeks advice from the clinician, but also "reality testing" and reassurances that her efforts, responses, and feelings (especially negative feelings) are warranted, or at least understood.

2. **The helpless, overwhelmed single parent.** The clinician becomes aware that this parent is not simply looking for good advice but for someone else to lean on, to make the hard decisions and to take over the responsibility that has become incapacitating. Parental isolation and depression are especially frequent concomitants.

3. **Child behavioral disorders.** These are particularly likely to emerge when the child is pushing the parent to provide unmet needs or when the parent's sense of concern, guilt, or exhaustion regarding the child renders behavioral management ineffective. Behavior disorders in the child may also be symptomatic of ongoing conflict between separated parents.

4. **The child who takes on a parentified helper role.** The child's adoption of a parental role may be necessary and adaptive for the family, while providing rewards for the child connected with their new and special position with the parent. On the other hand, such a role may infringe on the individual sociodevelopmental needs and growth of the child.

5. **The child who becomes the parent's companion and confidant.** The key issue here concerns the boundaries between parent and child—whether each has her or his own friends, activities, rights of privacy, and freedom to disagree or express anger with the other.

6. **Issues related to the absent parent.** Children must come to terms with developmentally staged personal dilemmas regarding who the absent parent was, is, and will be to them. Special difficulties and challenges exist for the child when the parents' relationship remains conflictual, as well as when the child has entirely lost contact with a parent who was formerly close.

7. **The adolescent single parent and the three-generation household.** This "kinship family" provides crucial social support, shared child rearing, and other resources. There are, however, likely to be intrinsic tensions between the grandparent(s) and the teenage parent. These most predictably center on issues of parental authority for the young child and personal autonomy for the adolescent. The nature of the grandparents' support for their daughter or son and whether they realistically and flexibly encourage the growth of her or his competencies is an important question to address.

8. **The introduction of a new adult into the household.** Whether a friend, relative, or potential future mate, the arrival of a new adult into an established single-parent household is a major event. Its meaning to the child is shaped by his own developmental stage and past events and patterns. The potential for the child to feel displaced, intruded on, or disregarded is substantial. Long-term adaptation requires that the parent display her or his intention to remain the head of the household, in charge not only of the children but also in overseeing the authority and responsibilities that are delegated to the new adult.

II. **Management.**

A. **Empathy with the issues.** The primary care clinician is often called on to hear, understand, and validate the concerns and responses of the single parent. Most common to these parents is the sense of aloneness in the consuming and awesome task of child rearing. It is an attitude of respect for this experience that becomes the clinician's first and most important tool.

- The clinician's direct inquiry of the parent (e.g., "You have a lot to juggle. How is it going?" or "How are you doing balancing everybody's needs? How about your own?") opens the door to establishing this basis of understanding and respect.

B. **Monitoring the needs of the child.** In order to monitor the needs of the child in the single-parent family, the clinician must remain mindful of the challenges confronting the child and assess his or her adaptation to them. As always, behavioral patterns, school performance, social functioning, and overall sense of happiness and confidence are the best indicators of the child's adaptation to stress. However, in some children signs of difficulty may not be obvious. For example, the child's anxious loyalty to a single parent or the parent's own urgent or unmet needs may keep either from acknowledging the stressful influences that impinge on the child. The child's needs may come into direct conflict with those of his or her parent (e.g., a parent's new adult relationship that takes away time with the child). Thus, it falls to the clinician to initiate, with the child as well as the parent, an exploration of the potential problems and issues. Directly asking the child about daily routines such as sleep patterns, home responsibilities, daily schedule, and school achievement will often open the door to an exploration of stress and poor adaptation.

C. **Supporting the parent.** With rare exceptions, support for the child requires support for the parent. The clinician can encourage and support a parent by simply valuing her or his efforts. Advocacy for clearly established generational boundaries and effective parental authority may help clear away some of the hesitancy and doubt the parent is experiencing. Concern for the parent as a person, with individual needs and goals, may encourage her to seek an effective network of social support.

For the single parent who comes across as helpless and overwhelmed and seems to be pushing for a truly dependent relationship, simple empathy, validation, and good advice are not enough. The clinician may experience the urge to rescue the parent in some way or, alternatively, to run away from such expressed neediness. Advice and helpful ideas offered by the clinician may be met with a disparaging "yes, but" response from the parent.

• For such parents, re-describing expressions of helplessness in terms of particular dilemmas introduces the possibility of choice and action (e.g., "It sounds as if you are dealing with a lot, and your child's behavior sounds particularly difficult right now, for both of you. Tell me your ideas for handling it"). By resisting the impulse to provide the answers and by encouraging and organizing the parent's own efforts at problem solving (e.g., "What will be the effect on your child of such a plan? How about on you and on your goals for yourself as a parent in the short term and in the long term?"), the clinician's role shifts from that of the fantasized rescuer to that of an understanding yet realistic coach. Additionally, reminding the parent of her or his demonstrated competencies, especially those that contradict the current perceptions of helplessness, may bolster self-efficacy and hopefulness.

BIBLIOGRAPHY

For Parents

Books

Wallerstein J, Blakeslee S. *What About the Kids? Raising Your Children Before, During, and After Divorce.* New York: Hyperion Press, 2003.

Websites

www.ParentsWithoutPartners.org. An international, nonprofit, educational organization for single parents and their children, founded in 1957. The site provides educational information, resources, meeting information, and a Website for children.
www.Parenthood.com. An educational site devoted to a broad spectrum of parenting issues.

For Professionals

Allmond B, Tanner JL, Gofman H. Shifts in the Traditional Family. In *The Family Is the Patient: Using Family Interviews in Children's Medical Care (2nd ed)*. Baltimore: Williams & Wilkins, 1999, pp. 331–350.
American Academy of Pediatrics. Family pediatrics. *Pediatrics* 111(suppl):1541–1587, 2003.
McLanahan S, Sandefur G. *Growing Up with a Single Parent: What Hurts, What Helps.* Cambridge, MA: Harvard University Press, 1994.

96

Stepfamilies

Margorie Engel
John S. Visher*

I. Description of the problem.

A. Epidemiology.

- Almost 16 million children live in a stepfamily relationship according to the U.S. Census Bureau (2000). This number does not include the many stepfamilies formed by a child's noncustodial parent, stepfamilies with college-age and adult stepchildren, families where an unwed mother married a man who is not the biological father of her child, cohabiting stepfamilies, or gay and lesbian households in stepfamily-like relationships.

- The prefix "step" denotes connection between members of a family by the remarriage of a parent and not by blood. Approximately 65% of all remarriages create a stepfamily, while 35% of all remarriages are created by childless couples. Therefore, it is important to note that the words "remarriage" and "stepfamily" are not synonymous, especially when reading re-divorce statistics.

- It is estimated that by the year 2010, the stepfamily relationship will be the most common type of American family.*

B. Stresses for children.

1. **Multiple changes.** Stepchildren come into their stepfamily with a history of multiple changes related to their parents' divorce that may put some of the children at risk. Life in a stepfamily brings another set of changes. When a residential move occurs, some obvious ones include leaving a familiar home, neighborhood, school, and best friends. More subtle changes include the new status of being the eldest or youngest child in the family, of no longer being the only child, and of sharing time, attention, and intimacy with a parent who previously had no competing emotional ties.

   - The new stepfamily adults, often caught up in their own personal happiness, may not be fully aware of their children's feelings about all of these changes. Processing change postdivorce usually takes 3–5 years; the remarriage occurs on average 2–3 years post divorce and may explain the child's heightened resistance to the new set of changes.

   - In the short run, divorce is usually painful for a child although new and extensive research indicates the long-term effects may have been exaggerated. Comprehensive studies indicate not all children experience change and loss to the negative degree often implied. In terms of general well-being, a significant percentage of children not only survive the breakup and remarriage, they thrive. As young adults, they emerge from divorce and stepfamilies with enhanced functioning—not despite the things that happened to them during the divorce and after, but because of them.

2. **Loyalty conflicts.** Loyalty conflicts are inevitable. An emotional connection to a stepparent may be experienced as a betrayal of the parent who is not living in the household. The absent parent is usually considered to be physically available to the child on a periodic basis. Loyalty conflicts are also present following parental abandonment or death when a child's parent remains present only in memory.

3. **Loss of control.** Feeling a loss of control may be at the root of much of the anger and depression in children and often predates life in a stepfamily. The adults have chosen to make major changes in their lives, oftentimes for the better; the children have had those changes imposed on them.

4. **Stepsiblings.** The presence of stepsiblings may exacerbate the stresses that accompany stepfamily life. Feelings of sibling rivalry, jealousy, insecurity, and the fear that a sibling may be more loved, are often more intense in a stepfamily. Noncustodial children may be offered special treats or exempted from the house rules that resident children must follow. Grandparents may give their grandchildren more

---

*Prior to her death in 2001, Emily Visher, PhD, contributed a portion of this stepfamily information to a chapter in the first edition of *Behavioral and Developmental Pediatrics*.

lavish gifts than those given to their stepgrandchildren. If a baby is born into the stepfamily, sibling jealousy might be magnified by the fear that the "mutual child" may be more loved by the adults. Conversely, the birth may help to solidify the stepfamily because the new baby is biologically related to all of the children and adults. It is certainly true that many stepsiblings develop close bonds, united by their common experience of many family changes.

C. Children's responses.

1. **Preschool.** The stress of a remarriage may cause some preschoolers to cling to parents and to regress behaviorally. In the stage of magical thinking, they may believe that their angry thoughts already have led to or will lead to family disruption. They may also harbor thoughts that they can magically reunite the divorced parents.

2. **School age.** School-aged children are often angry about their powerlessness to halt the changes in their lives. They may counter these feelings of helplessness by imagining that they caused the breakup of the marriage—a fantasy that at least offers some influence over a situation they cannot control. They may still wish that their parents were together and fantasize that if they are "good," their parents will be reunited, or that if they are "bad" or "sick," their parents will come together to help. As a result, when divorced parents do work together for the benefit of the child, children may unrealistically anticipate that short-term togetherness will lead to long-term reunion.

   • Children at this stage are rarely able to express these feelings verbally and are likely to act out their anger and guilt. They may have tantrums at home, fight with siblings or classmates, develop psychosomatic symptoms, become accident prone, start failing in their schoolwork, or even try to break up the new marriage. Conversely, they may respond by behaving with an angelic virtue, following all the rules and making no obvious waves, so that their inner turmoil remains concealed.

3. **Adolescence.** Adolescents present special difficulties for the stepfamily. They are caught up in their own issues of identity and autonomy, making the new relationships even more difficult to accept. Teen sexuality is burgeoning at the very time they enter a household that is, inevitably, highly sexualized by the newness of the adult marriage. The residential presence of close-in-age stepsiblings or stepparent of the opposite sex can also create sexual tensions.

   • Often an independent teenage child of a single parent is pressured, after the parent's remarriage, to return to a more childish stage of dependency. Teenagers who are used to being a parent's confidant and the "man" or "woman" of the house find themselves losing that favored status when they are expected to become "children" again. This may accelerate their drive to separate from the parents or a desire to live in the home of the other parent.

D. Stress for couples in stepfamilies. Adult couples in stepfamilies must also deal with many strong emotions. Loyalty to their children predates the stepfamily and may create conflicts with the new spouse. Parents may attempt to please the children at all costs in order to compensate for the many family changes. They may also avoid forming a solid bond with a new spouse because they mistakenly feel that to do so would be experienced as a betrayal of their relationships with their children. This, in turn, frequently conflicts with the needs of the new spouse, who may understandably feel like an outsider in an established household.

II. Helping children.

A. General principles.

1. **Accept the child's feelings.** While always validating a child's feelings, from a developmental perspective, children can be taught empathetic skills from early childhood onward and are cognitively capable from around the age of 5. The research on adolescent stepchildren's initiation of conflict with stepparents prescribes emphasizing empathetic skills on the part of children, just as we emphasize this with adults.

2. **Reassure the child (repeatedly, if necessary) that he is not responsible for the dissolution of the parents' marriage.**

3. **Stress that the child is a worthwhile, special person, no matter what decisions parents have made about their own lives.**

4. **Help the child put feelings into words rather than into negative behaviors.** Encourage verbal expression. For example, "A lot of children feel very angry when they have to share a room with stepbrothers or stepsisters. Maybe you feel that way sometimes."

5. **Encourage the child to communicate with parents and stepparents.** The clinician can do this by talking to the family as a group or by asking a child privately for

permission to communicate specific information to the adults. For example, discussing with the parents a child's feeling that a stepsibling is being favored or distress over parents' fighting.

6. **Provide support to the parents and stepparents.** Research strongly suggests that the psychological well being of children depends more on the functioning of the family than the type of family.

B. **Teenagers.**

1. **The acting out of sexual attraction between stepsiblings can be minimized by having the family adopt a dress code, making appropriate bedroom arrangements, and providing adequate supervision.** Adults also need to be aware of and deal with their sexual feelings toward a stepchild who may appear to be a younger version of their spouse.

2. **Adolescents are often reluctant to become an active member of the stepfamily because of their developmental drive for independence and autonomy and the primacy of their peer relationships.** While remaining open to shared activities, the adults need to allow adolescents to maintain their independence from the stepfamily and to integrate at their own pace. In some cases, the teenager chooses to move out in order to find his identity. It is important to remember and acknowledge that children living in stepfamilies are integral members of two separate households.

3. **Divided loyalties may make the adolescent act out in a negative way toward the stepparent.** The parent must emphasize to the adolescent the need to always act in a respectful, if not warm, manner toward the stepparent.

4. **The stepparent may never be able to serve as a parent to the adolescent.** Other types of relationships, such as adult friend or confidant, can play equally important and rewarding roles for both adolescent and stepparent.

III. **Helping adults.**

A. **The couple.**

1. **The adults almost always have unrealistically high expectations of what their new family will be like.** Such misconceptions can be avoided by anticipatory guidance and by directing them to sources of information that provide realistic information about stepfamily life, especially in the early phases. They can also talk with other, more experienced remarried parents and stepparents. Stepfamily life education, especially the comprehensive program *Smart Steps for Adults and Children in Stepfamilies*, is recommended for all stepfamily members.

2. **Communicate to stepfamily members acceptance of their family as a valid entity, not a flawed version of the nuclear family.** Reassure them that their struggles are not unique but are an expected part of the complex task of creating a stepfamily, a task that usually takes several years. The first couple of years are typically chaotic!

3. **Remind the parent and stepparent that a strong relationship with one another is not a betrayal of their children.** All children need a solid bond between the adults in the household, especially to allay fears that the stepfamily will dissolve in the way that their previous family did. They also need a model of a couple working well together, including appropriate conflict resolution, to help them as they grow up and begin to form adult relationships of their own.

B. **Stepparenting.**

1. **The best advice is, "Don't try to be an instant parent."** The foundation of good relationships is a supply of positive, shared memories. Authoritative parental relationships need time to build; with older children, there may not be enough time for this to fully materialize before they leave home as young adults.

2. **While stepparents often serve as parents in significant ways, they are additional parent figures and not replacements for a deceased or absent parent.** A stepparent is another reliable adult who can fill some of the child's needs for economic and emotional support along with child-rearing tasks at home and in the child's world outside the home. Stepparents may be relieved to learn that there are many different yet satisfactory roles they can play in their stepchildren's lives, support-system roles that depend on the ages and needs of the children as well as the desires of the stepparent. For example, a stepparent can be a parent to a young child, a friend to an older child, or a confidant to a teenager and adult stepchild.

3. **Adults may come into a new marriage with very dissimilar parenting experiences.** It is helpful to supply information about child development, correct misconceptions, and, in some cases, recommend that the couple take parenting and stepfamily dynamics courses together.

IV. Questions frequently asked by stepfamily adults.

A. What do children call a new stepparent? "Mother" and "father" (or variations on these) are more than just names; they describe relationships. It is not helpful to encourage or insist on such terms when a relationship has not yet developed or when the child feels uncomfortable using the name. All but the youngest children may initially feel that by calling the stepparent "Mommy" or "Daddy," they are forsaking the absent parent.

- What children call their stepparents often progresses through different stages. At first, the child may call the stepparent by his or her first name. Later, it might become "Daddy John" or "Mommy Mary." The important point is that for both child and adult the name feels comfortable and does not imply a rejection of the absent parent. Many stepfamilies find that nicknames for stepparents are a comfortable compromise for everyone.

B. What do stepparents do about discipline? Discipline is a major source of tension in most stepfamilies with young children. Frequently a parent unrealistically expects a new spouse to discipline the children effectively. Children, however, do not view a new stepparent as someone with the instant authority to set limits on their behavior. The best approach is for the two adults to work out house rules together and, at least initially, leave the enforcement of those rules to each child's parent. It may take several years with young children (longer with older children) for the stepparent to have sufficient emotional authority to discipline the child effectively.

C. How do stepfamilies deal with the absent parent? When adults criticize a child's other parent or use children as messengers or spies in unresolved hostilities, it prevents the development of successful stepfamily relationships. Children feel that criticism and anger toward any parent are also directed at them. It hurts them to hear negative comments about a parent they love. The clinician can help by showing parents how this behavior harms children and by supporting the children's desire not to be involved in conflicts between their parents. Encourage parents to verbally give children permission to care about *all* of the adults in their lives, with no need to choose sides, take part in a battle, or be responsible for the happiness of a parent who is left behind while they spend time in their other home.

D. How long does it take to feel like a family? Adults and children feel like a family when they identify themselves as part of a system to which they all belong, where they feel comfortable, and where their basic needs are met. The time it takes to feel that way varies but is almost always much longer than the adults expect. With young children, the process of settling down takes at least 18–24 months; with older children, it may take 5–7 years.

E. Should children continue to see the noncustodial parent? Children in stepfamilies usually do better if they can maintain ties to both of their parents as long as no physical or emotional risk is involved. When children move back and forth between households, it is easier if the adults collaborate as a parenting coalition. A parenting coalition is a limited alliance, formed to promote the welfare of the children. It is a cooperative rather than a competitive relationship and is based on an understanding that all the adults are important to the children. Another successful parenting style is parallel parenting, used when the divorced parents are unable to collaborate. When each household has distinct yet consistent ways of functioning, the child adjusts to the different behaviors, activities, and expectations.

F. What can make the children's "dual citizenship" easier? When children have just returned from visiting their other parent, they need transition time. It usually works better if the adults inform children about what happened while they were away instead of interrogating them about what happened in their other home. In each home, children need a space of their own: a separate room, part of a room, or even a closet or drawer where personal belongings are kept. Particularly helpful is a house rule that nothing in a child's private space can be touched without that child's permission.

- Some children might be disturbed over the differences in rules between the two households and others may use those differences as a weapon to play one household against the other. Nevertheless, children do eventually learn that codes of acceptable behavior differ between households (just as they differ between home, school, and the homes of friends). What matters is to know the rules in each location and to abide by them. Children accept this most readily if they have some input into the creation of rules in the stepfamily household and if the parents are not defensive about the rules the adults have established. Finally, it is important to keep the consequences for misbehavior within the household where it occurred. An infringement of one household's rules should not affect time spent or activities in the other household.

BIBLIOGRAPHY

For Stepfamilies

Organizations and Programs

Stepfamily Association of America 650 J Street, Suite 205 Lincoln NE 68508 1-800-735-0329 SAA@SAAfamilies.org www.SAAfamilies.org

Stepfamily Life Education Program Adler-Baeder F. *Smart Steps for Adults and Children in Stepfamilies: A six-week research-based educational program designed for use in a professional or support group environment.* Lincoln, NE: SAA Families Press.1-800-735-0329(Program also available in Spanish. Christian supplement: *Growing in Wisdom.*)

Websites

The Stepfamily Association of America. Research-based information, education, support, and advocacy to stepfamily members and the professionals who serve them; home page includes a search feature. www.SAAfamilies.org

Your Stepfamily Online. SAA's official online magazine for today's evolving stepfamily. www.yourstepfamily.com

Step Together. A chapter of the Stepfamily Association of America; provides "virtual" support. www.steptogether.org

Stepfamilies-International. Stepfamily information and resources including popular conference presentation and discussion topics. www.stepfamilies-international.org

Stepping Stones Counseling Center, "We not only work with stepfamily issues, we face them every day in our personal lives." www.stepfamilies.com

Books on General Stepfamily Dynamics

Bernstein AC. *Yours, Mine, and Ours: How Families Change When Remarried Parents Have a Child Together.* New York: Scribner, 1989..

Bray JH, Kelly J. *Stepfamilies: Love, Marriage, and Parenting in the First Decade.* New York: Broadway Books, 1998.

Deal RL. *The Smart Stepfamily: Seven Steps to a Healthy Family.* Bloomington, MN: Bethany House, 2002.

Engel M. *Stepfamily Financial Management Booklet Series.* Lincoln, NE: SAA Families Press, 2001.

Estess PS. *Money Advice for Your Successful Remarriage.* Cincinnati, Ohio: Betterway Books, 1996.

Lauer R, Lauer J. *Becoming Family: How to Build a Stepfamily That Really Works.* Minneapolis, MN: Augsburg Fortress, 1999.

Visher E, Visher J. *How to Win as a Stepfamily.* New York: Brunner/Mazel, 1991.

Books for Children

Berman C. *What Am I Doing in a Stepfamily?* Secaucus, NJ: Lyle Stuart, 1982.

Holyoke N. *Help! A Girl's Guide to Divorce and Stepfamilies.* Middleton, WI: The Pleasant Company Publications, 1999. (Ages 9–12)

Rogers F. *Let's Talk About It: Stepfamilies.* New York: GP Putnam's Sons, 1997. (Ages 4–8; by Fred Rogers of *Mr. Roger's Neighborhood*)

Lumpkin P. *The Stepkin Stories: Helping Children Cope with Divorce and Adjust to Stepfamilies* Wilsonville, OR: BookPartners, 1999. (Age under 10).

Bullard L. *Trick-or-Treat on Milton Street.* Carolrhoda Books, 2001.

Haughton E. *Rainy Day.* Carolrhoda Books, 2000.

Holub J. *Cinderdog and the Wicked Stepcat.* Morton Grove, Ill.: Albert Whitman & Co, 2001.

For Adolescents

Block JD, Bartell SS. *Stepliving for Teens.* Price Stern-Sloan, 2001.

Prilik PK. *Becoming an Adult Stepchild: Adjusting to a Parent's New Marriage.* Washington, DC: American Psychiatric Press, 1998.

Webber R. *Split Ends: Teenage Stepchildren.* Australian Council of Educational Research (SAA 800-735-0329; 1997.)

For Stepparents

Annarino KL. *Stepmothers and Stepdaughters: Relationships of Chance, Friendships for a Lifetime.* Berkeley, CA: Wildcat Canyon Press, 2000.

Burns C. *Stepmotherhood: How to Survive Without Feeling Frustrated, Left Out, or Wicked.* New York: Three Rivers Press, 2001.

Keenan BM. *When You Marry a Man With Children: How to Put Your Marriage First and Stay in Love.* New York: Pocket Books, 1992.

Lutz E (Foreword by Dr. Margorie Engel). *The Complete Idiot's Guide to Stepparenting.* New York: Alpha Books, 1998.

McBride J. *Encouraging Words for New Stepmothers.* Ft Collins, CO: CDR Press, 2001.

Norwood PK (with T Winender). *The Enlightened Stepmother: Revolutionizing the Role.* New York: Avon, 1999.

Oxhorn-Ringwood L, Oxhorn L (with Krausz MV). *Stepwives: 10 Steps to Help Ex-wives and Stepmothers End the Struggle and Put the Kids First.* New York: Fireside/Simon & Schuster, 2002.

Thoele SP. *The Courage to Be a Stepmom: Finding Your Place Without Losing Yourself.* Berkeley, CA: Wildcat Canyon Press, 1999.

For Professionals

Hetherington E. *For Better or For Worse: Divorce Reconsidered.* New York: Norton, 2002.

Mahoney MM. *Stepfamilies and the Law.* Ann Arbor: University of Michigan Press, 1994.

Visher E, Visher J. *Stepfamilies: A Guide to Working with Stepparents and Stepchildren.* New York: Brunner/Mazel, 1979.

Visher E, Visher J. *Old Loyalties, New Ties: Therapeutic Strategies with Stepfamilies.* New York: Brunner/Mazel, 1988.

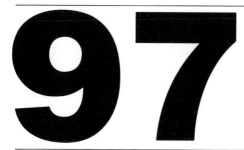

Television

Victor C. Strasburger

I. **Description of the issue.** Children and teens spend more time watching television (TV) than doing any other activity except for sleeping—an average of 3 hours or more per day. By the time today's children reach age 70 years, they will have spent 7–10 years of their lives watching TV.

- Children are especially vulnerable to the influence of TV. According to social learning theory, children and adolescents learn from watching their parents and other adults model certain behaviors. Certainly, there are no more attractive role models than on TV, discussing everything from sex and alcohol to food and careers. TV gives young people secret glimpses into the adult world and serves as a powerful teacher, shaping attitudes and influencing behavior.
- According to the cultivation effect, heavy viewers of TV tend to believe that the TV world is real and that people in everyday life should behave accordingly. The medium also exerts a powerful displacement effect: 3 hours a day spent viewing TV is 3 hours a day lost from schoolwork, reading, and exercise.

II. **Areas of concern.** Practitioners should familiarize themselves with the specific areas of concern with regard to TV content.

A. **Violence.** According to the National TV Violence Study (conducted from 1996 to 1998), children's TV is more violent than adult's TV. In addition, one quarter of the violent interactions feature guns. The average child views 10,000 murders, rapes, and assaults per year on TV. Violence is frequently portrayed as either humorous or as an acceptable solution to a complex problem, particularly for the "good guy." Scientific studies suggest that a heavy diet of TV violence may lead to aggressive behavior in certain susceptible children and teens. In one study, for example, children became more violent in their play after TV was introduced into their community. They also exercised less and were less creative in their play. In another remarkable 22-year study, a heavy diet of violent programming at age 8 years or younger correlated significantly with more aggressive behavior at ages 19 years and 30 years.

B. **Commercialism.** Children view 20,000 commercials per year. This is especially problematic for young children under age 8 years, who do not understand the difference between programming and commercials, or do not understand that commercials do not always tell the truth. Children influence $188 billion of their parents' spending each year plus spend about $155 billion of their own money. An estimated $12 billion a year is now spent on advertising and marketing to children alone.

C. **Overweight.** Numerous studies demonstrate a link between the amount of TV viewed and the prevalence of overweight in children. TV displaces more active activities and gives children and teens unhealthy ideas about nutrition. Snack food, fast food, and heavily sugared cereals are most frequently advertised. TV characters rarely engage in nutritious eating practices.

D. **Sexuality.** TV has become the leading sex educator in America today. This occurs in part because parents are reluctant to discuss sex or birth control with their children, and because the majority of schools no longer offer comprehensive sex education programs. On primetime TV, 75% of shows contain sexual content, but only 10% mention the risks or responsibilities of sexual activity or the need for contraception. Children and teens view an estimated 15,000 sexual references and innuendoes a year. Ads for condoms or birth control pills are extraordinarily rare on network TV. Experts attribute the high teenage pregnancy rate in the United States to three key factors: (1) inadequate access to birth control, (2) ineffective sex education in school, and (3) inappropriate media portrayals of human sexuality.

E. **Alcohol.** American children and teens view 2,000 beer commercials per year. Most of the ads try to create the illusion that drinking alcohol is normative behavior and that people who do so are more successful, happier, and sexier. For every antidrug public service announcement (PSA) on TV, there are an estimated 25–50 beer commercials.

Most PSAs deal only with marijuana, cocaine, inhalants, or heroin, not with alcohol—the leading killer of American teenagers today.

F. **Rock music and music videos.** Despite the fact that rock music lyrics have become sexier and more violent since the 1950s, there are no data to show that such lyrics have a negative behavioral impact. Indeed, in one study only 30% of young people even knew the lyrics to their favorite songs, and their ability to decipher the meaning of the lyrics was age-dependent. Music videos, on the other hand, have become extremely popular and are more likely to have a demonstrable impact. Although many music videos are harmless "performance videos" (of the band playing), others are concept videos that often tell a story replete with sexual imagery, violence, and sexism.

III. **Advice and guidance for families.**

A. **The American Academy of Pediatrics (AAP) recommends that parents limit their children's total media time to no more than 1–2 hours per day and that infants under the age of 2 years should not be routinely watching TV.** The easiest way to accomplish this is to counsel parents of 6–12-month-olds about the potential harmful effects of TV on children and to advise them to set strict limits from the outset.

B. **The AAP recommends that parents control which shows their children watch and that they watch TV with their children.** Studies show that parents can override any potentially harmful effects of TV programming by discussing objectionable material with their children.

C. **Primary care providers should counsel parents to avoid placing a TV set in a child's bedroom.** Currently, one fourth of young children, one third of older children, and more than half of teenagers have a TV set in their own bedroom. Control over TV viewing is impossible under such circumstances.

D. **Advising parents not to use the TV as "an electronic babysitter" is probably unrealistic. Rather, parents should be counseled to use the videocassette recorder to control what and when their child is viewing.** An easy way to put the issue into perspective for parents is through the following analogy: *"No parent would allow a stranger into his or her home to teach his or her child for 3 hours a day (especially a stranger who is obsessed with sex, violence, and commercialism). Yet that is precisely what TV is doing."*

E. **Primary care clinicians should periodically take a detailed TV history (how many hours watched per week, what shows, is there a TV set in the child's room, etc.).** Media history forms are available online from the AAP.

F. **Clinicians and parents need to familiarize themselves with the high-quality, low-cost videotapes that are available.** For preschoolers, the Rabbit Ears series of classic children's stories, narrated by Hollywood stars, with music by well-known performers, is an outstanding alternative to the usual network fare. The Coalition for Quality Children's Media is a nonprofit organization that rates videos for children and produces a quarterly newsletter. Another excellent nonprofit newsletter for parents is *Parents' Choice*, which reviews videos, programming, magazines, and books for children.

G. **Clinicians need to work with schools and with parents to emphasize the need for media education.** Teaching children how to view media can help mitigate any negative effects, and such programs are common in other developed countries.

H. **Feedback—both negative and positive—to the networks, the cable companies, and the Federal Communications Commission is critically important in trying to improve the quality of programming for children.** The networks estimate that one letter represents 10,000 viewers.

BIBLIOGRAPHY

For Professionals

Organizations

Center for Media Education
2120 L Street NW, Suite 200
Washington, DC 20037
202-331-7833
www.cme.org
Center for Media Literacy
3101 Ocean Park Blvd, Suite 200
Santa Monica, CA 90405
1-800-228-4630
www.medialit.org

Federal Communications Commission (FCC)
445 12th St. SW
Washington, DC 20554
1-888-CALL-FCC
www.fcc.gov
New Mexico Media Literacy Project
6400 Wyoming Blvd
Albuquerque, NM
505-828-3129
www.nmmlp.org
Parents' Choice Foundation
201 West Padonia Road, Suite 303
Timonium, MD 21093.
www.parents-choice.org

Publications

American Academy of Pediatrics. Policy Statements (all published in *Pediatrics*):Media Violence (108:1222-1226, 2001)Children, Adolescents, and TV (107:423-426, 2001)Sexuality, Contraception, and the Media (107:191-194, 2001)Media Education (104:341-343, 1999)Impact of Music Lyrics and Music Videos on Children and Youth (98:1219-1221, 1996)Children, Adolescents, and Advertising (95:295-297, 1995)

Strasburger VC. Children and TV advertising: Nowhere to run, nowhere to hide. *J Develop Behavioral Pediatr* 22:185–187, 2001.

Strasburger VC, Wilson BJ. *Children, adolescents, and the media.* Thousand Oaks, CA: Sage, 2002.

Wallack L, Diaz I, Dorfman L, et al. *News for a Change: An Advocate's Guide to Working with the Media.* Thousand Oaks, CA: Sage, 1999.

Twins

Jessie R. Groothuis

I. Description of the issue.

A. Epidemiology.

1. Twins occur in approximately 1 in 80 pregnancies.
2. Monozygotic twins occur with uniform frequency (3.5/1,000 births) and are not appreciably influenced by race, maternal age, or other known factors.
3. The incidence of dizygotic twins (the result of multiple ovulation) increases with maternal age, greater parity, in African populations, and with the use of fertility drugs. Dizygotic twins are genetically no more alike than nontwin siblings.
4. The observed increase in perinatal mortality in twins appears to be primarily due to the incidence (over 40%) of prematurity. Monozygotic twins are at a greater disadvantage for perinatal morbidity and death than are dizygotic twins. This is due to a higher incidence of lethal anomalies and an increased risk for transfusions in monozygotic twins.

II. Advice to parents of twins.

A. Infant twins.
Parents of infant twins need support and advice regarding organization, feeding, individualization and separation issues, and stress management. Ideally, discussion of these issues should begin *before* the birth of the twins. It is an excellent idea to refer expectant parents to a local Mother of Twins Club for advice and support both before and after delivery.

1. **Organization.** Efficient organization of the household and anticipatory preparation for caregiving tasks are essential for twin families. Parents should try to recruit outside help in the first weeks after the birth.
   - Parents should have enough essentials such as bottles, baby clothes, and diapers. A diaper service may be less expensive than disposable diapers for two babies.
   - Parents can buy either a twin stroller or two less expensive umbrella folding-type strollers, which can be clamped together. Two infant car seats will be necessary. Parents do not need to buy double sets of infant clothing. Infant twins can sleep in bassinets or even in a bed with bolsters rather than in two expensive cribs.
   - Organizing daily activities is very important to reduce stress. It may be helpful to make charts for feeding and other essential daily activities (a daily bath for the babies is not essential).
   - Parental time, both alone and spent with other family members, should be planned.

2. **Feeding.** Feeding infant twins can be very stressful. This may be due to specific feeding problems with premature or small-for-gestational-age twins or simply because it takes so long to feed two babies.
   - Twins may be breast-fed simultaneously, which will cut down on feeding time or the parents can awaken the second twin to feed after the first is fed.
   - Many mothers will elect to bottle-feed their twins at least some of the time. Whenever possible, two adults should be enlisted so that both twins are held for feedings. When this is not possible, the mother or other caregiver should prop one twin up against a leg or across the lap while holding the second infant so that both may be fed simultaneously.
   - Individualized demand feedings should be discouraged.
   - When babies advance to solid foods, freezing large quantities of food at one time will cut down on the work of meal preparation.

3. **Separation and individuation.** Facilitating separation and individuation of twins is important. Whereas a single infant bonds primarily to his or her mother, a twin also develops a strong tie to his or her twin. Problems with separation and individuation may be compounded if twin children are always treated as a single unit by family and friends (this is particularly the case with monozygotic twins). Table 98-1 outlines parental behaviors that will promote successful individualization of twins, and Table 98-2 presents questions for assessing the level of individualization of each twin.

Table 98-1 Parental behavior promoting individualization of twins

Choose different-sounding names.
Do not dress twins alike all of the time.
Use individual names when referring to twins.
Take twins on separate excursions.
Spend quality time alone with each twin.
Refer to other twin as "your brother/sister" or by his or her name.
Provide separate bedrooms as space allows.
Praise individually.
Discipline individually.
Do not leave twins to entertain each other for extended time periods.
Encourage frequent opportunities for individualized contact with other adults, siblings, and
  peers.
Provide toys according to individual preferences, needs, and interests.
Expect that twins' behavior should differ most of the time, and approve of differences.
Expect twins to think differently, and approve of differences.
Encourage relatives and friends to treat twins as two individuals (e.g., individualize gifts and
  social activities).

4. **Stress.** Stress is a particular problem for families with young twins and most parents
of twins report that the first year is very exhausting and difficult. Parents of twins
are faced with the difficulty of how to divide their attention between twins in order
to meet their individual needs. In extreme instances, the increased stress may be
evidenced by the fact that child abuse and neglect are significantly higher in families
with twins. While it is tempting to shuttle the family with two crying infants out of
the office as quickly as possible, it is important to allow sufficient time to question
parents carefully about stress and their coping ability. This may require having someone take the twins out of the examining room to provide a quiet environment to
discuss parental needs and other issues involving care and management of the twins.

5. **Acute illness.** Common childhood infectious illnesses frequently occur in both twins
concurrently. It is advisable to warn the family of the inevitability of the other twin
becoming ill if one twin develops an infectious disease. Consequently, caregivers
should give instructions for both twins, even if only one is ill. The clinician can minimize additional stress by counseling against the use of separation measures (such as
separate feeding utensils), which are extra work and do not prevent disease spread.

B. **Preschool twins.**

1. **Language delays.** Monozygotic twins (in the absence of perinatal risks) should
achieve developmental milestones at about the same time. Young twins may be delayed in many aspects of speech and language including delayed onset of speech, poor
articulation, decreased speech production, and deficient sentence construction and

Table 98-2 Assessment of twins' level of individualization

Does he or she cry if the other twin cries?
Who is his or her main source of comfort? (It should be the parents.)
Does he or she think his or her mirror image is the twin (after age 15–18 months)?
Does he or she engage in excessive imitation games with the twin?
Does he or she only respond to his or her own name (not the twin's) when called?
Is he or she frequently upset when the other twin is disciplined or upset?
Is there a "twin language"? Do the twins speak at an appropriate developmental level?
Is the developmental level appropriate for each twin?
Is he or she excessively upset when separated from the twin?
School-aged twins
Are the twins afraid to be separated (e.g., at school, overnight stay)?
Do the twins enjoy dressing differently?
Are the twins excessively jealous of the co-twin's friends?
Do the twins exhibit either excessive competition or total lack of competition with each other?
Do the twins have age-appropriate peer relationships and social activities?
Does each twin have individual interests, hobbies, and goals?

usage. The reasons for language delay in young twins are unclear and do not seem to reside in the greater pre- and perinatal biologic problems. Recent focus on three distinct, but possibly overlapping, areas of the family environment includes: reduced opportunity for extended verbal interaction with parents, increased interaction between twins, and competition between twins. In competing for adult attention, twins may adopt strategies such as speaking quickly and omitting whole syllables to get their information across more quickly.

2. **Discipline.** Disciplining twins poses a unique challenge. It is important to remind parents to discipline each twin appropriately and separately. There is a temptation to discipline both twins even when only one misbehaves, increased by the fact that the "good" twin will often attempt to do what the "bad" twin just got punished for. Biting is a particularly common observation among twins. The type of discipline used should be no different from that suggested for singleton children. Twins should not be compared to each other in terms of behavior (e.g., "Why aren't you good like your twin?").

3. **Toilet training.** Twins may toilet train at a somewhat later age than singleton children. Parents should delay toilet training until the twins are truly interested and can verbalize this interest. Parents should be sensitive to individual twin preferences and refrain from comparing their twins or encouraging excessive competition between them. Some twins will prefer to train together; others will do better when trained separately.

4. **Siblings.** Twins attract a great deal of attention, and siblings should not be neglected. Twins may also actively exclude nontwin siblings from their activities. Health care providers should encourage parents to set up outings that include only one twin and the nontwin sibling(s) or siblings alone. Activities should be planned where all siblings can interact equally together (e.g., music, sport activities, etc.).

C. **School-aged twins.**
1. **School entry.** Entry into school is a major step in separation from family, and it may be the first time that twins are separated from each other. Parents, teachers, and school administrators need to anticipate the particular difficulties twins may encounter when they first enter school.

2. **Classroom placement.** "Twins in School", a country-wide Australia school project, is the first to survey large numbers of parents and teachers to determine what has (or has not) worked in the education of twins.
   - It is often advisable to have twins with very different abilities assigned to different classrooms to decrease intertwin dependency; to accelerate individual independent, academic, and social growth; and to discourage excessive comparison by teachers and peers. Emotional or psychological problems may occur when one twin performs better than the other.
   - If twins seem anxious about classroom separation, having them carry a picture of their twin or permitting occasional visits to their twin's classroom may be helpful.
   - If twins experience significant academic and emotional problems because of classroom separation, placement in one classroom for a period of time may be necessary.
   - Separation does not need to be permanent; cases where it is (or is not) working can always be reversed in the next year. A partial separation, such as placement into separate work groups within a classroom, may encourage independence.

3. **Social relationships.** School is an important place for social growth and peer relationships. The initiation of separate social relationships may be particularly difficult for twins and for their parents. Twins should be encouraged to have their own friends and develop individual and separate social experiences. Decisions about individual dress and hairstyles should be left to the twins themselves. It must be emphasized to parents and to schools that the social and educational process must be individualized for each twin. Comparisons should be actively discouraged.

BIBLIOGRAPHY

For Parents

Organization

National Organization Mother of Twins Club
P.O. Box 23188

Albuquerque NM 87192-1188
505-275-0955

Publications

Gromada ??. *Mothering Multiples: Breastfeeding and Caring for Twins or More.* Schaumburg, IL:
La Leche League International, 1999.
Double Talk (published bimonthly); P.O. Box 412, Amelia OH 45102; 513-231-8946
Twins Magazine www.twinsmagazine.com

For Professionals

Gleeson C, Hay DA, Johnston CJ, et al. Twins in School. *Acta Genet Med Gemellol* 39:231–244,
1990.
Klein BS. *Not All Twins Are Alike: Psychological Profiles of Twinship.* Westport, CT: Praeger,
2003.
Siegel SJ, Siegel MM. Practical aspects of pediatric management of families with twins. *Pediatr
Rev* 4:8–12, 1982.
Hay DA, Prior M, Collett S, et al. Speech and language development in preschool twins. *Acta Genet
Med Gemellol* 36:213–223, 1987.

I. **Description of the problem.** The term *vulnerable child* is used to refer to any instance in which parents, because of earlier events, perceive their children to be abnormally susceptible to illness or death. The term *vulnerable child syndrome* was coined by Green and Solnit (1964) to describe children with severe behavioral and learning problems who had experienced serious illnesses or accidents early in childhood. Although these children had recovered fully, their parents continued to view them as especially prone to illnesses and death. It was the continuing, overprotective, enmeshed relationship between parent and child that adversely affected the child's psychological development.

- This classic description represents the extreme end of a spectrum. Less severe experiences can also heighten parents' anxieties and cause them to perceive their children to be at increased risk for illness or death. Similarly, there is a wide spectrum of developmental and behavioral outcomes: some children have severe problems, and others have few apparent ill effects. The term vulnerable child syndrome should be reserved only for cases meeting the criteria in Table 99-1.

A. **Epidemiology.** It is unknown to what extent the vulnerable child syndrome accounts for psychopathology among children.
  - In a community-wide study of 1,095 children ages 4–8 years, 10% of children were categorized as "perceived vulnerable." In that study, 21% of all the mothers reported that they had had prior fears that their child might die.
  - A number of studies have demonstrated an increased sense of vulnerability among mothers who are unmarried, less educated, and of lower socioeconomic status.

B. **Etiology.** A number of different factors have been reported to contribute to parental perceptions of vulnerability (Table 99-2) . In general, the earlier in a child's life that an event occurs, the more likely it is to enhance the parent's perception of the child as vulnerable. The translation of parental fears into childhood behavioral problems is a complex process. Most are believed to result from distortions in the normal development of a sense of separateness, independence, and self-esteem.

II. **Making the diagnosis.**

A. **Presentation.** The most important factor in managing the vulnerable child is early identification. This should be a consideration in a child with any of the following.
  1. A child who is brought frequently to the clinician with minor medical complaints.
  2. Recurring symptoms that may be psychosomatic, such as headaches or stomachaches.
  3. Behavioral problems or school learning difficulties.
  4. Parents who are having difficulty separating from their children.

B. **History: Key clinical questions.** Sensitive history taking begins the therapeutic process by conveying to the parent a sense of understanding and empathy. The clinician should ask questions that lead to an understanding of the parent's sense of vulnerability.
  1. *"To understand your child better, I need to know more. Let's go right back to the beginning. Let's start with your pregnancy."* This allows a more complete history that can focus on factors contributing to perceptions of vulnerability.
  2. *"What did the doctors tell you might happen? Did you at any time fear that the child might not make it?"* This type of question should be asked whenever a parent reports a problem, particularly during the pregnancy, delivery, and early childhood, no matter how minor it might appear.
  3. *"That must have been very frightening for you."* Whenever parents report something that might have been particularly worrisome to them, an empathic response will encourage them to talk further about their fears.
  4. *"How often do you leave him or her with a babysitter?"* Try to assess the parents' level of comfort in separating from their child by asking questions about the use of babysitters and their level of worry when apart from the child. Other questions should include information about other separation difficulties (e.g., when the child first started daycare or school).

Table 99-1 Diagnostic criteria for the vulnerable child syndrome

1. An event early in the child's life that the parent considered to be life-threatening.
2. The parent's continuing unrealistic belief that the child is especially susceptible to illness or death (often associated with frequent telephone calls and visits to the clinician for trivial symptoms).
3. The presence of a behavioral or learning problem in the child.

III. **Management.**

A. **Prevention.** The clinician must realize that any event or illness, even one considered to be medically insignificant, may have a very different meaning and implications for the parent. The clinician needs to take time to understand parents' beliefs and fears and address these appropriately. This may occur, for example, when a colicky infant's formula is changed. Some parents might interpret the change as implying that the child has a gastrointestinal abnormality. By explaining that colic is a self-limited condition affecting normal infants and by reinforcing this concept by changing back to the original formula within a few weeks, the clinician should be able to prevent the development of perceptions of vulnerability. When a child who is hospitalized for an acute illness is ready for discharge, the clinician should emphasize to the parents that recovery is or will be complete, that no special precautions will be necessary after a certain time, and that the child is no more vulnerable to illness than other children.

B. **Treatment.** Once it is recognized that parental perceptions of vulnerability are affecting a child's behavior or development, the following approach should be taken.

1. **After taking a complete history and performing a conspicuously meticulous physical examination, the clinician should give a clear statement that the child is absolutely physically sound.** He or she should not use equivocal comments such as, "He doesn't look too bad" or "I can't find anything wrong."

2. **Help the parents to understand and accept the notion that the child is considered special by the family and that this derives from their response to earlier events.** It may be helpful to explain the vulnerable child syndrome and describe it as a known entity. However, the clinician should be careful about labeling it as a "syndrome," which might have a stigmatizing implication for some parents.

3. **Support the parents in dealing with the child more appropriately** by setting consistent limits, discontinuing patterns of infantilization and overprotectiveness, dealing more effectively with problems of separation, and being less panicked about the child's somatic complaints.

4. Although these problems can usually be managed by the primary care clinician, a mental health referral may be necessary if the parents are unable to accept this approach.

Table 99-2 Antecedents of the vulnerable child

Preexisting
    Death of a relative or previous child early in life
    Prior miscarriage or stillbirth
Pregnancy related
    Pregnancy complications (e.g., vaginal bleeding)
    Abnormal screening results (e.g., abnormal alpha-feto protein)
    Delivery complications
Newborn period
    Prematurity
    Neonatal illness or complications
    Congenital abnormalities
    Hyperbilirubinemia
    False-positive results of screening (e.g., phenylketonuria)
Early childhood
    Excessive crying, colic, spitting up
    Any serious illness
    Admission to hospital for such things as "to rule out sepsis"
    Self-limited infectious illnesses (e.g., croup, gastroenteritis)

BIBLIOGRAPHY

Carey WB. Psychological sequelae of early infancy health crises. In Swartz JL, Swartz LH (eds), *Vulnerable Infants*. New York: McGraw-Hill, 1977.

Forsyth BWC, Canny PF. Perceptions of vulnerability 3½ years after problems of feeding and crying behavior in early infancy. *Pediatrics* 88:757–763, 1991.

Green M. Vulnerable child syndrome and its variants. *Pediatr Rev* 8:75–80, 1986.

Green M, Solnit AJ. Reactions to the threatened loss of a child: A vulnerable child syndrome. *Pediatrics* 34:58–66, 1964.

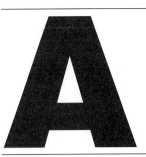

Clinicians interested in using the Pediatric Symptom Checklist (PSC) should obtain detailed information at http://psc.partners.org/psc about administration, scoring, and interpretation before using it in practice.

Scoring overview:

1. Each item is rated as never, sometimes, or often present and scored 0, 1, and 2, respectively.
2. The total score is the sum of all item scores (range = 1–70).
3. Test authors recommend using a cutoff score of *28 or higher* for children ages 6–16 years, and *24 or higher* for children ages 4–5 years.
4. A positive score suggests a need for further evaluation by a qualified health or mental health professional. Approximately 1 in 20 children with a behavior problem will be missed on this screen (false negative).

Pediatric Symptom Checklist for School-Aged Children

Please mark under the heading that best fits your child:	Never	Sometimes	Often
1. Complains of aches or pains	–	–	–
2. Spends more time alone	–	–	–
3. Tires easily, little energy	–	–	–
4. Fidgety, unable to sit still	–	–	–
5. Has trouble with a teacher	–	–	–
6. Less interested in school	–	–	–
7. Acts as if driven by a motor	–	–	–
8. Daydreams too much	–	–	–
9. Distracted easily	–	–	–
10. Is afraid of new situations	–	–	–
11. Feels sad, unhappy	–	–	–
12. Is irritable, angry	–	–	–
13. Feels hopeless	–	–	–
14. Has trouble concentrating	–	–	–
15. Less interest in friends	–	–	–
16. Fights with other children	–	–	–
17. Absent from school	–	–	–
18. School grades dropping	–	–	–
19. Is down on himself or herself	–	–	–
20. Visits doctor with doctor finding nothing wrong	–	–	–
21. Has trouble with sleeping	–	–	–
22. Worries a lot	–	–	–
23. Wants to be with you more than before	–	–	–
24. Feels he or she is bad	–	–	–
25. Takes unnecessary risks	–	–	–
26. Gets hurt frequently	–	–	–
27. Seems to be having less fun	–	–	–
28. Acts younger than other children his or her age	–	–	–
29. Does not listen to rules	–	–	–
30. Does not show feelings	–	–	–
31. Does not understand other people's feelings	–	–	–
32. Teases others	–	–	–
33. Blames others for his or her troubles	–	–	–
34. Takes things that do not belong to him or her	–	–	–
35. Refuses to share	–	–	–

Jellinek MS, Murphy JM, et al. Pediatric symptom checklist: screening school-age children for psychosocial dysfunction. *J Pediatr* 1988;112:201–209.

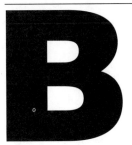

Child Development in the First Five Years

Child Development in the First Five Years

SOCIAL	SELF-HELP	GROSS MOTOR	FINE MOTOR	LANGUAGE
Shows leadership among children	Goes to the toilet without help	Swings on swing, pumping by self	Prints first name (four letters)	Tells meaning of familiar words
Follows simple game rules in board games or card games	Usually looks both ways before crossing street	Skips or makes running "broad jumps"	Draws a person that has at least three parts—head, eyes, nose, mouth, etc.	Reads a few letters (five)
	Buttons one or more buttons	Hops around on one foot, without support	Draws recognizable pictures	Follows a series of three simple instructions
Protective toward younger children	Dresses and undresses without help, except for tying shoelaces			Understands, concepts—size, number, shape
		Hops on one foot, without support	Cuts across paper with small scissors	Counts five or more objects when asked "How many?"
Plays cooperatively, with minimum conflict and supervision	Washes face without help		Draws or copies a complete circle	Identifies four colors correctly
Gives directions to other children		Rides around on a tricycle, using pedals		Combines sentences with the words "and," "or," or "but"
	Toilet trained Dresses self with help	Walks up and down stairs, one foot per step	Cuts with small scissors	Understands four prepositions—in, on, under, beside
Plays a role in "pretend" games—mom-dad, teacher, space pilot	Washes and dries hands	Stands on one foot, without support	Draws or copies vertical (|) lines	Talks clearly—is understandable most of the time

Child Development in the First Five Years *(continued)*

SOCIAL	SELF-HELP	GROSS MOTOR	FINE MOTOR	LANGUAGE
Plays with other children—cars, dolls, building				
"Helps" with simple household tasks	Opens door by turning knob	Climbs on play equipment—ladders, slides	Scribbles with circular motion	Talks in two–three word phrases or sentences.
Usually responds to correction—stops	Takes off open coat or shirt without help	Walks up and down stairs alone	Turns pages of picture books, one at a time	Follows two part instructions
Shows sympathy to other children, tries to comfort them				
	Eats with spoon, spilling little	Runs well, seldom falls		Uses at least ten words
Sometimes says "No" when interfered with	Eats with fork	Kicks a ball forward	Builds towers of four or more blocks	Follows simple instructions
Greets people with "Hi" or similar	Insists on doing things by self such as feeding	Runs	Scribbles with crayon	Asks for food or drink with words
Gives kisses or hugs	Feeds self with spoon	Walks without help	Stacks two or more blocks	Talks in single words
Wants stuffed animal, doll, or blanket in bed	Lifts cup to mouth and drinks	Stands without support	Picks up two small toys in one hand	Uses one or two words as names of things or actions
Plays pattycake	Picks up a spoon by the handle	Walks around furniture or crib while holding on		Understands words like "No," "Stop," or "All gone"
			Picks up small objects—precise thumb and finger grasp	
Plays social games, peek-a-boo, bye-bye		Crawls around on hands and knees		Word sounds—says "Ma-ma" or "Da-da" as name for parent
Pushes things away he/she doesn't want		Sits alone ⋯ steady, without support	Picks up object with thumb and finger grasp	Wide range of vocalizations (vowel sounds, consonant–vowel combinations)
Reaches for familiar persons	Feeds self cracker	Rolls over from back to stomach	Transfers toy from one hand to the other	Responds to name—turns and looks
Distinguishes mother from others	Comforts self with thumb or pacifier	Turns around when lying on stomach	Picks up toy with one hand	Vocalizes spontaneously social
Social smile	Reacts to sight of bottle or breast	Lifts head and chest when lying on stomach	Looks at and reaches for faces and toys	Reacts to voices. Vocalizes, coos, chuckles

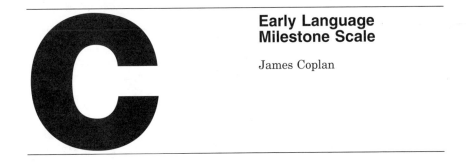

Early Language Milestone Scale

James Coplan

The Early Language Milestone Scale, second edition (ELM Scale-2) is designed primarily as a structured history of speech and language development, to be used by clinicians with varying degrees of expertise in early child development. The scale may be administered by either a pass-fail or a point-scoring method. The pass-fail method separates children into two groups: the slowest 10% with respect to speech and language development ("fail") and everyone else ("pass"). The point-scoring method yields age-, percentile-, and standard score equivalents for all possible point scores. The pass-fail method is recommended when screening large numbers of low-risk subjects; the point-scoring method is recommended when examining children who are at high risk for the presence of developmental delay or when evaluating a child with a known developmental disability. Complete instructions and pads of scoring forms are available from PRO-ED, 8700 Shoal Creek Boulevard, Austin TX 78758.

Reprinted with permission from PRO-ED, 8700 Shoal Creek Blvd., Austin, TX 78758.

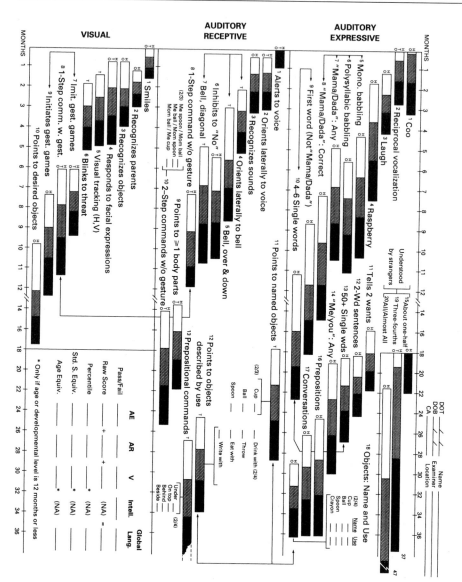

I. General Instructions

25% 50% 75% 90%   Percentage of Children
↓   ↓   ↓   ↓   Passing Item

Item may be elicited by

H = History
T = Direct Testing
O = Incidental Observation

- Always start with H, where allowed.
- Child passes item if passed by any of the allowable means of elicitation for that item.
- Basal = 3 consecutive items passed (work down from age line).
- Ceiling = 3 consecutive items failed (work up from age line).

II. Auditory Expressive (AE)
A. Content

AE 1. Prolonged musical vowel sounds in a sing-song fashion (ooo, aaa, etc.), not just grunts or squeaks.

AE 2. H: Does baby watch speaker's face and appear to listen intently, then vocalize when the speaker is quiet? Can you "have a conversation" with your baby?

AE 4. H: Blow bubbles or give "bronx cheer"?

AE 5. H: Makes isolated sounds such as "ba," "da," "ga," "goo," etc.

AE 6. H: Makes repetitive string of sounds: "babababa," or "lalalalala," etc.

AE 7. H: Says "mama" or "dada" but uses them at other times besides just labelling parents.

AE 8. H: Child spontaneously, consistently, and correctly uses "mama" or "dada," just to label the appropriate parent.

AE 9, AE 10, AE 13. H: Child spontaneously, consistently, and correctly uses words. Do not count "mama," "dada," or the names of other family members or pets.

AE 11. H: Uses single words to tell you what he/she wants. "Milk!" "Cookie!" "More!" etc. Pass = 2 or more wants. List specific words.

AE 12. H: Spontaneously, novel 2-word combinations ("Want cookie" "No bed" "See daddy" etc.) Not rotely learned phrases that have been specifically taught to the child or combinations that are really single thoughts (e.g., "hot dog").

AE 14. H: Child uses "me" or "you" but may reverse them ("you want cookie" instead of "me want cookie," etc.)

AE 17. H: "Can child put 2 or 3 sentences together to hold brief conversations?"

AE 18. T: Put out cup, ball, crayon, & spoon. Pick up cup & say "What is this? What do we do with it? (What is it for?)" Child must name the object and give its use. Pass = "drink with," etc., not "milk" or "juice." Ball: Pass = "throw," "play with," etc. Spoon: Pass = "Eat" or "Eat with," etc., not "Food," "Lunch." Crayon: Pass = "Write (with)," "Color (with)," etc. Pass item if child gives name and use for 2 objects.

B. Intelligibility

AE 15, AE 19, AE 20. "How clear is your child's speech? That is, how much of your child's speech can a stranger understand?"

—Less than one-half
—About one-half (AE 15)   Pick one
—Three-fourths (AE 19)   (H, O)
—All or Almost All (AE 20)

To score:
If less than one-half: Fail all 3 items in cluster.
If about one-half: Pass AE 15 only.
If three-fourths: Pass AE 19 and AE 15.
If all or almost all: Pass all 3 items in cluster.

III. Auditory Receptive (AR)

AR 1. H, T: Any behavioral change in response to noise (eye blink, startle, change in movements or respiration, etc.)

AR 2. H, T: What does baby do when parent starts talking while out of baby's line of sight? Pass if any shift of head or eyes to voice.

AR 3. H: Does baby seem to respond in a specific way to certain sounds (becomes excited at hearing parents' voices, etc.)?

AR 4. T: Sit facing baby, with baby in parent's lap. Extend both arms so that your hands are behind baby's field of vision and at the level of baby's waist. Ring a 2"-diameter bell, first with 1 hand, then the other. Repeat 2 or 3 times if necessary. Pass if baby turns head to the side at least once.

AR 5. T: See note for AR 4. Pass if baby turns head first to the side, then down, to localize bell, at least once. (Automatically passes AR 4.)

AR 6. H: Does baby understand the command "no" (even though he may not always obey)? T: Test by commanding "(Baby's name), no!" while baby is playing with any test object. Pass if baby temporarily inhibits his actions.

AR 7. T: See note for AR 4. Pass if baby turns directly down on diagonal to localize bell, at least once. (Automatically passes AR 5 and AR 4.)

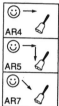

AR 8. H: Will your baby follow any verbal commands <u>without</u> you indicating by gestures what it is you want him to do ("Stop" "Come here" "Give me" etc.)? T: Wait until baby is playing with any test object, then say "(Baby's name), give it to me." Pass if baby extends object to you, even if baby seems to change his mind and take the object back. May repeat command 1 or 2 times. If failed, repeat the command but this time hold out your hand for the object. If baby responds, then pass item, V 8 (1-step command with gesture).

AR 9. H: Does your child point to at least 1 body part on command? T: Have mother command baby "Show me your..." or "Where's your..." without pointing to the desired part herself.

AR 10. H: "Can child do 2 things in a row if asked? For example 'First go get your shoes, then sit down'?" T: Set out ball, cup, and spoon, and say "(Child's name), give me the spoon, then give the ball to mommy." Use slow, steady voice but do <u>not</u> break command into 2 separate sentences. If no response, <u>then</u> give each half of command separately to see if child understands separate components. If child succeeds on at least half of command, then give each of the following: "(Child's name), give me the ball and give mommy the spoon." May repeat once but do not break into 2 commands. Then "Give mommy the ball, then give the cup to me." Pass if at least two 2-step commands executed correctly. (Note: Child is credited even if the order of execution of a command is reversed.)

AR 11. H: Place a cup, ball, and spoon on the table. Command child "Show me/where is/give me... the cup/ball/spoon." (If command is "Give me," be sure to replace each object before asking about the next object.) Pass = 2 items correctly identified.

AR 12. T: Put cup, ball, spoon, and crayon on table and give command "Show me/where is/give me... the one we drink with/eat with/draw (color, write) with/throw (play with)." If the command "Give me" is used, be sure to replace each object before asking about the next object. Pass = 2 or more objects correctly identified.

AR 13. Put out cup (upside down) and a 1" cube. Command the child "Put the block under the cup." Repeat 1 or 2 times if necessary. If no attempt, or if incorrect response, then demonstrate correct response, saying, "See, now the block is <u>under</u> the cup." Remove the block and hand it to the child. Then give command "Put the block <u>on top of</u> the cup." If child makes no response, then repeat command 1 time but do not demonstrate. Then command "Put the block <u>behind</u> the cup," then "Put the block <u>beside</u> the cup." Pass = 2 or more commands correctly executed (<u>prior</u> to demonstration by examiner, if "underneath" is scored).

IV. Visual

V 1. H: "Does your baby smile—not just a gas bubble or a burp but a real smile?" T: Have parent attempt to elicit smile by any means.

V 2. H: "Does your baby seem to recognize you, reacting differently to you than to the sight of other people? For example, does your baby smile more quickly for you than for other people?"

V 3. H: "Does your baby seem to recognize any common objects by sight? For example, if bottle or spoon fed, what happens when bottle or spoon is brought into view <u>before</u> it touches baby's lips?" Pass if baby gets visibly excited, or opens mouth in anticipation of feeding.

V 4. H: "Does your baby respond to your facial expressions?" T: Engage baby's gaze and attempt to elicit a smile by smiling and talking to baby. Then scowl at baby. Pass if any change in baby's facial expression.

V 5. T: Horizontal (H): Engage child's gaze with yours at a distance of 18". Move slowly back and forth. Pass if child turns head 60° to left and right from midline. Vertical (V): Move slowly up and down. Pass if child elevates eyes 30° from horizontal. Must pass both H & V to pass item.

V 6. T: Flick your fingers rapidly towards child's face, ending with fingertips 1–2" from face. Do not touch face or eyelashes. Pass if child blinks.

V 7. H: Does child play pat-a-cake, peek-a-boo, etc., in response to parents?

V 8. T: See note for AR 8 (always try AR 8 first; if AR 8 is passed, then automatically give credit for V 8).

V 9. H: Does child spontaneously initiate gesture games?

V 10. H: "Does your child ever point with index finger to something he/she wants? For example, if child is sitting at the dinner table and wants something that is out of reach, how does child let you know what he/she wants?" Pass <u>only</u> index finger pointing <u>not</u> reaching with whole hand.

D

Temperament

Your Child's Temperament

1. **Sensitivity:** Is your child sensitive to noises, temperature changes, lights, smells, and the texture of things? Does your child react strongly to loud noises or bright lights? Does he/she startle when the phone rings?

1	2	3	4	5
Usually not sensitive				Very sensitive

2. **Regularity:** Does your child normally eat and sleep the same amount each day?

1	2	3	4	5
Always				Never

3. **Activity:** Does your child have lots of energy? Is your child always on the go?

1	2	3	4	5
Quiet				Active

4. **Intensity:** Does your child have strong dramatic reactions to situations? When happy, does your child laugh loudly or does he smile and giggle softly and briefly?

1	2	3	4	5
Mild reaction				High intensity/ Dramatic

5. **Approach/Withdrawal:** What is your child's first and usual reaction to new people, new situations, or new places?

1	2	3	4	5
Outgoing				Slow to warm-up

6. **Adaptability:** Does you child adapt quickly to changes or new places, like visiting friends or relatives? Is it difficult for your child when there is a new routine, new person, or new activity?

1	2	3	4	5
Adapts quickly				Adapts slowly

7. **Persistence:** Does your child stick with things even when frustrated?

1	2	3	4	5
Gets "locked in"				Can stop

8. **Distractability:** Is your child very aware and easily distracted by noises and people? Can you distract your child from playing with things he/she shouldn't touch by giving a different toy?

1	2	3	4	5
Easily distracted				Not easily distracted

9. **Mood:** How often is your child happy and in a good mood vs. feeling negative or serious?

1	2	3	4	5
Usually positive				Often negative or serious

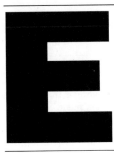

	Social	Self-Help	Gross motor	Fine motor	Language
Birth	Responds positively to feeding and comforting.	Alert: interested in sights and sounds.	Kicks legs and thrashes arms.	Looks at objects or faces.	Cries.
1 mo.	Social smile.	Responds to voices: turns head toward a voice.	Raises head and chest when lying on stomach.	Follows moving objects with eyes.	Cries in a special way when hungry.
2 mos.	Recognizes mother.	Reacts to sight of bottle or breast.	Holds head steady when held sitting.	Holds objects put in hand.	Makes sounds—ah, eh, ugh. Laughs.
3 mos.	Recognizes most familiar adults.	Increases activity when shown toy.	Makes crawling movements.	Shakes rattle.	
4 mos.	Interested in his or her image in mirror—smiles, playful.	Reaches for objects.	Turns around when lying on stomach.	Puts toys or other objects in mouth.	Squeals. Ah-goo.
5 mos.	Reacts differently to strangers.		Rolls over from stomach to back.	Picks up objects with one hand.	Makes razzing sounds—gives you the "raspberry."
6 mos.	Reaches for familiar persons.	Looks for object after it disappears from sight—for example, looks for toy after it falls off tray.	Rolls over from back to stomach.	Transfers objects from one hand to the other.	Babbles. Responds to his/her name, turns and looks.
7 mos.	Gets upset and afraid if left alone.	Anticipates being lifted by raising arms.	Sits without support.	Holds two objects, one in each hand, at the same time.	Makes sounds like da, ba, ga, ka, ma.

	Social	Self-Help	Gross motor	Fine motor	Language
8 mos.	Plays "peek-a-boo."	Feeds self cracker or cookie.	Crawls on hands and knees.	Uses forefinger to poke, push, or roll small objects.	Makes sounds like ma-ma, da-da, ba-ba.
9 mos.	Resists having a toy taken away.		Pulls self to standing position.	Picks up small objects using only finger and thumb.	Imitates speech sounds that you make.
10 mos.	Plays "patty-cake."		Sidesteps around playpen or furniture while holding on. Or walks.	Picks up two small objects in one hand.	Understands single words like bye-bye and nite-nite.
11 mos.	Shows or offers toy to adult.	Picks up spoon by handle.	Stands alone well.	Puts small objects in cup or other container.	Uses Mama or Dada specifically for parent.
12 mos.	Imitates simple acts such as hugging or loving a doll.	Removes socks.	Climbs up on chairs or other furniture.	Turns pages of books a few at a time.	Says one word clearly.
13 mos.	Plays with other children.	Lifts cup to mouth and drinks.	Walks without help.	Builds tower of 2 or more blocks.	Shakes head to express "No." Hands object to you when asked.
14 mos.	Gives kisses.	Insists on feeding self.	Stoops and recovers.	Marks with pencil or crayon.	Asks for food or drink with sounds or words.
15 mos.	Greets people with "Hi" or similar.	Feeds self with a spoon.	Runs.	Scribbles with pencil or crayon.	Says 2 words besides Mama or Dada. Makes sounds in sequences that sound like sentences.
18 mos.	Sometimes says "No" when interfered with.	Eats with a fork.	Kicks a ball. Good balance and coordination.	Builds tower of 4 or more blocks.	Uses 5 or more words as names of things.
21 mos.					Follows a few simple instructions.

Reprinted with permission from Harold Ireton. Behavior Science Systems, Inc.,

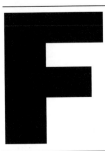

Socioemotional Development of Infants and Children: Themes and Behaviors

Stanley Greenspan

By 3 Months: Regulation and Interest in the World
Developmental Goals
- Can be calm.
- Recovers from crying with comforting.
- Is able to be alert.
- Looks at one when talked to.
- Brightens up to appropriate experiences.

Clinical Observations
- Shows an interest in the world by looking at (brightening) or listening to (turning toward) sounds. Can attend to a visual or auditory stimulus for 3 or more seconds.
- Can remain calm and focused for 2 or more minutes at a time, as evidenced by looking around, sucking, cooperating in cuddling, or other age-appropriate activities.

By 5 Months: Forming Relationships (Attachments)
Developmental Goals
- Shows positive loving affect toward primary caregiver (and other key caregivers).
- Shows full range of emotions.

Clinical Observations
- Responds to social overtures with an emotional response of pleasure (e.g., smile, joyful vocalizations).
- Can display negative affect (e.g., frown, negative vocalizations, angry arm or leg movements).

By 9 Months: Intentional Two-Way Communication
Developmental Goals
- Interacts in a purposeful (i.e., intentional, reciprocal, cause-and-effect) manner.
- Initiates signals and responds purposefully to another person's signals.

Clinical Observations
- Responds to caregiver's gestures with intentional gestures of his or her own (e.g., when caregiver reaches out to pick up infant, infant may reach up with own arms; a flirtatious caregiver vocalization may beget a playful look and a series of vocalizations).
- Initiates intentional iterations (e.g., spontaneously reaches for caregiver's nose, hair, or mouth; uses hand movements to indicate wish for a certain toy or to be picked up).

By 13 Months: Developing a Complex Sense of Self
Developmental Goals
- Sequences a number of gestures together and responds consistently to caregiver's gestures, thereby forming chains of interaction (i.e., opens and closes a number of sequential circles of communication).
- Manifests a wide range of organized, socially meaningful behaviors and feelings dealing with warmth, pleasure, assertion, exploration, protest, and anger.

Clinical Observations
- Strings together three or more circles of communication (interactions) as part of a complex pattern of communication. Each, unit or circle of communication begins with an infant behavior and ends with the infant's building on and responding to the caregiver response. For example, an infant looks and reaches for a toy (opening a circle of communication); caregiver points to the toy, gestures, and vocalizes, "This one?"; infant nods, makes a purposeful sound, and reaches further for toy (closing a circle of communication). As the infant explores the toy and exchanges vocalizations, motor gestures, or facial expressions with the caregiver, additional circles of communication are opened and closed.

By 18 Months: Increasingly Complex Sense of Self
Developmental Goals
- Comprehends, communicates, and elaborates sequences of interaction that convey basic emotional themes.

Clinical Observations

- Has the ability, with a responsive caregiver, to open and close 10 or more consecutive circles of communication (e.g., taking caregiver's hand and walking toward refrigerator, vocalizing, pointing, responding to caregiver's questioning gestures with more vocalizing and pointing; finally getting caregiver to refrigerator, getting caregiver to open door, and pointing to the desired food.)
- Imitates another person's behavior and then uses this newly learned behavior to convey an emotional theme (e.g., putting on daddy's hat and walking around the house with a big smile, clearly waiting for an admiring laugh).

By 24 Months: Representational Capacity of Emotional Ideas

Developmental Goals

- Creates mental representations of feelings and ideas that can be expressed symbolically (e.g., pretend play and words).

Clinical Observations

- Can construct, in collaboration with caregiver, simple pretend play patterns of at least one "idea" (e.g., doll hugging or feeding the doll).
- Can use words or other symbolic means (e.g., selecting a series of pictures, creating a sequence of motor gestures) to communicate a need, wish, intention, or feeling (e.g., "want that"; "me toy"; "hungry!" "mad!").

By 30 Months: Greater Representational Elaboration of Emotional Themes

Developmental Goals

- Can elaborate a number of ideas in both make-believe play and symbolic communication that go beyond basic needs (e.g., "want juice") and deal with more complex intentions, wishes, or feelings (e.g., themes of closeness or dependency, separation, exploration, assertiveness, anger, self-pride, or showing off).
- Creates pretend dramas with two or more ideas (e.g., dolls hug and then have a tea party). The ideas need not be related or logically connected to one another.
- Uses symbolic communication (e.g., words, pictures, motor patterns) to convey two or more ideas at a time in terms of complex intentions, wishes, or feelings. Ideas need not be logically connected to one another.

By 36 Months: Emotional Thinking

Developmental Goals

- Can communicate ideas dealing with complex intentions, wishes, and feelings in pretend play or other types of symbolic communication that are logically tied to one another.
- Distinguishes what is real from unreal and switches back and forth between fantasy and reality with little difficulty.

Clinical Observations

- In pretend play, involves two or more ideas that are logically tied to one another but not necessarily realistic (e.g., "The car is visiting the moon" [and gets there] "by flying fast"). In addition, the child can build on an adult's pretend play idea (i.e., close a circle of communication). For example, the child is "cooking a soup" and the adult asks what is in it. The child says, "rocks and dirt" or "ants and spiders."
- Engages in symbolic communication that involves two or more ideas that are logically connected and grounded in reality: "No go to sleep. Want to watch television." "Why?" asks the adult. "Because not tired." Child can close symbolic circles of communication (e.g., child says, "Want to go outside." Adult asks, "What will you do?" Child replies, "Play.").

By 42–48 Months: Emotional Thinking

Developmental Goals

- Is capable of elaborate, complex pretend play and symbolic communication dealing with complex intentions, wishes, or feelings.

Clinical Observations

- Engages in "how," "why," or "when" elaborations, which give depth to play and communication. (Child sets up castle with an evil queen who captured the princess. Why did she capture the princess? "Because the princess was more beatiful." When did she capture her? "Yesterday." How will the princess get out? "You ask too many questions.")
- Deals with causality in a reality-based dialogue. ("Why did you hit your brother?" "Because he took my toy." "Any other reason?" "He took my cookie.")
- Distinguishes reality and fantasy. "That's only pretend"; "That's a dream. It's not real.")
- Uses concepts of time and space. (Caregiver: "Where should we look for the toy you can't find?" Child: "Let's look in my room. I was playing with it there." Caregiver: "When do you want the cookies?" Child: "Now." Caregiver: "Not now; maybe in 5 minutes." Child: "No. Want it now!" Caregiver: "You can have the cookie in 1, 2, or 5 minutes." Child: "OK. One minute.")

BIBLIOGRAPHY

1. Greenspan S. *Building healthy minds: the six experiences that create intelligence and emotional growth in babies and young children.* New York: Perseus Publishing, 1999.

2. Greenspan S. *Infancy and early childhood: the practice of clinical assessment and intervention with emotional and developmental challenges.* Madison, Conn.: International Universities Press 1992.

3. Greenspan S. Clinical assessment of emotional milestones in infancy and early childhood. *Pediatr Clin North Am* 1991; (38)6, 1371–1385.

4. Greenspan S. Greenspan N. *First feelings: milestones in the development of your baby and child.* New York: Penguin Books, 1985.

5. Greenspan S. Greenspan N. *The essential partnership: how parents and children meet the emotional challenges of infancy and childhood.* New York: Penguin Books, 1989.

Index